D0915334

OXFORD MEDICAL PUBLICATIONS

Coronary Heart Disease Epidemiology

Coronary Heart Disease Epidemiology

From Aetiology to Public Health

Edited by

MICHAEL MARMOT

Department of Epidemiology and Public Health
University College and Middlesex School of Medicine, London
and
Department of Epidemiology and Population Sciences
London School of Hygiene and Tropical Medicine

and

PAUL ELLIOTT

Department of Public Health and Policy
London School of Hygiene and Tropical Medicine

OXFORD NEW YORK TORONTO MELBOURNE
OXFORD UNIVERSITY PRESS
1992

Oxford University Press, Walton Street, Oxford OX2 6DP
Oxford   New York   Toronto
Delhi   Bombay   Calcutta   Madras   Karachi
Petaling Jaya   Singapore   Hong Kong   Tokyo
Nairobi   Dar es Salaam   Cape Town
Melbourne   Auckland
and associated companies in
Berlin   Ibadan

Oxford is a trade mark of Oxford University Press

Published in the United States
by Oxford University Press, New York

© Michael Marmot, Paul Elliott,
and the contributors listed on p. xxi–xxiv, 1992

A catalogue record for this book is available from the British Library

Library of Congress Cataloging in Publication Data
Coronary heart disease epidemiology : from aetiology to public health
/ edited by Michael Marmot and Paul Elliott.
(Oxford medical publications)
Includes bibliographical references.
1. Coronary heart disease–Epidemiology.   I. Marmot, M. G.
II. Elliott, P. (Paul)   III. Series.
[DNLM: 1. Community Health Services.   2. Coronary Disease–
–epidemiology.   3. Risk Factors.   WG 300 C8233]
RA645.C68C67   1992   614.5'912—dc20   92–13139
ISBN 0–19–262124–6

Set by Footnote Graphics, Warminster, Wilts
Printed in Great Britain
by Bookcraft (Bath) Ltd,
Midsomer Norton, Avon

Preface

The idea for this book took shape in the editors' minds as a tribute to the work of Geoffrey Rose. We considered whether the book might be a collection of pieces by former students, friends, and colleagues—a good deal of overlap in these categories—and whether it might cover the topics to which Geoffrey Rose contributed. It quickly became apparent that such an effort would be a textbook of coronary heart disease epidemiology and prevention.

The aim of the book is not simply to review knowledge of well-established factors. A book on coronary heart disease must include them, but there are any number of reviews by expert committees and government bodies. Rather, our aim is to look forward, equipped with lessons learnt from the past. Thus we included major areas of new work that hold great promise for future knowledge. The authors, each at the forefront of his/her field, took seriously the charge to be topical or fresh, and reflect current thinking. The results are up-to-date personal accounts, rather than simply comprehensive reviews. The aim was to cover the frontiers of work on aetiology, on appropriate methodology, and on application of scientific knowledge to the development of policy.

A book that started life as a Festschrift and ended as a textbook might have posed a conflict of interest: should the invited contributors be Geoffrey Rose's friends and colleagues or should they be acknowledged experts in the field? In the event, there was no conflict. These two categories overlapped to a high degree. Our considerable dilemma was in having an embarrassment of riches from which to choose. We offer our profound apologies to those whom the pressures of space excluded.

Geoffrey Rose's work reflects, and often led, the progress of a whole field of scientific endeavour. His work covered the epidemiology of coronary heart disease, including studies within a single population and international studies, important areas of methodological development, trials to test preventive strategies, and the application of epidemiological and other knowledge to the development of public health policy for the prevention of this widespread disease. The sub-title of this book, *From aetiology to public health*, and its contents cover this spectrum. They exemplify the use and application of epidemiological research: to go from studies of aetiology to implementing public health policies and evaluating their effects.

For many of us, a significant development of recent years has been Geoffrey Rose's transition from epidemiology to public health. His initial position was 'pure': the epidemiologist should assemble the facts and leave them to others to act on. The danger in becoming an activist was seen to be loss of scientific 'objectivity'. There was also no particular reason to believe that people who were good at research were also good at effecting and implementing policy change. A natural transition, however, was to move to using epidemiological insights to plan public health strategies. The promotion by the World Health Organization (WHO) of the population approach to heart disease prevention began with Geoffrey Rose's chairmanship of the 1982 WHO Expert Committee on the Prevention of Coronary Heart Disease.

This provides an instructive model. It does not suggest that epidemiologists must become public health activists—they may if they are so inclined—but that they should use their knowledge to inform and analyse public health policy decisions.

This informs the structure of the book. A brief introduction sets the scene by (a) charting changes that have occurred in coronary heart disease mortality, following its emergence in countries undergoing economic development and other changes, and (b) giving an overview of the contribution of epidemiology to development of knowledge on aetiology and occurrence of coronary heart disease. The next part, on aetiology, starts with a chapter by Stamler summarizing evidence on the established risk factors and providing the knowledge base on which the newer developments, covered in this part, are built. Up-to-date accounts of the main areas of current research in coronary heart disease epidemiology are then given. The final part of the book is, appropriately, on public health—appropriate not only because an important purpose of epidemiological research is to improve the public health, but because this is an exciting and developing field of which we shall see much more in the future. This field has progressed to the point where scientific debate takes place alongside debates about the translation of research findings into health policy. It is to be expected, therefore, that there would not be complete accord. Some disagreement is to be found among authors, which reflects cogently argued current policy positions.

The book is aimed at two groups of readers: those interested in an up-to-date view of coronary heart disease epidemiology, and those who will appreciate that coronary heart disease serves as an instructive example of the application of research to the formation and evaluation of public health policy. We anticipate that this would serve as a reference work for medical students and as a text for postgraduate students and practitioners of epidemiology and public health, but would also be read by those actively concerned with prevention of cardiovascular disease.

We wish to acknowledge the special contribution of Gaye Woolven who, in effect, served as an executive editor for the book. It has been a pleasure to work with Oxford University Press in producing this volume.

June 1991   M.M.
London   P.E.

Foreword

Professor Kalevi Pyörälä

Progress in the field of epidemiology and prevention of cardiovascular diseases during the last decades has been enormous, beginning with epidemiological studies on the occurrence of coronary heart disease and hypertension and related factors in populations, and progressing through prevention trials and community demonstration projects to the development and application of preventive clinical practice and public health policy. This period of enormous progress coincides with the prime of the professional and scientific life of Professor Geoffrey Rose. However, this is not just a coincidence but, on the contrary, because Geoffrey Rose has been one of the forerunners in every step of this world-wide expedition.

Geoffrey Rose, like many other pioneers of cardiovascular epidemiology, received a thorough training in clinical medicine at St. Mary's Hospital, London, under the guidance of the famous Professor George Pickering. This gave him a solid background in the development of clinical methods applicable to studies of the occurrence of cardiovascular diseases and to the measurement of their risk factors in populations. This line of research commenced in 1959 when, as well as continuing his clinical work at St. Mary's Hospital, he joined the research staff of the London School of Hygiene and Tropical Medicine (LSH & TM). In 1960–1 he became acquainted with American cardiovascular epidemiology as Visiting Lecturer at the School of Hygiene and Public Health of the Johns Hopkins University, Baltimore. On his return to London, he became a Lecturer in Epidemiology at the LSH & TM (1961–2) and Senior Lecturer in Epidemiology in 1962–4. During the period 1964–70 he was Reader in Epidemiology at the University of London, and in 1970 he was appointed Professor of Epidemiology at St. Mary's Hospital Medical School. In 1977, following the death of Donald Reid, his teacher in epidemiology whom he deeply admired, he was invited to become Professor of Epidemiology at the LSH & TM. It is important to emphasize, however, that throughout this period and to the present day, he has kept in contact with clinical medicine as Honorary Consultant Physician at St. Mary's Hospital. This clinical attachment has been of great importance, because it has kept the direction of his epidemiological research in clinically relevant areas, facilitated his contacts with clinicians in research, and helped him in his communication with the medical profession as a teacher.

Geoffrey Rose's first epidemiological studies dealt with hypertension. One of the problems which he and his co-workers faced was the lack of a suitable instrument for the measurement of blood pressure in population studies: an ordinary sphygmomanometer leads to terminal digit preferences and potentially serious observer bias. He and his co-workers developed a modified instrument, the 'London School black box', which eliminated observer bias. This led others to the development of the so-called random-zero sphygmomanometer which is now the standard instrument in epidemiological studies on blood pressure. Various aspects of variability of blood pressure and variation of blood pressure measurement were addressed in that period in studies by Geoffrey Rose and his colleagues.

Generally accepted standardized methods for the diagnosis of coronary heart disease in population studies were not available at the beginning of the 1960s, when Geoffrey Rose started his work in this field. In 1962, in his paper 'The diagnosis of ischaemic heart pain and intermittent claudication in field surveys', he described a questionnaire which, under the name of the Rose Cardiovascular Questionnaire, has since then been used in population studies world-wide. This questionnaire has made his name known to everyone working in the field of coronary heart disease epidemiology. In 1960 Professor Henry Blackburn and his co-workers at the University of Minnesota, Minneapolis, had described a standardized coding system, the so-called Minnesota Code, for the classification of electrocardiographic abnormalities in population surveys. Geoffrey Rose adopted the Minnesota Code for British studies on coronary heart disease epidemiology and demonstrated that the coding could be reliably done by specially trained technicians. When the Research Committee of the International Society of Cardiology proposed that the World Health Organization (WHO) prepare a manual of methods for use in epidemiological studies of cardiovascular diseases, Geoffrey Rose and Henry Blackburn were asked to write it. This manual *Cardiovascular survey methods* was published in 1968 and has since been the first book to read for everyone who wants to become familiar with the basic methods used in epidemiological surveys on cardiovascular diseases. The second revised edition, written by Geoffrey Rose and Henry Blackburn jointly with Professor Richard Gillum (USA) and Professor Ronald Prineas (USA), was published in 1982.

The British prospective population studies initiated by Geoffrey Rose and his colleagues, in particular the Whitehall Study of London civil servants, made an important contribution to the understanding of the aetiology of coronary heart disease. While those studies were under way, the planning of the next step, risk factor intervention trials, was already in progress in the late 1960s. A controlled trial on smoking cessation was launched and preparations were started for a major international collaborative primary prevention trial, subsequently launched as the WHO European Collaborative Trial in the Multifactorial Prevention of Coronary Heart Disease and carried out under Geoffrey Rose's leadership by centres in Belgium, Italy, Poland, Spain, and the UK. Another, more recent, major international study in which Geoffrey Rose had an important role was the INTERSALT Study—the International Co-operative Study on the Relation of Electrolyte Excretion to Blood Pressure in Populations—which tested the hypothesis that there is a relationship between sodium intake and blood pressure. The plans for this study were developed under the leadership of Geoffrey Rose and Professor Jeremiah Stamler of the Northwestern University Medical School, Chicago, and its field survey comprising more than 50 population samples from 32 countries was carried out in 1985–6.

These are only a few examples from the wide scope of Geoffrey Rose's contributions to research in cardiovascular epidemiology and prevention. Alongside his impressive research activity, his contributions as a teacher and counsellor of young scientists are equally outstanding both nationally and internationally. A large number of physicians and scientists from the UK and other countries have had the privilege of studying under his guidance at the LSH & TM. The annual 10-Day International Teaching Seminars on Cardiovascular Epidemiology and Prevention, arranged since 1968 by the Section on Epidemiology and Prevention of the International Society and Federation of Cardiology, have been another important forum for Geoffrey Rose's international teaching activity. Geoffrey Rose, Professor Richard Remington (USA), Professor Jeremiah Stamler (USA), and Professor Rose Stamler (USA) formed the original core Faculty which created the spirit of these famous Seminars. Geoffrey Rose was the Chairman of the Seminar planning committee for 20 years. The number of Fellows accepted for each Seminar has been approximately 35 and the Faculty has consisted of seven or eight members. Until now more than 700 physicians or biomedical scientists from over 70 countries throughout the world have participated in these seminars. The 10-Day International Teaching Seminars have created a world-wide network of friendship between scientists, and these contacts have frequently led to collaborative international research. Two major international studies initiated as an outcome of these Seminars have already been mentioned: the WHO European Collaborative Trial in the Multifactorial Prevention of Coronary Heart Disease was initiated through connections created at the 3rd Seminar, held in Blessington, Ireland, in 1970, and the INTERSALT study was initiated at the 15th Seminar, held in Tuohilampi, Finland, in 1982. I had the privilege of being a participant of the first 10-Day Seminar, held in Makarska, Yugoslavia, in 1968, and that Seminar changed the direction of my professional and scientific life, as these seminars have done for many other physicians and scientists since then. The majority of the current leaders in the field of cardiovascular epidemiology are former Fellows of the 10-Day Seminars. The example of the 10-Day International Teaching Seminars has stimulated the initiation of regional and national teaching seminars and courses, while the International Teaching Seminars have continued to attract large numbers of qualified applicants. A shift of generation has recently taken place in the core Faculty and the Seminar planning committee, and it will be a demanding and challenging task for the new leaders of the Seminar activity to develop it further and to retain in a changing world the spirit created by the outstanding pioneer core Faculty!

Based on his vast experience in the teaching of epidemiology to clinicians, Geoffrey Rose has performed an important service for the students of this field by writing excellent and concise books which introduce beginners to the world of epidemiology. The book *Cardiovascular survey methods* has already been mentioned, but two other books written jointly with Professor David Barker of the University of Southampton, *Epidemiology in medical practice* and *Epidemiology for the uninitiated*, are also widely used throughout the world.

Translation of scientific information into preventive practice and public health policy has now become a reality, but this has been a slow and complex process needing the active participation of leading scientists. Movement in this direction started in the USA with Professor Jeremiah Stamler and Professor Frederick H. Epstein being among the first leading scientists to raise their voices and emphasize the need for a wide scope of action directed to the whole community, in addition to the clinical–individual approach. The momentum of the development of strategies for cardiovascular disease prevention was substantially increased in 1979 when Geoffrey Rose stepped out of his chamber of 'pure' epidemiologist–scientist and published his famous paper 'Strategy of prevention: lessons from cardiovascular disease' in which the terms 'high risk strategy' and 'mass strategy' were introduced. 'Mass strategy' was later renamed 'population strategy', and this became a key term in the further development of preventive strategies in the 1980s. In 1981 Geoffrey Rose chaired the WHO Expert Committee Meeting on Coronary Heart Disease, and the report of that Expert Committee, as well as the report of a subsequent WHO Expert Committee Meeting on Community Prevention and Control of Cardiovascular Diseases, held in 1984 and also chaired by Geoffrey Rose, has given clear guidelines for the development of national plans and programmes for coronary heart disease prevention. Such work is now in progress in many countries.

Geoffrey Rose has also played leading roles in international scientific organizations. In 1978–82 he was the Chairman of the Section on Epidemiology and Prevention and a member of the Scientific Board of the International Society and Federation of Cardiology. He was one of the founding members of the Working Group on Epidemiology and Prevention of the European Society of Cardiology and in 1979–80 was its first Chairman. As a brilliant lecturer he has over the years been a welcome keynote speaker at major international meetings on cardiovascular epidemiology and prevention. He is an honorary member or medallist of several scientific societies and organizations in his home country and other countries. In 1991, his contributions were additionally recognized in the UK by the award to him by the Queen of a high honour, Commander of the Order of the British Empire (CBE).

Finally, a personal note about the man behind these achievements. I first met Geoffrey Rose in 1968 at the 1st 10-Day International Teaching Seminar in Cardiovascular Epidemiology and Prevention, held in Makarska, Yugoslavia. I got to know him more intimately when I served as the Secretary of the Section on Epidemiology and Prevention of the International Society and Federation of Cardiology from 1974 to 1982 and succeeded him as the Chairman of the Section in 1982–6. His scientific thinking, his methods of leading and carrying out research, and his unusual ability to express his thoughts in spoken and written words have had an immense influence on my own development as scientist. Beyond that I have got to know Geoffrey Rose outside his professional world, and ties of fond friendship have developed between us. Warm kindness, integrity, humanity, and strong faith in God are those personal characteristics which have enabled him to be of great support to his friends and co-workers in times of distress and doubt. The picture of Geoffrey Rose would not be complete without drawing in the warm personality of Ceridwen, his wife and companion on their lifelong expedition. We all thank you for what you have been for us and wish you well!

Foreword

Professor Sir Stanley Peart

I first really began to be aware of Geoffrey Rose when he was a Registrar and then Senior Registrar at St. Mary's Hospital about 1954–5, but I did not know him very well. You must understand that I was a Lecturer in Medicine with very definite interests and they did not coincide with those of Geoffrey. When young, he seemed quite austere, and since I rarely talked to him I never penetrated this apparent shell. The reputation as a lay preacher did not immediately seem any reason for me to make greater efforts, even if my background as a Mary's student who liked rugby football and much that went with it might suggest a fertile field in which Geoffrey might test his talents. The 'Loneliness of the long distance runner' might also be apposite as this was his favourite sporting occupation.

Bill Miall was another who was associated with the Medical Unit just after the war when he was House Physician, and he was also to make his own considerable contribution to epidemiology. Both owe their interest in the subject to the influence of George Pickering, who had initiated the first really adventurous quantitative attack on the inheritance of blood pressure and had shown the continuity of distribution of this measurement in large populations. Both Geoffrey and Bill contrasted in their styles with the somewhat Rabelaisian approach of George, but this combination of opposites was tremendously successful.

I then lost sight of Geoffrey until I myself returned to St. Mary's, and, of course, particularly after George Pickering went to Oxford in 1956. This was when I first made the acquaintance of that delightful man Donald Reid, who is, I have to say, my favourite epidemiologist. He was a Highland Scot with a wicked sense of humour. He had been in the RAF as a neuropsychiatrist, a title used no doubt to distinguish them from the other bunch of somato-psychiatrists, and had survived a pneumonectomy, with psyche intact, for what turned out to be a benign lesion, despite the initial diagnosis. Interestingly enough, Geoffrey also served in the RAF as a neuropsychiatrist, the only flaw that I can find in his career. Donald Reid and I discussed how Geoffrey could be given a joint academic appointment between the LSH & TM and St. Mary's, since he clearly wanted to maintain his clinical links, despite much portentous advice against following such a potentially disastrous course, from those who shall be nameless, however eminent. Only the pure in heart and mind and population statistics can enter this Kingdom, but Donald and Geoffrey knew otherwise, and I was not inclined to put too much weight on advice from one such that I met on Hampstead Heath running backwards up a hill in army boots. And so, starting as a Lecturer and then a Senior Lecturer at LSH & TM, a joint appointment with the Medical School was born, and consultant responsibility for the care of patients on the Medical Unit went along with all the other epidemiological interests.

He progressed smoothly to take on the Chair of Epidemiology at St. Mary's and our personal clinical links were further strengthened. Even his move to the Chair of Epidemiology at the LSH & TM did not disturb the maintenance of some of his clinical work, and so it has continued to the present.

What is equally important has been the continuation of that link over the years by shared junior appointments, proving that there is more than one approach to epidemiology and that an appropriate balance between the individual needs of patients and wider epidemiological interests is not only possible, but desirable. The debt that I owe to Geoffrey and all his young men and women was shared by generations of medical unit staff. It was brought up best at our Death and Discharge Meeting each Friday morning. No loose statement passed unchallenged, precise quantitation was required, and anecdotal medicine, while tolerated with a quiet smile, was countered by extensive data and references to fuller studies which often refuted the individual conclusions. He educated us all in the most delightful way, and it has been the longest and most valued of associations.

He realized that his clinical aptitudes might be less sharp as time passed and other duties pressed, but all the staff knew that this was just part of his self-critical approach, and I just made sure that we did not assign two epidemiologists to run one clinical service. But there was more to come, since much to my surprise, and more to his, we were to work together on the Medical Research Council Trial in Hypertension, where Bill Miall added to the old St. Mary's group. Geoffrey was a real stalwart, and the benefit of his combination of clinical acumen and epidemiological skills showed through in the discussions and, of course, this has characterized all his epidemiological work, since he knows the clinical and human implications of the studies he has proposed. Just occasionally he has had doubts about this division, but even when he took on the Chair at the LSH & TM he persevered and our reward, as well I hope as his, has been the clear demonstration to the students at Mary's and at the LSH & TM that this is a productive and desirable way of life.

Finally I should describe the lowest point, as far as I know, in Geoffrey's life. I was on a ward round at St. Mary's when I received a telephone message telling me that he was in High Wycombe Hospital following a road traffic accident. This proved, of course, that even though he knew the risks of riding mopeds he was prepared to disregard them, but regrettably not the car that hit him. A quick trip to High Wycombe revealed the traditional picture of overhead frames with limbs attached in plaster and tubes into and out of every orifice and what is now called multisystem failure, but he is made of tough stuff and even when he developed an arteriovenous connection and pulsating exophthalmos he never complained, at least in my hearing. He might have done if he had heard our neurosurgical colleagues discussing floating a piece of muscle on a thread up the carotid to the ophthalmic artery so as to block it. That suggestion was talked out, much to everyone's relief, and, in any case, nature was kind and decided to shut the pathway while normal service was resumed in all other parts. Geoffrey's inner strength was truly revealed and added to our already considerable admiration.

Over the years I have appreciated his sceptical, sometimes acerbic, comments and have noted how his ability to inject a humorous aside has grown. His self-deprecatory remarks are never borne out by the facts. He is truly an unusual combination of physician and epidemiologist who has demonstrated to the world that this approach is rewarding, and the world has responded by recognizing his merit. In so doing he has created his own Rose School which includes not only his younger students, but also his older colleagues.

January 1991

Contents

PUBLIC HEALTH

Contributors

K. Ball
Department of Community Medicine, Horace Joules Hall, Central Middlesex Hospital, London.

D. J. P. Barker
MRC Environmental Epidemiology Unit, Southampton General Hospital.

E. Barrett-Connor
Department of Family and Community Medicine, School of Medicine, University of California, USA.

H. Blackburn
Division of Epidemiology, School of Public Health, University of Minnesota, USA.

B. P. M. Bloemberg
Department of Epidemiology, National Institute of Public Health and Environmental Protection, The Netherlands.

C. J. Bulpitt
Division of Geriatric Medicine, Hammersmith Hospital, London.

M. L. Burr
MRC Epidemiology Unit (South Wales), Cardiff.

J. Elford
Department of Public Health and Primary Care, Royal Free Hospital, School of Medicine, London.

P. Elliott
Department of Public Health and Policy, London School of Hygiene and Tropical Medicine, London.

P. C. Elwood
MRC Epidemiology Unit (South Wales), Cardiff.

F. H. Epstein
Department of Social and Preventive Medicine, University of Zurich, Switzerland.

W. R. Harlan
National Institutes of Health, Bethesda, MD, USA.

W. P. T. James
Rowett Research Institute, Aberdeen.

S. Johansson
Department of Medicine, University of Göteborg, Sweden.

J. V. Joossens
St. Raphael University Hospital, Leuven, Belgium.

W. B. Kannel
National Heart Institute, Framingham, MA, USA.

H. Keen
Department of Medicine, Guy's Hospital, London.

H. Kesteloot
Department of Epidemiology, St. Raphael University Hospital, Leuven, Belgium.

K.-T. Khaw
Clinical Gerontology Unit, New Addenbrooke's Hospital, University of Cambridge.

M. Kornitzer
Ecole de Santé Publique, Brussels, Belgium.

D. Kromhout
National Institute of Public Health and Environmental Protection, The Netherlands.

L. H. Kuller
Graduate School of Public Health, University of Pittsburgh, USA.

D. R. Labarthe
School of Public Health, University of Texas, USA.

B. Larsson
Sahlgrens Hospital, Göteborg, Sweden.

B. Lewis
St Thomas' Hospital, London.

T. A. Manolio
National Institutes of Health, Bethesda, MD, USA.

M. G. Marmot
Department of Epidemiology and Public Health, University College and Middlesex School of Medicine, London and Department of Epidemiology and Population Sciences, London School of Hygiene and Tropical Medicine.

P. M. McKeigue
Department of Epidemiology and Population Sciences, London School of Hygiene and Tropical Medicine.

T. W. Meade
MRC Epidemiology and Medical Care Unit, Northwick Park Hospital, London.

A. Menotti
Laboratory of Epidemiology and Biostatistics, Istituto Superiore di Sanita, Rome.

J. N. Morris
Department of Public Health and Policy, London School of Hygiene and Tropical Medicine, London.

M. F. Oliver
Wynn Institute for Metabolic Research, London.

C. Osmond
MRC Environmental Epidemiology Unit, Southampton General Hospital.

S. J. Pocock
Department of Epidemiology and Population Sciences, London School of Hygiene and Tropical Medicine.

N. R. Poulter
Department of Epidemiology and Public Health, University College and Middlesex School of Medicine, London.

A. Ralph
Rowett Research Institute, Aberdeen.

R. D. Remington
University of Iowa, USA.

B. M. Rifkind
National Heart, Lung, and Blood Institute, Bethesda, MD, USA.

G. Rose
Department of Epidemiology and Population Sciences, London School of Hygiene and Tropical Medicine.

P. S. Sever
Department of Clinical Pharmacology, St. Mary's Hospital Medical School, London.

A. G. Shaper
Department of Public Health and Primary Care, Royal Free Hospital, School of Medicine, London.

D. Simpson
Action on Smoking and Health, London.

J. Stamler
Department of Community Health and Preventive Medicine, Northwestern University, Chicago.

R. Stamler
Department of Community Health and Preventive Medicine, Northwestern University, Chicago.

P. M. Sweetnam
MRC Epidemiology Unit (South Wales), Cardiff.

T. Theorell
National Institute for Psycho-social Factors and Health, Stockholm, Sweden.

S. G. Thompson
Department of Epidemiology and Population Sciences, London School of Hygiene and Tropical Medicine, London.

H. Tunstall-Pedoe
Cardiovascular Epidemiology Unit, Ninewells Hospital, Dundee.

N. J. Wald
Department of Environmental and Preventive Medicine, St. Bartholomew's Hospital, London.

L. Wilhelmsen
Department of Medicine, Ostra Hospital, Sweden.

D. A. Wood
National Heart and Lung Institute, Royal Brompton National Heart and Lung Hospital, London.

INTRODUCTION

1

Coronary heart disease: rise and fall of a modern epidemic

Michael Marmot

It has been common to characterize coronary heart disease (CHD) as a disease of affluence. This may have been a reasonable description as CHD reached epidemic proportions in Western countries. It does not serve sufficiently to describe the present picture of CHD world-wide:

- CHD is emerging as a major cause of death in developing countries;
- CHD rates are rising in many countries of Central and Eastern Europe;
- CHD rates are falling in the wealthy countries of Europe, North America, and Australasia;
- CHD rates have continued to fall from a low level in Japan;
- within wealthy countries, CHD is now more common among the less wealthy groups;
- the decline in CHD in the UK and the USA has occurred faster among higher socio-economic groups.

Rather than characterize CHD as a disease of affluence, it is more accurate to say that differences in CHD between and within countries can only be understood with reference to the social, cultural, and economic features of those societies. The challenge is to find general ways of describing these trends in order to understand the social, economic, and cultural forces that determine them.

It is particularly instructive to review the three contrasts of Western Europe, 'Eastern' Europe, and Japan. The case that will be made here, that CHD is related to economic changes in society, in no way negates the importance of life-style: smoking, food patterns, exercise. These may well be part of the reason underlying broad societal changes in the rate of occurrence of CHD. A review of CHD trends suggests three broad classes of factors at work: nutrition, cigarette smoking, and other factors related to economic development.

Because it is such a major cause of death, the rise and fall of CHD is intimately bound up with changes in life expectancy. These will be reviewed first.

LIFE EXPECTANCY AND THE RISE AND FALL OF CHD

In regions of the world where CHD rates are high, e.g. Western Europe or North America, in general, the higher the rate of CHD the higher is the mortality from all causes. This is in part because CHD is such an important contributor to the total death rate, but also because there is a correlation between mortality from CHD and mortality from other causes. This is true for regions within a country, such as regions of England and Wales or states of the USA, social classes within a country (OPCS 1978), time trends, and, to a lesser extent, differences between European countries (Uemura and Pisa 1988).

Taking into account the 165 countries reviewed by Preston and Nelson (1974), there is an inverse association between CHD and all-cause mortality. Countries with low CHD mortality are most usually developing countries with high mortality from infectious disease. In the most general sense, this corresponds to the epidemiological transition (Omran 1971). As the toll of infectious disease mortality declines, it is replaced by a different pattern of chronic diseases: predominantly cardiovascular disease and cancer. This transition or health development is broadly related to the level of economic development. There are examples of poor countries where infectious disease mortality has declined, but as yet, does not appear to have been replaced by an increasing burden of chronic disease. More usually, the rise of CHD goes with economic development. In mature industrial economies, so too does the fall.

The epidemiological transition was well under way in the UK in the 1920s. In 1921, CHD and cancer combined caused approximately the same number of deaths as infectious diseases. By 1931 chronic diseases had become the major causes of death in both men and women (Davey Smith and Marmot 1991).

The decline of infectious disease mortality had a considerable impact on life expectancy. From 1922 to 1984 in England and Wales, life expectancy at birth increased from 55.6 to 71.6 years in men and from 59.6 to 77.6 years in women. This rapid improvement is mostly the result of reduction in infant mortality. Figure 1.1 shows that, at age 45, the increase in life expectancy over this 60 year period was only 3.9 years for men and a more impressive 6.7 years for women. This rather modest improvement at middle age reflects the rise of chronic disease mortality, particularly CHD and lung cancer. This rise was more marked in men than women, and hence men had a smaller rise in life expectancy. During the early part of this rise in CHD and lung cancer, in the 1930s, life expectancy at age 45 actually fell. After a long period when middle-age life expectancy was impressive for its relative lack of improvement, there was an increase of 1.8 years in

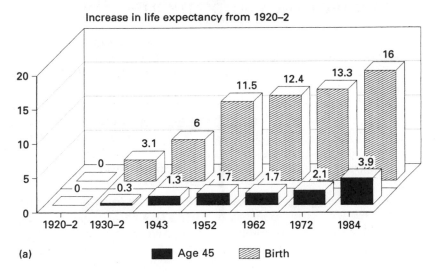

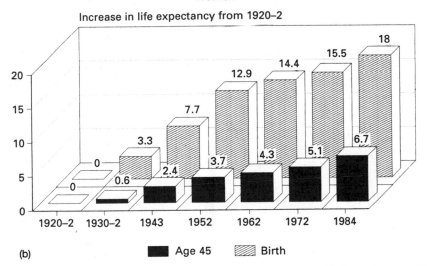

Fig. 1.1 Increase in life expectancy in England and Wales at birth, and at age 45, compared with 1920–2: (a) men; (b) women.

only 12 years. This can be attributed to the fact that the epidemics of CHD and lung cancer, although still major causes of death, have passed their peak and are now on the way down. This is illustrated in Fig. 1.2 which shows the decline in CHD mortality in England and Wales and other European countries over the period 1970–85. Such declines have affected

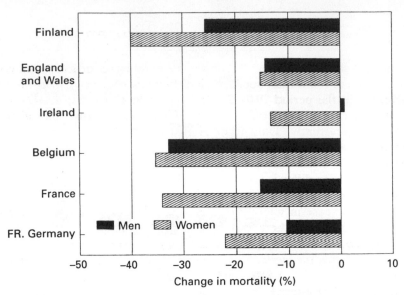

Fig. 1.2 Changes in CHD mortality (per cent) in Western Europe: 1970–85 age-standardized figures, men and women age 30–69. (From Uemura and Pisa 1988.)

other countries, notably the USA, Canada, Australia, New Zealand, and Japan (see below).

In passing, it may be noted that these data on life expectancy provide an answer to those who question the extent to which the rise in CHD and lung cancer could be attributed to changes in diagnostic fashion. At a time of decline in infectious disease mortality there was an actual decrease in life expectancy at middle age. Some causes of death had to be increasing. These were CHD and lung cancer.

The general picture then is of a sharp rise in CHD mortality that occurred at a time of economic development and sharp falls that occur as development in the affluent countries continues. 'Economic development' is used in a loose sense. During the 1930s, in England and Wales the decline in infant mortality rate was what would be expected with development. However, this was the time of the Great Economic Depression. This no doubt brought economic hardship to many, as presumably did 'developments' in Eastern Europe during the 1970s and 1980s. Nevertheless these conditions that appear to be associated with increasing CHD rates were likely to have been different from those more extreme conditions which characterize rural poverty in developing countries, or urban poverty in the UK in the nineteenth century—situations where the CHD rates are low.

EAST AND WEST EUROPE

Figure 1.3 shows trends in CHD rates for another set of European countries, those of the former socialist bloc. In all cases, among men the rates increased in the period 1970–85. In each of these countries, except the former German Democratic Republic (GDR), all-cause mortality increased concurrently. Data from Hungary and Czechoslovakia, for example, show that life expectancy decreased through this period. The picture for CHD is like that of Western Europe up until the 1950s and 1960s. What appears to differ is the decline in life expectancy at birth in Eastern Europe. The difference is likely to relate to infant mortality. At the time of the steep increase in CHD in England and Wales, infant mortality was declining. Although there was little improvement in life expectancy in middle age, there was still an increase in life expectancy at birth. In Eastern Europe, the increase in CHD is not balanced by a decline in infant mortality.

If we ask why Eastern Europe should be going through an epidemiological picture like that of England and Wales in an earlier period, it is perhaps not fanciful to suggest that this reflects the relative state of economic development. Those countries may be at the point in industrialization and economic development that, in the West, corresponded to the upswing of the CHD epidemic before it reached its peak.

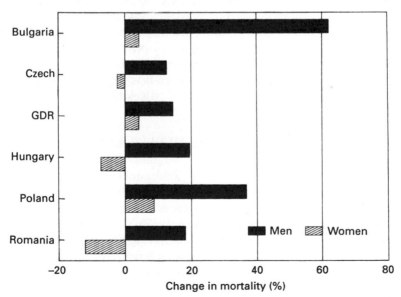

Fig. 1.3 Changes in CHD mortality (%) in Eastern Europe: 1970–85 age-standardized figures, men and women age 30–69.

Links between economic development and CHD

McKeown (1976) attributed the decline of infant mortality and infectious disease mortality that occurred with industrialization in England and Wales to improvements in nutrition. Adequate nutrition means largely adequate calories. Internationally, higher calorie consumption is related to lower mortality rates. The maintenance of adequate nutrition may have prevented an adverse effect on infant mortality of the high unemployment and poverty that existed in the 1930s in the UK (Winter 1983; Davey Smith and Marmot 1991).

Poor nutrition may also mean too much as well as too little. There has been controversy as to what has happened to fat intake, for example, in the UK and the USA during the twentieth century. The rise in consumption of polyunsaturates, in the USA since the 1960s and in the UK since the 1970s, may have played an important part in the decline in CHD (Marmot 1985). Data from food consumption surveys in the USA suggest that saturated fat intake declined from the 1960s (Stephen and Wald 1990). To what extent saturated fat intakes increased over the first half of the century before it decreased subsequently is unclear. Therefore the role of nutrition in causing the rise of ischaemic heart disease can be questioned. It may have played an enabling role. High intakes of saturated fat and consequent high mean levels of plasma cholesterol provide the conditions for a high population rate of heart disease. If these existed, some other factor(s) may be directly implicated in the increase in CHD.

An obvious candidate is cigarette smoking. Smoking increased relatively early in England and Wales. During the period of increased CHD, lung cancer was on the rise. This may well be in operation in Eastern Europe. As Kesteloot and Joossens report (Chapter 11 of this volume), smoking is highly prevalent in Hungary at a time when it is declining in frequency in many countries in Western Europe and North America.

COMPARISON WITH JAPAN

A rise in CHD rates is not an inevitable consequence of economic development, industrialization, and decline of infectious disease. Japan makes the case. Figure 1.4 contrasts mortality rates in Japan with those in England and Wales (Marmot and Davey Smith 1989). In middle age, all-cause mortality rates in Japan were higher than in England and Wales up to the early 1960s (Uemura and Pisa 1988). Japan's rates fell more steeply than those of England and Wales, and current rates are now considerably lower in Japan.

Over the last 25 years, trends in mortality in Japan have been more favourable for virtually all categories of mortality. For example, Japan has

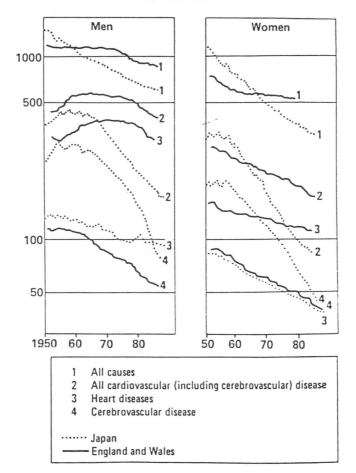

Fig. 1.4 Trends in mortality (age-standardized) among men and women aged 30–69 in Japan and in England and Wales, 1950–86.

had the highest rate in the world from stroke. Mortality from stroke has declined steeply. Despite dire warnings of the effect of industrialization and supposed Westernization, Japan escaped the CHD epidemic and has had among the lowest rates of heart disease of any industrialized country. But, as Fig. 1.4 shows, age-adjusted rates from this disease have also declined steeply, and to a greater extent than in England and Wales.

Given that infectious diseases were not replaced by CHD, there has been the expected effect on life expectancy (Table 1.1) (Marmot and Davey Smith 1989). At birth a Japanese boy could expect to live 75.2 years (assuming that today's mortality rates applied) compared with 71.5 years, for a boy born in England and Wales. The expectation of life of a girl born in Japan is now an astonishing 80.9 years compared with 77.4 years for a

Table 1.1 Life expectancy (years) of Japanese and of English and Welsh populations since 1955.

	Males		Females	
	At birth	At age 65	At birth	At age 65
Japan[1]:				
1955	63.6	11.8	78.8	14.1
1965	67.7	11.9	72.9	14.6
1975	71.7	13.7	76.9	16.6
1980	73.4	14.6	78.8	17.7
1986	75.2	15.9	80.9	19.3
England & Wales[2] [3]:				
1955	67.5	11.8	73.0	14.8
1965	68.5	12.1	74.7	15.8
1975	69.5	12.4	75.7	16.4
1980	70.4	12.8	76.6	16.8
1984–86	71.9	13.4	77.7	17.3

[1] Status and Information Department, Minister's Secretariat. Military and Health and Welfare, *Natal statistics 1965, 1986*. Tokyo Koser Token Kwokai, 1967–88. In Japan.
[2] Office of Health Economics. *Compendum of health statistics*, 6th ed. London OHE, 1987.
[3] Office of Population Censures and Surverys. *Monthly statistics*, 1986, London HMSO, 1989. (Series DH2).

girl born in England and Wales (Statistics and Information Department 1967–1988; OPCS 1989).

The speed with which life expectancy has increased is also impressive: 7.5 years for men and 8 years for women in the 21 years from 1965 to 1986. To put in perspective what this means, abolishing all heart disease and assuming that other causes of death did not increase in frequency would add 4.7 years to life expectancy in England and Wales. (I am grateful to Dr. Peter Boyle, IARC Lyons, for this calculation.) An improvement in life expectancy in a country that is equivalent to abolishing all heart disease and most cancer in 21 years is worthy of attention. This is what has happened in Japan.

Life expectancy is, of course, heavily influenced by mortality in the first year of life. Table 1.1 shows that, even at age 65, life expectancy has improved 4 years for men in Japan and 4.6 years for women since 1965 compared with 1.1 years and 1.4 years for men and women in England and Wales.

It seems reasonable to speculate that the same causes responsible for the rise and fall of CHD, with its impact on life expectancy, in Western Europe are operating in Eastern Europe, a generation later. Given the difference of the Japanese pattern, it is worth enquiring into the reasons behind

Japan's remarkable improvement in life expectancy. The lessons learnt may well have broader application (Marmot and Davey Smith 1989).

Genes?

CHD, like other epidemic diseases, relates closely to social conditions. Its frequency of occurrence has much more to do with the social and cultural features of a society than it does with the genetic make-up of the people who constitute that society. The two strongest general arguments for this are as follows. First, rapid changes have occurred in the rate of occurrence of CHD. In the USA, for example, death rates from CHD declined by 48 per cent between 1970 and 1985. In Japan, the reduction was 39 per cent in men and 30 per cent in women (Uemura and Pisa 1988). Gene frequencies do not change at that rate. Second, the differences between countries in rate of occurrence of CHD become blurred when people migrate. Migrants tend towards the rate of CHD of their country of adoption (Marmot *et al.* 1984*b*). Men of Japanese ancestry living in Hawaii have higher rates of CHD than do Japanese in Japan. Japanese in California have higher rates than those in Hawaii but less than the average for the USA (Marmot *et al.* 1975; Worth *et al.* 1975). Presumably they take on the life-style of the host country with its attendant disease consequences (Marmot and Syme 1976).

Medical care

Japan is not a high consumer of medical care. In 1980, Japan spent 6.4 per cent of gross domestic product on health care, not very different from the United Kingdom (5.8 per cent), and substantially less than the USA (9.5 per cent) and the Federal Republic of Germany (8.0 per cent). When prices are taken into account, by the use of 'purchasing power parities', Japan does spend more than the United Kingdom but less than Norway and France and about the same as Austria, the former Federal Republic of Germany, the USA, and the Netherlands (Parkin *et al.* 1989). These high expenditure countries all have shorter life expectancy than Japan.

It is not the amount spent that is of crucial importance but its effect. Charlton and Velez (1986) have examined mortality trends from 1951 to 1980 for a group of conditions which could be prevented by medical intervention. The countries included were Japan, England and Wales, USA, France, Italy, and Sweden. Japan started with by far the highest rate for these conditions in 1951 (largely due to stroke being included), and it showed the most dramatic decline of all the countries studied. However, unlike the other countries, Japan also showed a steep decline in mortality rates from causes not amenable to medical intervention. It started the period with the highest rate of such mortality, but by the late 1960s it had the lowest, and the downward trend continued subsequently.

The decline in Japan's mortality rates is of a magnitude and rapidity such as to make it unlikely that it could simply be explained by improvements in medical care.

Nutrition and smoking

Two-thirds of Japanese men smoke (Ueshima *et al.* 1987). This is extremely high by world standards. It is a puzzle as to why they do not therefore have high rates of CHD. In the Seven-Countries Study, smoking was a weak coronary risk factor in Japan, somewhat stronger in Southern Europe, and a strong risk factor in the USA (Keys 1980). It may be that the strength of smoking as a risk factor is related to the background level of risk as determined by diet and level of plasma lipids.

Dietary fat makes up less than 25 per cent of the Japanese diet compared with 42 per cent in the UK (Ueshima *et al.* 1987). The ratio of polyunsaturates to saturates is 1.1 compared with 0.34 in the UK. Fat intake may have increased in Japan, but it has a long way to go before it reaches 'Western' (or Eastern European) levels.

It may be that the coronary epidemic in the countries of Eastern Europe is related to high levels of smoking in the face of a high intake of saturated fat. In Japan, the high level of smoking takes place against a background low level of fat intake. This may help to explain why Japan appears to have carried off the balancing act of a decline in its 'own' diseases, stomach cancer and stroke, without taking on the West's diseases, CHD and cancer of the lung, colon, and breast.

Japanese diet may help to explain why CHD has not increased in Japan in the face of widespread smoking. It does not explain a dramatic 38 per cent *fall* in male CHD rates between 1970 and 1985. A decline in salt intake may be playing a role in the decline in stroke and, to a lesser extent, in CHD. But there must be other factors operating that have a large effect.

Economic forces

It was argued above that the rise and fall in CHD in Europe and North America was broadly related to economic development. The most dramatic change in Japan's circumstances in the post-war period has been its rise as an economic superpower.

There is a sharp contrast between Japan's economic performance and that of the UK during the period 1965–86 when Japan's life expectancy raced past that of the UK (Marmot and Davey Smith 1989). Japan's low inflation, high growth rate (4.2 per cent per annum (1965–87) compared with an OECD average of 2.3 per cent), and low unemployment are in sharp contrast with the UK's performance which is worse than the OECD average. Japan's gross national product (GNP) was lower than that of the UK in the 1970s but 50 per cent higher in 1987. In 1987, Japan ranked fourth in GNP per capita of OECD countries after Switzerland, the USA, and Norway.

Wilkinson argues that there is a relation internationally between income and life expectancy, but that the relation is stronger with measures of income distribution than with GNP (Wilkinson 1989). Japan, with the fastest rate of growth of any OECD country and now the fourth highest GNP, has the smallest relative differences in income between the top and the bottom 20 per cent of income groups (World Bank 1988). This might be part of the explanation as to why Japan's life expectancy has surpassed that of the UK (Marmot and Davey Smith 1989).

Work and social relations

Economic development brings wealth, but it also brings a change in the nature of working and social life. The Ni-Hon-San migrant study of men of Japanese ancestry living in Japan, Hawaii, and California produced evidence that the higher rate of CHD among Japanese in California was related to forgoing a Japanese life-style. Californian Japanese men had a higher fat diet and a higher mean serum cholesterol than men in Japan (Kato *et al.* 1973; Marmot *et al.* 1975; Nichaman *et al.* 1975). Independent of the level of serum cholesterol, men who were more traditionally Japanese, in the sense of retaining ties to a close-knit community, had a lower prevalence of CHD than men who were Westernized in their culture and social relations (Marmot and Syme 1976). This was consistent with the hypothesis put forward by Matsumoto (1970) that Japanese culture contains stress-reducing devices. He proposed that, in Japan, work provides social support and psychological security, as does the collective nature of Japanese society. These in turn may relate to protection from diseases such as CHD. This is consistent with a body of work relating social supports to protection from CHD and premature death (Berkman 1984). There is no evidence, despite popular fears in Japan, that this distinctive mode of social life is changing to resemble American culture. Westernization appears more confined to superficial aspects of life-style.

Karasek and Theorell (1990) have reviewed the influences that the psycho-social work environment may have on CHD risk. An impressive body of evidence suggests that work characterized by lack of control, little opportunity for development, and boring repetitive tasks is related to increased cardiovascular risk. We have speculated that perhaps this is less a feature of the Japanese work environment than it is of many Western countries (Marmot and Davey Smith 1989). This cannot be the whole story. Participation in the labour force and experience of work are not the same for women as for men. Against the primary importance of 'healthy' work as the determinant of long life expectancy is the favourable trend for women as well as for men.

In sum, the Japanese experience suggests that, to explain the broad trends in CHD, we may have to consider three classes of factors: nutrition, smoking, and economic factors that may exert their influence in a variety of ways.

SOCIO-ECONOMIC FACTORS

As noted, income inequalities appear to be more closely related to life expectancy than the overall income level, or wealth, of a society. Therefore it is important not only to examine how economic changes may be related to mortality changes for a whole society but to examine socio-economic subgroups within a society.

Social class differences within society

Social class differences in the rate of occurrence of disease are a manifestation of the socio-economic forces at work in causation. Currently, in many Western countries, there are social class differences in CHD mortality as there are in mortality from all causes (Marmot *et al.* 1987).

A potential problem with social class analysis is the measurement of class. Income or years of education are commonly used. In the UK, measurement of social class has traditionally been based on occupational prestige—the Registrar-General's social classes ranging from I (Professional) to V (Unskilled Manual). However, measures such as access to a car or home ownership (housing tenure) predict mortality in addition to social class based on occupation (Fox and Goldblatt 1982). That social class differences in mortality are not an artefact of the Registrar-General's social classes is shown by the Whitehall study of British civil servants (Fig. 1.5). Grade of employment shows a clear inverse relation with mortality—the lower the grade, the higher the risk. The smooth nature of the relationship

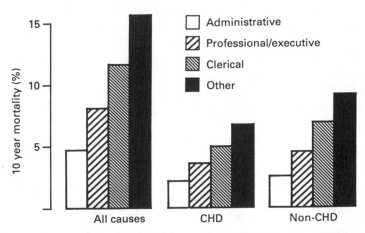

Fig. 1.5 Percentage of men dying in 10 years from all causes, from CHD, and from non-CHD by grade in the British Civil Service (age-adjusted figures)—the Whitehall Study. (From Marmot 1984*a*.)

is striking. It is not only the men at the bottom who are at increased risk, but the risk is spread throughout the range. Each grade of employment is associated with higher risk than the one above it (Marmot *et al*. 1984*a*). The gradient in mortality is the same for CHD as for death from other causes (Fig. 1.5). In Whitehall, classifying men by grade *and* whether they had access to cars or owned their home further spreads the risk (Davey Smith *et al*. 1990).

Time trends in social class differences

Although social class differences in CHD currently parallel those for mortality from all causes in the UK, it was not always thus. Changes in diagnostic fashion present difficulties in interpretation, but it appears that in the 1930s, when CHD was on the rise, it was more common in classes I and II than in the semi-skilled and unskilled classes IV and V (Marmot *et al*. 1978). The change-over had occurred by the early 1960s. Subsequently, as CHD rates have started to decline in the UK, there has been a marked decline in non-manual occupations and no decline at all among men in manual occupations or their wives (Marmot and McDowall 1986).

Social class differences in different cultures

The implication of the changing social class pattern of CHD is that the factors linking economic position to disease may change. This can be put together with the observation that, as economic development proceeds, CHD appears to increase, and as it proceeds further, it declines. It is as if CHD passes through society in a wave, affecting first the more privileged and subsequently the less privileged, declining first in those better off and presumably subsequently in the rest (Marmot and McDowall 1986). This is similar to the picture described previously for peptic ulcer (Susser and Stein 1962).

   The impact of social class in a society will therefore depend on other features of that society. This can be illustrated by the study of mortality in migrants to England and Wales. Migrants bring their pattern of disease with them. This then changes towards that of the host country. Among migrants to England and Wales, we see three social class patterns of mortality (Marmot *et al*. 1984*b*). Among immigrants from Ireland, there is the same pattern of inverse association with class as in England and Wales as a whole, but in each class the mortality rate for immigrant Irish is higher than the average rate for that class in England and Wales. Second, among immigrants from the Indian subcontinent there is little relation between class and mortality. Third, immigrants from the Caribbean show higher mortality rates in non-manual than in manual classes. This differing relation of mortality to class may be related to stages of economic development of the societies from which these different cultural groups come. The Afro-Caribbean picture is more like that of England and Wales in the 1930s, the South Asians like England and Wales in the 1950s, and the Irish similar to England and Wales now.

What we have described for CHD can be seen for a risk factor such as smoking (Fig. 1.6) (Yach 1990). In South Africa, the relation of class to smoking is different for different ethnic groups and is dependent on where those groups are in the socio-economic spectrum.

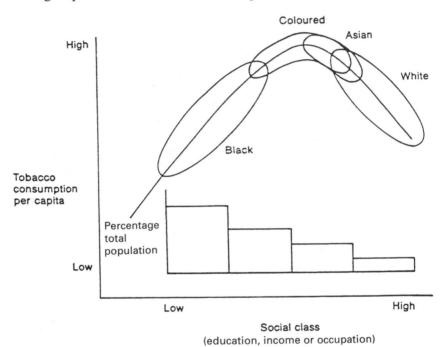

Fig. 1.6 Idealized summary of relation of social class to tobacco consumption among ethnic groups in South Africa. (From Yach 1990.)

Links between socio-economic position and CHD

This was extensively reviewed in the UK in the Black Report (Black *et al.* 1988) and will only be touched on here. Black and his colleagues suggested four possible types of explanation: artefact, social selection, culture/life-style, and material conditions. After detailed examination of the evidence, they rejected artefact and the possibility that social class differences are all due to 'selection' of unhealthier people into lower grades. Black favoured a materialist explanation, that social class differences in health are due to material conditions of life that show a correlation with income levels and wealth: housing, transport, and the environment. Whether we wish to class nutrition and smoking into life-style or material conditions, it is likely that they play a role. Barker's studies suggest that it may not only be conditions acting during adult life that are important. Circumstances *in utero* or in infancy may have a persisting effect on mortality rates throughout life (Barker 1989).

CONCLUSIONS

The trends in CHD listed at the beginning of this chapter point to the importance of social and economic forces in determining its rise and fall. It is useful to keep in perspective both the socio-economic differences between countries and those within.

Socio-economic differences within countries have come to assume such major importance that continued exploration of reasons underlying links between social position and CHD is likely to be fruitful. Investigation should fall into the broad classes discussed: material conditions, social environment including work and social life, nutrition, early environment, and life-style including smoking and exercise (Marmot *et al.* 1987; Marmot and Theorell 1988). Attention will have to be given not only to explanations of what 'risk factors' might account statistically for socio-economic differences in CHD within (and between) countries, but the prospects for changing them. Exploration is likely to fall into the same categories as those discussed in relation to Japan's health success: nutrition, work, and social environments. These have been reviewed (Marmot *et al.* 1987).

REFERENCES

Barker, D. J. P. (1989). The intrauterine and early postnatal origins of cardiovascular disease and chronic bronchitis. *J. Epidemiol. Community Health*, **43**, 237–40.

Berkman, L. F. (1984). Assessing the Physical Health Effects of Social Networks and Social Support. In *Annual review of public health* (eds L. Breslow, J. E. Fielding, and L. B. Lave), Annual Reviews Inc., Palo Alto, CA, pp. 413–32.

Black, D., Morris, J. N., Smith, C., Townsend, P., and Whitehead, M. (1988). *Inequalities in health: The Black report; The health divide*, Penguin Group, London.

Charlton, J. R. H. and Velez, R. (1986). Some international comparisons of mortality amenable to medical intervention. *Br. med. J.*, **292**, 295–301.

Davey Smith, G. and Marmot, M. (1991). Trends in mortality in Britain: 1920–1986. *Ann. Nutr. Metab.*, **35** (1), 53–63.

Davey Smith, G., Shipley, M. J., and Rose, G. (1990). The magnitude and causes of socio-economic differentials in mortality: further evidence from the Whitehall study. *J. Epidemiol. Community Health*, **44**, 260–5.

Fox, A. J. and Goldblatt, P. (1982). Longitudinal study. Socio-demographic mortality differentials. *Office of Population Censuses and Surveys Longitudinal Study. (O.P.C.S.L.S.)*, 1. A Publication of the Gov. Statistical Service.

Karasek, R. and Theorell, T. (1990). *Healthy work: stress, productivity, and the reconstruction of working life*, Basic Books, New York.

Kato, H., Tillotson, J., Nichaman, M., Rhoads, G. G., and Hamilton, H. B. (1973). Epidemiologic studies of coronary heart disease and stroke in Japanese men living in Japan, Hawaii and California: serum, lipids and diet. *Am. J. Epidemiol.*, **97**, 372–85.

Keys, A. (1980). In *Seven countries: a multivariate analysis of death and coronary heart disease*, Harvard University Press.

Marmot, M. G. (1985). Interpretation of trends in coronary heart disease mortality. *Acta Med. Scand. (Suppl.)*, **701**, 58–65.

Marmot, M. G. and Davey Smith, G. (1989). Why are the Japanese living longer? *Br. Med. J.*, **299**, 1547–51.

Marmot, M. G. and McDowall, M. E. (1986). Mortality decline and widening social inequalities. *Lancet*, **i**, 274–6.

Marmot, M. G. and Syme, S. L. (1976). Acculturation and coronary heart disease in Japanese-Americans. *Am. J. Epidemiol.*, **104**, 225–47.

Marmot, M. G. and Theorell, T. (1988). Social class and cardiovascular disease: the contribution of work. *Int. J. Health Serv.*, **18**, 659–74.

Marmot, M. G., Syme, S. L., Kagan, A., Kato, H., and Cohen, J. B. (1975). Studies of coronary heart disease and stroke in Japanese men living in Japan, Hawaii and California: prevalence of coronary and hypertensive heart disease and associated risk factors. *Am. J. Epidemiol.*, **102**, 514–25.

Marmot, M. G., Adelstein, A. M., Robinson, N., and Rose, G. (1978). Changing social class distribution of heart disease. *Br. Med. J.*, **2**, 1109–12.

Marmot, M. G., Shipley, M. J., and Rose, G. (1984a). Inequalities in death— specific explanations of a general pattern. *Lancet*, **i**, 1003–6.

Marmot, M. G., Adelstein, A. M., and Bulusu, L. (1984b). Lessons from the study of immigrant mortality. *Lancet*, **i**, 1455–8.

Marmot, M. G., Kogevinas, M., and Elston, M. A. (1987). Social/economic status and disease. *Annu. Rev. Public Health*, **8**, 111–37.

Matsumoto, Y. S. (1970). Social stress and coronary heart disease. *Millbank Mem. Fund Q.*, **48**, 9–36.

McKeown, T. (1976). In *The role of medicine*, Nuffield Provincial Hospitals Trust, London.

Nichaman, M. Z., Hamilton, H. B., Kagan, A., Sacks, S., Greer, T., and Syme, S. L. (1975). Epidemiologic studies of coronary heart disease and stroke in Japanese men living in Japan, Hawaii and California: distribution of biochemical risk factors. *Am. J. Epidemiol.*, **102**, 491–501.

Omran, A. R. (1971). The epidemiologic transition. *Milbank Mem. Fund. Q.*, **49**, 509–38.

OPCS (1978). *Occupational mortality 1970–1972*, HMSO, London.

OPCS (1989). *Mortality statistics 1986 (Series DH2)*, HMSO, London.

Parkin, D. W., McGuire, A. J., and Yule, B. F. (1989). What do international comparisons of health care expenditures really show? *Community Med.*, **11**, 116–23.

Preston, S. H. and Nelson, V. E. (1974). Structure and change in causes of death: an international summary. *Popul. Stud.*, **28**, 19–51.

Statistics and Information Department, Ministers Secretariat (1967–1988). *Vital statistics 1965–1986*, Kosei Tokei Kyokai, Tokyo.

Stephen, A. M. and Wald, N. J. (1990). Trends in individual consumption of dietary fat in the United States, 1920–1984. *Am. J. Clin. Nutr.,* **52,** 457–69.

Susser, M. and Stein, Z. (1962). Civilisation and peptic ulcer. *Lancet,* **i,** 115–18.

Uemura, K. and Pisa, Z. (1988). Trends in cardiovascular disease mortality in industrialised countries since 1950. *World Health Statist. Q.,* **41,** 155–78.

Ueshima, H., Tatara, K., and Asakura, S. (1987). Declining mortality from ischaemic heart disease and changes in coronary risk factors in Japan, 1956–1980. *Am. J. Epidemiol.,* **125,** 62–72.

Wilkinson, R. G. (1989). Class mortality differentials, income distribution and trends in poverty 1921–1981. *J. Soc. Pol.,* **18,** 307–35.

Winter, J. M. (1983). Unemployment, nutrition and infant mortality in Britain, 1920–1950, in J. M. Winter (ed.), *The working class in modern British history*, Cambridge University Press.

World Bank (1988). *World development report 1988.* Oxford University Press.

Worth, R. M., Rhoads, G., Kagan, A., Kato, H., and Syme, S. L. (1975). Epidemiologic studies of coronary heart disease and stroke in Japanese men living in Japan, Hawaii and California: mortality. *Am. J. Epidemiol.,* **102,** 481–90.

Yach, D. (1990). Tobacco-induced diseases in South Africa. *Int. J. Epidemiol.,* **14,** 1122–3.

2

Contribution of epidemiology to understanding coronary heart disease

F. H. Epstein

Understanding a disease means being able to explain its clinical and pre-clinical manifestations in terms of the responsible pathobiological mechanisms and to account for its occurrence in different populations and social groups within the community. In this context, epidemiology has played a crucial role in understanding coronary heart disease (CHD) and has provided a model, only beginning to be applied, for the potential contributions of epidemiology towards the prevention of other non-communicable disorders. Epidemiology is both a science and a method. It has contributed to the study of CHD on both levels. Surgeon Rear-Admiral Sheldon Dudley, in his presidential address to the Section of Epidemiology and State Medicine of the Royal Society of Medicine, has spoken of ecology as an 'attitude of mind' (Dudley 1936–7). Epidemiology, being in one of its metamorphoses human or medical ecology, is also an attitude of mind. As such, it has extended the clinical horizon to include the picture of health and disease in the community and it has influenced clinical scientists in their study designs. Epidemiology has become an integral part of the interdisciplinary approaches towards understanding CHD.

HISTORICAL BACKGROUND

It might almost seem as if CHD epidemiology started with a 'big bang' around 1948, shortly after the end of the Second World War. This is certainly true for epidemiological research in this field as a deliberate effort under the term 'epidemiology'. The beginnings reach back into the last century, particularly under the description 'geographical pathology'. It is a sobering experience to read the contributions of Aschoff and, especially, Anitschkow in the Proceedings of the Conference on Geographical Pathology held in the Netherlands in 1934 in which a good many of the currently accepted causes of atherosclerosis and its main clinical consequence, CHD, are foreshadowed (*Deuxième Conférence Internationale de Pathologie Géographique* 1934). The question why CHD epidemiology came over the horizon so suddenly and so forcefully in the brief period between 1947 and 1949 is part of the mystery of creative ideas and falls outside the present task of describing the impact of the studies conducted over the past 45 years which led to present knowledge and understanding.

Two great currents can be distinguished: the era of prospective studies which started in the late 1940s, and the era of intervention studies, with explorations in the 1960s, which started with full force in the early 1970s. The first era culminated in the discovery of CHD risk factors. These had become so firmly established, within a remarkably short period of time, by the early 1960s that preventive trials to test their cause and effect relationship to the disease were called for as an imperative need. The two eras overlap. The first era rose to a peak in the late 1960s and declined in the 1970s as the emphasis shifted to the second era of intervention studies, but has emerged from this partial eclipse during the last decade. This resurgence related to deepening of knowledge concerning established and search for new risk factors. The second era reached its peak around 1980 and has maintained its level, with a shift from large-scale to more clinical types of trials. Alongside these randomized trials involving individuals, intervention projects concerned with entire communities have gained in prominence.

In parallel with the developments just outlined, geographical differences in the frequency of CHD have continued to be in the centre of interest. They revolve around the question of why the disease is more common in some parts of the world and why secular mortality trends are steeper in some countries than others. In more recent years, there have been intensive efforts to explain the unexpected downward trends in CHD mortality in a number of countries.

During the past decade, the problem of how preventive cardiovascular care can be organized most effectively for individuals and on the community level—the matter of the high risk and population strategies of prevention—has moved more and more into the foreground. The issue is not strictly concerned with understanding CHD and will therefore not be further discussed here, being covered elsewhere in this book. However, those strategies are at the core of the question of why understanding CHD is essential for the practice of preventive cardiology.

So far this brief historical review has dealt with the interrelationships between CHD and its precursors within their epidemiological context. Investigations into the epidemiology of the precursors themselves have been of equal importance. The basic studies into the determinants of serum lipid levels within the broader field of lipid metabolism rank first and foremost not only in number but because of their direct relationship to the development of atherosclerosis from youth into older ages. The presence of cholesterol in atherosclerotic lesions has been known since 1843, and there were numerous studies on the role of cholesterol in atherogenesis prior to the Second World War (Epstein 1990). However, it is beyond question that Ancel Keys, whose pioneering research started in the late 1940s, was chiefly responsible for the wide interest in the 'cholesterol hypothesis' as it developed into the 'cholesterol theory'. Keys himself traced back some of this history (Keys 1953, 1975, 1983), but a full account of his contributions remains to be written, not only in terms of his own work but the wave of research by others which he stimulated. Keys' contributions span from nutritional experiments under controlled metabolic conditions to extensive international epidemiological field studies. During the intervening years, an enormous amount of data have been accumulated to identify the nutritional determinants of serum lipids, including cholesterol, and their interaction with genetic dispositions is beginning to be understood. This knowledge, based to a considerable extent on epidemiological studies, had an important impact on nutritional science in general and forms the basis of nutritional counselling as one cornerstone of CHD prevention programmes in the community and of nutritional advice in medical practice.

Epidemiology has also played an important part in understanding the determinants of blood pressure. It is of interest that the pioneers in epidemiological research were not always professional epidemiologists. Keys' original training was in human biology, and the first epidemiological study of blood pressure was promoted by Sir George Pickering, the renowned clinical scientist. It would be fair to say that a large part of current knowledge on the distribution of blood pressure levels and its determinants in different populations comes from epidemiological observations, opening the way for the control of hypertension by non-pharmacological means. Epidemiological investigations have also contributed substantially to the identification of the factors influencing glucose intolerance and diabetes. Similar advances in the emerging field of thrombogenesis and haemostasis as precursors of heart attacks are being made.

The strength of the epidemiological approach lies partly in its ability to identify not only risk factors for CHD but to determine their relative importance singly and in combination in the population at large. It also permits a quantitative estimate of how much of the disease can be accounted for in terms of known risk factors and what proportion may remain to be explained. This knowledge is important for the practice of preventive cardiology, public health planning of preventive services, and for the design of research still needed.

The achievements of cardiovascular disease epidemiology during recent decades give reason for much satisfaction and provide hope that these approaches will continue to be useful. As new methods are being developed, it will be possible to identify persons at increased risk with greater precision and to focus the need for preventive measures more sharply for the purposes of the high risk strategy. Further knowledge is going to be gained as to how preventive services can be established most effectively in the community. Community programmes for the prevention of cardiovascular diseases will be linked with programmes for the prevention of other chronic diseases, moving toward comprehensive approaches for the preservation of health (Epstein and Holland 1983).

LESSONS FROM CHANGES OVER TIME

Around 1950, the view was still widely held that atherosclerosis, as often as not called arteriosclerosis, is a degenerative condition and an inevitable concomitant of aging. It was recognized from autopsy studies that the extent of lesions may vary greatly from one individual to another, but this was attributed to constitutional rather than environmental differences. With the advent of epidemiology around this time, there was an intensified attempt to show that the increasing mortality from 'arteriosclerotic heart disease' in the preceding years could not be explained solely by changing fashions of death certification but reflected a true change, with the implication that environmental factors were responsible. Alongside the information from international mortality statistics, Morris's report (Morris 1951), based on autopsy records at the London Hospital, that ischaemic heart disease but not atherosclerotic lesions had become more common over time received much attention.

International mortality statistics since 1950, despite the changes in World Health Organization (WHO) nomenclature of causes of death certification, left no reasonable doubt that death from CHD was increasing in most Western countries. It came as a totally unexpected surprise in the 1970s that the trend had reversed in the USA and some other countries. This constitutes an important epidemiological contribution to understanding CHD because upward or downward secular changes in mortality are amongst the most persuasive pieces of evidence that disease occurrence is strongly influenced by environmental changes.

LESSONS FROM CROSS-CULTURAL VARIATIONS

Geographical variations in disease frequency constitute further convincing evidence for the relationship between life-styles and the disorders largely due to atherosclerosis. They were discussed at the Conference on Geographic Pathology in 1934, mentioned earlier. At the same conference, reference was also made to variations related to social class and occupation, investigated intensively since, which can also be attributed to environmental conditions. The term 'life-style', which came to be extraordinarily useful, was first used by Keys in the early 1950s. The suggestion that geographical differences in mortality are correlated with differences in dietary fat consumption and therefore with serum cholesterol levels was made by Keys (1953), opening up a field of research which has remained prominent. The Seven Countries Study, started by Keys in 1958, is the single most convincing piece of evidence that not only CHD mortality but also its incidence are associated with differences in fat consumption and serum cholesterol levels (Keys 1980). On the basis of a large number of studies around the world, it can no longer be questioned that marked differences in life-styles, particularly in regard to diet, run parallel with corresponding differences in CHD frequency. The fact that differences in CHD mortality, particularly within Europe, can exist in the absence of marked dietary differences does not in any way run counter to the view just expressed; it merely means that there are regional differences which must be due to other influences. Nor do these findings indicate that dietary changes in a favourable direction could not further reduce CHD frequency in countries with already relatively low risk.

Migrant studies constitute another approach to understanding geographic variations. The first of three prominent examples is the British–Norwegian–United States Migrant Study, initiated primarily by the late Professor D. D. Reid who preceded Professor Rose in the position from which he has now retired. It is one of Reid's many contributions towards creating foundations of chronic disease epidemiology and was published posthumously (Feinleib *et al*. 1982). The second example, the Japan–Honolulu–San Francisco Study, provided strong evidence that life-style is a key determinant of CHD risk (Robertson *et al*. 1977). Thirdly, in the Tokelau Island Study, a pioneering effort was made by Dr I. A. M. Prior to understand the changes in health which occur when populations move from their native habitat, in this case a remote Pacific island, to an industrialized society, in this case New Zealand (Wessen 1992). Cultural transition can, of course, take place without migration. The resulting increase in CHD frequency expected to occur in Third World countries falls in this category.

Epidemiological pathology has great potential but is hampered by the difficulties in obtaining adequate numbers of autopsies of deceased persons which are reasonably representative. Nevertheless, there are notable examples. The International Atherosclerosis Project showed marked differences in the extent of atherosclerotic lesions, comparing South American countries, the USA, and Europe (Geographic pathology of atherosclerosis 1968). These differences could be correlated with differences in diet and serum cholesterol. While the extent of arterial lesions and the frequency of CHD differed, severe lesions had to be present for death due to coronary disease to occur. A WHO Project in several countries provided similar data, especially on geographical differences in young persons (Atherosclerosis in five towns 1976). A number of studies, though not cross-

F. H. Epstein   25

cultural, have provided data on the correlation between lesions and risk factors (Oslo, Bogalusa, Framingham, Hawaii). A community-based study in New Orleans has given insight into differences in the extent and type of lesions in black and white people (Strong *et al.* 1980). An important study of the evolution of lesions at younger ages is under way in the USA and other countries. These studies have strengthened the view that the geographical differences in mortality are real since they reflect structural changes in the coronary and other arteries.

PREDICTING CHD

The outstanding single achievement of CHD epidemiology is no doubt the development of the risk factor concept. When the first wave of prospective studies was started in the late 1940s, it could hardly be anticipated that 20 years later it would be possible to predict the disease in overtly healthy people with such accuracy and power. It is often said that individual prediction lacks precision, but is there any other chronic disease, with the exception of lung cancer in smokers, which can be predicted with anything like the precision attainable for CHD? In fact, two of the three major risk factors, serum cholesterol and blood pressure, were already firmly established within less than 10 years, while the evidence for smoking was strongly suggestive (Measuring risk of coronary heart disease 1957). The term 'risk factor' first appeared in a Framingham publication in 1961 (Kannel *et al.* 1961). There were two more waves of prospective studies, not counting a considerable number of cross-sectional studies during the earlier years. The second wave started around 1960, while the third wave, consisting in part of follow-up observations on persons initially screened for participation in the large primary prevention trials, has covered the last 10–15 years. The prospective studies carried out over the years are very numerous. There are about 30 such studies in Europe and the Mediterranean area, around 25 in the USA, and some five in other parts of the world.

Considering the diversity of the populations included in these approximately 60 studies and the differences in their methodology, it is most remarkable that they all tell essentially the same story. Serum cholesterol, blood pressure, and smoking stand out as the major risk factors and carry the largest population-attributable risk. The importance of other risk factors, when measured, has also been generally confirmed; while the relative risk they carry may be relatively slight or their prevalence in the population comparatively low, their accumulated risk may approach that of the major risk factors. It would not have been possible to evaluate the many interacting and competing risk factors without powerful new biostatistical techniques, and great credit is due to those responsible for their development.

What are the limits of predictive power? It is now possible to identify 20 per cent of the population in which close to 60 per cent of the future events of CHD will occur. Perhaps this latter percentage, which is already very high, can be improved with the inclusion of new risk factors, in particular those related to thrombogenesis and genetic markers. Improvement of prediction for individuals would also require the development of more effective screening techniques. However desirable even more powerful prediction of disease would be, it could never replace the need for a population strategy of prevention because, amongst other reasons, the ultimate aim of prevention must be to create a new future generation of people in whom risk factors are less common.

Epidemiology has not only contributed the methods of predicting CHD but has developed the concept of 'tracking' of risk factors which aims to identify as early as possible in life those who will develop elevated risk factor levels in adulthood. Powerful methods of tracking would permit the institution of preventive measures before risk factors have already become too high, instead of waiting until they attain a level which should never have been reached in the first place and then lowering them when it is already too late. Efforts to improve tracking methods are under way. The matter of atherosclerosis as a childhood disorder and of early prevention will be touched upon in the next section.

PREVENTING CHD

The advent of the era of intervention studies, defined earlier, is tied closely to the emergence of risk factors and their power of prediction. When there remained no doubt in the 1960s that risk factors did indeed predict disease risk, it became urgently necessary to test whether lowering of risk factor level would lower the risk of CHD—whether, in fact, the relation between risk factors and risk was causal. A number of preliminary studies, notably the National Diet–Heart Study (1968) in the USA, were carried out in the 1960s, followed by full-scale intervention studies in the 1970s, as reviewed elsewhere (Epstein and Pyörälä 1987). It was expected with confidence that these controlled trials would give a decisive and definitive answer, not fully realizing at first that a number of unforeseen practical problems may reduce their power in providing unequivocal results. The fact that the primary prevention trials taken as a whole, whether viewed singly or in terms of a meta-analysis, have yielded positive results in the face of problems apt to limit their power gives added confidence in the validity of the results. There is no evidence at the present time that preventive measures, while lowering the risk of CHD, increase the risk of other disorders. Furthermore, the case for the primary prevention of CHD does not rest on the results of preventive trials alone but derives, in addition, from collateral evidence, such as the observations on cross-cultural differences and their relation to life-styles, the solid indications from clinical, pathological, and experimental investigations that CHD risk factors and the disease are causally related, and the remarkable consistency of the data from observational studies. The results of the large number of secondary prevention studies likewise support the concept of the cause and effect relationship between risk factors and risk.

Trials like those considered so far, in which individuals are randomized to experimental and comparison groups, lend themselves best to drawing inferences on causality. On the other hand, intervention projects in which the comparison is between entire communities with and without intervention programmes reflect better the impact of preventive measures on the population as a whole and, as such, also suggest causal links. A 'half-way house' between the two designs are trials in which circumscribed social or occupational groups are randomized, like the WHO European Trial (WHO 1989). In community projects, it generally takes longer for risk factor changes to show a demonstrable effect on mortality and morbidity because it takes time to mobilize the population to take part in the prevention effort. Evaluation is also made more difficult in countries where CHD is already declining 'naturally'. Nevertheless, the results of ongoing projects to date indicate the effectiveness of community-wide programmes in lowering risk factors and demonstrate, in some, a decline in mortality. Even in randomized trials, it may take longer than anticipated for effects on mortality to become evident (Multiple Risk Factor Intervention Trial Research Group 1990).

Over the years, increasing attention is being given to the fact that atherosclerosis starts early in life and therefore that prevention must also begin early. The matter has already been considered in connection with identifying risk carriers in youth. However, the ultimate aim must be to establish life-styles in youth which will ensure optimal risk factor levels throughout life. Projects with these aims are underway (WHO 1990).

CONTRIBUTIONS FROM EPIDEMIOLOGICAL METHODOLOGY

Standardization of methods is a prerequisite for the conduct of epidemiological studies and intervention trials, to ensure consistency of measurement over the course of the study and comparability between studies. Furthermore, methods used in clinical research may not be feasible in field studies, so that they have to be adapted for epidemiological purposes or it may be necessary to develop new methods. This is part and parcel of epidemiological research, but it could not be anticipated that these standardized methods would also find wide application in cardiological investigations. Major examples are the Minnesota Code for reading electrocardiograms, the Rose Questionnaire for the interpretation of chest pain and the diagnosis of angina pectoris, and methods for the unbiased measurement of blood pressure. Epidemiological studies have drawn attention to laboratory variation and error, leading, amongst others, to Lipid Standardization Programmes which have influenced clinical chemistry. Questionnaires have been developed for the assessment of psycho-social factors, the measurement of physical activity, and a variety of other purposes which have been found useful outside epidemiological research. A milestone along this road has been the 'Rose–Blackburn Manual', published by the WHO, which has provided guidelines for the application and use of standardized epidemiological methods in cardiovascular epidemiology (Rose and Blackburn 1968).

Epidemiological terms like specificity, sensitivity, and predictive power are now being used in clinical research for comparing, say, invasive and non-invasive methods to detect coronary artery lesions. Clinical investigators have also been influenced by epidemiologists in the design of experiments, paying attention to the problem of choosing experimental and control subjects from comparable populations, or in the use of multivariate biostatistical techniques. These examples serve to illustrate the extent to which epidemiological and clinical research have moved closer together.

IMPACT ON MEDICAL PRACTICE AND PUBLIC POLICY

Over the course of the years, cardiologists and medical practitioners in general in many countries have become increasingly aware of the importance of CHD risk factors and their significance for the prevention of the disease. At the same time, the public has become increasingly aware of this message. Heart associations, cardiac societies, and other professional organizations have helped in the dissemination of this knowledge. Governmental agencies in a number of countries have joined in the effort by appointing expert committees to prepare official reports and issuing recommendations. The WHO has played a key role during the last four decades in calling together experts to issue scientific progress reports, and major studies have been and are being conducted under its aegis. At the present time, hardly any argument exists about the need to detect and protect persons at increased risk, but there remains some opposition to the view, shared by most workers in the field, that preventive measures, especially those concerned with nutritional habits, must be extended to the entire population. There is still a long road to travel, more in some countries than others, in order to establish healthier life-styles in the population and preventive cardiology in the daily practice of medicine, but the basic foundations have been solidly laid.

UNDERSTANDING CHD—INSIGHTS FROM EPIDEMIOLOGY

The outstanding single message provided by epidemiology consists in having established a scientific basis for the recognition that CHD, as an epidemic condition in the population, is mostly due to environmental influences, thus opening the way for prevention. This is not to belittle the importance of genetic predispositions in modifying individual susceptibility. However, on both the community and individual level, the disease is caused as much or more by what we do than by what we are. The view is crystallized in the concept of 'life-style', a component of the social environment. Life-style is the first step in the chain which leads over the risk factors to the clinical events. Life-style determines risk factor levels, against the background of genetic variation. It is the confluence of clinical, pathological, experimental, and, last but not least, epidemiological evidence which attests to the causal relation between risk factors and the diseases primarily due to athero-sclerosis. Furthermore, evaluation of the epidemiological data permits an estimate of how much of the disease is 'explained' by the known risk factors and how much remains to be discovered, with the conclusion that a larger proportion is known than unknown. All this reasoning is mostly based on epidemiological findings because only population-based data allow extrapolations which reflect the general validity of the results.

The entire risk factor concept is derived from epidemiological observations. It has been instrumental in bringing cardiovascular epidemiology to the attention of the medical profession and the public. There is a good reason because the concept is not merely theoretical but has immediate applications in the practice of medicine both for the individual and on community level. Its acceptance is gratifying since risk factors provide the key to prevention. Guidelines for the reduction of risk factors have been derived from epidemiological and clinical studies, including indications for pharmacological treatment when life-style alterations have been shown to be insufficient. Data on the distribution and prevalence of risk factors in different populations and social groups, essential for health planning and as a background for the practice of preventive cardiology, quite apart from their bearing on aetiology, come from epidemiological research.

Cardiovascular epidemiology has had a marked impact on cardiologists and practising physicians in general. To an increasing degree, curative and preventive practice are being seen as a continuum. Population-based studies have provided a picture of how CHD in its various stages from latent to clinically overt manifestations presents itself in the community, making it possible to detect and treat the disease earlier and to give more effective emergency care. Although it sounds strange today, one of the truly outstanding American cardiologists, some 25 years ago during a meeting at the National Heart Institute in Bethesda, expressed great surprise when told by the epidemiologist present that over half of CHD deaths occur outside the hospital; he knew only how many deaths occurred after admission! This illustrates, as an example, how the intense current preoccupation with sudden death was influenced by epidemiological findings. It has already been mentioned how epidemiological approaches and methods have been useful to clinical investigators in the design of studies and their interpretation. The amazing phenomenon of the rise and fall of CHD mortality in various countries has also attracted much attention amongst cardiologists and provided common ground with epidemiologists.

The understanding of CHD epidemiology has been greatly furthered by primary and secondary prevention studies, including clinical trials in their classical form, large unifactorial and multifactorial intervention studies, and community projects. The results, seen as a whole, have been encouraging, have yielded estimates of the effectiveness of preventive measures, and have made decisive contributions towards understanding their determinants. The trials have also helped clinicians and epidemiologists to understand each other and, as in other areas of mutual interest, to bring them closer together.

CONCLUSION

In this bird's eye review, very few persons have been mentioned by name. The temptation to give credit to all the many workers primarily responsible for specific achievements was great, but it seemed impossible to be selective and fair at the same time. The problem was somewhat reduced because so many of the investigators are contributors to this book, though a good many more regrettably remain anonymous. It would not be inappropriate, however, to single out the man to whom this book is dedicated. Geoffrey Rose has carried out observational studies, conducted preventive trials, contributed to methodology, assumed leadership in applying research findings to prevention in the community, deliberately built bridges between epidemiology and clinicians, and has been a teacher of epidemiology. Thus he himself has covered most of the spectrum of epidemiological endeavour. His unique stature derives from having added to new knowledge a profound understanding of its scientific and social significance.

In the beginning, reference was made to epidemiology as an 'attitude of mind'. In closing, an early example of this attitude may be mentioned. Eighty-five years ago, Sir James Mackenzie, a founding father of modern cardiology, wrote on arteriosclerosis: 'In recent articles on this subject there is one very important aspect which has not been considered—that is the beginning of the conditions that lead on to arteriosclerosis. The case is generally considered when already the mischief is done, and the cause can usually be attributed to an agency that suits the particular fancy of the examining medical man' (Mackenzie 1906). To remedy the situation, Mackenzie attempted, towards the end of his life in 1921, the first long-term investigation of CHD (Mackenzie 1926). It gives reason for satisfaction that his vision is now being turned into action, based on better understanding.

REFERENCES

Atherosclerosis of the aorta and coronary arteries in five towns (1976). *Bull. WHO*, **53**, 485–645.

Deuxième conférence internationale de pathologie géographique, Utrecht (1934). Oosthoek, Utrecht.

Dudley, S. F. (1936–7). The ecological outlook on epidemiology. *Proc. R. Soc. Med.*, **30**, 57–70.

Epstein, F. H. (1990). Die historische Entwicklung des Cholesterin-Atherosklerose-Konzepts. *Ther. Umsch.*, **47**, 435–42.

Epstein, F. H. and Holland, W. W. (1983). Prevention of chronic diseases in the community—one-disease versus multiple-disease strategies. *Int. J. Epidemiol.*, **12**, 135–7.

Epstein, F. H. and Pyörälä, K. (1987). Perspectives for the primary prevention of coronary heart disease. *Cardiology*, **74**, 316–31.

Feinleib, M., Lambert, P. M., Zeiner-Henriksen, T., Rogot, E., Hunt, B. M., and Ingster-Moore, L. (1982). The British–Norwegian migrant study—analysis of parameters of mortality differentials associated with angina. *Biometrics* (Suppl.), **38**, 55–71.

Geographic pathology of atherosclerosis (1968). *Lab. Invest.*, **18**, 465–653.

Kannel, W. B., Dawber, T. R., Kagan, A., Revotskie, N., and Stokes, J., III (1961). Factors of risk in the development of coronary heart disease—six-year follow-up experience. *Ann. Intern. Med.*, **55**, 33–50.

Keys, A. (1953). Atherosclerosis—a problem in newer public health. *J. Mount Sinai Hosp.*, **20**, 118–39.

Keys, A. (1975). Coronary heart disease—the global picture. *Atherosclerosis*, **22**, 149–92.

Keys, A. (1980). *Seven countries—a multivariate analysis of death and coronary heart disease*. Harvard University Press.

Keys, A. (1983). From Naples to seven countries—a sentimental journey. *Prog. Biochem. Pharmacol.*, **19**, 1–30.

Mackenzie, J. (1906). Arterio-sclerosis. *Br. Med. J.*, **1**, 319.

Mackenzie, Sir James (1926). *The basis of vital activity, being a review of five years' work at the St. Andrews Institute for Clinical Research*, Faber and Gwyer, London.

Measuring the risk of coronary heart disease in adult population groups—a symposium (1957). *Am. J. Public Health*, **47** (4, Part 2), 1–64.

Morris, J. A. (1951). Recent history of coronary disease. *Lancet*, **i,** 1–7, 69–73.

Multiple Risk Factor Intervention Trial Research Group (1990). Mortality rates after 10.5 years for participants in the Multiple Risk Factor Intervention Trial. *J. Am. Med. Assoc.*, **263,** 1795–801.

National Diet–Heart Study (1968). *Circulation,* **37** (Suppl. 1).

Robertson, T. L., Kato, H., Rhoads, G. G., Kagan, A., Marmot, M., Syme, S. L., Gordon, T., Worth, R. M., Belsky, J. L., Dock, D. S., Miyanishi, M., and Kawamoto, S. (1977). Epidemiologic studies of coronary heart disease and stroke in Japanese men living in Japan, Hawai and California. Incidence of myocardial infarction and death from coronary heart disease. *Am. J. Cardiol.,* **39,** 239–49.

Rose, G. A. and Blackburn, H. (1968). *Cardiovascular survey methods*, WHO, Geneva.

Strong, J. P., Johnson, W. D., Oalman, M. C., Tracy, W. P., Newman, W. P., III, Rock, W. A., Malcolm, G. T., Koknatur, M. G., and Toca, V. (1980). Community pathology of atherosclerosis and coronary heart disease in New Orleans; relationship of risk factors to atherosclerotic lesions. In *Atherosclerosis V* (eds A. M. Gotto, Jr., L. C. Smith, and B. Allen), pp. 719–24, Springer Verlag, New York.

Wessen, A. F. (ed.) (1992). *Tokelau: migration and health in a small Polynesian society*, Oxford University Press.

WHO (1989). *WHO European Collaborative Trial in the multifactorial prevention of coronary heart disease*, WHO, Copenhagen.

WHO (1990). Prevention in childhood and youth of adult cardiovascular disease: time for action. Report of a WHO Expert Committee. *Tech. Rep. Ser.* 792, WHO, Geneva.

AETIOLOGY

3

Established major coronary risk factors

J. Stamler

Knowledge and Human power are synonymous, since ignorance of the cause frustrates the effect . . . Now the true and lawful goal of the sciences is none other than this: that human life be endowed with new discoveries and powers.

Francis Bacon
Novum Organum 1620

Don't crowd diseases point everywhere to deficiencies of society? One may adduce atmospheric or cosmic conditions or similar factors. But never do they alone make epidemics. They produce them only where due to bad social conditions people have lived for some time in abnormal situations.

Epidemics of a character unknown so far appear, and often disappear without traces when a new culture period has started. Thus did leprosy and the English sweat. The history of artificial epidemics is therefore the history of disturbances of human culture. Their changes announce to us in gigantic signs the turning points of culture into new directions.

Epidemics resemble great warning signs on which the true statesman is able to read that the evolution of his nation has been disturbed to a point which even a careless policy is no longer allowed to overlook. . .

Rudolf Virchow (Ackerknecht 1953)

There are no such things as pure and applied science—there are only science and the application of science.

Louis Pasteur (Dubos 1960)

[I am] . . . a man whose invincible belief is that Science and Peace will triumph over Ignorance and War, that nations will unite not to destroy, but to build, and that the future will belong to those who will have done most for suffering humanity.

Louis Pasteur (Dubos 1960)

The focus of this chapter is on four established major risk factors: 'rich' diet, diet-related above-optimal levels of serum total cholesterol (TC) and blood pressure (BP), and cigarette smoking (CIG). These have been shown to be centrally involved in the multifactorial causation of severe atherosclerotic disease, its complications, and its multiple clinical manifestations—first and foremost the epidemic of coronary heart disease (CHD) in Western industrialized countries. The extensive scientific knowledge on these risk factors and their aetiological role is the solid foundation of the combined population-wide and high risk strategy for the primary prevention and control of this epidemic (Katz *et al*. 1958; Stamler 1967; NHLBI 1981; WHO 1982, 1990; Stamler *et al*. 1985; NCEP 1988, 1990; NRC 1989).

Of the four established major risk factors, two—'rich' diet and cigarette smoking—are aspects of life-style that became mass phenomena in the twentieth century in Western industrialized countries. The other two— above-optimal levels of serum cholesterol and of blood pressure—are endogenous traits prevalent in a majority of the adult population of these countries as a result of mass consumption of a 'rich' diet. *The population-wide eating pattern is the key in three of these four established major risk factors*.

All four of these risk factors are designated *established* because substantial amounts of data from many disciplines have demonstrated their significant role in the aetiology of epidemic CHD. They are designated *major* for three reasons: their high prevalence in populations, particularly in Western industrialized countries, their strong impact on coronary risk, and their preventability and reversibility, primarily by safe improvements in population life-styles, from early childhood on. (Age and male gender are known risk factors, but are not amenable to influence and hence are not designated major; diabetes is a known risk factor, but of lower prevalence than cigarette smoking and elevated TC and BP in most populations, and hence is not designated major.)

'Rich' diet is pivotal among these four—the primary and essential cause of the coronary epidemic. Without it there is no epidemic even with high prevalence of smoking. Only in populations consuming a 'rich' diet and exhibiting its metabolic consequences does the important adjuvant (secondary) role of smoking in the aetiology of severe atherosclerotic disease become manifest on a large scale. 'Rich' diet is a habitual fare high in animal products and processed animal products, high in total fat, hydrogenated fat, and separated (visible) fat, high in cholesterol and saturated fat, high in refined and processed sugars, high in salt, high in alcohol for many in the population, high in caloric density, in 'empty' calories, and in ratio of calories to essential nutrients, low in potassium, fibre, and often other essential nutrients, and high in total calories for a low level of energy expenditure in the era of the automobile, television, and mechanized work. This eating pattern and smoking are unprecedented twentieth-century mass exposures—'. . . disturbances of human culture' (Virchow) (Ackerknecht 1953)—to which the human species is not adapted by evolution. 'Rich' diet produces above-optimal population mean levels of TC and BP from childhood on, for most people a rise in TC and BP from youth to middle age, low prevalence of optimal levels in the middle-aged and older population, and high prevalence (progressively through adulthood) of

hypercholesterolaemia and high blood pressure (HBP). Along with sedentary habit, 'rich' diet accounts for the emergence of obesity as a common
trait in the population from childhood on, and of consequent unfavourable patterns of glycaemia and uricaemia, including progressively higher
prevalence of non-insulin-dependent diabetes mellitus in middle-aged and
older population strata. Moreover, because of its high cholesterol content,
'rich' diet is significantly and independently related to long-term risk of
mortality from coronary, cardiovascular, and all causes over and above its
unfavourable effects on TC and BP.

HISTORICAL OVERVIEW

Most of the research leading to identification of the major risk factors and
elucidation of their role in the aetiology of the atherosclerotic diseases was
performed in the nineteenth and twentieth centuries, but there are roots
reaching back to the 1700s. Thus, in 1727 Brunner described the necropsy
findings in the aorta of his 75-year-old father-in-law, Johann Jakob Wepfer
(1620–95), discoverer of the relationship of cerebral haemorrhage to
apoplexy. Wepfer's aorta was severely atherosclerotic, and Brunner noted:
'The internal coat in several places was ruptured, lacerated and rotten like
fruit . . .' (Stamler, 1967, p. 42). In 1755 Albrecht von Haller, in a brief
essay, also commented on aortic plaques (Stamler 1967, p. 42). On opening into these at autopsy he found a yellow mush effusing between the
muscular fibres and the intima. He described this material as soft and
pultaceous, not dissimilar to that seen in atheromata. (The word 'atheroma'
is derived from the Greek *athere*, meaning mush or gruel. It had been in
use since the ancient Greek writers to describe any closed sac or cyst of
non-inflammatory origin filled with gruel-like material.) von Haller noted
that the same aorta exhibited multiple plaques, some of which were harder
and drier, i.e. undergoing fibrotic, cartilaginous, and osseous metaplasia.
He inferred that a gradual progression took place from the soft state of
atheroma to final bone-like plaque. Thus his special contribution was to
focus attention on the softening process (or accumulation of 'mush') as of
primary significance in atherosclerosis.

In the latter half of the eighteenth cntury, 'The coronary arteries entered
medical thought and literature with the belief held by a brilliant group of
English medical men, Jenner, Hunter, Fothergill, and Parry, that those
vessels were closely associated with angina pectoris . . .' (Dock 1939;
Moriyama *et al*. 1971, p. 326). Jenner described the findings at post-
mortem examination of Hunter, who died suddenly at St. George's Hospital
in 1793 after a 20 year history of recurrent anginal episodes. (At least one
of them was too persistent to be called stable angina nowadays—possibly
unstable angina or myocardial infarction?) The undersurface of the left

auricle and ventricle revealed two areas nearly an inch and a half square which were of a white colour, with an opaque appearance, and entirely distinct from the general surface of the heart. These two areas were covered by an '. . . exudation of coagulating lymph . . . The coronary arteries had their branches which ramify through the substance of the heart in the state of bony tubes . . .' (Moriyama *et al*. 1971, p. 327). In 1740, Krell had published a treatise on hardening of the coronary arteries (Moriyama *et al*. 1971, p. 323). He stated that the incrustations generally spoken of as ossifications were not bony but of a tophaceous nature, and were derived from atheromatous matter. He made the further point that this induration was not confined to senility but might occur at any period of life.

In the eighteenth century also the compound now known as cholesterol was first described, having been precipitated in crystalline form from alcoholic extracts of gallstones (Stamler 1967, p. 44). In 1816, Chevreul named it, again from the Greek *chole*, bile, and *steros*, solid. In 1838 Lecanu showed that it was present in human blood, and in 1843 Vogel showed that it was present in atherosclerotic plaques (Stamler 1967, p. 44). In 1857 Mettenheimer noted that the lipoidal 'mush' was doubly refractive because of the presence of cholesterol esters (Stamler 1967, p. 44).

During the second half of the nineteenth century, the microscopic studies of cellular pathology, initiated by Virchow and his colleagues, led to the delineation of atherosclerosis as a specific pathological entity in the generic grouping of the arterioscleroses (Windaus 1910). This advance stemmed from the elucidation of the unique morphological characteristics of the atherosclerotic plaque, i.e. the demonstration that the mushy gruel-like material—the hallmark of the lesion—was an accumulation of lipids, including free and esterified cholesterol. This delineation in turn led to the posing of critical questions. At what stage of atherogenesis does cholesterol-lipid deposition occur? Is this an early primary event or a late secondary event? What is the source of this cholesterol-lipid? Is it derived from blood cholesterol-lipid? What are the relationships among cholesterol-lipid in the diet, the circulating blood, and the lesion? All these questions were posed with more or less clarity by the turn of the present century, and pathogenetic theories were formulated (Stamler 1967, p. 44).

In the first decade of the twentieth century, the biochemist Windaus demonstrated that atherosclerotic aortas contained six to seven times more free cholesterol, and 20–26 times more cholesterol esters than normal aortas. Over the course of a quarter-century, he also carried out decisive work on the chemical formula and structure of cholesterol (Stamler 1967, p. 44).

Late in the nineteenth and early in the twentieth century, clinical investigators went a step further in elucidating relationships. They showed that several disparate diseases—hypothyroidism, the nephrotic syndrome, essential familial xanthomatosis (as it was then called), diabetes mellitus—were all characterized by prolonged hypercholesterolaemia and premature severe atherosclerosis (Stamler 1967, p. 47). These observations linked *level* of blood cholesterol and atherogenesis. In the 1920s, with the emergence of clinical cardiology as a medical speciality and the diagnosis in living patients of myocardial infarction (MI), this link was reinforced and extended by studies showing that people recovered from MI had higher mean serum cholesterol levels than those of controls (Stamler 1967, pp. 47, 49). These reports also noted that hypertension and diabetes were more common in post-MI patient than in controls, and that the great majority of MI cases were men.

In 1908–12, Ignatowski, Anitschkow, and their colleagues achieved the experimental production of atherosclerosis (Anitschkow 1933), accomplished initially by feeding rabbits animal products, in an experiment on the effect of dietary protein on the kidney; thus the finding of atherosclerosis was serendipitous. The investigators noted that the sera of their rabbits, which were fed eggs, milk, and meat, were grossly hyperlipidemic and that the arterial lesions were laden with cholesterol and fat. They inferred that the high cholesterol-lipid content, rather than the high protein content, of their experimental diets might be responsible and verified this in subsequent studies by feeding diets supplemented with pure cholesterol and fat. In the 1920s this group also showed that atherosclerosis could be produced by long-term feeding of diets supplemented with only small amounts of cholesterol, inducing only slight elevations of serum cholesterol, i.e. massive hypercholesterolaemia and organ cholesterolosis were not prerequisites for experimental atherogenesis (Anitschkow 1933).

The many animal studies that followed included those of Leary (1941), which led him to infer that cholesterol-lipid-laden foam cells played a pivotal role in atherogenesis. He concluded that, in experimental animals and in people on diets high in cholesterol and fat leading to increased plasma cholesterol levels, these cells, formed from reticulo-endothelial scavenger macrophages in liver, spleen, adrenal gland, lung, etc., entered the circulating blood and crossed arterial intima to form foam-cell cushions or atheromata, the initial lesions of atherosclerosis. Breakdown of foam cells and release of their cholesterol-lipid stimulated arterial cell responses, with resultant formation of atherosclerotic plaques.

Late in the nineteenth century and early in the twentieth century 'geographical pathology' also emerged as a research discipline. Reports were published on populations in Africa, Asia, and Latin America with much less atherosclerotic disease than was prevalent in Europeans. These were, in the main, studies by European investigators who were discharging medical responsibilities in the colonies. In the early 1930s Rosenthal (1934) reviewed 28 such papers then extant and formulated this inference: '. . . In no race for which a high cholesterol intake (in the form of eggs, butter and milk) and fat intake are recorded is atherosclerosis absent . . . Where a high protein diet is consumed, which naturally contains small quantities of cholesterol, but where the neutral fat is low, atherosclerosis is not prevalent'. Raab (1932) arrived at similar conclusions based on his survey of this literature. Snapper (1941), describing his experience in China, also emphasized the association between a habitual diet of mainly vegetarian foods, low in cholesterol and fat, and rarity of atherosclerotic disease. Kuczynski (1925) reported on an Asian population at the opposite end of the dietary spectrum—nomadic Kirghiz plainsmen who habitually consumed large amounts of meat and milk. He noted a high incidence of obesity, premature extensive atherosclerosis, contracted kidney, apoplexy, and arcus senilis. Their urbanized kinsmen, subsisting on more varied fare, did not exhibit such severe vascular diseases. In relation to the famine and severe shortage of dietary fats in Germany immediately after the First World War, Aschoff (1924) noted post-mortem evidence for regression of atherosclerosis. During the early decades of the twentieth century, several reports also appeared on isolated preliterate populations (e.g. in Africa and Asia) with low BPs and with little or no rise in BP with age, or HBP, or hypertensive cardiovascular disease (Shaper 1974). Common characteristics of these populations were leanness and predominantly vegetarian diets low in salt.

In summary, by the 1930s seminal contributions had been published by investigators from all over the world using every method of medical research—gross and microscopic pathology, biochemical pathology, clinical investigation, animal experimentation, and epidemiology (geographical pathology). Nutritional factors, particularly dietary cholesterol-fat and also caloric imbalance with consequent obesity, had been implicated in the aetiology of atherosclerotic disease, and at least in experimental animals had been shown to influence serum lipids, although this relationship remained obscure for the human species. The scientific roots for the rapid growth of knowledge were deep and variegated. Once the constraints of the Great Depression and the Second World War were removed, a resurgence of research quickly developed, relying on all that had gone before and rapidly going beyond it. Again, it involved every methodology. The scope of this investigative effort during the first post-war decade is reflected, at least in part, by the bibliographies of two monographs of the 1950s co-authored by the present writer—the first with 713 references and the second with 787 references, the great majority of them original papers published during those years (Katz and Stamler 1953; Katz *et al.* 1958).

In animal experimental studies, hypercholesterolaemia and atherosclerosis of all grades of severity, coronary as well as aortic, were induced by cholesterol-fat feeding (either alone, or in combination with another intervention, e.g. methionine deficiency, hypothyroidism) in virtually every species available to the laboratory—avian and mammalian, omnivorous, herbivorous, or carnivorous, including primates. In the presence of the nutritional prerequisites for atherogenesis, i.e. a cholesterol-fat-supplemented diet, other traits, exogenous and endogenous, were shown to influence the atherosclerotic process significantly (Katz and Stamler 1953; Katz *et al*. 1958). For example, in chickens with minimal hypercholesterolemia due to feeding mash containing 0.25 per cent cholesterol plus 5 per cent fat, but not in chickens fed plain mash, BP elevation induced by adding salt to feed resulted in intensified atherogenesis. Also, both exogenous and endogenous oestrogens were shown to prevent and reverse coronary atherosclerosis induced by cholesterol-fat feeding. Such findings underscored both the key role of dietary cholesterol-fat and the multifactorial nature of the aetiology of atherosclerotic disease, including (as in the experiments on feeding both cholesterol-fat and salt) the importance of multiple nutritional factors.

These years also witnessed the demonstration in several species that arterial plaques gradually regressed after discontinuation of an atherogenic diet. Possible implications for man of all these advances were virtually self-evident. To deny them either required evidence—not available—that man was exceptional and hence that the animal findings were not relevant, or rejection of the principles of experimental medicine established by the work of Claude Bernard, Charles Darwin, Louis Pasteur, and other nineteenth-century giants on the unity of the animal kingdom and the relevance of animal research for the aetiology, pathogenesis, prevention, and treatment of human disease.

During this post-war decade, important developments also came from biochemical and biophysical laboratories. The ultracentrifuge method for the study of proteins was modified to accomplish flotation of plasma lipoproteins, their separation into several classes, and their quantification. Extensive data were published on their patterns, on factors influencing them, both exogenous (including nutrition) and endogenous, and on their relationships to atherosclerosis in experimental animals and man (Katz and Stamler 1953; Katz *et al*. 1958).

The demonstration with isotopes that *the* characteristic of living organisms was a dynamic equlibrium, i.e. a steady state achieved by constant turnover of molecular constituents and not a static state, and the development of tracer methodology with use of multiple isotopes were extensively applied in atherosclerosis research. Results included the demonstration that cholesterol in atherosclerotic plaques was significantly derived from the circulating cholesterol-bearing lipoproteins of the plasma. The painstaking task of identifying the sequential steps in the biological synthesis of cholesterol from acetate, and their enzymatic regulation, was carried forward (Bloch 1965).

Clinical investigation demonstrated that serum total cholesterol, S_f 12–20 (low-density) lipoproteins (LDL), and S_f 20–100 (very low density) lipoproteins (VLDL) were higher in men with a history of MI than in healthy controls, with differences in mean levels greater at younger ages (Lawry *et al.* 1957). In metabolic ward studies, it was shown that, with maintained weight loss, serum TC, LDL, intermediate density lipoprotein (IDL), and VLDL all underwent marked sustained reduction (Katz *et al.* 1958, pp. 48–9, 82–3). This also resulted when people were isocalorically fed diets low in total fat and cholesterol. It was also shown that dietary neutral fats differed in their influences on serum cholesterol, i.e. saturated fats raised TC whereas unsaturated fats did not, and polyunsaturated fats from both plant and fish sources lowered TC (Katz *et al.* 1958, pp. 50–60). Short-term clinical studies in those years also indicated that high fat meals induced decreased fibrinolysis and increased blood coagulability, measured *in vitro* (Katz *et al.* 1958, pp. 48–9, 82–3).

Finally, this decade witnessed the emergence of cardiovascular epidemiology as a robust independent discipline, fruitfully linked with clinical medicine, physiology, biochemistry, and pathology. Early on, several reports were published relating mass nutritional deprivation and other lifestyle changes during the Second World War (for example in the Low Countries, Scandinavia, and the USSR) to changes in population serum lipids, blood pressure, thrombo-embolic disease, atherosclerosis at autopsy, and/or national mortality rates from cardiovascular diseases (Katz and Stamler 1953; Katz *et al.* 1958, p. 30). By the time of the Second World Congress of Cardiology in 1954, sufficient work was in progress in several countries to make possible an international symposium, with published *Proceedings* edited by Ancel Keys and Paul Dudley White (Keys and White 1956). Papers reported on the rarity of severe coronary atherosclerosis and the low incidence of CHD throughout adulthood in both men and women in Japan, in contrast with the USA, and on the low mean serum cholesterol levels in Japanese farmers, industrial workers, and clerks, in contrast with Japanese physicians and Japanese–Americans (Nisei) in Hawaii and Los Angeles. These findings were related to the habitual diet of most Japanese, which was high in vegetable products and low in total lipid. The data on social class differences and on migrants, consonant with old and new findings in other populations (Rosenthal 1934; Katz *et al.* 1958, pp. 24–6), indicated that population genetics could not be a crucial determinant of large inter-population differences in mean TC levels and in atherosclerotic disease.

Japan was quickly recognized to be remarkable among industrialized countries because of its low CHD rates, and became a focus of research endeavour. Its high death rates from stroke also received attention, and were related to high salt intake. Contrasting group mean levels of TC were also reported for healthy young adult and middle-aged southern Italian men compared with English, Swedish, and American men, and again were shown to correlate with mean dietary lipid intake (Katz *et al.* 1958, pp. 24–6). Striking contrasts—confirming those reported by classical geographical pathology—were also found in studies of Bantu compared with Europeans in South Africa and with Americans, and in rural Guatemalan handicraft and agricultural workers compared with urban Guatemalan and American business and professional men (Katz *et al.* 1958, pp. 20–4). The mean percentage of calories from total fat and from animal fat and the mean serum TC were all much lower in the Bantu and the rural Guatemalans compared with the others; mean serum TC was low at both age 30 and age 45 among the Bantu (167 and 179 mg/dl) in contrast with the higher levels of Americans (192 and 236 mg/dl) and the greater slope with age. Correspondingly, based either on clinical or post-mortem findings, atherosclerotic CHD was rare in the Bantu and the rural Guatemalans, but common in the other groups.

In agreement with these international cross-population findings, it was found that in the USA pure vegetarians—habitually eating fare devoid of cholesterol, lower in saturated fat, and higher in unsaturated fat than omnivores—had a mean serum cholesterol level 28 per cent lower than that of omnivores.

In 1953, data were published on the high prevalence of coronary atherosclerosis in young American soldiers killed in Korea, in contrast with its rarity in Koreans (Enos *et al.* 1953). Later in the decade, in relation to the establishment of the US National Heart Institute and the transformation of the American Heart Association from a professional organization to a voluntary health agency, attention was focused on the increase in cardiovascular mortality rates for middle-aged white American men in the period from 1920 to 1955, despite declines in mortality from stroke and from the infectious heart diseases (Moriyama *et al.* 1958). It was concluded that this trend was due to rising CHD mortality rates, and environmental exposures which may have been responsible were noted.

In these years, also, four reports were published on international ecological analyses using data from the Food and Agricultural Organization (FOA) on national per capita nutrients and from the World Health Organization (WHO) on national CHD mortality rates for industrialized countries (Katz *et al.* 1958, pp. 28–30). Several dietary constituents had significant positive correlations with CHD death rates in univariate analyses, including total calories and percentage of calories from total fat, animal fat, and animal protein; the percentage of calories from vegetable fat, vegetable protein, and carbohydrate had significant negative correlations with CHD death rates. None of these initial reports gave data on dietary cholesterol and CHD death rates, despite the compelling evidence from animal experimentation on the critical role of dietary cholesterol in the aetiology of severe atherosclerosis. When such analyses were performed in subsequent years, a significant positive relationship was shown in not only univariate but also bivariate (controlled for other dietary constituents) analyses (Stamler 1979; Liu *et al.* 1982).

During this post-war decade, there was a completely new development in cardiovascular epidemiology of major importance: the undertaking of long-term prospective within-population studies. In the latter 1950s, these investigations reported their first findings, relating several characteristics of individuals at baseline to CHD incidence and/or mortality during the next 3–5 years—in particular, in one or more studies, high serum TC, high LDL, high BP, obesity, cigarette smoking, and sedentary occupation (Morris *et al*. 1953; Gofman *et al*. 1956; AJPH 1957; Hammond and Horn 1958; Katz *et al*. 1958; Stamler *et al*. 1960). These data on the prognostic implications of these traits focused attention on their high prevalence in the middle-aged population, and in the USA it was noted that high mean values of serum cholesterol, systolic and diastolic blood pressure (SBP and DBP), and relative weight were present in middle-aged men and women from all samples of the general population under study, irrespective of geographical locale, ethnicity, or socio-economic status. Relative weight was shown to be related to both BP and TC, but it was also clear that the high cholesterol, high saturated fat *composition* of the habitual diet was playing a key role in determining population serum lipid–lipoprotein patterns. The prospective data also led to the recognition that observed values in populations of apparently healthy people—their means ± 2.0 standard deviations—were not a sound basis for identifying 'normal' values. In addition, they stimulated interest in the definition of *optimal* values associated with low probabilities of developing cardiovascular disease over the years.

Based on all these concordant findings and discussions about their implications for coping with rising CHD rates, publicly described as epidemic in onslaught, the term *risk factor* began to be used in the late 1950s to describe traits assessed to be aetiologically significant in predisposing people to heart attack and stroke (Stamler *et al*. 1959). Concurrently, researchers in the UK, Finland, and the USA undertook the first trials on ability to achieve primary or secondary prevention of CHD by diet means, and the present author initiated the first trial involving multifactorial intervention to control all the major risk factors (Katz *et al*. 1958; Stamler 1967). All these, with small sample sizes due mainly to limited funding and with other design flaws, were in retrospect pilot projects, but they were also pioneering undertakings that set the stage for later trials and for population-wide preventive efforts. At the end of this eventful decade, in 1959, the first statement was addressed to the public on the risk factors—(1) obesity, (2) elevated blood cholesterol level, (3) elevated blood pressure, (4) excessive cigarette smoking, and (5) heredity—and the possibility of safely influencing the first four of them and thereby of preventing heart attacks and strokes (White *et al*. 1959). The initiators of this statement were senior American cardiologists, cardiovascular researchers, and medical statesmen, several of them Past Presidents of the American Heart Association.

Not long after this 'Statement on arteriosclerosis', the American Heart Association (AHA) published its first reports on the possibility of preventing the atherosclerotic diseases by not smoking and by improving eating habits. Its statement, 'Dietary fat and its relation to heart attacks and strokes' summarized the research evidence on all the major risk factors, and then reviewed dietary recommendations—decreased intake of cholesterol, saturated fat, and (for overweight people) calories, and partial replacement of saturated fats by unsaturates, including polyunsaturates—aimed at '. . . a considerable alteration in the cholesterol level in the blood with the use of acceptable diets' (AHA 1961). In paragraphs under the heading 'Who in particular should modify fat content of his diet?', this report concluded:

Most persons in the United States who are overweight . . . Men with a strong family history of atherosclerotic heart or blood vessel disease, who have elevated blood cholesterol levels, an increase in blood pressure, are overweight and/or who lead sedentary lives of relentless frustration . . . Those people who have had one or more atherosclerotic heart attacks. . .

Thus, this was a recommendation directed at tens of millions of higher-risk American adults. It was a fitting culmination of more than a decade of major research that led to the pin-pointing of the major risk factors as important causes of the epidemic atherosclerotic diseases. It launched nationwide efforts in the USA for their prevention, primary and secondary, with reliance first and foremost on safe improvements in life-styles.

These first two statements on prevention of the atherosclerotic diseases did not explicitly present a population-wide approach. That came a few years later, when the AHA updated its statements, in the Report on the Primary Prevention of the Atherosclerotic Diseases by the Inter-Society Commission for Heart Disease Resources, in Scandinavian public health statements (ISCHDR 1970; Stamler 1979, 1981; NHLBI 1981), and as a *combined population-wide and high risk strategy* in the seminal report of the WHO Expert Committee on the Prevention of Coronary Heart Disease (WHO 1982).

FOUR ESTABLISHED MAJOR RISK FACTORS—PRESENT STATUS

Space limitations preclude even a brief survey of prodigious research output during the 1960s, 1970s, 1980s, to the present. Such a survey would not be feasible even if the writer were to ignore the important contributions of animal experimentation, pathological investigation, and molecular and cell biology, and confine himself to epidemiology. Suffice it here to note highlights from cross-population and within-population epidemiological research, and to call attention to extensive bibliographies, generally not all-encompassing, in monographs and reviews published from 1981 to 1991 (NHLBI 1981; WHO 1982, 1990; Stamler *et al.* 1985; NCEP 1988, 1990; NRC 1989).

Cross-population studies

By 1981, the literature included publications on five types of cross-population (ecological) investigations:

(1) at least 12 analyses of FAO–WHO data on relationships between national nutritional and mortality patterns;

(2) analyses of autopsy findings from different countries, and factors related to these findings, including comprehensive data from the International Atherosclerosis Project on over 31 000 decedents from 15 cities and countries, two of them highly industrialized (New Orleans and Oslo), and the other 13 non-industrialized low income areas in Africa, the Far East, and Latin America;

(3) field investigations of population samples in different countries, including the Seven Countries Study led by Ancel Keys;

(4) international studies on effects of migration, including the Ni-Hon-San Study on Japanese in Hiroshima and Nagasaki and Japanese-Americans in Hawaii and California;

(5) comparisons of populations within countries (NHLBI 1981).

During the most recent decade, several more reports have been published from such cross-population studies. All of them are consistent in finding relationships between population nutritional patterns, particularly dietary cholesterol-lipid, population mean serum lipids, and/or population CHD rates. Some also encompassed data on such variables as cigarette use, BP–HBP, and diabetes, and found them to be associated with CHD rates across populations.

A comment on this ecological aspect of epidemiological research may be useful. It has been asserted that such investigations serve only the purpose of formulating hypotheses for further research with the implication that they have no other relevance in regard to central issues of causation. This is unsound, since *every* analysis relating one variable to another is by its nature based on a question, i.e. at that stage it is already the exploration of a hypothesis. Studies of this type, like *all* other studies using whatever methodology, have their strengths and weaknesses, their possibilities and limitations, as discussed elsewhere (Stamler 1989). They should no more be 'put down' than any other type of investigation. In judging the crucial issue of aetiology of major chronic diseases, one must assess the *totality* of the data—nothing else suffices.

Specifically as to cross-population ecological studies, it has been argued that when cross-population data show significant positive relationships and within-population data based on individuals do not, it is likely that the former, rather than the latter, are valid reflections of the real world (Hegsted 1985). When *within*-population studies are conducted in a way to minimize methodological limitations in *that* type of research, findings of across- and within-population studies are likely to be concordant. A case in point is the relation of dietary lipid to serum cholesterol. A significant positive association was demonstrated decades ago in ecological studies across populations (as well as in animal experiments and clinical intervention studies), but not for individuals in within-population studies. For years this seemingly irreconcilable contradiction cast doubt on the validity of the relationship—until it was shown that there was marked within-individual day-by-day variation in eating patterns making it difficult to characterize individuals validly within more or less homogeneous groups and to rank them in regard to nutrient intake (Liu *et al.* 1978). It was soon recognized that this was at the root of the 'negative' findings in within-population studies. Lack of appreciation of this problem and of other sources of bias accounts for several false negative reports of within-population studies on dietary lipid and serum cholesterol, and on dietary lipid and CHD. As is now more widely understood, this methodological problem is soluble by in-depth procedures for assessing diets of individuals and/or by study designs involving very large sample size (INTERSALT 1988, 1989).

Within-population studies

A review published in 1981 cited 57 papers on within-population studies reporting multivariate analyses on the combined impact of the major risk factors on CHD risk (NHLBI 1981). It presented prospective data from more than 65 cohorts in 23 countries on four continents, reflecting a remarkable world-wide expansion of epidemiological research during the 1960s and 1970s. In the last 10 years, many of these studies have continued long-term surveillance of their cohorts and have reported additional results, including data based on 15, 25, 30, or more years of follow-up. In addition, other within-population investigations have been undertaken and have presented findings, for example on the MONICA cohorts in 26 countries, on the ARIC Study cohorts in the USA, and on the Chinese cohorts in the PRC–USA Co-operative Study on Cardiovascular and Cardiopulmonary Epidemiology.

Most of the studies reporting multivariate analyses on baseline traits and CHD risk have dealt with only three of the four established major risk factors, i.e. serum cholesterol, blood pressure, and cigarette smoking, but not diet. Only a small minority of these studies, far too few unfortunately, had resources permitting them to undertake assessments of the eating patterns of their individual participants. Some did this several years after their baseline examination, with consequent possible bias, for example due to change in diet by participants made aware at entry of high serum cholesterol and/or high blood pressure (Shekelle *et al.* 1982). Some used only a single 24 hour dietary recall with consequent sizeable error in classification (arraying) of individuals (e.g. on dietary cholesterol-fat intake) and marked attenuation in observed associations (e.g. between dietary lipid and TC, CHD) (Liu *et al.* 1978). Only a few studies evaluated eating habits of their participants at entry, hence at a relatively bias-free point, and with in-depth methodology, for example multiple 24 hour dietary recalls or Burke-type comprehensive standardized interviews on usual dietary pattern with cross-checks (Burke 1947; Stamler and Shekelle 1988), to permit reasonably valid ranking of individuals with regard to nutrient intake.

Among the within-population prospective investigations reporting data on TC, BP, and CIG, one is of special value because of its enormous sample size of 361 662 men aged 35–57 years at baseline, who were screened by standardized methods in 18 US cities in 1973–5 for the Multiple Risk Factor Intervention Trial (MRFIT) (Neaton *et al.* 1984; Stamler *et al.* 1986). (No diet data were collected.) Prospective findings on the mortality of this cohort are now available based on 12 years of follow-up. The particular merit of these data is their precision; owing to the very large sample size, confidence intervals around mortality rates are very narrow.

Table 3.1 gives age-adjusted CHD mortality rates per 10 000 person-years for the cohort without a history of diabetes or MI at baseline, stratified by baseline cigarette use and quintiles of TC and SBP. At every level of SBP, risk of CHD death rises progressively and markedly with higher serum cholesterol for both non-smokers and smokers. Optimal serum cholesterol is less than 182 mg/dl (<4.7 mmol/l). For non-smokers in the highest TC quintile, compared with the lowest TC quintile, relative risk ranges from 2.45 to 4.00, depending on SBP; for smokers, it ranges from 2.30 to 2.96. Similarly, at every TC level, risk rises progressively and markedly with higher SBP for both non-smokers and smokers. Optimal SBP is less than 118 mmHg. For non-smokers in the highest SBP quintile, compared with the lowest SBP quintile, relative risk ranges from 2.70 to 4.42, depending on TC; for smokers, it ranges from 2.46 to 3.36. Findings are similar with DBP in such analyses instead of SBP, but the range of relative risk is greater with SBP than with DBP, indicating that SBP is even more strongly related to CHD risk than is DBP (Stamler *et al.* 1989). Optimal diastolic pressure is less than 76 mmHg. Only 3 per cent of this total cohort are in the lowest risk group, i.e. non-smokers with serum cholesterol less than 182 mg/dl (<4.7 mmol/l) and systolic pressure less than 118 mmHg (Table 3.1). Owing to the impact of contemporary unhealthy

Table 3.1 Baseline cigarette smoking, quintiles of serum cholesterol, systolic pressure and age-adjusted CHD mortality per 10 000 person-years

Serum TC (mg/dl)	Systolic pressure (mmHg)					
	<118	118–124	125–131	132–141	142+	Q5/Q1
Non-smokers						
<182	3.09	3.72	5.13	5.35	13.66	4.42
182–202	4.39	5.79	8.35	7.66	15.80	3.60
203–220	5.20	6.08	8.56	10.72	17.75	3.41
221–244	6.34	9.37	8.66	12.21	22.69	3.58
245+	12.36	12.68	16.31	20.68	33.40	2.70
Q5/Q1	4.00	3.41	3.18	3.87	2.45	—
Smokers						
<182	10.37	10.69	13.21	13.99	27.04	2.61
182–202	10.03	11.76	19.05	20.67	33.69	3.36
203–220	14.90	16.09	21.07	28.87	42.91	2.88
221–244	19.83	22.69	23.61	31.98	55.50	2.80
245+	25.24	30.50	35.26	41.47	62.11	2.46
Q5/Q1	2.43	2.85	2.67	2.96	2.30	—

Q5 is quintile 5; Q1 is quintile 1.
Mean follow-up is 11.6 years.
342,815 men free of heart attack and diabetes at baseline screened for the Multiple Risk Factor Intervention Trial (MRFIT).
Excluded from the total of 361 662 men were 8322 without a baseline SBP reading, 5440 with a baseline history of MI and 5625 with a baseline history of diabetes mellitus. Because some men had more than one of these exclusion factors, the total number of men excluded was 18 847.

life-styles, the problem of increased risk involves practically the whole population—it is not 'just' a problem for the 20 or 30 per cent of people at very high risk, but is a population-wide problem (WHO 1982).

For non-smokers, absolute CHD risk ranges from a low of 3.09 per 10 000 person-years for men in the lowest quintile of both TC and SBP to a high of 33.40 for men in the highest quintile of TC and SBP—a risk greater by a factor of almost 11 (Table 3.1). The problem is qualitatively similar but quantitatively much worse for cigarette smokers (Table 3.1). For example, for smokers in the highest quintiles of both TC and SBP, CHD death rate is 62.11, almost double that of non-smokers with these same high levels of cholesterol and pressure, and *20* times as high as the death rate in the lower risk group. Even with optimal serum cholesterol and pressure, CHD death rate is 10.37 in smokers compared with 3.09 in non-smokers, more than three times higher. For those with cholesterol 203–220 mg/dl and SBP 125–131 mmHg (the centre of the distributions), CHD death rate is 21.07 for smokers compared with 8.56 for non-smokers, 2.5 times greater.

Furthermore, the excess risk of CHD death attributed to TC and SBP is much greater for cigarette smokers than for non-smokers. Thus, for the highest quintile of TC and SBP, the excess risk compared with the lowest quintile is $33.40 - 3.09 = 30.31$ excess CHD deaths per 10 000 person-years for non-smokers compared with $62.11 - 10.37 = 51.74$ excess CHD deaths per 10 000 person-years for smokers, i.e. a 55 per cent higher excess risk (Table 3.1). This is the case even though relative risk is less for this stratum for smokers than non-smokers, i.e. $62.11/10.37 = 5.99$ compared with $33.40/3.09 = 10.81$. In terms of the extra number of CHD deaths due to above-optimal risk factors in the population, it is this excess risk that is important, both for the population as a whole (the public health challenge) and for individuals (the clinical challenge). Thus, for smokers with TC and SBP in the highest quintiles compared with the lowest risk stratum, excess risk is $62.11 - 3.09 = 59.02$ excess CHD deaths per 10 000 person-years or, for the 11.6 years of follow-up from baseline, 684.6 excess CHD deaths per 10 000 men. For those men of average age of about 48 years at baseline, there were about seven excess CHD deaths per 100 men during the subsequent 12 years. This problem of excess risk during the prime of life is further demonstrated by data from the US National Co-operative Pooling Project: over the years from age 40 to age 65, excess risk was 29 excess major CHD events (non-fatal plus fatal) per 100 men in the highest quintile of risk compared with men in the lowest quintile of risk based on entry TC, DBP, and CIG findings (Pooling Project Research Group 1978).

Table 3.2 presents data for 347 978 men screened by MRFIT, i.e the 342 815 in Table 3.1 plus 5163 men with a baseline history of drug-treated diabetes, all free at baseline of a history of heart attack. The data in Table 3.1 result from use of the classical epidemiological technique of multiple

Table 3.2 Proportional hazards regression summary for multiple risk factors for CHD death over an average follow-up of 12 years

Variable	Coefficient	Difference		Relative risk
Serum TC (mg/dl)	0.0064***	230 vs 190		1.29
SBP (mmHg)	0.0222***	138 vs 118		1.56
CIG/day	0.0230***	20 vs 0		1.58
Diabetes	1.1676***	Yes	No	3.21
Race	−0.0397	Black	White	0.96
Income	0.1328***	Low	High	1.14
Age (years)	0.0901***	50	45	1.57

347 978 men aged 35–57 years with no history of MI screened for the Multiple Risk Factor Intervention Trial (MRFIT).
*** $p < 0.001$.

cross-classification; those in Table 3.2 are from a multiple regression analysis with use of the Cox proportional hazards model. Findings by the two methods are similar in regard to the significant strong graded exponential independent relationship of TC, SBP, and CIG to 12 year CHD risk. These relationships of the three established major risk factors to CHD risk are also independent of the significant associations of age, diabetes, and income with CHD risk. While risk of CHD death is not significantly different for blacks and whites of this MRFIT cohort, risks of death from stroke, all cardiovascular disease (CVD), and all causes are significantly and independently higher for blacks than for whites in similar multiple regression analyses. The greater risk for low income compared with high income men in the MRFIT cohort prevails for CHD, stroke, CVD, and all-cause mortality.

As shown in Table 3,2, 12 year risk of CHD death is more than three times higher for men with a baseline history of drug-treated diabetes (DM) compared with non-diabetic men, but its prevalence is relatively low (1.5 per cent of this MRFIT cohort). The greater risk associated with diabetes is manifest at every level of TC, SBP, and CIG, and for diabetic men, as for non-diabetic men, risk is related to each of these factors. In addition, TC, SBP, CIG, and DM are significantly and independently related to risk over 12 years of death from stroke, CVD, and all causes, and to 12 year risk of CHD mortality for subgroups of the MRFIT cohort identified by ethnicity (Asian, black, Hispanic, white) or age. These four factors are also all significantly related to 12 year risk of CHD, CVD, and all causes of death for 5362 MRFIT men with a baseline history of hospitalization for heart attack. All these data are consistent with findings of studies conducted in many other countries including Australia, Belgium, Denmark, England, Finland, France, Germany, Israel, Italy, The Netherlands, Norway, Poland, Scotland, Spain, Switzerland, the USA, and the USSR.

The foregoing estimates of CHD risk attributable to TC, BP, and CIG are based on a one-time measurement of risk. Therefore, as impressive as they are, they are none the less *underestimates*, since they are not corrected for the limitation in validity of measurement inevitable with only one measurement (so-called regression–dilution bias), nor are they controlled for change in status over time (cessation of smoking, dietary change to lower TC and/or BP, etc.). Estimates are available of the even greater values for relative risk with correction for regression–dilution bias (MacMahon *et al.* 1990).

The conclusion as to the powerful impact of TC, BP, and CIG is further buttressed by data now available for both men and women of widely varying ages, for example from the Chicago Heart Association Detection Project in Industry (CHA) (Table 3.3). Note the similarity of the CHA and MRFIT data for middle-aged men (Tables 3.2 and 3.3). Note also the larger coefficients for TC and CIG for CHA men aged 25–39 compared

Table 3.3 Proportional hazards regression summary for multiple risk factors for CHD death over 15 years of follow-up for white men and women, by baseline age, screened for the Chicago Heart Association Detection Project in Industry

Age	No. of people	CHD	deaths	Multivariate coefficient and relative risk					
				TC 230 vs 190		SBP 138 vs 118		CIG/day 20 vs 0	
				Coeff.	RR	Coeff.	RR	Coeff.	RR
Men									
25–39	7873	57†	7.2‡	0.0158***	1.88	0.0187*	1.45	0.0342***	1.98
40–59	8515	458	53.8	0.0074***	1.34	0.0190***	1.46	0.0211***	1.52
60–74	1490	209	140.3	0.0042*	1.18	0.0144***	1.33	0.0175**	1.42
Women									
40–59	7082	123	17.4	0.0045*	1.20	0.0219***	1.55	0.0507***	2.76
60–74	1243	90	72.4	0.0066**	1.30	0.0171***	1.41	0.0294***	1.80

Persons without clinical CHD at baseline.
† Number of deaths.
‡ Rate/1000.
* $p < 0.05$; ** $p < 0.01$; *** $p < 0.001$.

with those aged 40–59, i.e. the greater relative risk for any given level of exposure to TC or CIG for young adult compared with middle-aged men. Note also the significant coefficients for men aged 60–74 years, and for women aged 40–59 and 60–74 years at baseline. While the size of the coefficients, and hence the relative risk, tends to decrease with age, *excess risk increases with age*, since for both men and women CHD mortality rates rise greatly with age, as shown in Table 3.3 for both sexes. The same finding prevails for the general population. Therefore, for men in the upper half of the population distribution of TC, SBP, and CIG, compared with men in the lower half, *excess risk* is as much as three times higher at age 65–69 than at age 45–49. How low are the rates for men and women in the stratum at very low risk in these cohorts, for example non-smokers with TC < 182 mg/dl (<4.70 mmol/l) and SBP < 118 mmHg (cf. Table 3.1)? Cohorts numbering in the thousands are too small to answer this question with reasonable precision, based on actual measurement. For example, with a 3 per cent prevalence of such people in this cohort, the 8515 men aged 40–59 in Table 3.3 would have only 255 men in this stratum. Before the data on men screened for MRFIT were available, epidemiological studies could attempt only to estimate rates for very low risk subgroups based on coefficients from multivariate regression analyses. However, the data on MRFIT men yield actual rates of high precision.

More detailed analyses of this matter are presented in Table 3.4. The criteria used there to select low risk men were physicians' classical clinical cut-points for normal BP, SBP < 120 mmHg, DBP < 80 mmHg, TC < 182 mg/dl (<4.70 mmol/l) (quintile 1, Table 3.1), non-smoking, and no history at baseline of DM or MI. Of the men screened for MRFIT, only 11 098 (3.1 per cent) met these criteria—given twentieth-century life-styles in Western industrialized countries, low risk people are rare by middle age. Note the low risk factor levels of these 11 098 men (TC=162 mg/dl [4.2 mmol/l], SBP=111 mmHg, and DBP=72 mmHg) and compare them with the levels for the 342 242 men making up the rest of the cohort (TC=216 mg/dl [5.6 mmol/l], SBP=131 mmHg, and DBP=84 mmHg, plus 38 per cent smokers, averaging 26 cigarettes/day) (Table 3.4). Compared with these latter 342 242 men, 12 year age-adjusted mortality rates for the low risk stratum were lower by 90 per cent for CHD, 79 per cent for stroke, 86 per cent for all CVD, 31 per cent for all cancer, 21 per cent for all non-CVD non-cancer deaths, and—the 'bottom line'—54 per cent for all causes of death. The findings are similar, with removal from the comparison cohort of 10 525 men at very high risk due to a history at baseline of drug-treated diabetes and/or of hospitalization for heart attack (Table 3.4). Note that with a low serum cholesterol of 162.4 ± 15.3 mg/dl (4.2 ± 0.4 mmol/l), the death rates from both cancer and non-CVD non-cancer causes were *lower* for the 11 098 men compared with the other strata, lending further support to the judgement that, for generally healthy

Table 3.4 Mean levels for baseline risk factors and age-adjusted mortality per 10 000 person-years by cause

Variable	Low risk men	Rest of cohort	Rest of cohort excluding men with MI or DM
No. of men	11 098	342 242	331 717
Mean TC (sd) (mg/dl)	162.4 (15.3)†	216.0 (38.8)	215.8 (38.5)
Mean SBP (sd) (mmHg)	111.0 (5.9)	130.6 (15.7)	130.5 (15.6)
Mean DBP (sd) (mmHg)	71.6 (5.5)	84.2 (10.4)	84.1 (10.4)
Cigarette smokers (%)	0	37.6%	37.6%
Mean CIG/Day, all	0	9.7 (14.9)	9.7 (14.9)
Mean CIG/Day, smokers	0	25.7 (13.6)	25.8 (13.6)
Mean age (sd) (years)	43.5 (6.3)	46.0 (6.4)	45.9 (6.4)
Mortality end-point			
CHD	22‡ 2.1§	8032 20.3	6659 17.5
Stroke	3 0.4	762 1.9	682 1.8
CVD	38 3.8	10 569 26.7	8927 23.4
Cancer	136 13.6	7751 19.6	7403 19.4
Non-CVD, non-cancer	104 9.5	4755 12.0	4259 11.1
All deaths	278 26.9	23 075 58.2	20 589 53.9

11 098 low risk men and other strata. Men screened for Multiple Risk Factor Intervention Trial (MRFIT). Excludes men with no baseline SBP measurement.
† Standard deviation.
‡ Number of deaths.
§ Age-adjusted death rate per 10 000 person-years. Mean follow-up 11.6 years.

persons, low serum TC is *not* related aetiologically to risk of neoplastic or other non-CVD diseases.

At this point it is relevant to re-emphasize that the eating habits of populations decisively determine their patterns for two established major risk factors, blood pressure and serum cholesterol, and to spell out briefly the specific aspects of habitual ('rich') diet that have been shown to influence these two risk factors. Lifetime intake of a diet high in sodium and low in potassium, and therefore with a high ratio of sodium to potassium, leads to a rise in BP from youth to middle age for most people. Given such diets, the BP problem is made worse by caloric imbalance and obesity, and by high alcohol intake. Similarly, high intakes of dietary cholesterol and saturated fat, compounded by obesity and low fibre intake, produce a rise in serum cholesterol for most people from youth to middle age.

In producing average levels of TC in the population that are 30 or 50–70 mg/dl above optimal, *both* dietary cholesterol and saturated fat (SF) intake are important, a fact still overlooked in some policy statements and deliberately obscured by the egg industry. For populations with a mean level of TC of about 240 mg/dl, a reduction of about two-thirds in SF intake, from 17 to 6 per cent of kilocalories (kcal), can be expected to produce a TC fall of about 27 mg/dl, and a reduction of about two-thirds in dietary cholesterol, from 240 to 80 mg/1000 kcal, can be expected to produce a TC fall of 13 mg/dl, i.e. declines of 11.2 per cent and 5.4 per cent respectively (Stamler and Shekelle 1988). A 1 per cent TC reduction is estimated to yield a 2 per cent fall in CHD risk (LRCP 1984; Stamler *et al.* 1986)— hence the importance of both dietary lipids. The role of dietary cholesterol looms even larger given its adverse influences on low density lipoproteins (LDL), and its possible unfavourable effects on intermediate density lipoproteins (IDL, remnant particles) and high density lipoproteins (HDL), and on risk of mortality over and above its TC effects (see below). Further, the influence on TC of preventing and controlling obesity needs greater attention. Data from both the National Diet–Heart Study and MRFIT clearly demonstrate that, for overweight men consuming a fat-modified diet, a weight loss of 5–7 kg produces a marked enhancement in TC reduction (NDHS 1968; Caggiula *et al.* 1981). That is, to follow the above example, instead of a TC fall of 40 mg/dl (16.7 per cent) from reduced saturated fat and cholesterol alone, a concomitant loss of 5–7 kg would yield a total TC fall of more than 54 mg/dl (> 22.5 per cent). Finally, the limited data available indicate that a 3 g/day increase of dietary water-soluble fibre intake yields a TC reduction of up to 3 per cent. With the goal of maximal decrease in CVD risk, the reduction of BP and TC made possible by the foregoing safe dietary approaches merits their implementation in both population-wide and individual preventive efforts.

'Rich' diet is an unprecedented twentieth-century mass exposure to which the human species is not adapted by evolution. It is the main cause not only of contemporary deleterious patterns of TC and BP in the population, but also of non-insulin-dependent diabetes, hyperuricaemia, and obesity. Moreover, its lipid component, in particular high dietary cholesterol intake, in addition to raising serum TC, has an effect on risk of mortality from CHD, CVD, and all causes *independent* of its adverse influence on TC (Table 3.5) (Shekelle and Stamler 1989; Stamler and Shekelle 1988, 1989). This finding, indicated by earlier animal experimental and cross-population (ecological) research, was demonstrated for individuals in several populations in the 1980s (Stamler and Shekelle 1988). The added impact of high dietary cholesterol on risk is substantial; for example, with habitual intake higher by 200 mg/1000 kcal/day, there is a 52 per cent greater long-term risk of CVD death for middle-aged American men (Table 3.5) and a 32 per cent greater risk of all-cause mortality.

Relative risks from such multivariate analyses are multiplicative. Thus comparison of two populations, with habitual mean cholesterol intake of 300 versus 100 mg/1000 kcal/day, mean TC of 230 versus 190 mg/dl, mean DBP of 85 versus 75 mmHg, mean CIG/day of 20 versus none yields the

Table 3.5 Proportional hazards regression summary for multiple risk factors for CVD death over 24 years of follow-up for 1897 men aged 40–56 years and free of CHD at baseline in the Western Electric Study

Variable†	Coefficient	Difference		Relative risk
Diet cholesterol (mg/1000 kcal)	0.0021*	300 vs 100		1.52
Serum TC (mg/dl)	0.0044***	230	190	1.19
DBP (mmHg)	0.0345***	85	75	1.41
CIG/day	0.0308***	20	0	1.86

Coefficients for all-causes mortality were:
Diet cholesterol 0.0014* TC 0.0024** DBP 0.0276*** CIG 0.0321*** age 0.0854***
† Mean of values at first and second annual examination. Also included in the analysis are age, family history of CVD, alcohol intake and alcohol intake squared, BMI, kcal/day, saturated fat, polyunsaturated fat, and major organ system disease.

estimate from the coefficients in Table 3.5 of a CVD relative risk (RR) of 4.74 for the highest compared with the lower risk cohort.

Of decisive importance is the inverse comparison: RR for the population with favourable levels compared with the population with high mean risk factor levels. Relative risk is the reciprocal of that given above: 1/4.74= 0.21, i.e. a CVD death rate lower by 79 per cent. The corresponding estimate for all-cause mortality is a death rate lower by 73 per cent. This means that the average life expectancy for 50 year old men is greater by about 14 years (e.g. 34 versus 20 additional years of life) (Stamler and Shekelle 1988, 1989). Similar estimates result from analyses based on other data sets for populations studied prospectively, including those cited here and others from several countries.

MULTIFACTORIAL TRIALS ON PRIMARY PREVENTION

Given the multiplicative impact of the established major risk factors—TC, BP, CIG, and 'rich' diet—and the recognition thereof more than 20 years ago (Stamler 1967; ISCHDR 1970), it might be anticipated that in the undertaking of randomized controlled trials (RCTs) to assess ability to influence CHD and CVD incidence and mortality, RCTs involving multi-factorial life-style intervention would have been given priority. In fact, this has not been the case. For various reasons, most trials have involved unifactor intervention, especially of drugs to lower BP of hypertensive persons, or of drugs to lower TC of hypercholesterolaemic persons (mainly to study secondary rather than primary prevention).

Results of such trials are reviewed elsewhere in this book. Here attention is focused on three multifactorial RCTs on primary prevention which were able, by long-term counselling of their intervention groups, to modify eating patterns (particularly dietary lipid composition) and thereby accomplish modest sustained reductions in TC, and to achieve smoking cessation in a modest proportion of their intervention group participants. These trials were the European Collaborative Trial of Multifactorial Prevention of Coronary Heart Disease, the Multiple Risk Factor Intervention Trial (MRFIT) in the USA, and the Oslo Study (Hjerrmann *et al.* 1981; Holme *et al.* 1985; WHO 1986; Rose 1987; Stamler 1988; MRFIT 1990). The first of these was unique in its multinational aspect (Belgium, Italy, Poland, UK), in its randomization of groups of men employed in 80 factories (rather than randomization of individuals), in its large sample size of 60 881 men aged 40–59 years, and in involving middle-aged men 'across the board' rather than high risk men only (WHO 1986; Rose 1987). MRFIT randomized 12 866 men aged 35–57 years assessed to be in the upper 10–15 per cent of CHD risk based on a multifactor score derived from TC, DBP, and CIG levels at first screen (MRFIT 1990). In addition to dietary and anti-smoking counselling for its intervention group, both these trials utilized antihypertensive drugs for men with HBP. The Oslo Study randomized 1232 non-hypertensive men aged 40–49 years, with very high TC (mean 328.9 mg/dl [8.5 mmol/l]): of whom 79 per cent were cigarette smokers; its intervention group was advised to reduce cholesterol and saturated fat intake and to stop smoking.

An in-depth discussion of the design considerations of such trials is not possible here, nor does space permit a review of their intervention experience and of the risk factor changes recorded in their intervention and control ('usual care') groups (Stamler 1988). Suffice it to note that all three achieved *modest*, not marked, sustained net differences between these two groups in the anticipated direction. As to end-point findings, in the European trial the cumulative 6 year incidence rate was lower for intervention than for control men for each of the three pre-defined end-points: fatal CHD, −6.9 per cent; non-fatal MI plus fatal CHD, −10.2 per cent; total mortality, −5.3 per cent. Regression analyses showed that the outcome for each of these end-points was significantly related to effects of intervention on risk factors, as assessed by multiple logistic function (MLF) scores across the 40 pairs of factories (intervention and control) ($p \le 0.05$) (WHO 1986; Rose 1987).

In the Oslo Study, with 8.5–10 years of follow-up, i.e. 3.5 years beyond the end of active intervention, the significant favourable outcome recorded at 5 years persisted for the 604 intervention men compared with the 628 control men—25 versus 45 with non-fatal MI + CHD death (the trial primary end point), i.e. rates of 41.4 versus 71.7 per 1000, lower by 42 per cent for the intervention group ($p = 0.02$). Moreover, deaths from all causes numbered 19 versus 31 (31.5 versus 49.4 per 1000), lower by 36 per cent for the intervention group ($p = 0.05$, single-tailed, not accounting for multiple comparisons) (Holme *et al.* 1985).

In MRFIT, with a mean follow-up of 10.5 years, i.e. 3.8 years after the end of intervention, rates for all three pre-defined mortality end-points were lower for the 6428 members of the special intervention (SI) group compared with the 6438 members of the usual care (UC) group by 10.6 per cent for CHD death ($p = 0.12$), 8.3 per cent for CVD death ($p = 0.16$), and 7.7 per cent for total mortality ($p = 0.10$) (MRFIT 1990). For death from acute MI, the SI rate was lower by 24.3 per cent ($p = 0.02$). For the subgroup of men without resting electrocardiogram (ECG) abnormalities at baseline, which numbered 9272 participants (4603 SI and 4670 UC) identified a priori for hypothesis testing, SI death rates were lower than UC rates by 21.1 per cent for CHD ($p < 0.05$) and by 15.7 per cent ($p < 0.05$) for all mortality.

In summary, the positive findings of these RCTs indicate that primary prevention can be achieved by even modest reduction in the four major risk factors, beginning in middle age. This was the consistent finding with multifactorial intervention—primarily improved nutrition and smoking cessation—even after decades of adverse exposure, including exposure at very high risk levels. It was the finding in all three RCTs not only for CHD, but also for mortality from all causes.

RISK FACTOR TREND IN GENERAL POPULATIONS

During the last three decades, official public policies for CHD primary prevention have been developed at the national level in several countries with the support of professional organizations, voluntary health agencies, etc., and efforts at implementation have been undertaken (White *et al.* 1959; AHA 1961; ISCHDR 1970; NHLBI 1981; Stamler 1981; WHO 1982, 1990; Stamler *et al.* 1985; NCEP 1988, 1990; NRC 1989). Experience over the last 150 years demonstrates that the solution of mass public health problems requires multifaceted sustained effective public health efforts *based on national government leadership and support*, and reaching into every corner of the nation. Therefore the national public policies promulgated for CHD prevention are important prerequisites for progress. Their scientific foundation is the knowledge on the four established major risk factors, and their cornerstone is the application of that knowledge. These public health endeavours were given an important boost by the 1982 *Report on the prevention of coronary heart disease* by a WHO Expert Committee under Geoffrey Rose's leadership, and by subsequent related WHO activity at the international and regional level (WHO 1982). Unfortunately, these efforts have been and continue to be woefully underfunded in every country, and are impeded by many-sided persistent opposition by special commercial interests—butter councils, egg boards, salt institutes, tobacco institutes, etc. Nevertheless, progress has been made in several countries, reflected in trends in general national statistics. In the USA, for example, annual national food balance sheet data show the following declines in per capita availability of foods high in cholesterol and/or saturated fats: eggs (egg yolks are the single most important source of dietary cholesterol in American fare) down from a high of 389/person/year in 1950 to 249/person/year in 1987 (−36 per cent); butter, down from 17 lb/person/year (7.7 kg) in 1940 to 5 lb/person/year in 1987 (−71 per cent); lard, down from 14 lb/person/year (6.4 kg) in 1940 to 2 lb/person/year in 1987 (−86 per cent); total milk fat solids, down from 33 lb/person/year (15.0 kg) to 21 lb/person/year in 1984 (−36 per cent); red meat, down from a high of 163 lb/person/year in 1970 to 144 lb/person/year in 1987 (−12 per cent) (Stamler 1979, 1981; NHLBI 1981; Stamler *et al*. 1985; US Bureau of the Census 1990, p. 124). Similar trends are shown in data from periodic in-depth surveys of US population samples (Stamler 1979; NHLBI 1981; Stamler *et al*. 1985). They indicate that the per capita dietary cholesterol intake of adult men decreased from about 750 mg/day in the late 1950s to about 450 mg/day in the 1970s (−40 per cent), SF decreased from about 17 per cent of kcal to about 14 per cent (−20 per cent), and polyunsaturated fats increased from about 4.0 per cent of kcal to about 6.5 per cent (+62 per cent). Trends for women were similar. Data are available indicating that decreases in dietary cholesterol and SF intakes have been greater among more educated than among less educated population strata (Stamler 1979; NHLBI 1981; Stamler *et al*. 1985).

In accordance with these trends in nutrient intake, multiple data sets, including those from serial national health surveys in 1960–2, 1971–4, and 1976–80, show declines in mean TC levels of American adults, again differentially, i.e. greater decreases for more educated than for less educated strata (Stamler 1979, 1981; NHLBI 1981; Stamler *et al*. 1985). Overall, the decline has been from a mean level of about 235 mg/dl in the late 1950s to about 215–220 mg/dl in the late 1970s.

Mean BP levels and rates of HBP in older Americans were lower in 1976–80 than in 1960–2 (Stamler 1979, 1981; NHLBI 1981; Stamler *et al*. 1985). Almost certainly, this trend is due mainly to increased antihypertensive drug treatment.

Prevalence of cigarette smoking also declined considerably in the USA during these decades. Whereas in 1965, the year after the landmark *Report to the Surgeon General on smoking and health* (Advisory Committee to the Surgeon General 1965), 50 per cent of adult men were cigarette smokers, by 1987 this proportion had declined to 32 per cent. Of all adult women, 32 per cent were smokers in 1965, and 26 per cent in 1987. Again, these trends varied considerably depending on educational attainment. Thus, for persons who did not complete high school, virtually no decrease in smoking prevalence was recorded—rates of 35 and 34 per cent. In contrast, the decline for college graduates was 43 per cent, from a prevalence rate of 28 per cent to one of 16 per cent (US Bureau of the Census 1990, p. 123).

These decades also witnessed sizeable increases in regular leisure time physical activity among American adults, once again more so among the more educated than among the less educated.

Such population-wide experiences in the USA and other countries show that it is possible, even with only limited resources and in the face of serious obstacles, to effect and sustain nationwide favourable trends in life-styles and life-style-related major risk factors. It is a reasonable inference that these trends have contributed in an important way to the declines in CHD, CVD, and all cause mortality in these countries. This inference is supported statistically by analyses of international data for industrialized nations, showing significant correlations between national *trends* of per capita dietary lipid (including dietary cholesterol) and *trends* of CHD mortality, and between national *trends* of per capita cigarette use and *trends* of CHD mortality (Byington *et al.* 1979). It is further supported in a particular way by the American experience. As noted above, trends of nutritional pattern, serum cholesterol, cigarette use, and leisure time exercise have all been more favourable for more educated than for less educated Americans. If changes in these traits have played a significant aetiological role in the marked decline in CHD, stroke, CVD, and all-cause mortality in the USA since the late 1960s, then the declines should be greater in the more educated than in the less educated. Five papers have been published on this matter, all of them with data showing greater decreases in mortality for the more educated (MLIC 1979; Enstrom 1983; Pell and Fayerweather 1985; Feldman *et al.* 1988; Rogot and Hrubec 1989). This is further evidence for the crucial role of the established major risk factors, but in the *ultimately decisive area—prevention in the general population.*

SUMMARY AND DISCUSSION

The evidence presented here builds on a huge body of research amassed over many years and from many scientific disciplines, testifying to the strength of the relationships of the established major risk factors to coronary risk. The 'rich' diet is pivotal among the risk factors and plays a primary and overwhelming role in the causation of epidemic CHD and CVD. The low prevalence in the population of truly low risk people poses a vital challenge and points to the large possibilities for prevention through substantial shifts downwards in the population levels of these risk factors by safe improvements in population life-styles, especially dietary habits, from early childhood on. Rose's concept of the 'sick' population neatly encapsulates this idea and illustrates the essentiality of a strategy of prevention which combines both population-wide and high risk components (Rose 1985).

Large problems persist on both sides of the Atlantic in regard to the scope and consistency of government efforts to implement policies, including food and nutrition policies, recognized as vital for the control and prevention of CHD, CVD, and other chronic diseases. In the USA, intakes of saturated fat and cholesterol, despite the declines, are still considerably above recommended levels, total fat intake remains high, prevalence of obesity has risen, and the national goal for 1990 of an adult mean serum cholesterol level under 200 mg/dl has not been achieved. At the international level, many industrialized countries registered little or no decline in CHD mortality during the 1970s and 1980s, and some recorded major increases. In several countries—the UK, the USA, and others—there is the further gnawing problem, so far essentially unaddressed, of the particularly unfavourable findings for the less educated and less affluent (as already noted for the USA). Clearly, systematic application in the population of knowledge on the four established major risk factors—by public health and medical care—is still limited everywhere. Much remains to be done at every level, from the top of government downwards. Despite the downturn in a few countries, the CHD epidemic continues, and on a world scale is vast.

As the *British Medical Journal* commented in a recent news article on the problems of the world's children: 'The sad fact is that 40 000 children die every day from easily preventable diseases. *The solution is one of will, not of technology . . .*' (Logie 1990, emphasis added). This is also true for CHD–CVD prevention.

POSTSCRIPT

This chapter was completed on 9 February 1991—24 days into the Gulf War. Leaders of the major powers, focused on waging war, have even less time than heretofore—and even less resources—to devote to prevention and control of epidemic diseases. Their will is elsewhere. But humanitarianism, and the goal of Bacon and Pasteur that science be applied to benefit mankind, can and must prevail, just as peace can and must prevail. The unremitting and skilful pursuit of these goals is the highest sign of objectivity and dedication in a medical scientist. Precisely because Geoffrey Rose epitomizes these qualities, it is a signal honour to write a chapter in this volume celebrating him.

ACKNOWLEDGEMENTS

It is a pleasure to express appreciation to the many colleagues who collected the baseline data on the 361 662 men who were screened for MRFIT (see Reference for a listing), to colleagues at the MRFIT Coordinating Center who collected and analysed the data on the vital status of these men, particularly James Neaton Ph.D., Joanna Shih MS, and Deborah Wentworth MS, and to fellow members of the MRFIT Editorial Committee, Marcus Kjelsberg Ph.D., Chairman, Jerome Cohen MD, Lewis Kuller MD, and Judith Ockene Ph.D. It is also gratifying to acknowledge the contribution of the many staff members and volunteers who accomplished the Chicago Heart Association Detection Project in Industry, particularly James A. Schoenberger MD, Richard B. Shekelle Ph.D., and Sue Shekelle MSW, and to express thanks to Alan R. Dyer Ph.D. who performed data analyses presented here. It is likewise a pleasure to acknowledge the role of Oglesby Paul MD, founder and for many years leader of the Western Electric Study, Mark Lepper MD, and Ann MacMillan Shryock MS, who played a decisive role in collecting the baseline nutrition data in 1957–9, and Richard B. Shekelle Ph.D. who performed the data analyses displayed here. The research data reported here were collected with support from the American Heart Association and its Illinois and Chicago affiliates, the Chicago Health Research Foundation, the Illinois Regional Medical Program, the National Heart, Lung, and Blood Institute, and many private donors. The author is also pleased to acknowledge the bibliographical assistance of Carolyn Majkowski BA. He is especially grateful to Rose Stamler MA, who carefully and critically read this paper, and made many valuable suggestions.

REFERENCES

Ackerknecht, E. H. (1953). *Rudolf Virchow—doctor, statesman, anthropologist*, University of Wisconsin Press, Madison, WI.

Advisory Committee to the Surgeon General (1965). *Smoking and health*, US Department of Health, Education, and Welfare, Public Health Service, Washington, DC.

AHA (American Heart Association, Central Committee for Medical and Community Programs) (1961). *Dietary fat and its relation to heart attacks and stroke*, American Heart Association, New York.

AJPH (American Journal of Public Health) (1957). Measuring the risk of coronary heart disease in adult population groups—a symposium. *Am. J. Public Health*, **47**, Part 2, 1–63.

Anitschkow, N. (1933). Experimental arteriosclerosis in animals. In *Arteriosclerosis* (ed. E. V. Cowdry), pp. 271–322, Macmillan, New York.

Aschoff, L. (1924). *Lectures in pathology*, Hoeber, New York.

Bloch, K. (1965). The biological synthesis of cholesterol. *Science,* **150,** 19–28.

Burke, B. S. (1947). The dietary history as a tool in research. *J. Am. Diet. Ass.,* **23,** 1041–6.

Byington, R., Dyer, A. R., Garside, D., Liu, K., Moss, D., Stamler, J., and Tsong, Y. (1979). Recent trends of major coronary risk factors and CHD mortality in the United States and other industrialized countries. *Proc. Conf. on the Decline in Coronary Heart Disease Mortality* (eds R. J. Havlik and M. Feinleib), pp. 340–79, NIH Publication 79–1610, National Institutes of Health, Bethesda, MD.

Caggiula, A. W., Christakis, G., Farrand, M., Hulley, S. B., Johnson, R., Lasser, N. L., Stamler, J., and Widdowson, G. (1981). The multiple risk intervention trial (MRFIT). IV. Intervention on blood lipids. *Prev. Med.,* **10,** 443–75.

Dock, G. (1939). Historical notes on coronary occlusion: from Heberden to Osler. *J. Am. Med. Ass.,* **113,** 563–8.

Dubos, R. (1960). *Pasteur and modern science*, Anchor Books, Garden City, NY.

Enos, W. F., Jr, Holmes, R. H., and Beyer, J. (1953). Coronary disease among United States soldiers killed in action in Korea. *J. Am. Med. Assoc.,* **152,** 1090–3.

Enstrom, J. E. (1983). Trends in mortality among California physicians after giving up smoking: 1950–79. *Brit. Med. J.,* **286,** 1101–5.

Feldman, J. J., Makuc, D. M., Kleinman, J. C., and Cornoni-Huntley, J. (1988). National trends in educational differentials in mortality. *Am. J. Epidemiol.,* **129,** 919–33.

Gofman, J. W., Andrus, E. C., Hanig, M., Jones, H. B., Lanffer, M. A., Lawry, E. Y. *et al.* (1956). Evaluation of serum lipoprotein and cholesterol measurements as predictors of clinical complications of atherosclerosis. Report of a cooperative study of lipoproteins and atherosclerosis. *Circulation,* **14,** 691.

Hammond, E. C. and Horn, D. (1958). Smoking and death rates—report on 44 months of follow-up of 187,783 men. *J. Am. Med. Assoc.,* **166,** 1159–72.

Hegsted, D. M. (1985). An overview of nutrition research. In *NIH Workshop on Nutrition and Hypertension* (eds M. J. Horan, M. Blaustein, J. B. Dunbar, W. Kachadorian, N. M. Kaplan, and A. P. Simopoulos), pp. 9–16, Biomedical Information, New York.

Hjerrmann, I., Velve-Byre, D. V., Holme, I., and Leren, P. (1981). Effect of diet and smoking intervention on the incidence of coronary heart disease: report from the Oslo Study Group of a randomised trial in healthy men. *Lancet,* **ii,** 1303–10.

Holme, I., Hjerrmann, I., Helgeland, A., and Leren, P. (1985). The Olso Study: diet and anti-smoking advice. Additional results from a five-year primary preventive trial in middle-age men. *Prev. Med.,* **14,** 279–92.

INTERSALT Cooperative Research Group (1988). INTERSALT: an international study of electrolyte excretion and blood pressure. Results for 24 hour urinary sodium and potassium excretion. *Br. Med. J.,* **297,** 319–28.

INTERSALT Cooperative Research Group (Guest ed. P. Elliott) (1989). The INTERSALT Study—an international cooperative study of electrolyte excretion and blood pressure: further results. *J. Hum. Hypertension,* **3,** 283–407.

ISCHDR (Inter-Society Commission for Heart Disease Resources Atherosclerosis Study Group and Epidemiology Study Group) (1970). Primary prevention of the atherosclerotic diseases. *Circulation,* **42,** A55–95.

Katz, L. N. and Stamler, J. (1953). *Experimental atherosclerosis*, C. C. Thomas, Springfield, IL.

Katz, L. N., Stamler, J., and Pick, R. (1958). *Nutrition and atherosclerosis*, Lea & Febiger, Philadelphia, PA.

Keys, A. and White, P. D. (1956). World trends in cardiology: I. Cardiovascular epidemiology. *Selected papers from Second World Congress and Twenty-Seventh Annual Scientific Sessions of the American Heart Association*, Hoeber-Harper, New York.

Kuczynski, B. (1925). Pathologische-geographische untersuchungen in der kirgesisch-dsungarischen steppe. *Klin. Wochenschr.*, **4**, 39.

Lawry, E. Y., Mann, G. V., Peterson, A., Wysocki, A. P., O'Connell, R., and Stare, F. J. (1957). Cholesterol and β-lipoproteins in the serum of Americans: well persons and those with coronary heart disease. *Am. J. Med.*, **22**, 605–23.

Leary, T. (1941). The genesis of atherosclerosis. *Arch. Pathol.*, **32**, 507–55.

Liu, K., Stamler, J., Dyer, A., McKeever, J., and McKeever, P. (1978). Statistical methods to assess and minimize the role of intra-individual variability in obscuring the relationship between dietary lipids and serum cholesterol. *J. Chron. Dis.*, **31**, 399–418.

Liu, K., Stamler, J., Trevisan, M., and Moss, D. (1982). Dietary lipids, sugar, fiber and mortality from coronary heart disease. Bivariate analysis of international data. *Arteriosclerosis*, **2**, 221–7.

Logie, D. (1990). The world summit for children. *Br. Med. J.*, **301**, 625.

LRCP (Lipid Research Clinic Program) (1984). The Lipid Research Clinics Coronary Primary Prevention Trial results: II. The relationship of reduction in incidence of coronary heart disease to cholesterol lowering. *J. Am. Med. Assoc.*, **251**, 365–74.

MacMahon, S., Peto, R., Cutler, J., Collins, R., Sorlie, P., Neaton, J., Abbott, R., Godwin, J., Dyer, A., and Stamler, J. (1990). Blood pressure, stroke, and coronary heart disease. Part 1. Prolonged differences in blood pressure: prospective observational studies corrected for the regression dilution bias. *Lancet*, **335**, 765–74.

MLIC (Metropolitan Life Insurance Company) (1979). Recent trends in mortality from cardiovascular diseases. *Statist. Bull. Metropolitan Life Insurance Co.*, **60**, 3–8.

Moriyama, I., Woolsey, T., and Stamler, J. (1958). Observations on possible causative factors responsible for the sex and race trends in cardiovascular-renal disease mortality in the United States. *J. Chron. Dis.*, **7**, 401–12.

Moriyama, I. M., Krueger, D. E., and Stamler, J. (1971). *Cardiovascular diseases in the United Staes*, Harvard University Press.

Morris, J. N., Heady, J. H., Raffle, P. A. B., Roberts, C. G., and Parks, J. W. (1953). Coronary heart disease and physical activity of work. *Lancet*, **ii**, 1053–7, 1111–20.

MRFIT (Multiple Risk Factor Intervention Trial Research Group) (1990). Mortality rates after 10½ years for participants in the Multiple Risk Factor Intervention Trial. Findings related to a priori hypotheses of the Trial. *Circulation*, **82**, 1616–28.

NCEP (National Cholesterol Education Program) (1988). Report of the NCEP Expert Panel on detection, evaluation and treatment of high blood cholesterol in adults. *Arch. Intern. Med.*, **148**, 36–69.

NCEP (National Cholesterol Education Program) (1990). *Report of the Expert Panel on population strategies for blood cholesterol reduction.* National Institutes of Health Publication No. 90–3046, US Department of Health and Human Services, Public Health Services, Washington, DC.

NDHS (National Diet–Heart Study Research Group): (1968). National Diet–Heart Study final report. *Circulation,* **37** (I), 1–428.

Neaton, J. D., Kuller, L. H., Wentworth, D., and Borhani, N. O., for the Multiple Risk Factor Intervention Trial Research Group (1984). Total and cardiovascular mortality in relation to cigarette smoking, serum cholesterol concentration, and diastolic blood pressure among black and white males followed for five years. *Am. Heart J.,* **108,** 759–69.

NHLBI (Working Group On Arteriosclerosis of the National Heart Lung, and Blood Institute) (1981). *Arteriosclerosis 1981,* Vol. 2, National Institutes of Health, Bethesda, MD.

NRC (National Research Council, Committee On Diet and Health, Food and Nutrition Board, Commission On Life Sciences) (1989). *Diet and health— implications for reducing chronic disease*, National Academy Press, Washington, DC.

Pell, S. and Fayerweather, W. E. (1985). Trends in the incidence of myocardial infarction and in associated mortality and morbidity in a large employed population. *New Engl. J. Med.,* **312,** 1005–12.

Pooling Project Research Group (1978). Relationship of blood pressure, serum cholesterol, smoking habit, relative weight and ECG abnormalities to incidence of major coronary events: Final report of the Pooling Project. *J. Chron. Dis.,* **31,** 201–306.

Raab, W. (1932). Alimentare faktoren in der enstehung von arteriosklerose und hypertonie. *Med. Klin.,* **28,** 487, 521.

Rogot, E. and Hrubec, Z. (1989). Trends in mortality from coronary heart disease and stroke among U.S. veterans: 1954–79. *J. Clin. Epidemiol.,* **42,** 245–56.

Rose, G. (1985). Sick individuals and sick populations. *Int. J. Epidemiol.,* **14,** 32–8.

Rose, G. (1987). European collaborative trial of multifactorial prevention of coronary heart disease. *Lancet,* **i,** 685.

Rosenthal, S. R. (1934). Studies in atherosclerosis: chemical, experimental and morphologic. *Arch. Pathol.,* **18,** 473–506, 660–98, 827–42.

Shaper, A. G. (1974). Communities without hypertension. In *Cardiovascular disease in the Tropics* (eds A. G. Shaper, M. S. Hutt, and Z. Fejfar), pp. 77–83, British Medical Association, London.

Shekelle, R. B. and Stamler, J. (1989). Dietary cholesterol and ischaemic heart disease. *Lancet,* **i,** 1177–9.

Shekelle, R. B., Stamler, J., Paul, O., Shryock, A. M., Liu, S., and Lepper, M. (1982). Dietary lipids and serum cholesterol level: change in diet confounds the cross-sectional association. *Am. J. Epidemiol.,* **115,** 506–14.

Snapper, I. (1941). *Chinese lessons to Western medicine.* Interscience, New York.

Stamler, J. (1967). *Lectures on preventive cardiology.* Grune & Stratton, New York.

Stamler, J. (1979). Population studies. In *Nutrition, lipids, and coronary heart disease* (eds R. I. Levy, B. Rifkind, B. Dennis, and N. Ernst), pp. 25–88, Raven Press, New York.

Stamler, J. (1981). Primary prevention of coronary heart disease: the last 20 years. *Am. J. Cardiol.*, **47**, 722–35.

Stamler, J. (1988). Risk factor modification trials: implications for the elderly. *Eur. Heart J.*, **9** (Suppl. D), 9–53.

Stamler, J. (1989). Opportunities and pitfalls in international comparisons related to patterns, trends and determinants of CHD mortality. *Int. J. Epidemiol.*, **18**, S3–18.

Stamler, J. and Shekelle, R. B. (1988). Dietary cholesterol and human coronary heart disease. The epidemiologic evidence. *Arch. Pathol. Lab. Med.*, **112**, 1032–40.

Stamler, J. and Shekelle, R. B. (1989). Lower dietary cholesterol and saturated fat intake, lower serum cholesterol, and expected effects on coronary risk and on longevity. *Lipid Rev.*, **3**, 89–96.

Stamler, J., Lindberg, H. A., Berkson, D. M., Shaffer, A., Miller, W., and Poindexter, A. (with the assistance of M. Colwell and Y. Hall) (1959). Epidemiological analysis of hypertension and hypertensive disease in the labor force of a Chicago utility company. In *Hypertension*, Vol. VII, *Drug action, epidemiology and hemodynamics—Proceedings of the Council for High Blood Pressure Research, American Heart Association* (ed. F. R. Skelton), pp. 23–50, American Heart Association, New York.

Stamler, J., Lindberg, H. A., Berkson, D. M., Shaffer, A., Miller, W., and Poindexter, A. (with the assistance of M. Colwell and Y. Hall) (1960). Prevalence and incidence of coronary heart disease in strata of the labor force of a Chicago industrial corporation. *J. Chron. Dis.*, **11**, 405–20.

Stamler, J., Stamler, R., and Liu, K. (1985). High blood pressure. In *Coronary heart disease* (eds W. E. Connor and J. D. Bristow), pp. 85–109, J. B. Lippincott, Philadelphia, PA.

Stamler, J., Wentworth, D., and Neaton, J. D. (1986). Is the relationship between serum cholesterol and risk of premature death from coronary heart disease continuous and graded? Findings in 356,222 primary screenees of the Multiple Risk Factor Intervention Trial (MRFIT). *J. Am. Med. Assoc.*, **256**, 2823–8.

Stamler, J., Neaton, J. D., and Wentworth, D. N. (1989). Blood pressure (systolic and diastolic) and risk of fatal coronary heart disease. *Hypertension*, **13**, 2–12.

US Bureau of the Census (1990). *Statistical abstract of the United States, 1990*, US Government Printing Office, Washington, DC.

White, P. D., Sprague, H. B., Stamler, J., Stare, F. J., Wright, I. S., Katz, L. N., Levine, S. L., and Page, I. H. (1959). *A statement on arteriosclerosis, main cause of 'heart attacks' and 'strokes'*, National Health Education Council, New York.

WHO (World Health Organization Expert Committee On the Prevention of Coronary Heart Disease) (1982). *Prevention of coronary heart disease*, WHO Tech. Rep. Ser. 678, WHO, Geneva.

WHO (World Health Organization European Collaborative Group) (1986). European collaborative trial of multifactorial prevention of coronary heart disease: Final report on the 6-year results. *Lancet*, **i**, 869–72.

WHO (WHO Expert Committee On Prevention In Childhood and Youth Of Adult Cardiovascular Disease) (1990). *Prevention in childhood and youth of adult cardiovascular diseases: time for action: Report of a WHO Expert Committee.* WHO Tech. Rep. Ser. 792, WHO, Genea.

Windaus, A. (1910). Über den gehalt normaler und atheromatoser aorten an cholesterin und cholesterinester. *Z. Physiol. Chem.*, **67**, 174.

4

The Framingham experience

W. B. Kannel

The epidemiological approach to unravelling the causes of coronary heart disease (CHD) has yielded a number of factors related to its occurrence which have come to be known as risk factors. The yield of these population studies has been bountiful indeed, identifying 246 risk factors in one or another study over the past four decades. The term 'risk factor', first proposed in the Framingham Study in 1961, has been variously defined. The often implied causal relationship requires acceptance of guilt by association. The actual likelihood of an aetiological relationship depends on the timing, strength, consistency, and biological rationale of the observed associations. The latter is usually derived from laboratory and clinical research (Kannel and Sytkowski 1987; Kannel 1990).

The Framingham Study indulged in analytical epidemiology which evolved progressively from the early 1950s, when simple counting and sorting were used, to discriminant function analysis (Cornfield 1962; Truett *et al.* 1967), multivariate logistic regression analysis, Walker–Duncan initiative procedures (Walker and Duncan 1967), and time-dependent variables introduced in a Cox proportional hazard model (Cox 1972). Wu and Ware (1979) incorporated history and multiple measurements into logistic models; Cox (1972) introduced semi-parametric proportional hazards, and we now use parametric non-proportional survival models. It is now acknowledged that CHD is a multifactorial process with no one factor strictly determinative, essential, or sufficient alone to produce the disease. In every instance, the risk associated with any factor has been found to vary according to the constellation of other risk factors present (Epstein 1979; Kannel 1990). This requires the use of multivariate risk assessments to determine the net and joint effect of risk factors. Use of a constellation of risk factors provides a substantially better prediction than any single factor. These multivariate statistical procedures are also useful in attaining an understanding of the pathogenesis of the disease and in devising means for prevention.

At the inception of the Framingham Study in 1948 application of an epidemiological approach to gain insight into the causes of cardiovascular disease was novel. However, this prospective epidemiological investigation has accumulated information on the incidence of cardiovascular disease, the undistorted full clinical spectrum in all who have it, clues to pathogenesis, the chain of circumstances leading to its occurrence, and its importance as a force of morbidity and mortality.

The risk factor concept evolved from epidemiological evidence relating suspected predisposing factors to subsequent development of cardiovascular disease. Upon quantification of the associated absolute, relative, and attributable risks associated with these contributors to cardiovascular disease, concepts of normal have changed from usual or average to optimal values compatible with long-term freedom from disease. Thus acceptable blood pressures and lipid values have been progressively revised downwards over the decades (ISCHDR 1984).

Because these observational spontaneous 'experiments' were not controlled trials, causal inferences are conjectural. However, the major risk factors seem to be aetiological because they are strong and dose-related, predictive in a variety of population samples, independent of other risk factors or mediated through them, pathogenetically plausible, and supported by clinical investigations and animal experiments (ISCHDR 1984).

INDIVIDUAL RISK FACTORS

Four decades of eidemiological research have identified innate and acquired cardiovascular risk factors which contribute to the major atherosclerotic disease outcomes (Kannel 1990). Non-trivial differences in their impact on specific cardiovascular events exist (Cupples *et al.* 1987). Whereas all the major cardiovascular risk factors contribute powerfully to CHD, for stroke, hypertension predominates and lipids play little role. For peripheral arterial disease cigarettes and glucose intolerance are most influential. For cardiac failure hypertension, left-ventricular hypertrophy (LVH), CHD, and diabetes are paramount (Cupples *et al.* 1987).

These common risk factors operate in both sexes at all ages but with different strengths. Diabetes and a low level of high density lipoprotein cholesterol (HDL-cholesterol) eliminate the female advantage over men (Kannel 1987). Cigarette smoking has a greater influence in men, and is non-cumulative and reversible on cessation (Kannel *et al.* 1984). Fibrinogen is a major independent risk factor for CHD, stroke, and peripheral arterial disease in both sexes (Kannel *et al.* 1987a).

Some risk factors, such as blood lipids, impaired glucose tolerance, and fibrinogen, diminish in impact with advancing age (Cupples *et al.* 1987; Kannel *et al.* 1987a; Harris *et al.* 1988). However, decreased risk ratios are offset by a high absolute risk resulting in a large excess risk. All risk factors are relevant in the elderly. Obesity and weight gain promote all the major atherogenic traits (Higgins *et al.* 1987), and physical indolence promotes risk factors and CHD at all ages (Kannel *et al.* 1985). Systolic blood pressure and isolated systolic hypertension are major risk factors (Kannel *et al.* 1980; Kannel 1986; Wilking *et al.* 1988). The ratio of total to HDL-cholesterol provides the best and most convenient lipid risk profile (Kannel 1983).

Risk factors seldom occur in isolation, and when they cluster they greatly augment the risk associated with any particular risk factor, making it necessary to deal with each risk factor as an ingredient of a cardiovascular risk profile.

MAJOR FINDINGS

The Framingham Study has successfully identified or documented several classes of contributors to cardiovascular disease. These include atherogenic personal attributes, living habits that promote these, signs of preclinical disease, and host susceptibility to these influences. The established atherogenic factors include the blood lipids, blood pressure, glucose intolerance, and fibrinogen.

The atherogenic potential for the serum total cholesterol has been shown to derive from the low denisty lipoprotein cholesterol (LDL-cholesterol) fraction which was found to be positively related to CHD incidence (Kannel 1983). HDL-cholesterol has been shown to be inversely related to CHD incidence consistent with its metabolic role in removing cholesterol from the tissues (Kannel 1983). Risk of CHD is independently related to each of these lipoprotein-cholesterol fractions. Reflecting this two-way traffic of cholesterol, the ratio of total to HDL-cholesterol has been established by the Framingham Study as an efficient lipid risk profile. This lipid profile appears more efficient at detecting coronary candidates than the LDL-cholesterol recommended by the US federal guidelines (Expert Panel 1988).

Hypertension, labile or fixed, systolic or diastolic in character, at any age in either sex, was shown to be an independent contributor to CHD incidence, whether mild or severe (Kannel *et al.* 1980; Kannel 1986; Wilking *et al.* 1988). The systolic pressure was shown to be as powerful a predictor of cardiovascular events as the diastolic pressure (Kannel *et al.* 1980). The importance of isolated systolic hypertension was established as a precursor of CHD and stroke. Despite the strong independent effect of blood pressure on CHD incidence, controlled trials have been inconclusive (MacMahon *et al.* 1986). The risk of hypertension varies widely depending on the amount of coexistent risk factors. The agents used in the trials have adverse metabolic effects on lipids and carbohydrate tolerance which may have cancelled the benefit of the reduction in blood pressure achieved (MacMahon *et al.* 1986). Since the excess risk of hypertension is concentrated in those with other risk factors, it is they who require vigorous antihypertensive therapy, and unless the risk profile is improved benefit cannot be expected.

The Framingham experience

Table 4.1 Risk of CHD in diabetics according to the level of other risk factors (50-year-old subjects): Framingham Study

	10-year percentage probability of CHD event					
Women	8	12	15	19	23	32
Men	5	8	12	18	25	44
High blood pressure	(No)[1]	(Yes)[2]	Yes	Yes	Yes	Yes
Cholesterol	(No)[3]	No	(Yes)[4]	Yes	Yes	Yes
Cigarette smoking	No	No	No	Yes	Yes	Yes
HDL-C	(No)[5]	(No)[5]	No	No	(Yes)[6]	Yes
ECG-LVH	No	No	No	No	No	Yes

[1] SBP = 120 mmHg; [2] SBP = 160 mmHg; [3] cholesterol = 165 mg/dl; [4] cholesterol = 240 mm/dl; [5] HDL-C = 58 mg/dl; [6] HDL-C = 34 mg/dl.
SBP, systolic blood pressure; HDL-C, HDL-cholesterol.

Insulin resistance, hyperinsulinaemia, and glucose intolerance have been cited as atherogenic (Reaven 1988). Diabetes or impaired glucose tolerance was shown to make a unique contribution to cardiovascular events with a greater impact on women than on men (Table 4.1). Diabetes, along with a poor ratio of total to HDL-cholesterol were each noted to eliminate the female advantage over men in propensity to atherosclerotic cardio-vascular disease (Kannel and McGee 1979). Diabetics were noted to have greater amounts of atherogenic risk factors than non-diabetics, including elevated blood pressure, increased ratio of total cholesterol to HDL-cholesterol, hyperuricaemia, elevated fibrinogen, and LVH. The impact of diabetes in atherosclerotic cardiovascular disease has not been entirely attributable to associated cardiovascular risk factors, indicating a unique effect. However, cardiovascular risk in diabetics was found to vary widely depending on concomitant cardiovascular risk factors (Table 4.1). A strong relationship between diabetes and cardiac failure, even adjusting for coexistent hypertension and other atherogenic risk factors, strongly suggests that diabetes directly damages the myocardium.

Both diabetics and hypertensive persons were found to be particularly prone to unrecognized myocardial infarction (MI), necessitating vigilance with routine periodic electrocardiogram (ECG) examinations. Diabetes was found to impose an added risk in persons who had already sustained MI, predisposing to recurrences and cardiac failure. Hypertension, obesity, insulin resistance, hyperinsulinaemia, hypertriglyceridaemia, and low HDL-cholesterol tend to coexist. All these factors accelerate atherogenesis and may be responsible for the increased propensity of either the diabetic or hypertensive patient to develop heart disease.

INDICATORS OF ACTIVE ATHEROGENESIS

The white blood cell count and the fibrinogen, within the normal range of values, both appear to indicate active lesions which may be unstable. There is an inflammatory response to cholesterol and other components of the atheroma in the arterial intima. The white blood cell count, in otherwise healthy persons, may indicate such accelerated atherogenesis. In any event, a number of prospective epidemiological studies have shown CHD incidence to be related to the antecedent white blood cell count (Ernst et al. 1987). In the Framingham Offspring Study white blood cell counts were obtained from 1393 men and 1401 women free of cardiovascular disease and aged 30–59 years. Over 12 years of follow-up there were 180 cardio-vascular events in men and 80 in women, of which 197 were coronary events. The white blood cell count was found to be significantly correlated with most of the established cardiovascular risk factors, most strongly with cigarette smoking and haematocrit. The 12 year age-adjusted incidence of cardiovascular disease in general and CHD in particular increased pro-gressively in each sex with each tertile increment in white blood cells over a three-fold range in men and a two-fold range in women. There was a net effect of white blood cells taking other cardiovascular risk factors into account. Each standard deviation increment in white blood cells in men was associated with a 42 per cent increment in CHD incidence. There was apparent interaction with cigarette smoking in men since the excess risk associated with a high normal white blood cell count was confined to non-smokers, in whom each increment of 1000 in white blood cells was associ-ated with a 32 per cent increment in cardiovascular disease in general and a 29 per cent increment in CHD in particular. The impact of white blood cells on risk rivals that of the other major risk factors.

Fibrinogen within the usual range of values was shown to be another major independent atherogenic risk factor, extending findings from else-where (Kannel et al. 1987a). The relationship of fibrinogen to peripheral arterial disease and cardiac failure was added to the demonstrated associa-tion with CHD and stroke. Significant age-adjusted relationships were noted for CHD, stroke, and peripheral arterial disease in men (Table 4.2). In women, a significant relationship to cardiac failure, but not to stroke, was also noted. Cardiovascular disease, CHD, and all-cause mortality were all related to fibrinogen in both sexes age-adjusted, which persists on adjustment for the standard risk factors. Fibrinogen was noted to enhance risk in the hypertensive and the cigarette smoker. About half the risk associated with cigarette smoking could be attributed to their higher fibrinogen values. There are now five prospective studies which document excessive cardiovascular events in association with elevated fibrinogen. Each standard deviation increase in fibrinogen is associated with a

Table 4.2 Risk of cardiovascular events associated with elevated fibrinogen: 16 year follow-up

Cardiovascular events	Age-adjusted 10 year rate per 1000		Risk ratio[1]	
	Men	Women	Men	Women
CHD	304	134	1.8***	1.7***
Stroke	95	51	2.6*	1.0†
Peripheral arterial disease	51	51	1.5	4.0*
Cardiovascular disease[2]	407	228	1.8***	1.7**

Framingham Study: subjects aged 45–84 years.
† NS; * $p < 0.05$; ** $p < 0.01$; *** $p < 0.001$.
[1] Risk ratio T_3/T_1 fibrinogen.
[2] Also include cardiac failure.

1.6-fold increase in CHD incidence, a risk ratio close to that observed for cholesterol.

LIVING HABITS

Certain elements of life-style were found to have a strong influence on the occurrence of cardiovascular disease. This life-style was typified by unrestrained weight gain, cigarette smoking, and sedentary habits (ISCHDR 1984; Kannel and Sytkowski 1987; Kannel 1990). Type A behaviour, characterized by an overdeveloped sense of time urgency, drive, and competitiveness, was noted to predispose to CHD and shown in the Framingham Study to apply to women as well as to men (Eaker *et al*. 1983). Men married to highly educated women were found to be at increased risk of CHD if their wives worked outside the home (Eaker *et al*. 1983).

The well-recognized contribution of diets rich in calories, saturated fat, and cholesterol to the occurrence of CHD was not confirmed by Framingham Study data, possibly because of too little variation in the relevant nutrients and imprecise methodology for dietary assessments.

Weight gain was shown to induce all the major cardiovascular risk factors and weight loss to improve them. Obesity-related risk factors include hypertension, glucose intolerance, insulin resistance, hypertriglyceridaemia, reduced HDL-cholesterol, hyperuricaemia, and elevated fibrinogen (Reaven 1988). Abdominal obesity was confirmed as a particularly atherogenic variety of adiposity (Higgins *et al*. 1987; Wilking *et al*. 1988; Bjorntnop 1985). Largely, but not entirely, as a result of promoted atherogenic risk factors, weight gain is associated with an increased incidence of cardio-vascular events (Higgins *et al.* 1987).

Exercise of moderate degree was found to have a protective effect against CHD in young and old men in the Framingham cohort at any level of other risk factors (Kannel *et al.* 1985). It is clearly useful as an adjunct to a comprehensive risk reduction programme because it raises HDL-cholesterol, helps lower blood pressure, improves glucose intolerance, and helps control obesity (Kannel *et al.* 1985).

Cigarette smoking was shown to be a powerful risk factor for athero-sclerotic cardiovascular disease. This is not unexpected since it lowers HDL-cholesterol, raises fibrinogen, aggregates platelets, decreases the oxygen-carrying capacity of the blood, and causes release of catecholamines making the myocardium more irritable (Kannel *et al.* 1984). These effects can and do precipitate coronary attacks and sudden deaths, particularly in coronary candidates who have other risk factors and a compromised arterial circulation. There is evidence suggesting that risk of cardiovascular events such as CHD and peripheral arterial disease can be halved in those who give up smoking compared with those who continue to smoke. This benefit is achieved regardless of how long persons have previously smoked.

Epidemiological data from the Framingham Study and elsewhere have shown a protective effect of alcohol intake for CHD. This benefit is not seen with alcohol abuse and does not apply for stroke, which may be adversely affected. Alcohol raises HDL-cholesterol, but this is offset by induced rises in blood pressure and triglyceride.

ECG PREDICTORS

ECG abnormalities at rest and during exercise were shown to indicate ischaemic myocardial damage and a compromised coronary circulation. ECG-LVH, intraventricular conduction disturbance, and non-specific re-polarization abnormality were all shown to be associated with increased risk of CHD. The Framingham Study established LVH as an important hazard in the evolution of cardiovascular disease (Kannel *et al.* 1987*b*). The important determinants of LVH in the population were shown to be blood pressure, body weight, alcohol intake, and glucose intolerance. Each con-tributes independently to the incidence of LVH.

ECG, X-ray, and echocardiographic indications of LVH are frequently encountered in the course of hypertension (Kannel *et al.* 1987*b*). They are not incidental to an attempt of the heart to cope with an increased work load as it exacts a penalty of a three-fold escalation of the risk associated with hypertension. All clinical manifestations of atherosclerosis occur at two to three times the general population rate in persons with ECG-LVH. Echocardiographic studies at Framingham also showed that anatomical evidence of LVH carries an increased risk with cardiovascular disease incidence proportional to the degree of ventricular hypertrophy, with no indication where compensatory hypertrophy leaves off and pathological hypertrophy begins.

ECG and anatomical (roentgenographic) versions of LVH were each found to influence risk of cardiovascular disease independently. The ECG version was more ominous than the roentgenographic version. It appears that anatomical and ECG indicators of LVH reflect different pathogenetic processes.

FAMILIAL FACTORS

Innate susceptibility was suggested in the Framingham cohort by showing that a family history of premature cardiovascular disease confers excess risk. Framingham Study siblings with a brother with documented CHD had more than double the risk of a CHD event which was not accounted for by shared risk factors (Snowden *et al.* 1982). Although CHD has been observed to cluster in families, there has been some question as to whether a positive family history is an independent risk factor. Framingham data were analysed to determine whether a parental history of death from CHD before age 65 was an independent risk factor for CHD of early or late onset (Schildkraut *et al.* 1989). A history of death due to CHD in parents of the cohort (non-documented) was found to be associated with a 30 per cent increased risk of CHD. The effect was stronger for an early CHD outcome— adjusted (relative risk of 1.5)—than for a late outcome (risk ratio of 1.2). This effect of parental history of CHD death on risk was not mediated by other risk factors. Findings were similar with a history of early CHD in either parent. For CHD occurring beyond the age of 60, maternal CHD death was a stronger predictor.

POST-MI RISK FACTORS

The role of the standard CHD risk factors in predicting the long-term risk of recurrent coronary events in survivors of MI was examined in the Framingham cohort (Wong *et al.* 1989). Age-adjusted analysis of 459 MI survivors showed the risk of reinfarction to be positively associated with blood pressure and serum cholesterol. Coronary death was strongly associated with blood sugar, systolic blood pressure, serum cholesterol, heart rate, and diabetes. In multivariate analysis, systolic blood pressure, serum cholesterol, and diabetes were independently predictive of reinfarction. Relative weight was inversely associated with reinfarction for reasons that are not clear. Systolic pressure, serum cholesterol, and diabetes persisted as independent predictors of coronary mortality in multivariate analysis.

Women appeared to be at higher risk of reinfarction and death than men following an MI. However, when adjustment was made for the effects of the aforementioned risk factors, women had only half the risk of death from CHD compared with men. Thus higher baseline risk factors in women MI survivors than in men tends to obscure the continued survival advantage of women following an MI. Thus, in persons recovered from an MI, standard risk factors continue to have relevance, particularly systolic pressure, serum cholesterol, and diabetes.

MULTIVARIATE RISK PROFILES

These predictions of disease are an estimation of disease probability in a stated time interval given a specified set of characteristics. This probability is always specific to the risk factors under consideration.

After four decades of epidemiological data from Framingham and elsewhere, the risk factor concept has become firmly established. CHD can now be predicted with reasonable accuracy from nothing more than ordinary office procedures and simple laboratory tests (Table 4.3). Trials have been undertaken to examine the prospects for primary prevention by correcting risk factors in coronary candidates. Whereas trials against elevated cholesterol have proved efficacious, those against hypertension have been disappointing, probably because of failure to improve the multivariate risk profile, including blood lipids (MacMahon *et al.* 1986).

Categorical assessments of risk according to the number of risk factors arbitrarily defined, while they do identify high risk persons, tend to overlook persons at high risk because of multiple marginal abnormalities. Since this segment of the population at risk provides most of the CHD candidates, it is important not to overlook them. To facilitate office and public health risk assessments, scoring systems have been devised in the form of handbooks, personal computer software, and small electronic calculators (Table 4.3).

STROKE PROFILE

A Framingham Stroke Risk Profile has been devised based on data on more than 500 strokes evolving in the cohort over 34 years of follow-up. The ingredients of the profile include cardiac disease, atrial fibrillation, systolic blood pressure, LVH, age, diabetic status, and cigarette smoking. The risk profile assigns a numerical weight to each item based on its contribution to stroke incidence. The sum total score of these values

Table 4.3 CHD risk factor prediction chart

1. Find points for each risk factor

Age (if female)

Age	Pts	Age	Pts
30	-12	47-48	5
31	-11	49-50	6
32	-9	51-52	7
33	-8	53-55	8
34	-6	56-60	9
35	-5	61-67	10
36	-4	68-74	11
37	-3		
38	-2		
39	-1		
40	0		
41	1		
42-43	2		
44	3		
45-46	4		

Age (if male)

Age	Pts	Age	Pts
30	-2	57-59	13
31	-1	60-61	14
32-33	0	62-64	15
34	1	65-67	16
35-36	2	68-70	17
37-38	3	71-73	18
39	4	74	19
40-41	5		
42-43	6		
44-45	7		
46-47	8		
48-49	9		
50-51	10		
52-54	11		
55-56	12		

HDL-cholesterol

HDL-C	Pts
25-26	7
27-29	6
30-32	5
33-35	4
36-38	3
39-42	2
43-46	1
47-50	0
51-55	-1
56-60	-2
61-66	-3
67-73	-4
74-80	-5
81-87	-6
88-96	-7

Total cholesterol

Total-C	Pts
139-151	-3
152-166	-2
167-182	-1
183-199	0
200-219	1
220-239	2
240-262	3
263-288	4
289-315	5
316-330	6

Systolic blood pressure

SBP	Pts
98-104	-2
105-112	-1
113-120	0
121-129	1
130-139	2
140-149	3
150-160	4
161-172	5
173-185	6

Other

Other	Pts
Cigarettes	4
Diabetic-male	3
Diabetic-female	6
ECG-LVH	9
0 pts for each NO	

2. Sum points for all risk factors

Age	+	HDL-C	+	Total C	+	SBP	+	Smoker	+	Diabetes	+	ECG-LVH	=	Point total

Note: *Minus points subtract from total.*

3. Look up risk corresponding to points total

Pts	Probability (%) 5 yr	Probability (%) 10 yr	Pts	Probability (%) 5 yr	Probability (%) 10 yr	Pts	Probability (%) 5 yr	Probability (%) 10 yr	Pts	Probability (%) 5 yr	Probability (%) 10 yr
≤1	<1	<2	10	2	6	19	8	16	28	19	33
2	1	2	11	3	6	20	8	18	29	20	36
3	1	2	12	3	7	21	9	19	30	22	38
4	1	2	13	3	8	22	11	21	31	24	40
5	1	3	14	4	9	23	12	23	32	25	42
6	1	3	15	5	10	24	13	25			
7	1	4	16	5	12	25	14	27			
8	2	4	17	6	13	26	16	29			
9	2	5	18	7	14	27	17	31			

4. Compare with average 10 year risk

Age	Probability (%) Women	Probability (%) Men
30–34	<1	3
35–39	<1	5
40–44	2	6
45–49	5	10
50–54	8	14
55–59	12	16
60–64	13	21
65–69	9	30
70–74	12	24

provides an estimate of the conditional probability of a stroke within a 10 year period of time. The profile should be helpful to physicians who are interested in knowing the urgency for treatment of predisposing factors and in motivating their patients to comply with preventive measures.

CHD PROFILE

A coronary risk assessment has also been devised which enables prevention-minded physicians to estimate the conditional probability of a CHD event in their patients from a constellation of risk factors determined by ordinary office procedures and simple laboratory tests (Kannel 1991). The score derived from multivariate regression coefficients allows physicians to judge the urgency for preventive management without overlooking persons at high risk because of multiple marginal risk factor abnormalities (Table 4.3).

THE FRAMINGHAM OFFSPRING STUDY

A study of the offspring of the Framingham cohort and their spouses was implemented. The objective was to examine familial aggregation of risk factors, secular trends in risk factors, and CHD incidence. This study has also enabled the Framingham Study to stay at the frontier of epidemiological research by adopting new technology. With the advent of non-invasive ultrasound techniques we can now evaluate the prognostic significance and determinants of anatomical myocardial hypertrophy, contractility, ejection fractions, and diastolic compliance. The study is now visualizing atherosclerotic plaques non-invasively to examine the relation of risk factors to lesions causing CHD and strokes. New laboratory methods have enabled us to refine further the blood lipid–CHD connection by investigating subfractions of LDL and HDL and their apoprotein make-up, lipoprotein LPa, and fibrinogen and platelet functions. Ambulatory monitoring is allowing an examination of blood pressure variation and ECG changes as people go about their daily lives.

SECULAR TRENDS

A decline in cardiovascular mortality over the past three decades in the USA is well documented, but the reasons for the decline remain unclear. The Framingham Study cohort was analysed to determine changes in risk factors and cardiovascular mortality over three decades (Sytkowski *et al.* 1990). The 10 year incidence of cardiovascular disease and death were examined in three groups of men, who were aged 50–59 years at baseline in 1950, 1960, and 1970, in order to evaluate the contribution of secular trends in the incidence of cardiovascular disease, risk factors, and medical care to the decline in mortality.

The 10 year cumulative mortality from cardiovascular disease in the 1970 cohort was 43 per cent less than that in the 1950 cohort and 37 per cent less than that in the 1960 cohort. Among the men who were free of cardiovascular disease at baseline, the 10 year cumulative incidence of cardiovascular disease declined by approximately 19 per cent from 190 per 1000 in the 1950 cohort to 154 per 1000 in the 1970 cohort, whereas the 10 year cardiovascular death rate declined by 60 per cent.

Significant improvements in risk factors for cardiovascular disease in men free from cardiovascular disease were found. In the 1970 cohort compared with the 1950 cohort a lower serum cholesterol, lower systolic blood pressure, and reduced cigarette smoking were found. These improvements appear to have had a greater influence on mortality from cardiovascular disease than on its incidence. The improvement in cardiovascular risk factors in the 1970 cohort appears to have been an important contributor to the 60 per cent decline in mortality noted. However, a decline in incidence of cardiovascular disease and improved medical interventions may also have contributed to the observed decline in mortality (Sytkowski et al. 1990).

PREVENTIVE IMPLICATIONS

The epidemiological data demonstrating the hazards of what was considered usual blood pressure and blood lipids prompted trials to examine the benefits of treating mild hypertension and hypercholesterolaemia. These trials and the development of a variety of pharmaceuticals, which, with different modes of action, can effectively lower blood pressure, raise HDL-cholesterol, and reduce LDL-cholesterol without inducing dangerous side-effects, have stimulated national guidelines for early detection and control of blood lipids and blood pressure. Trials of lowering cholesterol by drugs and diet have convincingly demonstrated benefits against CHD events, angiographically evaluated lesions, and xanthoma regression. The trials of antihypertensive treatment have been consistently successful in preventing strokes but have been disappointing against CHD (MacMahon et al. 1986). For the latter it appears that longer treatment with agents that do not adversely affect other features of the coronary risk profile are required.

Although rational, as features of a comprehensive risk reduction programme, controlled trial evidence showing the benefits of exercise, weight control, smoking abatement, and control of hyperglycaemia do not exist.

None the less, these can be recommended since they are also worthwhile for other reasons. Also, preventive management, as well as risk estimation, is likely to be optimal only if it is multifactorial and aimed at improving the risk profile. Preventive strategies should include public health measures to improve the ecology by shifting the entire distribution of risk factors to more favourable levels, health education to enable people to protect their own health, and preventive medicine for high risk candidates requiring drugs. Implementation of hygienic measures required, such as diet modification, exercise, smoking abatement, and weight reduction, require development of greater skills in behaviour modification.

REFERENCES

Bjorntorp, P. (1985). Regional patterns of fat distribution. *Ann. Intern. Med.,* **103,** 994–5.

Cornfield, J. (1962). Joint dependence of risk of coronary heart disease on serum cholesterol and systolic blood pressure: a discriminant function analysis. *Fed. Proc.,* **21,** 511–24.

Cox, D. R. (1972). Regression models and life tables. *J. R. Statist. Soc. Ser. B.,* **34,** 187–220.

Cupples, L. A., D'Agostino, R. B., and Kiely, T. (1987). *Some risk factors related to the annual incidence of cardiovascular disease and death. Framingham Study. 30-year follow-up.* NIH Publ. 87–2703, US Department of Commerce, National Technical Information Service, Washington, DC.

Eaker, E. D., Haynes, S. B., and Feinleib, M. (1983). Spouse behavior and coronary heart disease in men: prospective results from the Framingham Heart Study. II. Modification of risk in type A husbands according to the social and psychological status of their wives. *Am. J. Epidemiol.,* **118,** 23–41.

Epstein, F. H. (1979). Predicting, explaining and preventing coronary heart disease. An epidemiological view. *Mod. Concepts Cardiovasc. Dis.,* **48,** 7–12.

Ernst, E., Hammerschmidt, M. D., Bagge, U., Matrai, A., and Dormandy, J. A. (1987). Leukocytes and the risk of ischemic diseases. *J. Am. Med. Assoc.,* **257,** 2318–24.

Expert Panel (1988). Report of the national cholesterol education program expert panel on detection, evaluation and treatment of high blood cholesterol in adults. *Arch. Intern. Med.,* **148,** 36–9.

Harris, T., Cook, E. F., and Kannel, W. B. (1988). Proportional hazards analysis of risk factors for coronary heart disease in individuals aged 65 or older. The Framingham Heart Study. *J. Am. Geriatr. Soc.,* **36,** 1023–8.

Higgins, M., Kannel, W. B., Garrison, R., Pinsky, J., and Stokes, J., III (1987). Hazards of obesity. The Framingham Experience. *Acta Med. Scand. (Suppl.),* **723,** 23–36.

ISCHDR (Inter-Society Commission for Heart Disease Resources) (1984). Report: optimal resources for primary prevention of atherosclerotic disease. *Circulation,* **70,** 155A–205A.

Kannel, W. B. (1983). High density lipoproteins: epidemiologic profile and risks of coronary artery disease. *Am. J. Cardiol.*, **52,** 93–123.

Kannel, W. B. (1986). Hypertension: relationship with other risk factors. *Drugs (Suppl. 1),* 1–11.

Kannel, W. B. (1987). New perspectives in cardiovascular risk factors. *Am. Heart J.,* **114,** 213–19.

Kannel, W. B. (1990). Contribution of the Framingham Heart Study to preventive cardiology. Bishop lecture. *J. Am. Coll. Cardiol.,* **15,** 206–11.

Kannel, W. B. and McGee, D. L. (1979). Diabetes and glucose intolerance as risk factors for cardiovascular disease. The Framingham Study. *Diabetes Care,* **2,** 110–26.

Kannel, W. b. and Sytkowski, P. A. (1987). Atherosclerosis risk factors. *Pharmaceut. Ther.,* **32,** 207–35.

Kannel, W. B., Dawber, J. R., and McGee, D. L. (1980). Perspectives in systolic hypertension: the Framingham Study. *Circulation,* **61,** 1179–82.

Kannel, W. B., McGee, D. L., and Castelli, W. P. (1984). Latest perspective on cigarette smoking and cardiovascular disease: the Framingham Study. *J. Cardiac Rehab.,* **4,** 267–77.

Kannel, W. B., Wilson, P. W. F., and Blair, S. N. (1985). Epidemiologic assessment of the role of physical activity and fitness in development of cardiovascular disease. *Am. Heart J.,* **109,** 876–85.

Kannel, W. B., Wolf, P. A., Castelli, W. P., and D'Agostino, R. B. (1987a). Fibrinogen and risk of cardiovascular disease. The Framingham Study. *J. Am. Med. Assoc.,* **258,** 1183–6.

Kannel, W. B., Dannenberg, A. L., Levy, D. (1987b). Population implications of electrocardiographic left ventricular hypertrophy. *Am. J. Cardiol.,* **60,** 851–931.

Kannel, W. B. (1991). Using a coronary risk profile in office evaluations. *J. Myoc. Isch.,* **3,** 70–8.

MacMahon, S. W., Cutler, J. D., Furberg, C. D., and Payne, G. H. (1986). The effects of drug treatment of hypertension on morbidity and mortality from cardiovascular disease: a review of randomized trials. *Prog. Cardiovasc. Dis.* (Suppl. 29), 99–118.

Reaven, G. M. (1988). Banting Lecture 1988. Role of insulin resistance in human disease. *Diabetes,* **37,** 1595–607.

Schildkraut, J. M., Myers, R. H., Cupples, L. A., Kiely, D., and Kannel, W. B. (1989). Coronary risk associated with age and sex or parental heart disease in the Framingham Heart Study. *Am. J. Cardiol.,* **64,** 555–9.

Snowden, E. B., McNamara, P. M., Garrison, R. J., Feinleib, M., Kannel, W. B., and Epstein, F. H. (1982). Predicting coronary heart disease in siblings—a multivariate assessment. The Framingham Study. *Am. J. Epidemiol.,* **115,** 217–22.

Sytkowski, P. A., Kannel, W. B., and D'Agostino, R. B. (1990). Changes in risk factors and the decline in mortality from cardiovascular disease. The Framingham Heart Study. *New Engl. J. Med.,* **322,** 1635–41.

Truett, J., Cornfield, J., and Kannel, W. B. (1967). A multivariate analysis of the risk of coronary heart disease in Framingham. *J. Chron. Dis.,* **20,** 511–24.

Walker, S. H. and Duncan, D. B. (1967). Estimation of the probability of an event as a function of several independent variables. *Biometrics,* **54,** 167–79.

Wilking, S., Van, B., Belanger, A., Kannel, W. B., D'Agostino, R. B., and Sfiel, K. (1988). Determinants of isolated systolic hypertension. *J. Am. Med. Assoc.*, **260**, 3451–5.

Wong, N. D., Cupples, L. A., Ostfeld, A. M., Levy, D., and Kannel, W. B. (1989). Risk factors for long-term coronary prognosis after initial myocardial infarction: the Framingham Study. *Am. J. Epidemiol.*, **130**, 469–80.

Wu, M. and Ware, J. H. (1979). On the use of repeated measurements in regression analysis with dichotomous responses. *Biometrics*, **35**, 513–21.

5

The maternal and infant origins of cardiovascular disease

D. J. P. Barker and C. Osmond

This chapter presents evidence that retardation of growth during critical periods of development in fetal life and infancy is linked to the development of cardiovascular disease in adult life.

GEOGRAPHICAL STUDIES

Our own research began with the inability to explain the large geographical differences in death rates from cardiovascular disease in England and Wales. Variations in adult diet and cigarette smoking do not explain why the highest cardiovascular death rates are in industrial areas in the north and west of the country, and in some of the less affluent rural areas such as North Wales. Rates are low throughout the south and east, including London. It is a paradox that although the steep increase in coronary heart disease during this century has been associated with rising prosperity, the disease is now more common in poorer areas and in lower-income groups.

One possibility is that these differences in mortality derive not from the current environment but from the environment to which people were exposed during childhood. The existence of detailed records of infant mortality from the beginning of the century allows current death rates in any area of England and Wales to be compared with infant mortality rates 60 or more years ago. This comparison can be made with the country divided into 212 local authority groupings. The correlations between past infant mortality and current mortality from cardiovascular disease are remarkably strong, with the correlation coefficient being 0.73 (Barker and Osmond 1986). Infant mortality is a general indicator of an adverse environment, and these correlations permit only a conclusion that poor living conditions in childhood are a risk factor for cardiovascular disease—a conclusion first put forward by Forsdahl (1977), who found a similar geographical relation between infant and cardiovascular mortality in the counties of Norway.

The detailed infant mortality records in England and Wales allow neonatal mortality (deaths before 1 month of age) to be distinguished from post-neonatal mortality (deaths from 1 month to 1 year). This gives an important new insight, for, surprisingly, cardiovascular mortality is more closely linked to neonatal mortality (Barker *et al.* 1989*a*). In the past, neonatal mortality was high in places where many babies had low birthweight (Local Government Board 1910). High neonatal mortality was associated with high maternal mortality rates, which were found in places where women had poor physique and health (Campbell 1932). Therefore there is a geographical association between poor maternal physique and health, poor fetal growth, and high death rates from cardiovascular disease.

The recent fall in stroke mortality in the UK and many other Western countries is consistent with improvement in maternal health during the past century. To explain the rise in ischaemic heart disease it seems necessary to postulate two groups of causes, one associated with poor living standards and acting in infancy, and the other associated with prosperity and presumably linked to the Western diet.

FOLLOW-UP STUDIES

Further epidemiological exploration of the relation of early growth to cardiovascular disease requires studies of adults in middle and old age whose early development was recorded at the time. From 1911 onwards every baby born in Hertfordshire county was weighed at birth, visited periodically by health visitors throughout the first year, and weighed again at 1 year. The records for the whole county have been preserved, and it is therefore possible to trace men and women born around 60 years ago, and to relate their early growth to the occurrence of illness and death and the presence of known risk factors (Barker *et al.* 1989*c*).

In our first study we followed up 6500 men who were born in eight districts of the county between 1911 and 1930, all of whom were breastfed at birth. Table 5.1 shows standardized mortality ratios for coronary heart disease in these men, of whom 469 had died from the disease. The ratios fell steeply with increasing weight at 1 year, a trend not shown by deaths from non-circulatory causes. Coronary heart disease mortality also fell with increasing birthweight, although the relation was not as strong as that with weight at 1 year. Stroke mortality showed similar trends.

These findings pose the question of what processes link reduced fetal and infant growth with cardiovascular disease. We have interviewed and measured the blood pressures of 791 of the men who still live in the area of Hertfordshire where they were born. 573 (72 per cent) of these have also agreed to attend a clinic and give blood samples. Table 5.2 shows that mean systolic pressure fell with increasing birthweight. This is consistent with previous observations in men and women aged 36 years (Barker *et al.*

Table 5.1 Standardized mortality ratios for coronary heart disease according to weight at 1 year in 6500 men born during 1911–30

Weight at 1 year (lb)	Coronary heart disease		All non-circulatory disease	
≤18	100	(36)	74	(39)
−20	84	(90)	99	(157)
−22	92	(180)	74	(215)
−24	70	(109)	67	(155)
−26	55	(44)	84	(99)
≥27	34	(10)	72	(31)
All	78	(469)	78	(696)

Numbers of deaths in parentheses

Table 5.2 Mean systolic pressure in men aged 59–70 years

Birthweight (lb)	No. of men	Systolic pressure (mmHg)
−5.5	31	169
−6.5	95	166
−7.5	251	165
−8.5	233	163
−9.5	125	162
>9.5	56	162
All	791	164

1989*b*). Mean pressure was not related to weight at 1 year. This contrasts with the findings for mean plasma fibrinogen, measured by Dr T. W. Meade and his colleagues at Northwick Park. High plasma fibrinogen is a strong predictor of both coronary heart disease and stroke (Meade and North 1977; Meade *et al.* 1986). Levels fell with increasing weight at 1 year (Table 5.3). However, they did not fall with birthweight. Higher serum cholesterol was associated with failure of weight gain in infancy (Barker 1991*b*). The prevalence of impaired glucose tolerance fell as both birth-weight and weight at 1 year increased (Hales *et al.* 1991).

It could be argued that the relations shown in Tables 5.1–5.3 only demonstrate that an adverse early environment, indicated by lower weight gain, results in cardiovascular disease through the cumulative effects of a variety of influences acting during childhood and adolesence. We reject this. Blood pressure, fibrinogen, cholesterol, and impaircd glucose tolerance

Table 5.3 Mean plasma fibrinogen in men aged 59–70 years

Weight at 1 year (lb)	No. of men	Fibrinogen (g/l)
≤18	31	3.29
−20	73	3.16
−22	140	3.16
−24	145	2.99
−26	61	2.91
≥27	25	3.01
All	475	3.08

in the Hertfordshire men were not related to either current social class or social class at birth. The first three of these risk factors were specifically related either to birthweight or weight at 1 year. We interpret these relations as evidence of the long-term effects of an adverse environment during a critical period of growth *in utero* or in infancy, examples of so-called 'programming'. The adverse environment retards the weight gain of the fetus and irrecoverably constrains the growth of particular tissues—which tissues depends on the nature of the adverse influences and their timing. Both birthweight and weight at 1 year were strongly positively related to the men's adult height but were only weakly related to their body mass index. This suggests that processes linked to skeletal growth of a baby rather than fat deposition protect against cardiovascular disease. The phenomenon of 'programming' has been demonstrated in a range of structures and functions in experimental animals (Dubos *et al.* 1966; Winick and Noble 1966; Kahn 1968; Mott *et al.* 1991).

Adult influences add to those of the early environment. The highest mean blood pressures in the Hertfordshire men (172 mmHg) were in those in the lowest third of birthweight and highest third of body mass index; the lowest pressures (156 mmHg) were in men in the highest third of birthweight and the lowest third of body mass index. High mean plasma fibrinogen levels (3.29 g/l) were found in men who were current smokers and in the lowest third of weight at 1 year; low levels (2.77 g/l) were found in non-smokers in the highest third of weight at 1 year.

Birthweight is a summary measure of fetal growth which includes head size, length, and fatness. We now know that it greatly underestimates the relation between retarded fetal growth and blood pressure. In order to explore the association between measurements at birth and blood pressure we examined 449 men and women aged around 50 years who were born in one hospital in Preston (Barker *et al.* 1990). At the hospital, Sharoe Green, unusually detailed observations were made at birth. Table 5.4 shows the

Table 5.4 Mean systolic pressures (mmHg) of men and years according to birthweight and placental weight

Birthweight (lb)	Placental weight				
	−1.0	−1.25	−1.5		
−5.5	152	154	153		
	(26)	(13)	(5)		
−6.5	147	151	150	166	151
	(16)	(54)	(28)	(8)	(106)
−7.5	144	148	145	160	149
	(20)	(77)	(45)	(27)	(169)
>7.5	133	148	147	154	149
	(6)	(27)	(42)	(54)	(129)
All	147	149	147	157	150
	(68)	(171)	(120)	(90)	(449)

Numbers of people in parentheses
1 lb = 0.45 kg

mean systolic pressures according to birthweight and placental weight. There are opposing trends such that systolic pressure is lower by around 10 mmHg with increasing birthweight and is higher by around 12 mmHg with increasing placental weight.

Adjustment for gestation did not affect these trends. An important aspect of the findings is that most people with high systolic pressure were not unusually small at birth. Rather, their birthweights were within the normal range but did not match the weight of the placenta. A feature of babies born with the heaviest placentas, weighing more than 1.5 lb, among whom adult blood pressures were highest, was that they were asymmetrical at birth, being relatively short in relation to their head circumference. This suggests that one process linking fetal growth with adult blood pressure may be diversion of fetal cardiac output away from the trunk to favour the brain.

Large placental weight is associated with clinical hypertension in later life as well as higher mean blood pressure. Among the 449 men and women the risk of having treatment for hypertension was 3.7 times greater among those with placentas weighing more than 1.5 lb compared with those whose placentas weighed 1.0 lb or less.

The maternal influences which result in large placental size are largely unknown. In Preston only four out of 56 (7 per cent) babies born at term to mothers in social classes I and II had placentas exceeding 1.5 lb. This compares with 62 out of 254 (24 per cent) for mothers in the lower social classes. Our hypothesis is that the influence which links low social class large placental weight is poor maternal nutrition (Barker 1991*a*). idence in support of this comes from a recent study of 8684 births in Oxford, where iron deficiency anaemia was associated with heavier placental weight and a higher ratio of placental weight to birthweight (Godfrey *et al.* 1991).

CONCLUSION

Our findings show that retarded fetal and infant growth are strongly related to death from cardiovascular disease, and to its risk factors. We think that these long-term associations of retarded growth reflect restraint of tissue growth by an adverse environment during a critical period of fetal or infant development, so-called 'programming'. We suspect that programming occurs widely in human development and has an important effect on the development of degenerative disease. Long-term human studies now in progress will extend our knowledge of its occurrence and may give insight into the timing of critical periods.

The relation of early growth to risk factors and cardiovascular disease rates is continuous. Death rates fall progressively up to the highest values of infant weight (Table 5.1). Therefore it follows that, while an average birthweight is usual, it may not be optimal.

We have shown that the effects of programming interact with influences in the adult environment including body weight and cigarette smoking. The existence of programming does not imply that adult influences should be discounted, though in the past we have probably overestimated their importance.

Our findings are open to the interpretation that genetic influences which are immediately manifest as growth failure in early life reveal themselves in adult life through the occurrence of degenerative disease. However, studies of the birthweights of the first-born children of mothers and daughters suggest that genetic factors play only a small part in determining birthweight (Carr-Hill *et al.* 1987). Experiments in which newborn mice were randomly assigned to foster mothers show that individual variations in post-weaning growth rates are related more to the nutritional status of the foster mother than to the origins of the offspring (Dubos *et al.* 1966).

We favour an environmental explanation of our findings and suspect that maternal nutrition is important. More research is needed into the nutritional influences which, by regulating fetal and infant growth, determine cardiovascular disease in the next generation.

REFERENCES

Barker, D. J. P. (1991*a*). The intrauterine environment and adult cardiovascular disease. *Ciba Foundation Symp. 156. The childhood environment and adult disease*, pp. 3–16, Wiley, Chichester.

Barker, D. J. P. (1991*b*). The intrauterine origins of cardiovascular and obstructive lung disease in adult life. *J. R. Coll. Phys.*, **25**, 129–33.

Barker, D. J. P. and Osmond, C. (1986). Infant mortality, childhood nutrition, and ischaemic heart disease in England and Wales. *Lancet*, **i**, 1077–81.

Barker, D. J. P., Osmond, C., and Law, C. (1989*a*). The intra-uterine and early postnatal origins of cardiovascular disease and chronic bronchitis. *J. Epidemiol. Community Health*, **43**, 237–40.

Barker, D. J. P., Osmond, C., Golding, J., Kuh, D., and Wadsworth, M. E. J. (1989*b*). Growth in utero, blood pressure in childhood and adult life, and mortality from cardiovascular disease. *Br. Med. J.*, **298**, 564–7.

Barker, D. J. P., Winter, P. D., Osmond, C., Margetts, B., and Simmonds, S. J. (1989*c*). Weight in infancy and death from ischaemic heart disease. *Lancet*, **ii**, 577–80.

Barker, D. J. P., Bull, A. R., Osmond, C., and Simmonds, S. J. (1990). Fetal and placental size and risk of hypertension in adult life. *Br. Med. J.*, **301**, 259–62.

Campbell, J. M., Cameron, D., and Jones, D. M. (1932). *High maternal mortality in certain areas*. Ministry of Health Reports on Public Health and Medical Subjects No. 68, HMSO, London.

Carr-Hill, R., Campbell, D. M., Hall, M. H., and Meredith, A. (1987). Is birth-weight determined genetically? *Br. Med. J.*, **295**, 687–9.

Dubos, R., Savage, D., and Schaedler, R. (1966). Biological Freudianism: lasting effects of early environmental influences. *Pediatrics*, **38**, 789–800.

Forsdahl, A. (1977). Are poor living conditions in childhood and adolescence an important risk factor for arteriosclerotic heart disease? *Br. J. Prev. Social Med.*, **31**, 91–5.

Godfrey, K. M., Redman, C. W. G., Barker, D. J. P., and Osmond, C. (1991). The effect of maternal anaemia and iron deficiency on the ratio of fetal weight to placental weight. *Br. J. Obst. Gynaecol.*, **98**, 886–91.

Hales, C. N., Barker, D. J. P., Clark, P. M. S., Cox, L. J., Fall, C., Osmond, C., Winter, P. D. (1991). Fetal and infant growth and impaired glucose tolerance at age 64 years. *Br. Med. J.*, **303**, 1019–22.

Kahn, A. J. (1968). Embryogenic effect on post-natal changes in haemoglobin with time. *Growth*, **32**, 13–22.

Local Government Board (1910). *Thirty-ninth annual report 1909–10. Supplement on infant and child mortality*, HMSO, London.

Meade, T. W. and North, W. R. S. (1977). Population-based distributions of haemostatic variables. *Br. Med. Bull.*, **33**, 283–8.

Meade, T. W., Mellows, S., Brozovic, M., Miller, G. J., Chakrabati, R. R., North, W. R. S., Haines, A. P., Stirling, Y., Imeson, J. D., and Thompson, S. G. (1986). Haemostatic function and ischaemic heart disease: principal results of the Northwick Park Heart Study. *Lancet*, **ii**, 533–7.

Mott, G. E., Lewis, D. S., and McGill, H. C. (1991). Programming of cholesterol metabolism by breast or formula feeding. *Ciba Foundation Symp. 156. The childhood environment and adult disease*, pp. 56–76, Wiley, Chichester.

Winick, M. and Noble, A. (1966). Cellular responses in rats during malnutrition at various ages. *J. Nutr.*, **89**, 300–6.

6

Coronary risk factors in childhood

D. R. Labarthe

INTRODUCTION

This chapter concerns two of the established risk factors for coronary heart disease (CHD)—blood cholesterol concentration and blood pressure (systolic and diastolic). These factors are considered as they occur in the pre-adult period of life in relation to their occurrence in adulthood, where they are associated in a direct and immediate way with manifest CHD. There is wide variation among populations in mortality due to CHD, and this variation is determined to an important degree by differences in the distributions of the major risk factors among adults. Given these facts, the central focus of this review is the question: what are the earliest ages at which differences in population mean values of the major risk factors, corresponding to the differences observed in adults, are evident?

As background to discussion of this question, certain aspects of the natural history of CHD will be addressed. Then, some aspects of the distributions of cholesterol and blood pressure in pre-adult populations will be described. Several issues must be considered before answering the central question on the basis of this evidence, and these will be addressed in the discussion.

BACKGROUND

At least since 1950, mortality for men ascribed to heart disease, mainly to CHD, has differed several-fold between countries (roughly from 150 to 700 deaths/100 000/year). Such differences have been less marked and the rates typically much lower for women (roughly from 100 to 300 deaths/ 100 000/year) (Thom *et al.* 1985). Recognizing such population differences among men in the mid-1950s, Ancel Keys and colleagues organized the Seven Countries Study to test the hypothesis that dietary differences, along with several other factors, were the main determinants of these differences. Sixteen cohorts of men, aged 40–59 years at entry, in seven countries were examined and followed for subsequent CHD experience as well as mortality from any cause. The major determinants of population differences in CHD mortality included specific aspects of diet, as well as serum cholesterol concentration and systolic and diastolic blood pressure, in addition to other factors, as observed at the baseline examinations (Keys 1980).

Mortality for heart diseases has also varied within countries since 1950, with sharp increases being observed in the rates for some countries and equally sharp decreases elsewhere. Although this secular variation within countries has been striking, for men the relative positions of the countries with respect to heart disease mortality has not changed greatly as a result, for example countries with initially high rates have tended to continue to exhibit relatively high rates. For women, the secular variation in rates within countries has in some instances been as great as or greater than the initial differences between countries. The change in nearly every country has been downward; however, if there have been changes in the relative positions of the countries with respect to heart disease mortality for women, as the rates are in most cases relatively low such changes are not of major importance (Thom *et al.* 1985). The search for explanations of these marked secular trends and their variation between countries led to the establishment of the WHO MONICA Project, which is currently investigating the relation between trends in coronary mortality and concurrent trends in the major risk factors, indicators of medical care, and other possible determinants over the period from the mid-1980s to the mid-1990s (WHO MONICA 1988).

Cardiovascular diseases also account for a major proportion of all deaths in both developed and developing countries, and CHD is projected to become an increasingly important component of the mortality in developing countries in the coming decades. This is the anticipated result of increasing life expectancy and a decreasing burden of competing causes of death earlier in life, changes already evident in higher social strata within some developing countries (Dodu 1988).

The foregoing observations indicate that population differences in rates of coronary mortality are complex, having large geographical and temporal components, especially for men. This complexity is an important consideration in linking population differences in risk factor distributions of children to the occurrence of CHD in adults. Some further considerations follow.

CHD, appearing as an acute non-fatal or fatal clinical event, is a condition of adulthood with the highest rates found in men. Accordingly, the focus of much of the epidemiological investigation of CHD (as illustrated above by the Seven Countries Study) has been on men aged in the 40s and older, where coronary events are relatively common. Yet a strong theoretical basis has been established for the view that the pathogenesis of CHD, and of other complications of atherosclerosis occurring in adulthood, has its origin well before age 20 (McGill 1980).

This view underlies a longstanding interest in the epidemiology of the major risk factors as they occur before adulthood. It is also the basis for increasing optimism that interventions applied before adulthood may be effective in preventing atherosclerosis and its late complications, especially those interventions which would prevent the development of the major risk factors themselves if they were applied broadly throughout the population as a whole (Strasser's concept of 'primordial prevention') (Strasser 1978; WHO 1990). The validity of this concept of prevention rests in part on the answer to the present question as to whether there are, in childhood, population differences in risk factor distributions corresponding to the population differences in risk factors and coronary mortality among adults.

A final point to be considered as background to examination of the evidence concerns the expected magnitude of the differences in risk factor levels to be found in childhood if, in fact, there are such differences corresponding to those in adults. What are the differences in risk factor levels in adulthood among populations with marked differences in coronary mortality? To address this preliminary question, data obtained from the 10 year follow-up experience of the Seven Countries Study are presented in Table 6.1 (Keys 1980). For illustration, the three countries are represented whose combined cohorts experienced the lowest, the median, and the highest age-standardized coronary mortality (deaths per 10 000 men) of 6.0 (Japan), 20.3 (Italy), and 45.5 (Finland) over the first 10 years from the entry examination, a greater than seven-fold gradient in coronary mortality.

Table 6.1 Age-adjusted 10 year CHD mortality and selected risk factors at ages 40–44 and 55–59 (Seven Countries Study)

Country (CHD)	CHOL		SBP		DBP	
	40–44	55–59	40–44	55–59	40–44	55–59
Japan (6.0)						
Tanushimaru	167	168	120	138	68	78
Ushibuka	162	164	126	140	75	80
Italy (20.3)						
Crevalcore	194	204	136	157	84	90
Montegiorgio	192	198	128	142	78	83
Rome Railroad	207	204	135	143	86	90
Finland (45.5)						
East Finland	265	259	141	153	87	90
West Finland	248	251	133	143	80	82

CHD, CHD deaths/10 000 population/year, age-standardized, in men free of CHD at entry.
CHOL, median serum cholesterol (mg/100 ml) at entry.
SBP, median systolic blood pressure (mmHg) at entry.
DBP, median diastolic blood pressure, fifth phase (mmHg) at entry.
From Keys 1980.

The age-specific median values for serum cholesterol and systolic and diastolic blood pressure for the youngest and oldest 5 year age groups of men in each of the corresponding cohorts are also presented in the table. For cholesterol, there is a clear gradient between countries, with values (in mg/100 ml) in the 160s in Japan, in the 190s to 200s in Italy, and in the 240s to 260s in Finland. Notably, this gradient in median values for serum cholesterol is less than two-fold, a much narrower difference than that in mortality. The values are also about the same at the two age levels shown in the table for each cohort.

For both systolic and diastolic blood pressure, the median values are lower in Japan than in Italy or Finland, more clearly at ages 40–44 than at ages 55–59. However, the values in Finland are only some 10–15 per cent greater than the values in Japan for the younger men and the difference is still less for the older men. On the one hand, these observations for blood pressure reflect the recognized importance for population differences in coronary mortality of what might appear superficially to be rather modest differences in risk factor values. On the other hand, the between-population differences in median values of both these major risk factors, at the outset of a 10 year period of mortality experience, are less by about one order of magnitude than the mortality differences with which they are associated as major determinants. It might be expected that the differences in mean values of the risk factors observable in childhood, between high and low mortality populations, would be even less.

CHOLESTEROL

As reviewed in greater detail elsewhere, population differences in levels of blood cholesterol concentration during childhood have been investigated mainly in two distinct ways (Labarthe *et al.* 1991). First, populations have been compared on the basis of samples of children selected at one particular age. Second, comparisons have been made on the basis of the age-specific population mean values over several years of age. These are both cross-sectional approaches; such longitudinal data as are known to exist for different populations are not readily compared owing to fundamental differences in the designs of these studies.

For total cholesterol, Knuiman *et al.* (1980) examined boys aged 7–8 years in population samples in 16 countries in Europe, Africa, Asia, and North America. The use of a central laboratory for all lipid determinations and standardization of procedures for sample collection confers exceptional value upon the results, which demonstrate a continuous distribution of population mean values from about 130 mg/100 ml (Nigeria) to 190 mg/100 ml (Finland). From a subsequent more detailed study of boys aged 8–9 years in several of the same populations, mean values of 158 mg/100 ml in

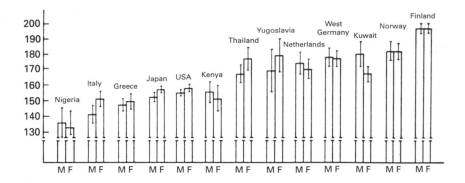

Fig. 6.1 Average cholesterol (mg/dl) for 13-year-olds with 95 per cent confidence limits. (From Wynder *et al.* 1981.)

Italy and 189 mg/100 ml in Finland were reported (Knuiman *et al.* 1983). Thus these observations indicate population differences in mean values for total cholesterol concentration which are apparent as early as ages 7–9 years.

Wynder *et al.* (1981) compared boys and girls at age 13 from 13 populations through the Know Your Body Project (Fig. 6.1). Here, mean values of total cholesterol concentration are presented, with a range from about 135 mg/100 ml (Nigeria) to 195 mg/100 ml (Finland), in close agreement with the results reported by Knuiman *et al.* (1980). Values for Japan and Italy were about 153 mg/100 ml and 142 mg/100 ml respectively for boys, and 158 mg/100 ml and 152 mg/100 ml respectively for girls, as read from the figure. A less marked pattern of variation was shown for 12 European populations at the same age (WHO 1990). Values for Northern Europe were highest, those for Southern Europe were lowest, and those for Central and Eastern Europe were intermediate.

The second approach, which examines the distributions of age-specific mean values between populations, can be illustrated by Fig. 6.2 which is based on a recent review of world-wide literature concerning surveys of cholesterol values in children (Labarthe *et al.* 1991). For illustration, data for boys from selected reports which represent a wide range of ages can be compared. The two populations with observations from birth indicate the marked increase in cholesterol which occurs in the first 2 years of life. In each population represented, the age pattern shows a peak value of mean total cholesterol concentration, with variation in the age at the peak value, from 8 to 11 years. Overall, these data indicate a pattern of cholesterol values which are lower for younger children, reach a peak at pre-teen ages, decrease in the early teenage years, and increase again in the mid-teens. This pattern is consistent among populations in its form, but there are

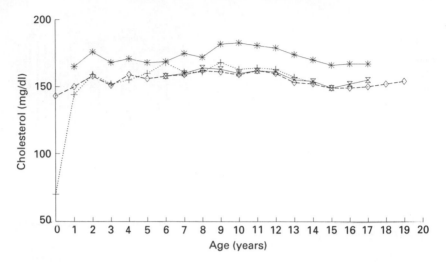

Fig. 6.2 Total cholesterol concentration by age for white North American males: + Bogalusa 1978; ◇ North America 1980; ∗ USA 1978 (HANES I); X̄ Muscatine 1978. (From Labarthe *et al*. 1991.)

differences between populations in the ages at which the inflection points occur. These four populations, all in North America, show smaller differences in absolute values at given ages than do analogous data from geographically and racially more diverse populations. For example, similar surveys in Finland and Japan suggest differences of 30–50 mg/100 ml in mean cholesterol concentration at each age from 5 to 15 years of age, but somewhat lesser differences by age 18. However, the independent nature of these surveys and therefore the lack of centralized laboratory determinations limits confidence in comparing these absolute values.

BLOOD PRESSURE

Analogous comparisons can be made for blood pressure. However, the standardization of measurement procedures is less, often very much less, than is possible for cholesterol determinations in a centralized laboratory. Therefore these comparisons must be qualified by the reservation that apparent population differences could, to an important degree, reflect measurement differences.

For systolic pressure, Wynder *et al.* (1981) present the results of studies in 15 countries for boys and girls aged 13 (Fig. 6.3). For boys, the range of values from lowest to highest is from about 103 to 118 mmHg, in Yugoslavia and Finland respectively. For girls, the extreme values are similar to those

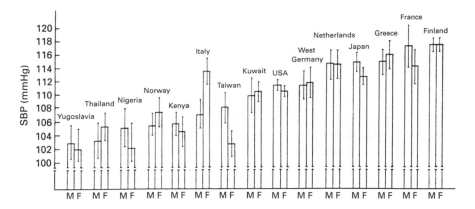

Fig. 6.3 Average systolic blood pressure (SBP) for 13-year-olds with 95 per cent confidence limits. (From Wynder *et al.* 1981.)

for boys and are found in the same two countries, although others (Nigeria and Taiwan) share approximately the same lowest value. The systolic pressures reported for Japan and Italy are 116 mmHg and 107 mmHg respectively for boys, and 113 mmHg and 114 mmHg respectively for girls. Diastolic pressures are not reported here.

Comparison of age distributions of blood pressure between populations has been reported previously on the basis of a review of some 129 published reports of surveys in childhood, described elsewhere in detail (Brotons *et al.* 1990). Such comparisons were stimulated some years ago by the provocative scheme through which Epstein and Eckoff (1967) summarized the age patterns of systolic pressure in adults, down to age 20, from surveys reported from around the world. From selected surveys of school-age populations, the age patterns can be illustrated as in Fig. 6.4 for systolic pressure for boys (Labarthe *et al.* 1989). Similar to the patterns for cholesterol, these exhibit some population differences in the ages at which the slopes of increments in pressure change, but these differences are less marked—either in fact or only in appearance because of blunting of the patterns by individual variation and measurement error—than those for cholesterol concentration. However, the main focus of attention for present purposes are the differences in absolute values at each age, which among these seven populations appear to be 10 mmHg or less up to age 14, and still less at older ages (where fewer populations are represented).

For fourth-phase diastolic pressure, a subset of four studies exhibits similar absolute differences in mean values at each age. For fifth-phase diastolic pressure, where five of these seven studies contribute, differences of 15 mmHg or greater are observed among the populations at ages from 7 to 13 years, narrowing to 10 mmHg at 13 years. For girls, the respective

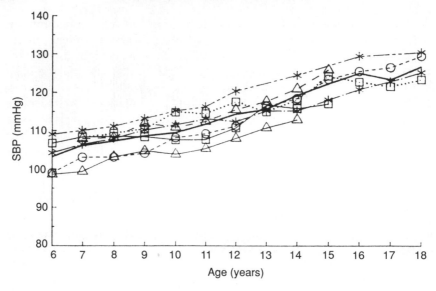

Fig. 6.4 Selected studies and pooled values. Mean values of systolic blood pressure (SBP) by age, males: —— pool; -○- the Netherlands; ·· □ ·· Greece; – – △ – – Yugoslavia 1; * Yugoslavia 2; – – – USA; —□— India; —△— China. (From Labarthe *et al.* 1989.)

patterns of the absolute differences at each age are similar. Overall, these results suggest closer similarity among populations for systolic pressure than for either measure of diastolic pressure, but it is not presently possible to exclude greater variation in methods of measurement of diastolic pressure as the basis for this impression.

DISCUSSION

The question under consideration is: What are the earliest ages at which differences in population mean values of the major risk factors, corresponding to those observed in adults, are evident? On the basis of the observations reviewed, several comments are needed before suggesting an answer. Some relate to both cholesterol and blood pressure, and one to blood pressure specifically.

First, the ages at which population comparisons can presently be made are limited. This is because studies in childhood typically include the school-age population, or only a portion of it, and not newborns, infants, or pre-school children, nor those who are beyond school age but not yet in the high risk age groups for coronary events. These are large and important gaps.

Second, the present data for children at ages 7–9 or 13 years must be interpreted with some caution. This is because population differences in risk factor values may reflect different tempos of growth and maturation, such that at a fixed age the subjects representing different populations are only in different phases of development of the risk factors, as in other respects. The broader cross-sectional comparisons demonstrate the basis for this concern, in that changes in population mean values of the risk factors with age are not 'synchronous' across populations. At the same time, however, they lend some confidence to the interpretation that, over age ranges of several years, there are differences in absolute mean values of the risk factors which are consistent and therefore are probably not mere artefacts.

Third, the children observed represent calendar periods and birth cohorts whose relation to the mortality experience and risk factor status of the Seven Countries Study cohorts, or current members of the corresponding age groups in the same national populations or any other group, is unclear. To have proposed as a point of reference the risk factor patterns from the Seven Countries Study was to oversimplify the problem by conveniently ignoring the large temporal variation in coronary mortality described earlier. This illustration of reference values may be justified, however, to the degree that the populations with highest and lowest coronary mortality, such as Finland (or the USA) and Japan, have generally remained far apart in rates, despite the marked within-population secular trends which were documented by Thom *et al.* (1985). But the expected correspondence of these rates, and of the related baseline risk factor measurements in the late 1950s, to the risk factor levels in children examined in the 1970s or 1980s is not necessarily close. To assume otherwise would beg the question.

Fourth, the observed differences among population mean values for cholesterol concentration and blood pressure are very similar for boys and girls. These population differences for girls do not correspond to differences in coronary mortality among women in different countries which are equivalent to those among men. Linkage of population levels of risk factors in childhood with adult mortality must be qualified by this difference between sex groups.

Fifth, specifically for blood pressure, the problem of measurement error due to different methods of procedure cannot be removed satisfactorily from the interpretation of apparent differences in mean values between populations. Unlike blood cholesterol concentrations, blood pressure cannot be measured in a central laboratory, even by use of hard-copy recording devices which do permit central reading. Local circumstances and matters of technique can still interfere unless strict training and certification of observers are employed; this has not been done to date in international comparative studies in children, although INTERSALT demonstrated its feasibility for a large multinational study of blood pressure in adults.

After these several qualifications, it might seem that little could be said in answer to the question posed. However, the comparative findings for cholesterol reported by Knuiman and colleagues strongly suggest that differences in this factor at ages 7–9 years are real. The magnitudes of the differences are approximately as great as those observed in the Seven Countries cohorts at the extremes of the mortality rates. The reported difference between the highest and lowest values at this age is greater than the difference between the maximum and minimum values observed from the pre-teen peak to the early teen low point in the age pattern of mean values by age, so that population differences in the tempo of development are not likely to be the whole explanation. Measurement differences can be essentially excluded. Collateral evidence indicates relations between these population differences and characteristics of diet (Knuiman *et al.* 1983). Further, they are consistent with differences observed at age 13 in the Know Your Body Project. Therefore one can conclude that real differences in population mean values of cholesterol concentration do occur as early as ages 7–9. Three questions remain. Do these differences continue throughout the ensuing years of life until the period of manifest coronary disease is reached? Are such differences detectable at earlier ages? What is the meaning, in adulthood, of these risk factor differences for girls, in contrast with those for boys?

For blood pressure, the interpretation of the observed differences at age 13 and in the school age years as early evidence of persistent population differences is weakened by some of the four considerations raised above. One cannot say with the same degree of confidence as for cholesterol values that the differences observed are either real or important, in the sense of being premonitory of such differences in adults. Differences in growth and maturation could explain the differences in blood pressure at a fixed age across populations, even though the differences appear to occur over a broad range of ages throughout the school-age group. However, the magnitudes of the differences are similar to those observed among the Seven Countries cohorts. Further, the measurement of systolic pressure is generally more reliable than is that of diastolic pressure, so that this component is less likely to reflect spurious differences. Thus it seems reasonable to conclude that these observations on blood pressure might represent true population differences in childhood which are antecedents of differences in population mean values in adulthood. In addition to the question of whether these are in fact real differences, the same questions remain as for cholesterol.

Concerning aetiology and public health, what are the implications of these conclusions? For the optimist, the foregoing argument may seem an unduly cautious affirmation of the relation between risk factor levels in childhood and those in adulthood. For the nihilist, it may appear to go too far beyond the face value of the evidence. In the author's view, the observations reviewed here lend support to the concept of primordial prevention in suggesting that children in populations with historically high rates of coronary mortality will tend to have higher levels of the risk factors than children in populations with historically low rates. Accordingly, intervention to limit the upward progression of the population mean of cholesterol and systolic blood pressure with age is warranted in the former case, and intervention to preserve the more favourable risk factor distributions is desirable in the latter.

Meanwhile, further research on the main outstanding questions should be pursued. The choice of strategies for doing so is a topic in itself which cannot be elaborated upon here but depends on many of the considerations raised in the present discussion.

REFERENCES

Brotons, C., Singh, P., Nishio, T., and Labarthe, D. R. (1990). Blood pressure by age in childhood and adolescence: a review of 129 studies worldwide. *Int. J. Epidemiol.*, **18**(4), 824–9.

Christensen, B., Glueck, C., Kursterovick, P. *et al.* (1980). Plasma cholesterol and adolescents: the prevalence study of the Lipid Research Clinics Program. *Pediatr. Res.*, **14**, 194–202.

Dodu, S. R. A. (1988). Emergence of cardiovascular diseases in developing countries. *Cardiology*, **75**, 56–64.

Epstein, F. H. and Eckoff, R. D. (1967). The epidemiology of high blood pressure—geographic distributions and etiologic factors. In *The epidemiology of hypertension* (eds J. Stamler, R. Stamler, and T. N. Pullman), Grune & Stratton, New York.

Keys, A. (1980). *Seven Countries*, Harvard University Press.

Knuiman, J. T., Hermus, R. J. J., and Hautvast, J. G. A. J. (1980). Serum total and high density lipoprotein (HDL) cholesterol concentrations in rural and urban boys from 16 countries. *Atherosclerosis*, **36**, 529–37.

Knuiman, J. T., Westenbrink, S., van der Heyden, L., West, C. E., Burema, J., De Boer, H., *et al.* (1983). Determinants of total and high density lipoprotein cholesterol in boys from Finland, the Netherlands, Italy, the Philippines and Ghana with special reference to diet. *Hum. Nutr. Clin. Nutr.*, **37C**, 237–54.

Labarthe, D. R., Brotons, C., Singh, P., and Nishio, T. (1989). Epidemiology of blood pressure in childhood: an international perspective. *Semin. Nephrol.*, **9**, 287–95.

Labarthe, D. R., O'Brien, B., and Dunn, K. (1991). International comparisons of plasma cholesterol and lipoproteins. *Ann. N.Y. Acad. Sci.*, 108–119.

Lee, J. and Lauer, R. M. (1978). Pediatric aspects of atherosclerosis and hypertension. *Pediatr. Clin. North Am.*, **25**, 909–29.

McGill, H. C., Jr (1980). Morphologic development of the atherosclerotic plaque. In *Child prevention of atherosclerosis and hypertension* (eds R. M. Lauer and R. B. Shekelle), Raven Press, New York.

Scrinivasan, S. R., Prerichs, R. R., and Berenson, G. S. (1978). Serum lipids and lipoproteins in children. In *Pediatric Aspects* (ed. W. B. Strong), 85–110. Grune and Stratton, New York, NY.

Strasser, T. (1978). Reflections on cardiovascular diseases. *Interdisc. Sci. Rev.*, **3**, 225–30.

Thom, T. J., Epstein, F. H., Feldman, J., and Leaverton, P. E. (1985). Trends in total mortality and mortality from heart disease in 26 countries from 1950 to 1978. *Int. J. Epidemiol.*, **14**(4), 5120.

USA (1978). Total serum cholesterol levels of children 4–17, United States 1971–74. Department of Health and Welfare Publication No. (PHS) 78–1655, Series 11, No. 156. Government Printing Office, Washington, DC.

WHO (World Health Organization) MONICA Project Principal Investigators (1988). The World Health Organization MONICA project (monitoring trends and determinants in cardiovascular disease): a major international collaboration. *J. Clin. Epidemiol.*, **41**(2), 105–14.

WHO (World Health Organization) (1990). *Prevention in childhood and youth of adult cardiovascular disease: time for action*, WHO Tech. Rep. Ser. 792, WHO, Geneva.

Wynder, E. L., Williams, C. L., Laakso, K., and Levenstein, M. (1981). Screening for risk factors for chronic disease in children from fifteen countries. *Prev. Med.*, **10**, 121–32.

7

Blood pressure in the elderly

C. J. Bulpitt

This chapter reviews the relationship between mortality and systolic and diastolic blood pressure (SBP and DBP), which are both strongly related to coronary heart disease (CHD) and stroke. Blood pressure increases with age, but in industrialized countries average DBP in men peaks at age 50–60 and then plateaus and declines after age 65. This is true for both cross-sectional and cohort data in the Framingham Study (Kannel and Dawber 1974; Kannel 1984) (Fig. 7.1). SBP, on the other hand, continues to increase in cohort data, although it plateaus at age 70 in cross-sectional data presumably due to 'exhaustion of susceptibles'. The same data do not reveal the expected differences between cohort and cross-sectional data in women (Fig. 7.2), but DBP plateaus at age 55–65 and declines thereafter. SBP rises up to age 75, the extent of the data. In view of the different relationship between SBP and DBP and age, the relationship between both SBP and DBP and mortality is reviewed in three groups: the young and middle-aged (<60 years), the elderly (60–79 years), and the very elderly (80+years). In so doing, the relative importance of SBP compared with DBP in predicting mortality at different ages is considered, and the implications for treatment are discussed.

THE YOUNG AND MIDDLE-AGED

Darne *et al.* (1989) reviewed the studies comparing SBP and DBP and concluded that 'DBP is more strongly related to cardiovascular diseases before the age of 45; whereas SBP is more strongly related to cardiovascular diseases after the age of 45'. In the Framingham Study, CHD events (fatal and non-fatal) were related more to DBP than to SBP in men aged 35–44, although this was not true for women (Kannel *et al.* 1971). In view of the difficulties in adjusting for age when SBP is increasing with age much more than DBP (thus possibly giving a closer relationship between mortality and SBP if age standardization is not adequate), the stronger relationship over the age of 45 cannot be considered proven without further investigation. In men screened for the Multiple Risk Factor Intervention Trial (MRFIT) and aged 35–57 at entry, mortality after 6 years was adjusted for age,

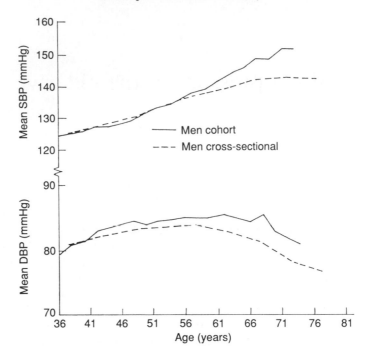

Fig. 7.1 Increase in SBP and DBP in men in the Framingham Study and according to both cohort and cross-sectional analyses (Shurtleff 1974). (From Bulpitt 1989.)

cigarettes per day, and serum cholesterol using the Cox Proportional Hazards model (Rutan *et al.* 1988). The relative risk (RR) for a one standard deviation increase in SBP (16 mmHg) or DBP (10 mmHg) was 1.7 and 1.8 respectively for stroke death, 1.4 and 1.3 respectively for CHD death, and 1.3 and 1.2 respectively for all-cause mortality.

For all levels of DBP, an increase in SBP conferred additional risk. This does not imply that SBP is more important than DBP, as for a given SBP risk increases with DBP. Such an analysis does imply that, for middle-aged men, SBP and DBP are equally good predictors of CHD mortality. However, Rutan *et al.* (1988) reviewed 16 studies and considered that 14 support a greater role for SBP. On the other hand, Dyer *et al.* (1982) examined the Chicago data, adjusted SBP and DBP to give them equal weight, and reported the relationship between mortality and the rescaled values SBP+DBP representing mean arterial pressure (MAP) and SBP−DBP representing pulse pressure. Pulse pressure was not related to mortality, indicating an equal contribution for SBP and DBP. Darne *et al.* (1989) employed a principal components analysis to give a steady component of BP equivalent to MAP and a pulsatile component analogous to pulse

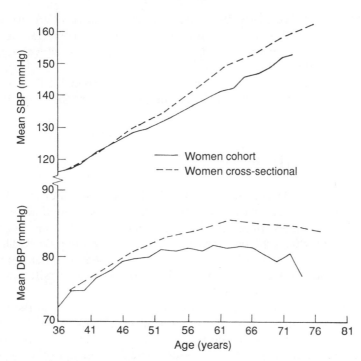

Fig. 7.2 Increase in SBP and DBP in women in the Framingham Study and according to both cohort and cross-sectional analyses (Shurtleff 1974). (From Bulpitt 1989.)

pressure. The steady component was a strong risk factor for cardiovascular mortality in both sexes, but the pulsatile component was only important in women and then it had a positive association with CHD but a negative relationship with stroke.

With the present evidence it must be concluded that MAP is of proven importance but the contribution of pulse pressure has yet to be determined. A blood pressure of 170/80 mmHg gives the same MAP and for all we know carries the same cardiovascular risk as 130/100 mmHg. The acid test in the young and middle-aged is whether or not lowering SBP is more important than lowering DBP.

In randomized controlled trials of antihypertensive treatment, SBP prior to treatment has proved to be a better predictor of mortality than DBP. In the Australian National Trial (Management Committee 1984) and the Hypertension Detection and Follow-up Program (1979), DBP did not predict mortality. This may be because of the very restricted entry range for DBP in these trials. In the placebo group of the Medical Research Council (MRC) trial both SBP and DBP at entry predicted mortality, and benefit from active treatment was reported for all entry levels of SBP and

DBP (Miall and Greenberg 1987; MRC Working Party 1988). As SBP is lowered when DBP is lowered and vice versa this information does not prove that both are lowered with benefit. Trials are required where SBP is lowered more than DBP and vice versa.

Thus it is possible that SBP is more important than DBP in younger subjects, but what about in the elderly? In these subjects SBP and DBP are less closely related.

THE ELDERLY (AGE 60–79)

Kannel *et al.* (1971) concluded that SBP is the best predictor of CHD mortality in the elderly. Such a conclusion depends on their ability to allow for the effect of age. Interestingly, they reported that at age 40, a 144 mmHg SBP produces the same risk of CHD as a 95 mmHg DBP. The SBP corresponding to a DBP of 95 mmHg at age 50 is 146 mmHg, at age 60 it is 155 mmHg, and at age 65 it is 158 mmHg. Lower levels of SBP appear to be relatively less important in the elderly.

In the European Working Party on High Blood Pressure in the Elderly (EWPHE), trial entry SBP predicted mortality and entry DBP did not, but a benefit in terms of a reduction in cardiovascular mortality was observed for all levels of entry SBP and DBP, with some possible fall-off in benefit at DBP < 95 mmHg (Amery *et al.* 1985). Interestingly, when DBP on 'treatment' was less than 90 mmHg, mortality increased (Staessen *et al.* 1989). However, this was equally true in the placebo and actively treated groups, and cannot have been an adverse effect of drug treatment. A similar increase was observed for treated SBP < 150 mmHg. The J-shaped curve when mortality is plotted against DBP has now been observed in many studies, usually in those including subjects with known ischaemic heart disease (Cruikshank 1988). Although there are theoretical considerations why it may be possible to lower blood pressure too far (and this may particularly be so with DBP (Strandgaard and Haunso 1987)), the existence of such a problem remains to be proved.

It could be argued that SBP is more important than DBP if the treatment of an elevated SBP in the absence of a raised DBP (isolated systolic hypertension (ISH)), proves more important than the treatment of a raised DBP in the absence of an elevated SBP (isolated diastolic hypertension (IDH)).

Isolated systolic hypertension

The prevalence of sustained ISH, defined as a consistent finding of SBP > 160 mmHg and DBP < 90 mmHg is approximately 3 per cent of men aged 60, 9 per cent of men aged 70, 7 per cent of women aged 60, and 13 per cent of women aged 70 (Bulpitt 1989). Two questions may be asked: for a given SBP how important is the DBP (e.g. 180/100 mmHg versus 180/ 80 mmHg (ISH)), and for a given MAP how important is the pulse pressure (e.g. 170/80 mmHg (ISH) versus 130/100 mmHg (both having an MAP of 110 mmHg))?

The response to the first question is almost certainly that the DBP will increase the risk for the subject with pressure 180/100 mmHg, rather than for the subject with pressure 180/80 mmHg. In response to the second question, patients with ISH do carry a higher risk with increasing MAP (Kannel *et al.* 1971; van den Ban *et al.* 1989) and the risk of ISH is well established (Colandrea *et al.* 1970; Kannel *et al.* 1980; Forette *et al.* 1982; Rutan *et al.* 1988), but three experimental studies of treating ISH have included only small numbers and have not shown a benefit from treatment (Coope 1987; O'Malley *et al.* 1988; Perry *et al.* 1989) Two large placebo-controlled trials are currently under way to examine the effects on stroke and cardiovascular morbidity from antihypertensive treatment in subjects aged over 60 years with SBP > 160 mmHg and DBP < 90–95 mmHg: the Systolic Hypertension in Elderly Persons (SHEP) trial (Perry *et al.* 1989) in the USA, and the Systolic Hypertension in Europe (SYST-EUR) trial organized by members of EWPHE (Staessen *et al.* 1990). It may well prove useful to treat ISH in the elderly.

Thus SBP is an important predictor of morbidity and mortality in the elderly, and this is true independently of DBP. DBP is also an important predictor of cardiovascular disease at age 65–74 for both stroke and CHD. Figure 7.3 illustrates the relationship between DBP and CHD deaths in the Framingham Study for both men and women (Shurtleff 1974; Bulpitt 1985). The relationship between DBP and CHD mortality is not impressive in women, but in men age 65–74 risk increases markedly with a DBP over 85 mmHg. For stroke (data not shown) an increase in events with increasing DBP was apparent in both men and women (Shurtleff 1974). The association between mortality and DBP in the elderly is all the more remarkable if we consider that DBP falls in the elderly and that *the fall may be greatest in those at most risk.*

THE VERY ELDERLY (OVER AGE 80)

In the very old neither SBP nor DBP have a positive association with mortality. Four European studies reported a higher mortality for lower levels of BP (Frant and Groen 1950; Bechgaard 1967; Fry 1974; Burch 1983). In a recent publication, Mattila *et al.* (1988) again reported this association in subjects over the age of 85. Table 7.1 gives the relative death rates for these subjects, of whom 82 per cent were women and whose average age was 88.4 years. The excess mortality is apparent for DBP less

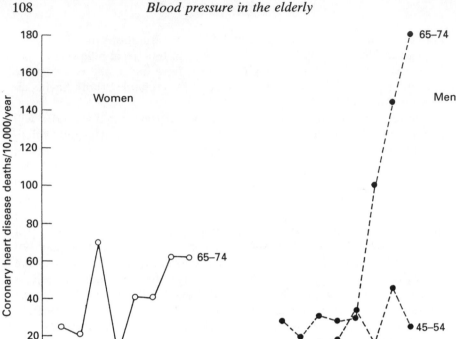

Fig. 7.3 CHD death rates in the Framingham Study according to DBP at entry: men and women aged 45–54 and 65–74 years (18 year follow-up) (Shurtleff 1974). (From Bulpitt 1985.)

than 80 mmHg and SBP less than 140 mmHg. The authors rejected the hypothesis that ill health causes a fall in blood pressure and subsequent mortality as the result appeared true for both those living at home and those in institutional care. However, it cannot be assumed that those at home are healthy, and it must not be concluded that lowering blood pressure in those with high levels would not be beneficial. A subject with a high blood pressure may have a strong myocardium, but reducing his or her blood pressure may, for all we know, prevent death from stroke and prolong a good survival even further.

If SBP and DBP changes from a positive to a negative indicator of risk, we should be able to identify an age at which this transition occurs. In a Californian retirement community, Langer *et al.* (1989) reported that, in men, the relationship between both SBP and DBP was positive when men and women aged 70–74 were followed for 10 years. However, men over the age of 75 (average age 78 years) showed an inverse pattern with high

Table 7.1 Relative death rate over 5 years for 561 persons (82 per cent women) over the age of 85 (average age 88.4 years) in Finland

DBP (mmHg)					
<70	70–79	80–89	90–99	100–109	≥110
1.39	1.32	0.88	0.74	0.84	0.55

SBP (mmHg)						
<120	120–139	140–159	160–179	180–199	≥200
4.55	1.69	0.93	0.71	0.76	0.67

From Mattila *et al.* 1988.

Blood pressure in the elderly

Table 7.2 Total mortality over 10 years for 246 men and 208 women over the age of 75 studied in a Californian retirement community

| | Ratio of observed to expected total mortality | | | | | | | |
| | DBP (mmHg) | | | | SBP (mmHg) | | | |
	<75	75–84	85–94	>95	<130	130–149	150–169	>170
Men	1.29	1.02	0.74	0.92	1.18	0.95	0.97	0.98
Women	0.79	0.95	1.22	1.14	0.74	0.76	1.13	1.21

From Langer *et al.* 1989.

risks at DBP < 75 mmHg and SBP < 130 mmHg (Table 7.2). In women over the age of 75 (average age 78 years) the positive relationship between SBP and total mortality persisted.

It would appear likely that risk inverts at about age 70 in men and age 80 in women. Women 10 years older than men have approximately the same cardiovascular mortality, and these data support the hypothesis that the inverse relationship develops at a certain high level of cardiovascular morbidity and mortality. One hypothesis to explain the data is that a damaged myocardium leads to both a low blood pressure and mortality. This may well explain the J-shaped curve for CHD mortality and DBP in younger persons. In the very elderly the low blood pressure may have many causes (mostly adverse), and the J-shaped curve for DBP in men becomes an inverse relationship between both DBP and SBP by the age of 70+ and in women over the age of 80. Again, this tells us nothing about the likely results of treatment, which may still prove beneficial in prolonging life in the very elderly hypertensive subject.

CONCLUSIONS

There has been much debate as to the relative importance of SBP and DBP as predictors of mortality and morbidity (Rutan *et al.* 1988; Bulpitt 1990), but little is known of the relative benefit to be obtained from treating elevated SBP versus DBP. The treatment of ISH and IDH may both provide clues to the puzzle. There is no doubt that ISH is an important predictor of mortality and morbidity (Colandrea *et al.* 1970; Kannel *et al.* 1980, 1981; Garland *et al.* 1983; Tverdal 1987; van den Ban *et al.* 1989). Whether or not this risk can be reduced in the elderly is being tested by two randomized controlled trials, the SHEP trial and the SYST-EUR trial.

IDH does not appear to have aroused the same interest as ISH. Perhaps this is because IDH has always been considered important and therefore uncontroversial, or maybe it has been considered a rarity. If we define IDH in the elderly as DBP > 90 mmHg and SBP < 160 mmHg, then IDH is much more common than ISH up to the age of 75 years. It is also more common in men (Bulpitt 1989). Between the ages of 60 and 70 the prevalence of IDH is between 5 and 9 per cent. As DBP decreases over the age of about 50 and SBP increases, IDH decreases with age. In view of lack of evidence to the contrary we may assume that IDH carries the same risk as the MAP and that the lack of a large pulsatile component makes little difference (Dyer *et al.* 1982; Darne *et al.* 1989).

At age 35–39 DBP may best predict death for CHD (Kannel *et al.* 1971; Tverdal 1987), but the importance of SBP *as a predictor* increases with age and at age 40–64 it is more important (Lichtenstein *et al.* 1985). Tverdal (1987) therefore suggested that the relative predictive strength of SBP and DBP may be dependent on age. However, this finding may have little practical application in the elderly. First, the fall in blood pressure without treatment may be the most important predictor of mortality, and in this instance DBP and SBP may be equally important, and, second, the epidemiological findings do not indicate whether it is better to reduce DBP rather than SBP in the elderly or vice versa.

REFERENCES

Amery, A., Birkenhäger, W., Brixko, R., Bulpitt, C. J., Clement, D., Deruyttere, M., *et al.* (1985). Efficacy of antihypertensive drug treatment according to age, sex, blood pressure, and previous cardiovascular disease in patients over the age of 60. *Lancet,* **i,** 1349–54.

Bechgaard, P. (1967). The natural history of benign hypertension: one thousand hypertensive patients followed for 26 to 32 years. In *Epidemiology of Hypertension* (eds J. Stamler, R. Stamler, and T. N. Pullman), p. 357, Grune & Stratton, New York and London.

Bulpitt, C. J. (ed.) (1985). The prognosis of essential hypertension. *Handbook of hypertension,* Vol. 6, *Epidemiology of hypertension,* pp. 344–58, Elsevier, Amsterdam.

Bulpitt, C. J. (1989). Definition, prevalence and incidence of hypertension in the elderly. In *Handbook of hypertension,* Vol. 12, *Hypertension in the elderly* (eds A. Amery and J. Staessen), pp. 153–69, Elsevier, Amsterdam.

Bulpitt, C. J. (1990). Is systolic pressure more important than diastolic pressure? *J. Hum. Hypertension,* **4,** 471–6.

Burch, P. R. J. (1983). Blood pressure and mortality in the very old. *Lancet,* **ii,** 852–3.

Colandrea, M. A., Friedman, G. D., Nichaman, M. Z., and Lynd, C. N. (1970). Systolic hypertension in the elderly: an epidemiologic assessment. *Circulation,* **41,** 239–45.

Coope, J. (1987). Hypertension in the elderly. *J. Hypertension,* **5,** S69–72.

Cruikshank, J. M. (1988). Coronary flow reserve and the J-curve relation between diastolic blood pressure and myocardial infarction. *Br. Med. J.,* **297,** 1227–30.

Darne, B. Girerd, X., Safar, M., Cambien, F., and Guize, L. (1989). Pulsatile versus steady component of blood pressure: a cross-sectional analysis and a prospective analysis on cardiovascular mortality. *Hypertension,* **13,** 392–400.

Dyer, A. R., Stamler, J., Shekelle, R. B., Schoenberger, J. A., Stamler, R., Shekelle, S., *et al.* (1982). Pulse pressure-III. Prognostic significance in four Chicago epidemiologic studies. *J. Chron. Dis.,* **35,** 283–94.

Forette, F., De La Fuente, X., Golmard, J. L., Henry, J. F., and Hervy, M. P. (1982). The prognostic significance of isolated systolic hypertension in the elderly: results of a ten year longitudinal survey. *Clin. Exp. Hypertension,* **4,** 1177–91.

Frant, R. and Groen, J. (1950). Prognosis of vascular hypertension. *Arch. Intern. Med.,* **85,** 727.

Fry, J. (1974). Natural history of hypertension. A case of selective non-treatment. *Lancet,* **ii,** 431–3.

Garland, C., Barrett-Connor, E., Suarez, L., and Criqui, M. H. (1983). Isolated systolic hypertension and mortality after age 60 years. *Am. J. Epidemiol.,* **118,** 365–76.

Hypertension Detection and Follow-up Program (1979). Five-year findings of the Hypertension Detection and Follow-up Program: I. Reduction in mortality of persons with high blood pressure, including mild hypertension. *J. Am. Med. Assoc.,* **242,** 2562–71.

Kannel, W. B. (1984). Hypertensive disease in the elderly: consequence of arteriosclerosis or blood pressure? In *Hypertonie im Alter: Normvariante oder Krankheit?* (eds M. Bergener and H. Grobecker), p. 31, Schattauer Verlag, Stuttgart and New York.

Kannel, W. B., Gordon, T., and Schwartz, M. J. (1971). Systolic versus diastolic blood pressure and risk of coronary heart disease. *Am. J. Cardiol.,* **27,** 335–46.

Kannel, W. B. and Dawber, T. R. (1974). Hypertension as an ingredient of a cardiovascular risk profile. *Br. J. Hosp. Med.,* **11,** 508.

Kannel, W. B., Dawber, T. R., and McGee, D. L. (1980). Perspectives on systolic hypertension: the Framingham study. *Circulation,* **61,** 1179–82.

Kannel, W. B., Wolf, P. A., McGee, D. L., Dawber, T. R., McNamara, P., and Castelli, W. P. (1981). The Framingham study. Systolic blood pressure, arterial rigidity, and risk of stroke. *J. Am. Med. Assoc.,* **245,** 1225–9.

Langer, R. D., Ganiats, T. G., and Barrett-Connor, E. (1989). Paradoxical survival of elderly men with high blood pressure. *Br. Med. J.,* **298,** 1356–7.

Lichtenstein, M. J., Shipley, M. J., and Rose, G. (1985). Systolic and diastolic blood pressures as predictors of coronary heart disease mortality in the Whitehall study. *Br. Med. J.,* **291,** 243–5.

Management Committee of the Australian National Blood Pressure Study. (1984) Prognostic factors in the treatment of mild hypertension. *Circulation,* **69,** 668–76.

Mattila, K., Haavisto, M., Rajala, S., and Heikinheimo, R. (1988). Blood pressure and five year survival in the very old. *Br. Med. J.,* **296,** 887–9.

Miall, W. E. and Greenberg, G. (1987). The Medical Research Council's Working Party on mild to moderate hypertension. In *Mild hypertension—is there pressure to treat?* Cambridge University Press.

MRC (Medical Research Council) Working Party (1988). Stroke and coronary heart disease in mild hypertension: risk factors and the value of treatment. *Br. Med. J.,* **296,** 1565–70.

O'Malley, K., McCormack, P., and O'Brien, E. T. (1988). Isolated systolic hypertension: data from the European Working Party on High Blood Pressure in the Elderly. *J. Hypertension,* **6,** S105–8.

Perry, H. M., Smith, W. M., McDonald, R. H., Black, D., Cutler, J. A., Furberg, C. D., *et al.* (1989). Morbidity and mortality in the Systolic Hypertension in the Elderly Program (SHEP) pilot study. *Stroke,* **20,** 4–13.

Rutan, G. H., Kuller, L. H., Neaton, J. D., Wentworth, D. N., McDonald, R. H., and McFate-Smith, W. (1988). Mortality associated with diastolic hypertension and isolated systolic hypertension among men screened for the Multiple Risk Factor Intervention Trial. *Circulation,* **77,** 504–14.

Shurtleff, D. (1974). Section 30. Some characteristics related to the incidence of cardiovascular disease and death: Framingham Study, 18-year old follow-up. In *An epidemiological investigation of cardiovascular disease: the Framingham Study* (eds W. B.Kannel and T. Gordon), DHEW Publ. (NIH) 74–599, National Institutes of Health, Bethesda, MD.

Staessen, J., Bulpitt, C. J., Clement, D., de Leeuw, P., Fagard, R., Fletcher, A. E., *et al.* (1989). Relation between mortality and treated blood pressure in elderly patients with hypertension: report of the European Working Party on High Blood Pressure in the Elderly. *Br. Med. J.,* **298,** 1552–6.

Staessen, J., Amery, A., and Fagard, R. (1990). Editorial review: Isolated systolic hypertension in the elderly. *J. Hypertension,* **8,** 393–405.

Strandgaard, S. and Haunso, S. (1987). Why does antihypertensive treatment prevent stroke but not myocardial infarction? *Lancet,* **ii,** 658–61.

Tverdal, A. (1987). Systolic and diastolic blood pressures as predictors of coronary heart disease in middle aged Norwegian men. *Br. Med. J.,* **294,** 671–3.

van den Ban, G. C., Kampman, E., Schouten, E. G., Kok, F. J., van der Heide, R. M., and van der Heide-Wessel, C. (1989). Isolated systolic hypertension in Dutch middle-aged and all-cause mortality: a 25-year prospective study. *Int. J. Epidemiol.,* **18,** 95–9.

8

Coronary heart disease in the elderly

W. R. Harlan and T. A. Manolio

INTRODUCTION

Remarkable progress has been made in the past 40 years in understanding the epidemiology of coronary heart disease (CHD), its pathogenesis, its treatment, and ultimately its prevention. The identification of the major CHD risk factors and the development of strategies for their modification have contributed substantially to the decline in CHD mortality rates. Until recently, most research has focused on middle-aged men, in whom the epidemic of atherosclerotic CHD has been so apparent and for whom the health and economic consequences have been so great. Considerably less information is available about the risk and course of CHD, and the potentials for its prevention, in older men and women.

In recent years, research in CHD has expanded to include older persons for several reasons. First, declining birth rates and increasing longevity have produced a shift in the demographics of industrialized countries to larger numbers of older persons. CHD is the leading cause of death in Americans aged 65 and older (NCHS 1990), and is the leading cause of hospitalization in those over 65 (Graves 1989). The increasing numbers of Americans living to age 65 and beyond, and the increasing survival after initial cardiovascular disease events at all ages (Feinleib and Gillum 1986), have combined to produce a dramatic increase in cardiovascular disease prevalence and mortality in those aged 65 and older.

These shifts, combined with improved and more elaborate medical care, have led to an increasing economic burden of health care costs in older persons. About one-third of American health care expenditures are attributed to those over 65 years, though they currently represent only about 11 per cent of the population. Despite the widely recognized decline in age-adjusted mortality from CHD, hospitalization rates and health care expenditures for cardiovascular disease have increased in the elderly (Wei and Gersh 1987). The declining case fatality rate of newly recognized CHD, the increased use of costly procedures in the elderly, and the increased longevity of the US population have led to an increase in the use of ambulatory, hospital, and chronic care services for CHD in this age group.

Finally, and perhaps most importantly, it has been recognized that CHD is neither an inevitable nor an irreversible consequence of aging. Even though coronary atherosclerosis is present at autopsy in up to 60 per cent of those aged 65 and older, one should not forget that it is *absent* in the remainder (Weisfeldt *et al.* 1988). Vigorous and active elderly persons are becoming recognized as being more the rule than the exception. The concept of 'premature' cardiovascular disease (as though 'mature' cardiovascular disease was somehow to be expected) has fallen into disrepute, as evidenced by the deletion of the term 'premature' from the mission statement of the American Heart Association. In addition, studies of subclinical markers such as echocardiography, ultrasonography, and arteriography have demonstrated that left-ventricular hypertrophy (LVH) and atherosclerosis may be reversible, or that their progression can at least be halted (Brown *et al.* 1990; Schulman *et al.* 1990). While these studies have been conducted as secondary preventive efforts in persons with established disease, with a minority of patients above 65 years of age, the extent of disease and the existence of clinical complications makes these patients comparable to older persons. These findings offer indirect but important evidence that cardiac enlargement and atherosclerosis are dynamic processes which are potentially modifiable through intervention on CHD risk factors. They lend support to the growing expectation that modification of risk can affect morbidity and mortality in the elderly as effectively as for younger persons.

CHARACTERISTICS OF CHD IN THE ELDERLY

Prevalence, mortality, and incidence

CHD prevalence in the elderly, estimated from the National Health Interview Survey, is 169/1000 in American men over age 65 and 113/1000 in American women over age 65 (Adams and Benson 1990). There has been a modest upward trend in CHD prevalence in the past decade for those over age 65. Rates of CHD mortality in the USA increase with age for black and white men and women, with rates for women lagging behind those for men by about 10 years (Figure 8.1). Although mortality rates have declined in all age groups, the percentage declines are greater in younger than in older persons regardless of race or sex (NCHS 1990). Unfortunately, there are few data on population-based CHD incidence rates and no reliable estimates can be made of changes in incidence.

Clinical manifestations

Several characteristics of CHD in the elderly differ from those common to younger patients. Presentation of clinical disease is often atypical, and may

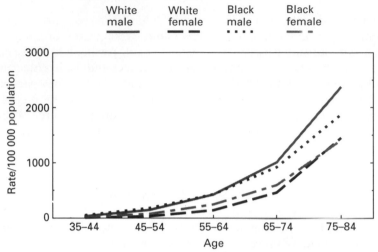

Fig. 8.1 Death rates for CHD by age, race and sex, USA, 1987. (From NCHS 1990.)

be associated with only minimal symptoms. Severe functional impairments, such as congestive heart failure or cognitive decline, may develop and progress slowly, so that patients and their families are only vaguely aware of them or consider them to be a normal concomitant of aging. Although the prevalence of coronary atherosclerosis increases with age, it is more often asymptomatic in older persons (Gersh 1986). In autopsy studies, the prevalence of fixed stenosis of at least 50 per cent in any of the coronary arteries approaches half of all elderly subjects who died from any cause (Gerstenblith *et al*. 1985), and rises to 78 per cent for those over 90 years (Waller and Roberts 1983). In contrast, clinically apparent disease (defined by the presence of angina or a history of myocardial infarction) occurs in only about 20 per cent of men and 12 per cent of women above 65 (Wei and Gersh 1987). Therefore symptomatic disease represents only a fraction of the true prevalence of CHD in the elderly (Gerstenblith *et al*. 1985).

The high prevalence of asymptomatic, often extensive, atherosclerosis in this age group may make determination of precipitants of overt disease, rather than risk factors for atherosclerosis, more important for the prediction of clinical disease in the elderly. Research in younger populations has often focused on factors leading to the development and progression of atherosclerotic lesions, such as increased blood pressure and adverse lipid profiles. In populations where atherosclerosis is already present, factors leading directly to interruption of blood flow to vital organs may be more important in the precipitation of clinical disease, and should be more readily detected than in younger populations. Such factors might include increased thrombosis (or inability to lyse clots) on atherosclerotic plaques, increased vasomotor tone or inability to dilate arterial wall contiguous to a plaque, decreased formation of collateral vessels, or impaired functional reserve due to preceding or coexistent disease. In addition, factors that affect one's *perception* of health or illness may become increasingly important in those whose symptoms may be minimal or atypical. Major life changes associated with aging, such as a serious illness or death of a spouse, change in daily activity from employment to leisure or retirement, or loss of ability to function independently, can all affect the presentation, treatment, and course of cardiovascular disease.

Subclinical disease in population-based studies

The growing application of highly sensitive non-invasive measures of subclinical disease promises to improve the identification of risk factors for the development and progression of atherosclerotic disease. Although non-invasive assessment of coronary arterial structure has yet to be developed and applied on a population basis, technologies such as peripheral arterial ultrasonography and echocardiography are providing important insights into the atherosclerotic process.

Thickness of the inner layers of the carotid arterial wall (intima plus media) can be reliably imaged with high frequency ultrasonography (Pignoli *et al*. 1986), and these measurements have been related to atherosclerosis in the carotid and coronary vasculature (Craven *et al*. 1990). Prevalence of significant intimal–medial thickening rises dramatically with age, from 14 per cent in men aged 42 years to 82 per cent at age 60 (Salonen *et al*. 1988). Population-based data from several large American studies soon to be published indicate that average arterial wall thickness and prevalence of significant stenosis increase progressively throughout adult life, well into the eighth decade. Intimal–medial thickness in women is less than in men at each age, lagging behind men by about 8 years. Conventional CHD risk factors such as hypertension, smoking, and dyslipidemia are associated with greater levels of intimal–medial thickening (Salonen *et al*. 1988). Ultrasonographic measurement of intimal–medial thickness will permit better discrimination of persons with and without atherosclerosis. This is of particular importance in studying elderly subjects, since they are more likely to have atypical or minimal symptoms. In addition, ultrasonography can be used as a surrogate end-point; several interventional studies are assessing whether modification of risk factors can halt progression or induce regression as measured by this technique.

LVH, whether measured by chest roentgenography, electrocardiography, or echocardiography, has long been recognized as being strongly associated with CHD morbidity and mortality (Levy *et al*. 1989). The prevalence of LVH is greater in men than in women and increases dramatically with age, although much of the age-related increase appears to result from concomitant disease (Dannenberg *et al.* 1989). Echocardiographic and Doppler measures demonstrate declines in left-ventricular function in the presence of hypertension and coronary disease, and with advancing age (Gardin *et al.* 1987). Echocardiography, like ultrasonography, provides important opportunities in population-based studies to detect and follow subclinical forms of heart disease and to assess the effects of interventions.

RISK FACTORS FOR CHD IN OLDER PERSONS

The conventional CHD risk factors documented for persons less than 65 years of age appear to be important for those over this age as well. However, the associated relative risks in many studies are attentuated in older persons, though the absolute excess risk is often greater. In the discussion of individual risk factors that follows, we examine the distributions of risk for older persons and assess the strength of these associations in older compared with younger persons, where these estimates are known. A separate chapter of this book (Chapter 7) is devoted exclusively to hypertension in the elderly, and it is not addressed here.

Serum lipids and lipoproteins

Total serum cholesterol and low density lipoprotein cholesterol (LDL-cholesterol) levels above age 65 are generally lower than at younger ages, and decline with increasing age (Fig. 8.2). This decline begins at approximately age 45 in men and age 65 in women, and is observed in both cross-sectional and cohort studies. While the cross-sectional data could reflect selective loss of individuals with high values at earlier ages, longitudinal declines may be related to the development of co-morbid conditions at older ages. Institutionalized or functionally impaired men and women have substantially lower levels of total cholesterol (Harris *et al.* 1992).

High density lipoprotein cholesterol (HDL-cholesterol) levels are on average about 0.26 mmol/l higher in women than in men throughout adult life and change little with age. Therefore the ratio of LDL-cholesterol to HDL-cholesterol is more salutary in women than in men at younger ages, but after menopause a continuing rise in LDL with unchanging HDL creates a less favourable profile.

An analysis of multiple studies of CHD development in older persons permits some comparisons of prediction of disease by serum lipid measurements before and after 65 years for men and women. Total serum cholesterol predicts CHD mortality in men above and below age 65, but the relative risk is lower in those aged 65 and older (1.32) compared with those under age 65 (1.74) (Manolio *et al.* 1992). As was so clearly demonstrated

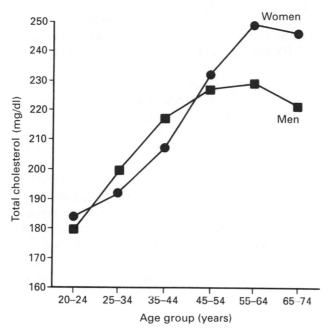

Fig. 8.2 Mean total cholesterol levels according to age and gender: NHANES II. (From Fulwood *et al.* 1986.)

in the Whitehall Study, however, the higher event rate in the older group translates to a greater absolute excess risk in older persons (Rose and Shipley 1986). This has implications for screening and CHD prevention; a larger proportion of older persons identified by cholesterol measurement will actually develop CHD, making screening and intervention more efficient in this age group. The associations with LDL are similar to those for total serum cholesterol in men, although fewer studies have measured LDL or HDL. HDL-cholesterol has an inverse association with CHD development in men, but as noted for total cholesterol, the relationship diminishes with age.

The association between total serum cholesterol and CHD in older women is considerably less strong and consistent than in older men or younger women (Manolio *et al.* 1992). Similarly, the relationship with LDL-cholesterol for older women is less consistent and robust. In contrast, HDL-cholesterol levels have a consistent inverse relationship with CHD risk, though the magnitude of this association is diminished in older women. Plasma triglyceride has a positive relationship in older women, but data are few and potential confounding factors have not always been considered.

The only salient conclusion from data in older women is that considerably more observational study of peri- and post-menopausal women is needed to clarify the relationships of serum lipids and lipoprotein sub-fractions to CHD development. Several large cohort studies currently in follow-up phases and interventional studies in progress should further delineate these relationships. A promising opportunity is presented by post-menopausal oestrogen replacement therapy, which has been shown to raise HDL-cholesterol and lower LDL-cholesterol levels. Several observational studies have reported that women using oestrogens have experienced 40–50 per cent fewer CHD events and lower overall mortality (Bush *et al*. 1987; Henderson *et al*. 1991). These studies lend strong support to the effect of oestrogen on decreased CHD mortality, but have been criticized because oestrogen users are generally women with higher socio-economic status and lower risk factor profiles. The potential adverse effects of oestrogens on breast and uterine cancer development are not precisely defined, but it should be recognized that these potential adverse effects are considerably less common than CHD. Randomized clinical trials are needed to determine the value in primary and secondary prevention of CHD and to balance the benefits against the risks of widespread use of such therapy.

Cigarette smoking

The prevalence of cigarette smoking among the elderly, as well as the number of cigarettes smoked per smoker per day, are the lowest of all adult age groups (Luepker 1986). This may be related to a survival effect, with the heaviest smokers dying at earlier ages, or to a decreased tolerance for nicotine with advancing age. As with elevated cholesterol levels, the risk ratio of CHD associated with smoking declines with increased age, leading some to conclude that vigorous efforts to promote smoking cessation in the elderly may not be justified. Although clinical trial evidence in the elderly are not available, observational data strongly support a survival benefit in those who stop smoking regardless of age. A recent US Surgeon General's report demonstrated beneficial effects on survival at all ages, and also emphasized the substantial risk reductions associated with smoking cessation in those with diagnosed CHD (USDHHS 1990). Considering that more than 7 million smokers are over age 60 in the USA, and that smoking is a major risk factor for six of 14 leading causes of death in those over 60, there is clearly a need for smoking cessation efforts targeted at older persons.

Factors associated with thrombosis and thrombolysis

The recognition that thrombosis is the most common precipitating cause of myocardial infarction has directed attention to factors determining the formation of clots and the endogenous lysis of clots. Evidence is accumulating that fibrinogen and factor VII in particular are strong and independent risk factors for CHD in middle-aged populations, though data in the elderly are scant. Levels of fibrinogen and factor VII appear to increase with age in the few data available in the elderly (Balleisen *et al.* 1985). Data from the Northwick Park Study suggest that relative risk associated with elevated fibrinogen diminishes with age, though data from the Framingham Study support the continued importance of fibrinogen in older men (Meade 1987; Kannel *et al.* 1987). Other factors related to thrombolysis, such as tissue plasminogen activator and plasminogen activator–inhibitor (PAI-l), have been associated with increased risk of unstable angina and myocardial infarction in clinical series, and assessments of these factors have been initiated in population-based studies. Because thrombosis is an important precipitating factor in clinically manifest coronary disease, endogenous factors related to thrombosis and thrombolysis are being investigated as a potential avenue for preventive interventions. The issue is even more important for elderly persons who are more likely to have the atherosclerotic 'substrate' on which clots may form. Several population-based studies currently under way will soon provide important new data on the distributions and risks associated with the thrombotic process in the elderly.

Other cardiovascular risk factors

Other risk factors have been described for middle-aged adults, but few data are available on the distributions and CHD risks in older persons of obesity, glucose intolerance, diet, physical activity, and behavioural and psycho-social factors. Observational studies and clinical trials, many of which have under-represented or excluded the elderly in the past, are needed to provide risk information on this growing segment of the population.

PREVENTIVE STRATEGIES IN OLDER PERSONS

What is the potential for CHD prevention in the elderly? Given the increased absolute risk associated with major CHD risk factors in the elderly, preventive efforts in this age group would be expected to provide greater benefit and be more efficient than efforts in middle age. Evidence documenting the potential for halting progression or even inducing regression of arterial lesions (Brown *et al.* 1990) supports the concept that atherosclerosis is not an immutable process, and that it is never too late to attempt to alter it. Trials in progress on modification of blood pressure, such as the Systolic Hypertension in the Elderly Program (SHEP), or elevated cholesterol levels, such as the Cholesterol Reduction in Seniors Program, are among the first to be performed in an exclusively elderly population. Although SHEP results on the treatment of isolated systolic hypertension will be available in mid-1991, it will be several years before adequate clinical trial evidence is available on modification of other risk factors. In the interim, it seems prudent to generalize the beneficial experience in middle-aged populations to the elderly, and to extend preventive intervention to modify conventional risk factors into this age group.

INTERVENTIONAL STRATEGIES IN OLDER PERSONS

Strategics and goals of treatment for clinically manifest CHD in the elderly differ little from strategies in younger populations. The benefits of beta blockade in older survivors of myocardial infarction were clearly demonstrated in the Beta-Blocker Heart Attack Trial (Hawkins *et al.* 1983), and use of aspirin and thrombolytics in the elderly is supported by data from the Second International Studies of Infarction Survival (ISIS-2 Collaborative Group 1988). Older persons can undergo coronary bypass surgery and percutaneous transluminal coronary angioplasty with somewhat elevated, but acceptable, mortality rates, and may experience fewer post-operative symptoms than their younger counterparts (Horneffer *et al.* 1987).

However, interventional strategies may be complicated in the elderly by the increased prevalence of other chronic disease and medication use. Optimal medical and surgical therapies for CHD may be contraindicated in patients with co-existing illnesses. Even the ability to modify established risk factors can be compromised, as they may occur in patients unable to tolerate antihypertensive medications because of adverse effects. The decline in functional reserve with age in almost every organ system, even in the absence of overt non-cardiovascular illness, leads to a higher risk of adverse effects from medications and a higher rate of complications from diagnostic and therapeutic procedures. Thus, not only is CHD more likely to present atypically and lead to more severe sequelae in the elderly, it is also more difficult to treat once it is recognized clinically.

Despite the difficulties of managing CHD in the elderly, several characteristics of this age group may facilitate management. Compliance with therapy is the highest of any age group, both because of an increasing appreciation of one's vulnerability to illness, and perhaps because of a greater trust in the medical care system than is often evident in younger groups. In addition, the elderly may have lower expectations of normal functional abilities with increasing age, and may be more willing to accept functional limitations without requiring extensive medical interventions. Interest in balancing life satisfaction against simple longevity is increasing, and may lead to a shift away from the traditional therapies that prolong life to those that maximize its quality. The combination of improved efficiency of risk reduction in the elderly as a group (because of their higher absolute risk) and the improved efficacy of risk reduction efforts in elderly individuals (because of their increased compliance) make this age group a particularly attractive one in which to concentrate preventive strategies.

SUMMARY

CHD does not appear to represent a remarkably different disease in the elderly, whether assessed in terms of pathogenesis, risk factors, course, or treatment, than that characteristic of middle-aged persons. A major impediment to the understanding of CHD in the elderly is the inadequacy of data in this age group. The associations between CHD and standard risk factors such as high blood pressure, serum total cholesterol, and cigarette smoking have appeared to weaken with increasing age. While this may be due to simple lack of statistical power, there may be other reasons as well. Those who survive to age 65 probably had lower risk profiles in youth, and with tracking might be expected to have lower risk profiles in later years as well. Since most CHD risk factors increase in prevalence with age, these 'survivors' may start from a lower initial level, or they may somehow be resistant to environmental effects that influence conventional risk factors. In addition, the increased risk of CHD associated with age, independent of known risk factors, leads to an increase in risk of disease for those with and without a given risk factor. Just as risk factors may be difficult to detect in a population with very low prevalence of disease, they may also be difficult to detect in one with a very high prevalence. Therefore the ability to detect an effect of a given risk factor above that associated with age may be diminished at extremes of age.

The development of atherosclerosis in women and its clinical manifestations lag behind those in men by 10–15 years in middle and late adult life at least until age 75 years. The increasing atherosclerosis and rate of clinical events in the years after menopause probably reflect an acceleration of the process already under way and more advanced in men. Because the data for women are relatively sparse, and because the later expression of events is often complicated by co-morbid conditions, there remain several unresolved issues about risk factors for CHD in older women. The continuation of several cohort studies and the development of data from more recent studies should resolve some of these questions. Considering the numbers of persons currently surviving into advanced age, the inadequacy of data available on them, and the potential for benefit of preventive and interventional strategies, the study of CHD in the elderly presents some of the greatest challenges to cardiovascular epidemiology since the intensive investigation of the epidemic of CHD began more than 50 years ago.

REFERENCES

Adams, P. F. and Benson, V. (1990). Current estimates from the National Health Interview Survey, 1989. *Vital Health Statist.,* **10,** 86.

Balleisen, L., Bailey, J., Epping, P. H., Schulte, H., and van de Loo, J. (1985). Epidemiological study on factor VII, factor VIII and fibrinogen in an industrial population. I. Baseline data on the relation to age, gender, body weight, smoking, alcohol, pill using and menopause. *Thromb. Haemost.,* **54,** 475–9.

Brown, G., Albers, J. J., Fisher, L. D., Schaefer, S. M., Lin, J. T., Kaplan, C., *et al.* (1990). Regression of coronary artery disease as a result of intensive lipid-lowering therapy in men with high levels of apoliproprotein B. *New Engl. J. Med.,* **323,** 1289–98.

Bush, T. L., Barrett-Connor, E., Cowan, L. D., Criqui, M. H., Wallace, R. B., Suchindran, C. M., *et al.* (1987). Cardiovascular mortality and noncontraceptive use of estrogen in women: results from the Lipid Research Clinics Program Follow-up Study. *Circulation,* **75,** 1102–9.

Craven, T. E., Ryu, J. E., Espeland, M. A., Kahl, F. R., McKinney, W. M., Toole, J. F., *et al.* (1990). Evaluation of the associations between carotid artery atherosclerosis and coronary artery stenosis: a case-control study. *Circulation,* **82,** 1230–42.

Dannenberg, A. L., Levy, D., and Garrison, R. J. (1989). Impact of age on echocardiographic left ventricular mass in a healthy population (the Framingham Study). *Am. J. Cardiol.,* **64,** 1066–8.

Feinleib, M. and Gillum, R. F. (1986). Coronary heart disease in the elderly: the magnitude of the problem in the United States. In *Coronary heart disease in the elderly* (eds N. K. Wenger, C. D. Furberg, and E. Pitt), p. 48, Elsevier, New York.

Fulwood, R., Kalsbeek, W., Rifkind, B., Russell-Briefel, R., Muesing, R., LaRosa, J., *et al.* (1986). Total serum cholesterol levels of adults 20–74 years of age. *Vital Health Statist.,* **11** (236).

Gardin, J. M., Rohan, M. K., Davidson, D. M., Dabestani, A., Sklansky, M., Garcia, R., *et al.* (1987). Doppler transmitral flow velocity parameters: relationship between age, body surface area, blood pressure and gender in normal subjects. *Am. J. Noninvas. Cardiol.,* **1,** 3–10.

Gersh, B. J. (1986). Clinical manifestations of coronary heart disease in the elderly. In *Coronary heart disease in the elderly* (eds N. K. Wenger, C. D. Furberg, and E. Pitt), pp. 276–97, Elsevier, New York.

Gerstenblith, G., Weisfeldt, M. L., and Lakatta, E. G. (1985). Disorders of the heart, In *Principles of geriatric medicine* (eds R. Andres, E. Bierman, and W. Hazzard), pp. 104–19, McGraw-Hill, New York.

Graves, E. J. (1989). National Hospital Discharge Survey: Annual Summary, 1987. *Vital Health Statist.,* **13,** 32.

Harris, T., Kleinman, J. C., Makuc, D. M., Gillum, R., and Feldman, J. J. (1992).

Is weight loss a modifier of the cholesterol–heart disease relationship in older persons? *Ann. Epidemiol.,* **2,** 35–41.

Hawkins, C. M., Richardson, D. W., and Vokonas, P. S. (1983). Effect of propranolol in reducing mortality in older myocardial infarction patients: the Beta-Blocker Heart Attack Trial experience. *Circulation,* **67** (Suppl. I), I-94–7.

Henderson, B. E., Paganini-Hill, A., and Ross, R. K. (1991). Decreased mortality in users of estrogen replacement therapy. *Arch. Intern. Med.,* **151,** 76–83.

Horneffer, P. J., Gardner, T. J., Manolio, T. A., Hoff, S. J., Rykiel, F. M., Pearson, T. A., *et al.* (1987). The effects of age on outcome after coronary bypass surgery. *Circulation,* **75** (Suppl. V), V-6–12.

ISIS-2 Collaborative Group (1988). Randomised trial of intravenous streptokinase, oral apirin, both, or neither among 17,187 cases of suspected acute myocardial infarction: ISIS-2. *Lancet,* **ii,** 349–60.

Kannel, W. B., Wolf, P. A., Castelli, W. P., and D'Agostino, R. B. (1987). Fibrinogen and risk of cardiovascular disease: the Framingham Study. *J. Am. Med. Assoc.,* **158,** 1183–6.

Levy, D., Garrison, R. J., Savage, D. D., Kannel, W. B., and Castelli, W. P. (1989). Left ventricular mass and incidence of coronary heart disease in an elderly cohort. *Ann. Intern. Med.,* **110,** 101–7.

Luepker, R. V. (1986). Feasibility of risk factor reduction in the elderly. In *Coronary heart disease in the elderly* (eds N. K. Wenger, C. D. Furberg, and E. Pitt, pp. 134–52, Elsevier, New York.

Manolio, T. A., Pearson, T. A., Wenger, N. K., Barrett-Connor, E., Payne, G. H., and Harlan, W. R. (1992). Cholesterol and heart disease in older persons and women: review of an NHLBI workshop. *Ann. Epidemiol.,* **2,** 161–76.

Meade, T. W. (1987). The epidemiology of haemostatic and other variables in coronary artery disease. In *Thrombosis and haemostasis 1987* (eds M. Verstraete, J. Vermylen, H. R. Lijnen, and J. Arnout), pp. 37–60. International Society on Thrombosis and Haemostasis and Leuven University Press, Leuven.

NCHS (National Center for Health Statistics) (1990). *Vital statistics of the United States, 1987,* Vol. II, Mortality, Part A, Public Health Service, Washington DC.

Pignoli, P., Tremoli, E., Poli, A., Oreste, P., and Paoletti, R. (1986). Intimal plus medial thickness of the arterial wall: a direct measurement with ultrasound imaging. *Circulation,* **6,** 1399–406.

Rose, G. and Shipley, M. (1986). Plasma cholesterol concentration and death from coronary heart disease: 10 year results of the Whitehall study. *Br. Med. J.,* **293,** 306–7.

Salonen, R., Seppanen, K., Rauramaa, R., and Salonen, J. T. (1988). Prevalence of carotid atherosclerosis and serum cholesterol levels in Eastern Finland. *Arteriosclerosis,* **8,** 1–5.

Schulman, S. P., Weiss, J. L., Becker, L. C., Gottlieb, S. O., Woodruff, K. M., Weisfeldt, M. L., *et al.* (1990). The effects of antihypertensive therapy on left ventricular mass in elderly patients. *New Engl. J. Med.,* **322,** 1350–6.

USDHS (US Department of Health and Human Services) (1990). *The health benefits of smoking cessation,* DHHS Publication (CDC) 90–8416, pp. 191–240, US Department of Health and Human Services, Public Health Services, Centers for Disease Control, Center for Chronic Disease Prevention and Health Promotion, Office on Smoking and Health.

Waller, B. F. and Roberts, W. C. (1983). Cardiovascular disease in the very elderly: analysis of 40 necropsy patients aged 90 years or over. *Am. J. Cardiol.,* **51,** 403–21.

Wei, J. Y. and Gersh, B. J. (1987). Heart disease in the elderly. *Curr. Prob. Cardiol.,* **12,** 1–65.

Weisfeldt, M. L., Lakatta, E. G., and Gerstenblith, G. (1988). Aging and cardiac disease. In *Heart disease* (3rd edn), (ed. E. Braunwald), pp. 1650–62, W. B. Saunders, Philadelphia, PA.

9

Regional variations in coronary heart disease in Great Britain: risk factors and changes in environment

A. G. Shaper and J. Elford

INTRODUCTION

There are striking regional variations in coronary heart disease (CHD) mortality in Great Britain, well recognized for many years and investigated in a variety of ways. A major approach has been to relate the mortality rates in towns in England, Wales, and Scotland to environmental data such as water quality. This has produced evidence of a strong negative correlation between water hardness and CHD mortality on a town or borough basis. However, although towns with soft water tend to have higher cardiovascular and CHD mortality than towns with hard water, there is a remarkably wide range of mortality present at any given level of water hardness. Recent studies of the 'water story' have shown that a number of environmental variables each make a separate and important contribution to explaining regional variations in cardiovascular and CHD mortality (Pocock *et al.* 1980). These include water hardness (negative), rainfall (positive), temperature (negative), and two indices of socio-economic status—car ownership (negative) and percentage manual workers (positive). Adjustment for these climatic and socio-economic differences considerably reduces the magnitude of the water hardness effect, which appears to be non-linear with an estimated 10–15 per cent excess of all cardiovascular deaths in areas of *very* soft water compared with areas of medium hardness. Beyond medium hardness no effect is seen on CHD mortality. Whether there really is a 'water factor' or whether it represents an environmental variable whose distribution closely resembles water hardness has yet to be determined. Whatever the outcome, the excess CHD mortality seems small when compared with the effects of such factors as cigarette smoking. Clearly, there are marked limitations to relating these ecological variables to town mortality, and there is a need to go beyond the crude scattergrams and correlations and among the people.

BRITISH REGIONAL HEART STUDY

The British Regional Heart Study (BRHS) set out to examine whether differences in the distribution of personal characteristics could be responsible for the marked regional variations in CHD and stroke in Great Britain. The study is based on the measurement of potential risk factors in middle-aged men drawn from general practices in 24 medium-sized towns in England, Wales, and Scotland (Shaper *et al.* 1981). Towns were chosen that reflected known geographical variations in mortality from cardiovascular disease and, whenever possible, were representative of the region in socio-economic terms (Shaper *et al.* 1981) (Fig. 9.1).

In 1978–80 a team of research nurses examined 7735 men aged 40–59 years (78 per cent response rate) using a standardized questionnaire and making physical measurements, taking blood samples for biochemical and haematological variables, performing electrocardiography (ECG), and measuring respiratory function. All the men, including those with evidence of CHD at screening, have been followed for both cardiovascular morbidity and all-cause mortality, with 99 per cent of the surviving men being traced to their current general practitioners at 9½–11 years after screening. The data acquired have allowed for *cross-sectional* studies of the prevalence of CHD in these men, of the interrelationships between the many variables measured, and between the prevalence of CHD and these variables. It has also allowed for a *prospective* study of major CHD events (heart attack, sudden death), stroke, and all-cause mortality, and thus for the assessment of the aetiological role of the many potential risk factors measured. Men were selected at random from the age–sex registers of each general practice and no exclusions were made on the grounds of cardiovascular or other forms of ill health or medical treatment. This inclusive policy provided a subgroup of men in whom the relationship between risk factors and new major CHD events in men with pre-existing CHD could be determined.

Prevalence of CHD

All men completed an administered questionnaire which included the World Health Organization (WHO) (Rose) enquiry into chest pain on exercise (angina) and severe prolonged chest pain (possible myocardial infarction). They were also asked whether a doctor had ever told them that they had any form of CHD. In addition, a three-orthogonal-lead electrocardiogram was carried out and analysed by computer. The prevalence of CHD, based on the chest pain questionnaire and ECG, averaged about 25 per cent, ranging from 17 per cent in Lowestoft to 30 per cent in Merthyr Tydfil, an almost two-fold difference similar to the difference in standardized

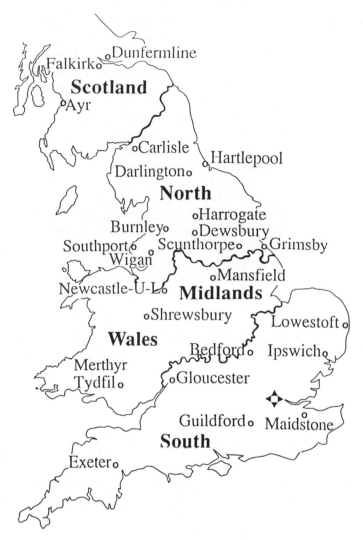

Fig. 9.1 Towns used in the BRHS.

mortality ratios (SMRs) for CHD in the 24 towns. There was a strong correlation ($r = 0.79$, $p < 0.0001$) between the prevalence rates and the SMRs, indicating that the routinely collected mortality data for CHD are not merely reflecting differing case fatality rates between the towns.

CHD and risk factors on a town basis

For the purposes of this review we have compared the prevalence of risk factors measured in 1978–80 with both the SMRs for CHD (1979–83) and the prevalence of CHD based on the WHO (Rose) questionnaire and ECG in the 1978–80 screening examination. The correlation with the town SMRs are stronger and statistically more significant than with the prevalence rates of CHD in the towns. On a *town* basis, CHD mortality was associated with both mean systolic and diastolic blood pressure (SBP and DBP) in the men examined at screening ($r = 0.57$ and $r = 0.54$), and even more strongly with the percentage of men with systolic or diastolic hypertension (≥ 160 mmHg, $r = 0.62$, and ≥ 90 mmHg, $r = 0.57$). There was a strong association with current cigarette smoking ($r = 0.59$), heavy drinking ($r = 0.66$), and the percentage of manual workers ($r = 0.55$). Physical activity (excluding occupational activity) was also strongly and negatively associated with CHD mortality ($r = -0.57$). All these associations were statistically highly significant. For mean blood cholesterol, high density lipoprotein cholesterol (HDL-cholesterol), plasma triglycerides, and body mass index (BMI) (kg/m^2), no associations of statistical significance were present.

It cannot be sufficiently strongly emphasized that the presence of an association between a variable and CHD mortality, even if strong and statistically significant, need not necessarily indicate causality and may well reflect the presence of other confounding variables. Similarly, the absence of an association in such ecological comparisons need not indicate that the variable is of no causal importance in the development of CHD, but merely that it does not apparently contribute to intertown variations in CHD mortality.

CHD and risk factors on an individual basis

While ecological relationships may be of considerable interest and provide important clues to aetiology, they are never sufficient in themselves to pronounce on causality. It is always necessary to go beyond the cross-sectional survey information to prospective (longitudinal, cohort) studies in order to determine the relative risks and the absolute rates of disease associated with each variable (Shaper *et al.* 1985). The initial univariate analysis does not take into account the fact that there are relationships between the risk factors, and that each true risk factor is making some separate (independent) contribution to the overall level of risk. Multiple logistic regression helps to determine the independent contribution of each *factor* to the risk of heart attack when all the factors are acting simultaneously.

To examine univariate risk, the distribution of each risk factor measured on 7735 men in the BRHS was ranked in ascending order and divided into five equal-sized groups, with approximately 1500 men in each group. The number of heart attacks occurring in each of the five groups during the follow-up period of 6.2 years was examined, and the relative risk between top and bottom fifth calculated.

Age

The youngest fifth ranged from 40 to 43 years and the oldest from 56 to 59 years. The relative risk of having a heart attack was 4.7 times greater in the older group than in the younger group. Age is clearly a useful and powerful indicator of risk, presumably as a proxy for exposure to all other factors.

Blood pressure

Across the range of SBP and DBP a relative risk of about 3.0 is found between the top and bottom fifths of the distribution. A two-fold risk of CHD is apparent at SBP levels of $\geqslant 148$ mmHg even after adjustment for other factors, with 40 per cent of men falling into this category. The top 20 per cent of the DBP range also carried a two-fold risk of a CHD major event.

Cigarette smoking

Current cigarette smokers of whatever quantity carried a three-fold risk of heart attack compared with men who had never smoked, and even ex-smokers still carried a two-fold risk. When 'smoking years' were used to compare risk between the top and bottom fifths, a 5.1 relative risk was found.

Blood cholesterol

Despite the lack of association on a town basis, there was a continuous increase in risk of heart attack with increasing total cholesterol concentration, with a relative risk of 3.1 between the lowest fifth (< 5.5 mmol/l) and the highest fifth ($\geqslant 7.2$ mmol/l).

HDL-cholesterol

HDL-cholesterol had a negative relationship with heart attacks, with a two-fold increase in risk in men in the lowest fifth of the distribution (< 0.93 mmol/l).

Triglycerides

Triglycerides showed a strong positive association which disappeared when adjusted for HDL-cholesterol and total cholesterol. However, current thinking on the primacy of HDL-cholesterol or plasma triglycerides suggests that the greater variability in triglyceride concentration may lead to marked underestimation of its importance *vis-à-vis* HDL-cholesterol (Davey Smith and Phillips 1990).

Body mass index

Although there is an increase in the rate of heart attack as BMI increases, with a relative risk of 1.8 between the top and bottom fifths, BMI has positive relationships with serum total cholesterol, blood pressure, and triglycerides, and a negative relationship with HDL-cholesterol. Adjustment for these relationships leaves BMI with no apparent relationship with heart attack. However, as the development of obesity is closely linked with the development of these other factors over a long period of time, it is unreasonable to regard obesity and overweight as being 'of no significance'.

Alcohol

Despite the strong regional relationship between heavy drinking and SMRs for CHD, the prospective study reveals no consistent relationship between alcohol intake and heart attacks (Shaper *et al.* 1987).

Town and individual relationship

Using the results of the prospective analysis as our basic measure of causality, it is evident that some factors which in a regional analysis appear to be of importance (e.g. alcohol) do not appear to be causally associated with heart attack rates. On the other hand, some variables which are not associated with heart attack on a regional basis are clearly of aetiological importance, namely total cholesterol, HDL-cholesterol and/or triglycerides, and BMI. The two factors which emerge as having both a strong regional relationship and a strong individual relationship with rates of heart attack are blood pressure (particularly SBP) and cigarette smoking. Blood cholesterol is almost certainly a fundamental factor in the origins of atherosclerosis and CHD, and average levels in men and women in the UK, at all ages and in every town in which it has been measured, are high (mean > 6.0 mmol/l) by international standards. While these levels are associated (causally) with a high level of susceptibility to CHD they are not responsible for regional variations in CHD.

Social class

Prevalence rates of CHD at screening were higher in manual workers. Recall of a doctor diagnosis of CHD was 40 per cent higher in the manual workers (4.4 and 6.1 per cent) and the prevalence of ischaemic ECG abnormalities was 25 per cent higher (6.5 and 8.1 per cent) (Pocock *et al.* 1987). The incidence of major CHD events over 5 years follow-up was 44 per cent higher in manual workers, and this was substantially contributed to by marked differences in cigarette smoking as well as higher levels of blood pressure, more obesity, and much lower levels of physical activity in leisure time. Adjustment for these differences left the manual workers with an overall 24 per cent excess of CHD major events, which was of marginal statistical significance ($p = 0.08$). As these analyses are based on single measures of risk factors, they may well fail to take into account adequately the real contribution of these factors to the social class difference.

Social class differences do not explain the two-fold difference in CHD mortality between towns in Southeast England and those in the North and Scotland. There appear to be other environmental factors which contribute to these regional variations even after adjustment for social class differences (OPCS 1986).

Blood groups

Towns with a higher prevalence of blood group O have higher incidence rates of heart attack in the BRHS study, and such towns tend to be in Scotland or the North of England (Whincup *et al*. 1990). In individual subjects, however, the incidence of heart attack was higher in men with blood group A than in those with other blood groups (relative risk 1.21, 95 per cent confidence interval 1.01–1.46). Total serum cholesterol was slightly but significantly higher in men with blood group A. No other risk factor, including social class, was related to blood group. It is evident that geographical differences in the distribution of blood groups do not explain geographical variations in CHD in the UK.

Explaining variation

In many studies concerned with regional variations in disease, complex statistical analyses are carried out in order to determine which factors are making independent contributions to the outcome and how much of the total incidence of disease can be 'explained' by the key independent factors. In CHD it is often said that the classical risk factors such as smoking, blood pressure, and blood cholesterol will in combination 'explain' only about 50 per cent of the variation observed. The assumption is then made that there must be another major factor or factors in existence which have not been measured (factor X). Such simplistic interpretations fail to take into account that single estimations of a factor cannot do more than act as a crude proxy for a lifetime exposure to varying levels of the factor. Were it possible to take a better measure of exposure by multiple and repeated measures over a lifetime, we might perhaps be nearer to better 'explanation' of variance. Another issue relates to the conceptual model that is used for reviewing the interactions between risk factors. Failure to think in terms of an appropriate model is likely to lead to simplistic statements about 'explaining the variance'.

The data we have presented show that several risk factors for CHD are operating during middle age in a way that strongly suggests causality. Several of these factors also appear to account to some extent for the regional variations in CHD mortality. From a preventive point of view it is of considerable concern to determine whether these effects are reversible in adult life, or whether they reflect a much earlier establishment of risk in younger adults, adolescents, or even children. It has even been suggested that the adult risk of CHD is irreversibly determined in infancy and possibly *in utero* (Barker 1990). Studying changes in the environment may reveal whether this results in a corresponding change in health (Haenszel 1970) and the risk of CHD. The BRHS has studied such changes by examining migration into and within Great Britain.

MIGRATION IN THE BRHS COHORT

All men were asked their place of birth and for how long they had lived in the town where they were examined. With this information they were allocated to three groups: non-migrants, internal migrants, and international migrants. The non-migrants ($n = 3144$) were born in the town where they were examined and had lived there for most, if not all, their lives. Internal migrants ($n = 4147$) were born in Great Britain, but not in their town of examination. On average these men had moved into their town of examination in their mid-twenties. The international migrants ($n = 422$) were born outside Great Britain and on average had moved into their town of examination in their late twenties. Information on the migration status of 22 men was not available.

Great Britain was divided into four zones according to the established geographic trend in cardiovascular mortality (Britton 1990). These four zones are the South of England (seven BRHS towns), the Midlands and Wales (four towns), the North of England (10 towns), and Scotland (three towns) (Fig. 9.1).

Migration and the risk of CHD

There was a pronounced gradient in the risk of CHD across the geographical zones not only for the cohort as a whole but also for each of the three migration categories—non-migrants, internal migrants, and international migrants. No matter where the men were born, those living in the South had the lowest risk and those living in Scotland the highest (Elford *et al.* 1989). The geographical trend in CHD risk was significant at the 5 per cent level for all men and for each separate migration category.

Which is more important for the risk of CHD in middle-age: where a person is born, or where that person lives in middle-age? To answer this question, we divided the country into two parts north and south of a line drawn between the Severn Estuary and the Wash. This is a well-established boundary between areas of high CHD mortality (to the north) and areas of relatively low mortality (to the south) (Britton 1990). *Internal* migrants were then classified as to whether they were born north or south of this divide.

Men born in the South of England who subsequently moved north experienced a higher CHD risk than men who remained in the South (7.3 versus 4.4/1000/year). Equally, men born in the 'rest of Great Britain' who moved south experienced a lower risk than those who stayed put (3.3 versus 7.9/1000/year) (Table 9.1). In fact, those who moved south faced a risk little different from that of people who had always lived there. Fitting a logistic model to the data in Table 9.1 confirmed that the geographical zone of examination was a more important determinant of the risk of heart attack than the geographical zone of birth.

Table 9.1 Risk of major CHD event during 6.5 years of follow-up by zone of examination and zone of birth for internal migrants only (events/1000/year)

Zone of birth	Zone of examination	
	South	Rest of Great Britain
South	4.4	7.3
Rest of Great Britain	3.3	7.9

Migration and blood pressure

There was almost a five-fold difference in the prevalence of hypertension ($\geqslant$160/90 mmHg) among the middle-aged men living in the 24 towns of the BRHS. Only 5 per cent of men examined in Shrewsbury were hypertensive compared with 24 per cent of those living in Dunfermline (Shaper *et al.* 1988). In general, the prevalence of hypertension was higher in the North of England and Scotland than in the South. The geographical gradient in blood pressure was found not only for the cohort as a whole, but also for non-migrants, internal migrants, and international migrants ($p < 0.05$) (Elford *et al.* 1990).

To assess the relative importance of factors acting early and later in life for geographical differences in blood pressure, internal migrants were classified according to their geographical zone of birth as well as their zone of examination (Table 9.2). Within each geographical zone of birth, i.e. looking along each row, men examined in the South of England had a lower mean SBP than those examined in Scotland. In general, men examined in the North had intermediate mean SBPs. Within each geographical zone of examination, i.e. looking down each column, there was no such consistent

Table 9.2 Mean SBP (mmHg) by zone of examination and zone of birth

	Zone of examination			
Zone of birth	South	Midlands & Wales	North	Scotland
South	141.7	137.9	145.1	156.7
Midlands & Wales	143.4	143.5	143.1	144.6
North	140.9	142.2	145.6	153.0
Scotland	143.1	138.0	143.9	147.7

gradient by zone of birth. Similar findings were obtained for DBP (Elford *et al*. 1990). No matter where they were born in Great Britain, men living in the South had lower mean blood pressure than men living in the North of England and Scotland. Fitting a multiple linear regression model to the data in Table 9.2 confirmed the importance of the geographical zone of examination, rather than the zone of birth, for adult blood pressure.

Factors present in adult life appeared to exert a stronger influence on the geographical gradient in blood pressure than those present around the time of birth or in childhood. This finding is consistent with studies of international migrants who, on moving from a relatively low to a relatively high blood pressure community, themselves experienced an increase in blood pressure (Beaglehole *et al*. 1977; Joseph *et al*. 1983).

Migration and height

Was the classification of internal migrants by their zone of birth and zone of examination able to distinguish accurately between influences acting early in the life-cycle and those acting later? We were concerned that we had simply created a classification that always opted for the place of examination no matter which variable was considered. Adult height is undoubtedly determined by genetic and early life influences, such as infant nutrition (Rona 1981). Consequently, we would expect adult height to be strongly influenced by where a person is born and brought up, rather than by where he or she ends up living in middle age. We examined geographical variations in height among the internal migrants, according to their zone of birth and zone of examination, to test the classification's ability to distinguish the two correctly.

Men born in Scotland were shorter, on average, than men born in the South of England, no matter where they ended up living. And men born in the Midlands and the North were of intermediate height, again irrespective of where they lived in middle age (Elford *et al*. 1990). Among the internal migrants, the place of *birth* was indeed the crucial determinant of adult height. Therefore this suggests that our classification of internal migrants by their zone of birth and zone of examination was able to discriminate between influences acting early in life and those present later in the life-cycle.

The geographical differential in height among the internal migrants in the BRHS throws into sharp focus the presence of earlier regional variations in both their prenatal and childhood environments, as well as geographical differences in their genetic make-up. However, those early-life factors which shaped their adult height did not exert the same influence on either the geographical gradient in CHD or the corresponding gradient in blood pressure. Instead, regional differences in both CHD and blood pressure were strongly influenced by factors acting later in life associated with the adult environment. These have already been described in the first part of this chapter.

THE CHILDHOOD ORIGINS OF ADULT CARDIOVASCULAR DISEASE

Forsdahl (1977) argued that 'a poor standard of living in early years followed by prosperity' may be a potential risk factor for adult CHD. In this and subsequent ecological analyses conducted in the USA (Buck and Simpson 1982) and England and Wales (Barker and Osmond 1986), it was argued that geographical differences in CHD reflected earlier regional differences in the prenatal and childhood environment. According to this hypothesis, men born into relative poverty in Scotland earlier this century would be more susceptible to factors related to affluence in later life than men born in the relatively prosperous South. This elevated susceptibility would be expressed as an increased risk of CHD in adult life. Furthermore, according to the hypothesis, people born in a relatively poor area who subsequently moved to a more affluent part of Great Britain would experience a higher incidence of CHD than those who had always lived in the more affluent area. Conversely, regardless of where they eventually settled, people born and raised in more affluent areas would suffer less adult heart disease. According to the hypothesis, among migrants the place of birth should be a more important determinant of CHD risk than the place of examination.

Migration into and within Great Britain provided the opportunity to test this hypothesis. We found that the place of examination, and not birth, was the crucial determinant of CHD risk. Consequently, our findings do not support the hypothesis that geographical differences in adult CHD reflect earlier regional variations in the prenatal and infant environment. On the contrary, our data confirm the importance of factors acting in adult life for the elevated rates of heart disease in the North of England and Scotland. Changes in blood pressure levels upon migration may have partially accounted for corresponding changes in CHD risk among those who moved.

CONCLUSION

Regional variations in the risk of CHD provide the epidemiologist with a remarkable opportunity for aetiological investigation. Risk factors which relate strongly to CHD incidence or mortality on a regional basis may not be implicated when the same factors are studied in individuals, and vice versa. Causality must be firmly based on strong relationships in individuals. The BRHS confirms the importance of cigarette smoking and hypertension in contributing to regional variations as well as to social class differences in CHD. Critical to the risk of CHD and the modification of such risk is the question of whether it is exposure to these risk factors in adult life only, exposure throughout life, or even exposure at much earlier periods which is critical. Migration into and within Great Britain by the BRHS men provides strong evidence for the importance of the adult environment in determining the risk of both hypertension and CHD. There is little support here for the hypothesis that hypertension or CHD are irreversibly determined *in utero* or in early infancy.

ACKNOWLEDGEMENTS

The British Regional Heart Study is a British Heart Foundation Research Group and is also supported by the Department of Health and The Chest, Heart and Stroke Association.

REFERENCES

Barker, D. J. P. (1990). The fetal and infant origins of adult disease. *Br. Med. J.,* **301,** 1111.

Barker, D. J. P. and Osmond, C. (1986). Infant mortality, childhood nutrition, and ischaemic heart disease in England and Wales. *Lancet,* **i,** 1077–81.

Beaglehole, R., Eyles, E., Salmond, C., and Prior, I. (1977). Blood pressure in Tokelauan children in two contrasting environments. *Am. J. Epidemiol.,* **105,** 87–9.

Britton, M. (ed.) (1990). Geographic variation in mortality since 1920 for selected causes. *Mortality and geography. A review in the mid-1980s, England and Wales.* Ser. DS No. 9, HMSO, London.

Buck, C. and Simpson, H. (1982). Infant diarrhoea and subsequent mortality from heart disease and cancer. *J. Epidemiol. Community Health,* **36,** 27–30.

Davey Smith, G. and Phillips, A. N. (1990). Declaring independence. Why we should be cautious. *J. Epidemiol. Community Health,* **44,** 257–8.

Elford, J., Phillips, A. N., Thomson, A. G., and Shaper, A. G. (1989). Migration and geographic variations in ischaemic heart disease in Great Britain. *Lancet,* **i,** 343–6.

Elford, J., Phillips, A. N., Thomson, A. G., and Shaper, A. G. (1990). Migration and geographical variations in blood pressure in Britain. *Br. Med. J.,* **300,** 291–5.

Forsdahl, A. (1977). Are poor living conditions in childhood and adolescence an important risk factor for arteriosclerotic heart disease? *Br. J. Prev. Social Med.,* **31,** 91–5.

Haenszel, W. (1970). Studies of migrant populations. *J. Chron. Dis.,* **23,** 289–91.

Joseph, J. G., Prior, I. A. M., Salmond, C. E., and Staley, D. (1983). Elevation of systolic and diastolic blood pressure associated with migration: the Tokelau Island migrant study. *J. Chron. Dis.,* **36,** 507–16.

OPCS (Office of Population Censuses and Surveys) (1986). *Registrar General's dicennial supplement on occupational mortality 1979–83,* HMSO, London.

Pocock, S. J., Shaper, A. G., Cook, D. G., Packham, R. F., Lacey, R. F., Powell, P., and Russell, P. F. (1980). British Regional Heart Study: variations in cardiovascular mortality, and the role of water quality. *Br. Med. J.,* **280,** 1243–9.

Pocock, S. J., Shaper, A. G., Cook, D. G., Phillips, A. N., and Walker, M. (1987). Social class differences in ischaemic heart disease in British men. Lancet, **ii,** 197–201.

Rona, R. J. (1981). Genetic and environmental factors in the control of growth in childhood. *Br. Med. Bull.,* **37,** 265–72.

Shaper, A. G., Pocock, S. J., Walker, M., Cohen, N. M., Wale, C. J., and Thomson, A. G. (1981). British Regional Heart Study: cardiovascular risk factors in middle-aged men in 24 towns. *Br. Med. J.,* **283,** 179–86.

Shaper, A. G., Pocock, S. J., Walker, M., Phillips, A. N., Whitehead, T. P., and Macfarlane, P. W. (1985). Risk factors for ischaemic heart disease: the prospective phase of the British Regional Heart Study. *J. Epidemiol. Community Health,* **39,** 197–209.

Shaper, A. G., Phillips, A. N., Pocock, S. J., and Walker, M. (1987). Alcohol and ischaemic heart disease in middle-aged British men. *Br. Med. J.,* **294,** 733–7.

Shaper, A. G., Ashby, D., and Pocock, S. J. (1988). Blood pressure and hypertension in middle-aged British men. *J. Hypertension,* **6,** 367–74.

Whincup, P. H., Cook, D. G., Phillips, A. N., and Shaper, A. G. (1990). ABO blood groups and ischaemic heart disease in British men. *Br. Med. J.,* **300,** 1679–82.

10

Methods in nutritional epidemiology

D. Kromhout and B. P. M. Bloemberg

INTRODUCTION

After the Second World War interest in the role of diet in the aetiology of coronary heart disease (CHD) increased greatly. Dietary surveys became an important component of large-scale epidemiological studies, for example the Seven Countries Study, the Western Electric Study, the Ireland–Boston Diet Heart Study, the Honolulu Heart Study, the London Busmen and Bank Clerks Study, and the Whitehall Study, to mention only a few. Characteristically, the dietary part of these epidemiological studies was carried out by nutritionists using traditional dietary survey methods, for example cross-check dietary history, dietary record, or 24 hour recall method. During the last decade there has been a boom in the interest of epidemiologists in the role of diet in the occurrence of other chronic diseases, for example different types of cancer. Owing to the low rate of occurrence of the different types of tumours, large populations had to be examined in order to have enough power to detect relations between dietary variables and disease outcome. This stimulated research into simple dietary survey methods that can easily be applied to large populations. The scepticism of nutritionists about the usefulness of these methods stimulated research into the validity and reproducibility of these methods carried out by nutritional epidemiologists. These validation studies provided insight into the usefulness of these methods in epidemiological studies.

Epidemiologists who try to analyse food intake data in relation to the occurrence of disease are confronted with several problems. If the data are analysed as foods, the question remains as to what nutrient or nutrients are responsible for any observed association. If data are analysed as nutrients, good quality computerized food tables should be available. If a nutrient is significantly associated with the disease of interest the question should always be asked as to whether the nutrient studied, or another highly correlated nutrient, or a (non-) nutritive substance which has not been studied, could be responsible for the observed association. These issues will be addressed in this chapter.

THE FOCUS OF NUTRITIONAL EPIDEMIOLOGY

Nutritional epidemiology is focused on the role of dietary variables in explaining differences in the occurrence of disease either between populations or between individuals. In traditional nutritional epidemiological studies information is gathered on food intake and this is related to the occurrence of disease. However, it is questionable whether this is the most profitable way of studying diet–disease associations; foods contain many nutrients and non-nutritive substances that are metabolized before they exert their influence on disease occurrence. Therefore there are advantages in studying associations between disease occurrence and biochemical variables as well as direct relations with dietary variables (Fig. 10.1). If an association is observed between a biochemical variable and a disease, the dietary determinants of this biochemical variable should be identified in the next phase of research. When this approach is chosen, close co-operation between nutritional epidemiologists, biochemists, physiologists, and clinical nutritionists is needed.

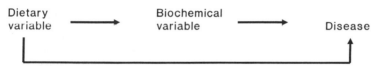

Fig. 10.1 Relations between dietary variables, biochemical variables, and disease occurrence.

An example of this approach is the Seven Countries Study, in which Keys and coworkers (Keys 1970) showed that saturated fat intake is a strong determinant of serum cholesterol and mortality from CHD. Recently, the food intake data of the 16 cohorts of the Seven Countries Study, collected during the baseline survey around 1960, have been recoded by one dietitian in a standardized way (Kromhout *et al.* 1989). Thereafter, food composites representing the average food intake of each cohort have been collected locally. These food composites have been chemically analysed in one laboratory and, amongst others, detailed fatty acid analyses were carried out. These data were used in analysing relations between the average intake of dietary fatty acids, the average serum cholesterol level, and the 25 year mortality from CHD in the 16 cohorts. These analyses showed that, in particular, saturated fatty acids with 12 and 14 carbon atoms were strongly associated with serum cholesterol. The sum of all saturated fatty acids was strongly related to 25 year mortality from CHD (Kromhout 1991). These results suggest that, as well as cholesterol metabolism, other mechanisms, such as the thrombogenetic effect of saturated fatty acids, may play a role in explaining differences in mortality from

CHD between populations. This example shows that, in addition to re-search on diet as a determinant of disease occurrence, research on the dietary determinants of biochemical intermediates may enhance our in-sight into the role of diet in the aetiology of disease.

DIETARY SURVEY METHODS

Dietary survey methods can be characterized by the way that food intake data are collected. This can be done using the record, interview, or food frequency methods (Bingham 1987) (Table 10.1). The record method is used if an investigator wants accurate information about food intake during a limited period, for example 1–7 days. If the usual food intake is of primary importance to an investigator, repeatedly collected food records during a certain time period can be used. The dietary information collected by this method can either be obtained by weighing all foods or by recording in household measures. Record methods are laborious and can only be used when a small number of persons are examined.

Table 10.1 The most commonly used dietary survey methods

Record	Interview	Food frequency
Precise weighing	Recall	Structured
Weighed inventory	Dietary	Open-ended
Record in	history	
household measures		

The interview methods can be divided into recall and dietary history methods. The most commonly used method is the 24 hour recall, which attempts to obtain a complete description of all foods eaten during the 24 hours preceding the interview. An important drawback is that no picture is obtained about the usual food intake of an individual but only a snapshot of the food intake during the previous day, although repeatedly collected 24 hour recalls can be used as an estimate of the usual food intake. Another approach is to ask the respondent to estimate his/her usual intake, as applied in dietary history methods. These methods provide information about the usual food intake of an individual during a consider-able period of time varying between 2 weeks and 1 year. The most exten-sive method in this category is the so-called cross-check dietary history method originally developed by Burke (1947). As well as information about the usual food consumption pattern during and between meals, the consumption of specific foods is checked either in combination with a 3-day record or by information on the quantities of various foods purchased per week for the whole family. This method is time consuming and can only be carried out in epidemiological studies of not more than about two thousand participants.

In nutritional epidemiology there is the need for simple methods that can be applied to large populations. Food frequency methods are very well suited for this purpose; they are characterized by the collection of information about the frequency with which certain foods are eaten during a specified period (Willett 1990). Structured questionnaires with a limited number of foods are most popular. The number of foods in the questionnaire is generally derived from large data bases or pilot studies in which complete information about food intake is collected. Only those foods that contribute substantially to the nutrients of interest are selected, so that the number of foods in the questionnaire can be limited to as few as 60 (Willett *et al*. 1985). In the more advanced food frequency methods, information about portion sizes is also collected using photographs. This approach does not provide information on the total diet and is therefore time- and population-dependent.

Food intake data are generally converted into nutrient intake by using food tables. However, the use of a food table introduces an additional source of error. The nutrient content of the same food can vary depending on food type, mode of cultivation, storage conditions, method of processing, method of preparation, etc. Therefore the samples of foods collected for chemical analyses should be as representative as possible. Only then can food tables be obtained with reasonable accuracy.

The source of errors introduced by the use of food tables can be overcome by chemical analyses of food samples. Chemical analyses are very expensive and therefore are not often used. The most economic method is the equivalent food composite technique, which is characterized by chemical analysis of the average food intake of the group studied so that no information is available about the variation of nutrient intake within the group. Therefore this methodology can only be applied when associations are studied at the group level. The equivalent composite method can also be used as a component of studies to validate the use of food tables.

This type of methodology was applied in the Seven Countries Study by analysing the content of nutrients and non-nutritive substances in food composites representing the average food intake of the 16 cohorts at the beginning of the Study. These data can be related to 25 year mortality from different chronic diseases in the 16 cohorts. Another application of this principle could be to analyse food composites representing the average food intake of cases and non-cases in a case-control or cohort study. In this way information can be obtained with respect to the validity of the nutrient content of foods in food tables.

VALIDITY AND REPRODUCIBILITY

In studying diet–disease relations information about the accuracy of dietary survey methods is needed. Accuracy has to do with the difference between the estimate and the true value of the parameter (the total error in the estimate)—high accuracy means small total error. Generally, accuracy is divided into two components: validity and reproducibility.

The validity of a method is assessed by comparing it with an independent method of unquestionable accuracy. Dietary survey methods of unquestionable validity do not exist. Information about the relative validity of dietary survey methods may be obtained by evaluating the method of interest with another generally accepted method designed to measure the same concept, for example comparing the 24 hour recall with the 1 day record method. Dietary survey methods can also be validated by comparing energy and nutrient intakes with a biochemical indicator of these intakes, for example 24 hour nitrogen in urine as an indicator of protein intake and total energy expenditure estimated by the double-labelled water technique as an indicator of total energy intake (Isaksson 1980; Livingstone *et al.* 1990). As well as the validity, the reproducibility of a dietary survey method is also of importance. A method is reproducible if two independent measurements give the same result in the same situation. Reproducibility studies using dietary survey methods estimating the current food intake, for example the 24 hour recall, are mainly influenced by the intra-individual variation in the intake of foods. The dietary history method, however, is based on the concept that the participant has to recall the foods consumed and to integrate this information to the usual food consumption pattern during at least the 2 weeks preceding the interview. Reproducibility studies using dietary history methods therefore provide information about the ability of the participant to give reproducible information on the usual intake of foods. The validity and reproducibility of different types of dietary survey methods will be discussed.

Dietary survey methods estimating the current food intake, for example 1 day or several days recording of food intake and 24 hour recall, do not give the same results for the average energy and nutrient intake of groups. Energy and nutrient intake tend to be underestimated by the 24 hour recall method (Bingham 1987). The 1 day record and the 24 hour recall method are not suited for estimating the usual food and nutrient intake of an individual because of the large intra-individual variation in the daily intake of certain foods. Examples are the intake of shellfish and liver. These foods are rich sources of cholesterol and are eaten infrequently in relatively large quantities. Therefore the intra-individual variation in these foods and in cholesterol intake is large (Marr and Heady 1986). This means that information about the usual food intake of an individual using these dietary survey methods can only be obtained when repeated measures during a period of, for example, a year are obtained.

Such a design has been used in a validation study comparing the validity of 14 repeated 24 hour recalls for the assessment of the usual energy and protein intake in 123 young adult women (van Staveren 1985). The validity was examined by comparing the mean daily energy intake with changes in body weight over a 14 month period and by comparing the mean daily protein intake with the protein intake assessed from nitrogen excretions in 14 collections of 24 hour urine. The results of this study showed that the 24 hour recall gives a valid estimate of the mean energy and protein intake of groups. Analyses on the individual level showed that 16 per cent of the subjects either consistently over- or under-reported their food intake.

Compared with the record, the cross-check dietary history method tends to overestimate energy intake (Bingham 1987). This could be due to the overestimation of infrequently used foods. The cross-check dietary history method is frequently used in case-control studies. It is essential in this type of study to estimate what the food intake of the cases was before the occurrence of the disease. It is therefore of interest to investigate the validity of the dietary assessment in both cases and controls with respect to their dietary habits in the past. Such a study has been carried out within the context of the Zutphen Study (Bloemberg *et al.* 1989*a*). Information was available on the food intake of 43 myocardial infarction patients and 86 healthy controls, collected in 1970 when all participants were free of disease. In 1985 information was collected on the current food intake of these subjects and they were also asked to estimate their food intake of 15 years previously. The retrospectively assessed food intake was compared with the actual food intake in 1970. Retrospectively, the energy intake was overestimated by approximately 300 kcal/day. The data collected in 1970 showed a significantly lower energy intake in myocardial infarction cases compared with controls. However, the retrospectively assessed energy intake data did not show a significant difference. The results of this study suggest that the power to detect a significant difference in energy intake between cases and controls was considerably reduced when dietary data were assessed retrospectively.

In reproducibility studies using the dietary history method the time interval between the measurements is crucial: it should not be too short so as to avoid recollection of the first interview, but should not be too long so as to prevent changes in food habits. Within the Zutphen Study it was shown that the differences in reproducibility estimations of different nutrients in elderly men were small when repeated dietary surveys were carried out 3 and 12 months after the initial survey (Bloemberg *et al.* 1989*b*). The ratios of the inter-individual and intra-individual variance were large for carbohydrates and small for preformed vitamin A. The larger this ratio, the higher is the probability to detect a relationship if one exists. The results of this study suggest that, for energy and most of the nutrients, the observed relation between a dietary variable and another risk factor was only slightly attenuated due to lack of reproducibility of the measurement of the dietary variables. Consequently, repeated application of the cross-check dietary history method in the case of low-order correlations, for example the association of saturated fat and serum cholesterol at the individual level, is of little help.

The Zutphen Study showed that the reproducibility differed for different foods (Bloemberg *et al.* 1989*b*). Bread, alcoholic beverages, milk, and sugar products were reproduced well. Potatoes, fruit, cheese, edible fats, and pastry were moderately well reproduced. Vegetables and meat were least reproducible. This has consequences for the design of future studies on diet–disease relations. Nutrients present in poorly reproduced foods should either be better estimated during the interview or another method should be used for their estimation.

The validity and reproducibility of a semi-quantitative food frequency questionnaire has been described by Willett *et al.* (1985). A 61 item questionnaire was administered twice at an interval of approximately 1 year. During the same period four 1 week dietary records were collected from the same 173 nurses. Overall, 48 per cent of the subjects in the lowest quintile and 49 per cent of the subjects in the highest quintile of the caloric adjusted intake computed from the dietary records were also in the lowest and highest quintile respectively of the questionnaire. The intra-class correlations were similar for the questionnaire and 1 week dietary record (range 0.41–0.79), indicating a similar reproducibility of both methods. These authors conclude that a simple self-administered questionnaire can provide useful information about individual intakes during a 1 year period. This conclusion may be overoptimistic because a substantial number of the subjects are misclassified in the distribution of the different nutrients.

The average total energy intake of these female registered nurses aged 34–59 years was about 1600 kcal/day with the record method and about 1400 kcal/day with the questionnaire (Willett *et al.* 1985). The average resting metabolic rate for women aged 30–60 years weighing 60 kg is about 1300 kcal/day (Shofield *et al.* 1985). This suggests that the energy intake is seriously underestimated in Willett's study. If the underestimation is proportional to energy intake, it may not influence associations between dietary variables and disease outcome. However, it has repeatedly been shown that underestimation is related to body mass index (van Staveren 1985; Prentice *et al.* 1986; Kromhout *et al.* 1988). Obese individuals tend to underestimate their energy intake. In the USA in particular, with its high prevalence of obesity, this may invalidate the results of dietary surveys.

In order to obtain a proper estimate of the strength of the association between dietary variables and disease occurrence, repeated measures of these variables are needed when dietary survey methods that estimate the current food intake are used. Using only one measure leads to an under-estimation of the strength of the association as a result of regression dilution bias (MacMahon *et al.* 1990). Therefore repeated measures of these variables in a subsample of the population surveyed are needed.

From the results of studies carried out so far it can be concluded that validation and reproducibility studies should always be a part of an epidemiological study investigating diet–disease relations. Semi-quantitative food frequency questionnaires can be validated against a large number of 24 hour recalls or 1 day records. The reproducibility of the questionnaire should be tested by repeating the questionnaire after 1 year. Objective measures of energy and protein intake obtained by the double-labelled water technique and measurement of nitrogen in 24 hour urine collections respectively should be obtained. Blood samples could be collected for validation of the intake of certain micronutrients, such as β-carotene. Only if these types of validation and reproducibility studies are carried out, will a good picture of the accuracy of semi-quantitative food frequency questionnaires be obtained. This strategy is already being put into practice in the international study on diet, cancer, and health being carried out in seven countries and co-ordinated by the International Agency for Reseach on Cancer, Lyon, France.

ANALYSES OF DIETARY DATA

Foods are complex substances containing a large variety of chemicals. These may be divided into the following categories: nutrients, additives, contaminants, chemicals formed during food preparation, natural toxins, and other natural substances. This means that analyses of food intake data restricted to nutrients do not cover all aspects of foods. Fortunately, most interest concerns associations between nutrient intake and the occurrence of disease, but in some instances the relation between non-nutritive substances and disease incidence may be of importance. An example is the frequently observed inverse relation between the intake of fruits and vegetables and the occurrence of lung, breast, colon, stomach, and pancreatic cancer. This may suggest that certain nutritive antioxidants, such as β-carotene and vitamin C, may be of importance in the aetiology of these diseases. However, it is possible that non-nutritive anticarcinogens present in these foods (e.g. indoles, phenols, and flavones) may be of importance in preventing these diseases. It could also be possible that the total anti-carcinogenic potential of these foods, for example the sum of nutritive antioxidants and non-nutritive anticarcinogens, is responsible for the preventive effect of vegetables and fruits. Therefore analyses of dietary intake data with respect to both foods and nutrients are of importance.

The attractiveness of analyses with respect to foods is that, if causality is established, they can be translated directly into preventive action. We observed an inverse relation between fish intake and 20 year mortality from CHD in the Zutphen Study (Kromhout *et al.* 1985). This inverse association has now been confirmed in several prospective studies carried out in countries with a relatively low fish consumption. In these cultures the consumption of one or two servings of fish per week could be of value in the prevention of CHD.

The problem of this type of analysis is that the responsible nutrient(s) or non-nutritive substances present in fish cannot easily be identified. There is substantial evidence that large amounts of $n-3$ polyunsaturated fatty acids, present in fish, influence lipid metabolism and thrombogenesis. However, there is no evidence that a small amount of fish will influence these mechanisms and could be responsible for a lower incidence of CHD among fish-eaters. This means that either $n-3$ polyunsaturated fatty acids influence the occurrence of CHD through other mechanisms or that other substances present in fish are at work.

Analyses with respect to nutrients are preferably guided by the results of experimental research. Experimental studies in humans have shown that saturated fatty acids, and particularly saturated fatty acids with 12–16 carbon atoms, have an elevating effect on serum cholesterol (Keys *et al.* 1965). All saturated fatty acids with more than 10 carbon atoms were shown to be thrombogenic in animal experiments (Hornstra 1991). The results of these experimental studies suggest that epidemiological studies should pay special attention to specific saturated fatty acids in relation to the occurrence of CHD.

It has been suggested that, before associations between dietary variables and disease outcomes are analysed, adjustment for energy intake should be carried out (Willett and Stampfer 1986). The rationale for this approach is that energy balance could be an important determinant of disease. If this is the case, such an adjustment is justified. However, an unbiased estimate of energy intake is needed, which is difficult to obtain particularly in obese subjects (van Staveren 1985; Prentice *et al.* 1986; Kromhout *et al.* 1988). If a priori information has shown that the association between a certain nutrient and a disease is stronger than that between energy intake and the disease, such an adjustment is not justified.

A problem that frequently occurs in nutritional epidemiological studies is multicollinearity. The different energy-containing nutrients are strongly correlated. A person with a high energy intake will generally have a high intake of protein, fat, and carbohydrate. The reverse is true for a person with a low energy intake. In statistical analysis of these types of data, the researcher should always be guided by what is known from experimental and clinical studies. If, for instance, a strong inverse association exists between saturated fat and starch intake and both are related to CHD incidence in an observational study, the association between saturated fat intake and CHD is more likely to be causal than is that between starch intake and CHD: there is much more evidence from experimental and clinical studies that saturated fat is the causal agent.

Another way of addressing this issue of multicollinearity is to carry out a large prospective study. In this study, stratified analyses could be carried out analysing strata with subjects who have a low or a high saturated fat intake and, for instance, a low starch intake relative to CHD incidence. In this way it is possible to study the effect of saturated fat on disease occurrence in the context of a low starch diet.

A relation between a dietary variable and a risk factor or disease occurrence can only be studied if the variation in the dietary variable is sufficiently large. In populations with a homogeneous diet this will be a problem. We have already reported that within the Seven Countries Study saturated fatty acids are an important determinant of differences in long-term mortality from CHD between the 16 cohorts. Within the Zutphen Study no association was found between the intake of saturated fat and mortality from CHD. This may be due to the fact that variation in saturated fat intake in the Zutphen men was relatively small, for example mean=18 per cent of energy and SD=3 per cent of energy, compared with a range from 3 to 22 per cent energy between the different cohorts of the Seven Countries Study (Keys 1970).

In the Seven Countries Study information on food intake of all individuals of five cohorts in Finland, Italy, and the Netherlands in the period around 1970 was collected using the cross-check dietary history method. The same methodology was used in dietary surveys carried out in Italy and the Netherlands in 1965. All these data have been coded recently in a standardized way. Fifteen year mortality data are available for the more than 3000 men aged 50–69 around 1970, so that diet–disease relations can be analysed at the individual level. The major advantage of this data-base is that information about intra- and inter-individual variation is available. By using cohorts established in different countries, a large between person variation will also be available in food and nutrient intake. This enhances the probability of detecting significant associations between dietary variables and mortality from different diseases.

SUMMARY

Nutritional epidemiological studies are confronted with several problems. A gold standard for estimating food intake does not exist. In order to obtain insight into the true food intake, different dietary survey methods including semi-quantitative food frequency questionnaires should be applied at the same time in validation and reproducibility studies. Within prospective investigations, validation and reproducibility studies should be carried out repeatedly during the course of the follow-up. In this way it will be possible to obtain information about the different sources of error of food intake assessment. This type of data will enable investigators to analyse diet–disease relations in the most optimal way.

REFERENCES

Bingham, S. (1987). The dietary assessment of individuals; methods, accuracy, new techniques and recommendations. *Nutr. Abstr. Rev., Ser. A,* **57**, 705–42.

Bloemberg, B. P. M., Kromhout, D., and Obermann-de Boer, G. L. (1989*a*). The relative validity of retrospectively assessed energy intake data in cases with myocardial infarction and controls (the Zutphen Study). *J. Clin. Epidemiol.,* **42**, 1075–82.

Bloemberg, B. P. M., Kromhout, D., Obermann-de Boer, G. L., and van Kampen-Donker, M. (1989*b*). The reproducibility of dietary intake data assessed with the cross-check dietary history method. *Am. J. Epidemiol.,* **130**, 1047–56.

Burke, B. S. (1947). The dietary history as a tool in research. *J. Am. Diet. Assoc.,* **23**, 1041–6.

Hornstra, G. (1991). Unpublished observations.

Isaksson, B. (1990). Urinary nitrogen output as a validity test in dietary surveys. *Am. J. Clin. Nutr.,* **33**, 4–5.

Keys, A. (1970). Coronary heart disease in seven countries. *Circulation,* **41**, (Suppl. 1), I-1–211.

Keys, A., Anderson, J. T., and Grande, F. (1965). Serum cholesterol response to changes in the diet. IV. Particular saturated fatty acids in the diet. *Metabolism,* **14**, 776–87.

Kromhout, D. (1991). Unpublished observations.

Kromhout, D., Bosschieter, E. B., and De Lezenne Coulander, C. (1985). The inverse association between fish consumption and 20-year mortality from coronary heart disease. *New Engl. J. Med.,* **312**, 1205–9.

Kromhout, D., Saris, W. H. M., and Horst, C. H. (1988). Energy intake, energy expenditure, and smoking in relation to body fatness: the Zutphen Study. *Am. J. Clin. Nutr.,* **47**, 668–74.

Kromhout, D., Keys, A., Aravanis, C., Buzina, R., Fidanza, F., Giampaoli, S., Jansen, A., Menotti, A., Nedeljkovic, S., Pekkarinen, M., Simic, B. S., and Toshima, H. (1989). Food consumption patterns in the 1960's in seven countries. *Am. J. Clin. Nutr.,* **49**, 889–94.

Livingstone, M. B. E., Prentice, A. M., Strain, J. J., Coward, W. A., Black, A. E., Barker, M. E., McKenna, P. G., and Whitehead, R. G. (1990). Accuracy of weighed dietary records in studies of diet and health. *Br. Med. J.,* **300**, 708–12.

MacMahon, S., Peto, R., Luther, J., Collins, R., Sorlie, P., Neaton, J., Abbott, R., Godwin, J., Dyer, A., and Stamler, J. (1990). Blood pressure, stroke and coronary heart disease. Part 1. Prolonged differences in blood pressure. Prospective observational studies corrected for regression dilution bias. *Lancet,* **335**, 965–74.

Marr, J. W. and Heady, J. A. (1986). Within- and between person variation in dietary surveys: Number of days needed to classify individuals. *Hum. Nutr. Appl. Nutr.,* **40A,** 347–64.

Prentice, A. M., Black, A. E., Coward, W. A., Davies, H. L., Goldberg, G. R., Murgatroyd, P. R., Ashford, J., Sawyer, M., and Whitehead, R. G. (1986). High levels of energy expenditure in obese women. *Br. Med. J.,* **292,** 983–7.

Shofield, W. N., Shofield, C., and James, W. P. T. (1985). Basal metabolic rate. *Hum. Nutr. Appl. Nutr.,* **39C** (Suppl. 1), 5–41.

van Staveren, W. A. (1985). *Food intake measurements: their validity and reproducibility.* Ph.D. Thesis, Agricultural University, Wageningen, pp. 94–115.

Willett, W. (1990). *Nutritional epidemiology,* Oxford University Press.

Willett, W. and Stampfer, M. J. (1986). Total energy intake: implications for epidemiologic analyses. *Am. J. Epidemiol.,* **124,** 17–27.

Willett, W., Sampson, L., Stampfer, M. J., Rosner, B., Bain, C., Witschi, J., Hennekens, C. H., and Speizer, F. E. (1985). Reproducibility and validity of a semi-quantitative food frequency questionnaire. *Am. J. Epidemiol.,* **122,** 51–65.

11

Nutrition and international patterns of disease

H. Kesteloot and J. V. Joossens

The problem of nutrition and mortality is primarily one of reliability of the data. Mortality is sensitive to classification errors, but mortality from all causes and life expectancy in industrialized countries are not. Nutrition of a population is difficult to assess correctly over either short or long time periods. Instantaneous measurement of nutrition (1 day, 1 week) is influenced by many factors, among them the large day-to-day variation in intake and/or interviewing errors. The estimation of nutritional changes occurring in a population over many decades is also difficult (Bingham 1990).

The overall reliability of mortality data among countries, and especially that of coronary heart disease (CHD), can be tested by comparing it with mortality from all causes. More refined analyses of the trend patterns of CHD mortality are possible by checking the trends in different classification categories of mortality in the same country and for the same sex, for example comparing CHD trends with total cardiovascular and non-CHD–non-cerebrovascular mortality. The rationale behind this is that if deaths are systematically misclassified a compensatory error must occur in one or more other classification categories (Joossens and Kesteloot 1989). In general, it can be said that CHD values since 1968 are reliable.

On the other hand it is possible to check the reliability of nutrition data in a given population by comparing multiple surveys from the same population. Such sets of data are available for, among others, England and Wales, the USA, Finland, and Belgium. Nutritional data from different populations can also be approximated by levels and trends of different causes of mortality. The selection of those causes of mortality is based on known relationships—causal or non-causal—with foods, nutrients, or other factors. In Western countries lung cancer mortality can be used as a rough surrogate for cigarette smoking, colon cancer mortality for saturated fat intake (Carroll and Khor 1975; Weisburger and Wynder 1987), breast cancer mortality for total fat intake (Rose *et al.* 1986), rectal cancer mortality (Joossens and Kesteloot 1990; Tuyns *et al.* 1988) and CHD mortality (National Research Council 1989, pp. 159–201) for the ratio of polyunsaturated to saturated fats (P/S), and stroke or stomach cancer mortality for salt intake (Joossens and Kesteloot 1988). The mortality data from these causes can also be used for comparing trends.

Finally, results from nutritional survey data can be compared between countries with food disappearance data from the Food and Agricultural Organization (FAO) (Food Balance Sheets 1984). Although the FAO data are more susceptible to errors and give generally higher values, because wasted food is also included, they are helpful for making hypotheses about nutrition and mortality. FAO data and national disappearance data have been used extensively all over the world; they are generally consistent with survey data (Bingham 1990; Kesteloot *et al.* 1991) and for many countries they are the only available source.

METHODS

Mortality data are derived from World Health Organization (WHO) publications (1950–89). The data from Belgium (1987) were provided by the National Institute of Statistics. Data from 1950 to 1988 are presented for all-cause, cardiovascular, and total cancer mortality (5th–9th revisions of International Classification of Diseases (ICD) for 10 representative countries where survey data on fat and/or salt intake are available). The data on fats from Portugal are derived from FAO data (1979–81) because of lack of survey data. CHD and stroke mortality data for 1968 onwards are taken from the 8th and 9th revisions of the ICD because the data from earlier revisions are less reliable.

All data are age adjusted between ages 45 and 74 years by the direct method using as weights those proposed for the European population (Doll *et al.* 1970). Change in mortality per year and per million population from 29 industrialized countries (Joossens and Kesteloot 1989) are estimated in each country from the slope of the linear regression of mortality with time, using the available data from the 8th and 9th revisions of the ICD between 1968 and 1988. Only average values of both sexes are presented in the figures because of limitations of space. FAO data from 1979 to 1981 are standardized to a constant energy intake. Correlations with available mortality data (averages of 3 or less years between 1984 and 1987) are presented for 36 countries (Kesteloot *et al.* 1991).

RESULTS AND DISCUSSION

Data for all-cause, CHD, stroke, and cancer mortality are given in Figs 11.1–11.3 for nine representative countries where we have survey data on

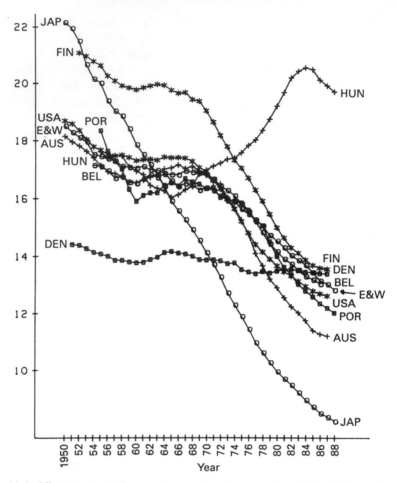

Fig. 11.1 All-cause mortality per thousand in nine countries, 1950–88 (age adjusted 45–74 years, mean of both sexes). The data have been smoothed by 5 year means.

fat and/or salt intake. The mortality data of the Netherlands are not shown, although nutritional data are available. Their CHD mortality data are similar to those from England and Wales, but at a lower level.

Data from nutrition surveys and the trends and levels of mortality for various causes in 10 countries are presented in Tables 11.1–11.3. Data on life expectancy from birth and on the change of life expectancy between 1967 and 1987 are given in Table 11.1. Intercorrelations of CHD and stroke mortality with FAO data are given in Table 11.4.

Table 11.1 shows that two major nutritional changes have occurred over the last 20 years. First, there was a marked increase in polyunsaturated fat (PUFA) in Australia (Baghurst *et al.* 1988), the USA (National Research

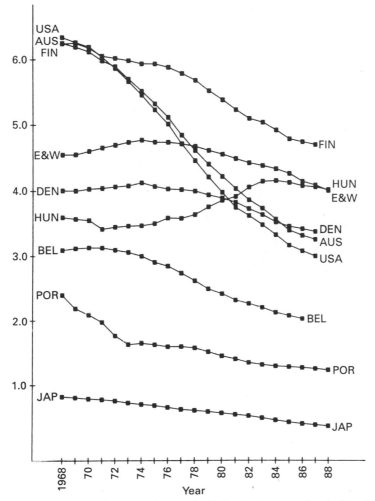

Fig. 11.2 CHD mortality per thousand, 1968–88. Presented as in Fig. 11.1.

Council 1989, pp. 54–6), and Belgium (Joossens *et al.* 1989; Joossens and Kesteloot 1990), and a smaller one in Finland (Pietinen 1990) and in England and Wales (Coronary Heart Disease Prevention 1988). In Belgium, PUFA intake increased by 200–300 per cent, more in the north than in the south (Joossens *et al.* 1989), and in Finland it increased by 67 per cent although it started from much lower values (Pietinen 1990). Although the level of PUFA in the Netherlands is relatively high, it has not changed since 1960 (Kromhout *et al.* 1990). In Denmark the most important change is a marked increase in total fat from 30 per cent of energy in the 1950s to nearly 42 per cent (Dyerberg 1986; Haraldsdóttir *et al.* 1986; Trygg, personal

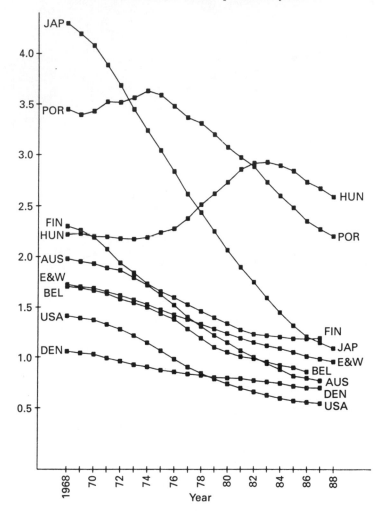

Fig. 11.3 Cerebrovascular mortality per thousand, 1968–88. Presented as in Fig. 11.1.

communication) combined with a low P/S ratio and a high saturated fat intake. The same happened in Hungary, but with a still higher saturated fat intake of 27 per cent of energy and a P/S ratio 10 times lower than in Japan (Biró 1989). In Japan fat intake has increased over the last 50 years from 5 per cent to 22 per cent (Ueshima 1989); the latter value could be near the optimal level (Weisburger and Wynder 1987). The P/S ratio decreased by 40 per cent during the same time period.

A second nutritional change is the decrease in salt intake which has occurred almost everywhere, most probably because of the mass introduction of refrigerators. Salt intake has changed dramatically in Japan

Table 11.1 Levels and trends of nutrients compared with life expectancy

	Australia	Finland	Japan	Portugal	Belgium	USA	England & Wales	Netherlands	Denmark	Hungary
	1985	1982	1987	1980	1980–84	1985	1986	1985	1977	1986
Total fat[a]	38.9 ↓	38.0 ↓?	22.2 ↑↑	29.0	42.4 ↑	42.0=?	42.7=	39.9 ↓↓	42.0 ↑↑	42.3 ↑↑
Saturated fat[a]	15.8 ↓	19.0 ↓	4.8 ↑	13.1	17.6 ↓	15.5 ↓	17.7 ↓	17.2 ↓	22.3 ↑	27.1 ↑↑↑
Polyunsaturated fat[a]	6.5 ↑↑↑	5.0 ↑↑	5.4 ↑	15.9	7.9 ↑↑	7.5 ↑↑↑	6.2 ↑↑	6.3=	5.5 ↑	2.9=?
P/S ratio	0.41 ↓	0.26 ↑↑↑	1.10 ↓↓	1.20	0.45 ↓↓	0.48 ↑↑↑	0.35 ↓	0.37	0.24 ↑	0.11 ↓↓
Salt excretion[b] (mmol/day)	~150 ↓	181 ↓↓↓	258 ↓↓↓	257 ↓↓	173 ↓↓	155 ↓?	188 ↓?	164 ↓	157 ↓?	243 ↓?
Life expectancy 1987 or 1988	76.5	74.8	78.9	74.1	75.4	75.1	75.6	77.0	75.0	70.2
Changes in life expectancy between 1967 and 1987	+5.5	+5.3	+7.0	+7.6	+4.6	+4.7	+3.6	+3.2	+2.1	+0.7

[a] In per cent of energy
[b] Adjusted to 13.7 mmol of creatinine; data from INTERSALT (1988), except for Australia.
All values are averages of both sexes. The fat intake was obtained in the indicated year. The countries are ranked according to changes in all-cause mortality (Table 11.2).

Table 11.2 Annual change in mortality in deaths per million

	Australia	Finland	Japan	Portugal	USA	Belgium	England & Wales	Netherlands	Denmark	Hungary
All-causes***	−371***	−362***	−355***	−299***	−281***	−270***	−206***	−157***	−30**	+210***
Total cardiovascular	−295***	−225***	−220***	−183***	−232***	−159***	−120***	−88***	−68***	+74***
CHD	−184***	−93***	−24***	−30***	−206***	−76***	−31***	−53***	−41***	+48***
Stroke	−76***	−64***	−181***	−92***	−54***	−56***	−43***	−32***	−19***	+41***
Total cancer	+11***	−44***	−19***	+4	+13***	+6	−5*	−1	+32***	+62***
Lung cancer	+8***	−16***	+11***	+13***	+25***	+17***	−10***	+9***	+26***	+38***
Colon cancer	+2**	+1*	+5***	−2	−2***	−2***	−2***	+1*	+2*	+5***
Rectal cancer	+0.4	−0.3	+0.4**	−3***	−3***	−4***	−2***	−3***	−2***	+6***
Stomach cancer	−9***	−20***	−44***	−21***	−4***	−15***	−12***	−13***	−11***	−24***
Breast cancer p	+2*	+2	+3***	+6***	+0.2	+10***	+6***	−0.3	+4*	+10***

Estimated from the available years of the 8th and 9th revision of ICD between 1968 and 1988 and ranked according to change in all-cause mortality. Age adjusted to the European population between age 45 and 74 years. Average of males and females.
* $p < 0.05$; ** $p < 0.01$; *** $p < 0.001$.

Table 11.3 Level of mortality in deaths (per million) in last available year

	Australia 1987	Finland 1987	Japan 1988	Portugal 1988	USA 1987	Belgium 1987	England & Wales 1988	Netherlands 1987	Denmark 1987	Hungary 1988
All-cause	11 130	13 530	8480	12 200	12 750	12 235	12 880	11 100	13 600	19 380
Total cardiovascular	4758	6838	2632	4601	5250	4278	5743	4224	5064	8992
CHD	3232	4640	514	1410	2989	1880	3995	2580	3447	4069
Stroke	788	1246	1126	2192	618	825	988	652	752	2548
Total cancer	3851	3567	3282	3240	4171	4533	4583	4441	4857	5453
Lung cancer	928	999	543	473	1382	1373	1326	1330	1345	1446
Colon cancer	409	152	203	211	360	302	322	338	364	364
Rectal cancer	138	108	141	116	64	143	176	108	219	265
Stomach cancer	155	311	749	539	109	222	270	269	171	507
Breast cancer p	630	504	191	520	713	850	910	841	896	667

Age adjusted to the European population between age 45 and 74 years. Average of males and females. The countries have been ranked according to changes in all-cause mortality (Table 11.2).

Table 11.4 Correlation coefficients between mortality, average of maximum three available years (1984–7), and FAO nutritional data (1979–81) standardized for energy intake

	Total fat	Animal fat	Vegetable fat	Cereals
CHD	0.23	0.46**	−0.40*	−0.38*
Stroke	−0.66***	−0.56***	−0.25	0.68***
Lung cancer	0.43**	0.54***	−0.15	−0.38*
Colon cancer	0.58***	0.63***	−0.02	−0.63***
Rectal cancer	0.12	0.34*	−0.39*	−0.09
Stomach cancer	−0.69***	−0.58***	−0.29	0.79***
Breast cancer p	0.76***	0.76***	0.09	−0.82***

Average of men and women, 36 countries.
The correlations between cereals and total fat, animal fat, and vegetable fat are −0.93, −0.85, and −0.24 respectively.
* $p < 0.05$; ** $p < 0.01$; *** $p < 0.001$.

from the extremely high values observed in the 1950s in 24 h urine samples (Sasaki 1964) with a mean of 360 mmol NaCl/day. A maximum of 1040 mmol/day was observed in a farmer by Takamatsu (1955). In 1979, Ikeda *et al.* (1986), using duplicate food sample analysis, found a mean value of 225 mmol/day, ranging between 205 and 290 mmol/day in subsamples. The INTERSALT Study (INTERSALT 1988) found 187 mmol/day in Japan, which was confirmed by the Cardiac Study (Yamori 1989) with a value of 187 mmol/day and a range in seven centres of 137–256 mmol/day. Those observations contradict the statements of Kono *et al.* (1983) and Howson *et al.* (1986) who found no consistent decrease in salt intake in Japan. However, the latter used the less reliable food supply data of the Japanese government, whereas the former used either 24 h urine or duplicate sample analysis. The mass introduction of refrigerators in Japan in the 1960s was probably the major cause of this decline. In 1960, 9 per cent of households owned a refrigerator, and this increased to 91 per cent in 1970 and to more than 99 per cent from 1977 onwards (Hirayama 1984). Because of the low body weight and height values of the Japanese, the urinary values should be multiplied by a factor of approximately 1.3 to compare them with Western populations. In Belgium, salt intake decreased by 29 per cent from 1966 to 1986 in middle-aged persons (INTERSALT 1988; Joossens and Kesteloot 1991) and by 26 per cent in the elderly (Joossens and Kesteloot 1991). In Finland an important decrease in 24 h salt excretion has been observed from about 400 mmol/day in the 1950s to 157 mmol/day now (Pietinen 1982, 1990). Salt intake also decreased markedly in Portugal (Miguel and de Pádua 1980; INTERSALT 1988). Salt intake is somewhat lower in the USA–133 mmol/day according to INTERSALT (1988)—and this is in agreement with their relatively low stroke rates and very low stomach cancer levels (Table 11.2). If the trends of stroke and stomach cancer mortality in the USA (Acheson 1966; Joossens and Geboers 1981) can be equated with changes in salt intake (Joossens *et al.* 1971; Joossens and Kesteloot 1988), then salt intake already started to decrease in the 1920s, probably because of the mass introduction of ice boxes and refrigerators. The most important conclusion from the INTERSALT study is that the level of salt intake is a major determinant of the increase in blood pressure with age at the population level.

Figures 11.1–11.3 and the mortality trends and levels given in Tables 11.2 and 11.3 reveal important changes in mortality. In Japan and Portugal the decrease in cardiovascular mortality is mainly due to the decrease in stroke consistent with changes in stomach cancer rates and in salt intake, and enhanced by higher animal protein intake and by mass treatment of hypertension. This is consistent with the finding that among seven regions in Japan a significant correlation exists between life expectancy or stomach cancer and 24 h salt excretion (Yamori 1989). On the other hand, the decreasing cardiovascular mortality in Australia and the USA is primarily due to decreasing CHD, whereas in Finland, Belgium, and England and Wales both decreasing CHD and stroke are important. The Netherlands and Denmark show only a small decrease in cardiovascular mortality, but a major difference between these two countries is a substantial decrease in all-cause mortality in the Netherlands compared with a minimal decrease in Denmark. The latter observation clearly indicates that declines in mortality do not reflect advances in medical and surgical technology and in pharmacology in a technologically advanced country like Denmark. In 1987 the level of total mortality in Finland in the given age group was slightly lower than that in Denmark, whereas in 1952 total mortality in Finland was 47 per cent higher than that in Denmark (Fig. 11.1). In Hungary, there is an increase in mortality where still high, but probably decreasing, levels of salt intake (198 mmol/day (INTERSALT 1988)) are accompanied by an increasing total fat, saturated fat, and very low PUFA intake. However, since 1984 improving mortality data are seen in Hungary for stroke, cardiovascular disease, and all causes (Fig. 11.1), but less so for CHD (Fig. 11.2) and not at all for cancer. The increase in cancer mortality in Hungary is in agreement with the concept that saturated fat is a strong promoter of cancer.

Smoking habits also play an important role, exemplified by the results in Finland and in England and Wales. Only four of 29 countries have decreasing lung cancer rates in males since 1968: Finland, England and Wales, Scotland, and Austria, with annual gradients in deaths per million of -38, -37, -27, and -19 respectively. In females the annual gradients are $+6$, $+16$, $+31$, and $+5$ respectively, leaving only three countries—Finland, England and Wales, and Austria—with decreasing lung cancer rates for both sexes together. As a result, total cancer mortality is decreasing significantly in Finland and to a smaller degree in England and Wales (Table 11.2). The decrease in total cancer mortality in Japan is due to the substantial decrease in stomach cancer (Table 11.2).

The results for rectal cancer (Table 11.2) in the USA and Belgium in comparison with those in Hungary are consistent with the finding of a positive association with saturated fat and a negative association with PUFA (Table 11.4). Epidemiological evidence also points in that direction (Tuyns *et al.* 1988). Experimental evidence, however, points to a detrimental influence of vegetable PUFA in colon cancer and to a favourable influence for olive oil and fish fat (Reddy and Sugie 1988). No data are available on experimental rectal cancer.

Three separate studies in Belgium have demonstrated the existence of a highly significant relationship between the level of saturated fat intake and the total serum cholesterol level (Joossens *et al.* 1966; Kesteloot *et al.* 1987, 1989). The level of PUFA intake has a small but significant lowering effect on the high density lipoprotein cholesterol level. In Belgium the level of saturated fat correlates positively with all-cause and cardiovascular mortality, while the level of PUFA intake correlates negatively (Joossens *et al.* 1989). For stroke the evidence is weaker but the influence of saturated fat and PUFA on blood pressure (Puska *et al.* 1983) and on clotting mechanisms (Hornstra 1990) has been demonstrated in clinical, epidemiological, and experimental research. No clinical trial has ever been done on the relationship between salt intake and stroke, probably because of the lack of economic incentive.

It is not possible, when using available data such as those observed here, to prove causal relationships between food and/or nutrients and given causes of mortality. However, the data do allow us to generate hypotheses which cannot be derived from clinical observations and that can be checked yearly over long periods of time. One conclusion can already be drawn: changes in mortality over the last 20 years reflect much more changes in nutrition and smoking habits than advances in medical science. How otherwise could we explain how in 1987 Cubans had a similar life expectancy to Americans (74.8 versus 75.1 years), that since 1967 Portugal has had the highest increase in life expectancy among 36 countries, and that Denmark has had almost the lowest increase (only five East European countries scored less).

The role of environmental pollution, though real, is frequently overestimated. The highest life expectancy in East European countries is seen in one of the most polluted areas, namely the former German Democratic Republic: 72.9 years with an increase of 2.1 years from 1967 to 1987 (compare with Hungary, a much less polluted country, in Table 11.1). This is an argument for the thesis that internal pollution is more important than external pollution. The study offers support to the concept that nutrition is the most important determinant of life expectancy within and between populations.

REFERENCES

Acheson, R. M. (1966). Mortality from cerebrovascular disease in the United States. In *Cerebrovascular disease epidemiology* (ed. K. Kost), pp. 23–40, Public Health Monogr. 76, Department of Health, Education and Welfare, Washington, DC.

Baghurst, K. I., Crawford, D. A., Worsley, A., and Record, J. (1988). The Victorian Nutrition Survey—intakes and sources of dietary fats and cholesterol in the Victorian population. *Med. J. Aust.,* **149,** 12–20.

Bingham, S. (1990). Patterns of lipid consumption in the United Kingdom. In *Lipids and health* (ed. G. Ziant), pp. 169–77, Excerpta Medica, Amsterdam.

Biró, G. (1989). Nutrition and cardiovascular risk: the Hungarian experience. *Acta Cardiol.,* **44,** 472–4.

Carroll, K. K. and Khor, H. T. (1975). Dietary fat in relation to tumorigenesis. *Prog. Biochem. Pharmacol.,* **10,** 308–53.

Coronary Heart Disease Prevention (1988). *Action in the UK, 1984–1987,* Bradleys, Reading.

Doll, R., Muir, C., and Waterhouse, J. (1970). *Cancer incidence in five continents,* Vol. II, Springer-Verlag, Berlin.

Dyerberg, J. (1986). Linolate derived polyunsaturated fatty acids and prevention of atherosclerosis. *Nutr. Rev.,* **44,** 125–34.

Food Balance Sheets (1984). 1979–81 average. Food and Agriculture Organization, Rome.

Haraldsdóttir, J., Holm, L., Højmark Jensen, J., and Møller, A. (1986). *Danskernes kostvaner 1985,* Levnedsmiddelstyrelsen, København.

Hirayama, T. (1984). Epidemiology of stomach cancer in Japan. With special reference to the strategy for the primary prevention. *Jap. J. Clin. Oncol.,* **14**(2), 159–68.

Hornstra, G. (1990). Effect of dietary lipids on some aspects of the cardiovascular risk profile. In *Lipids and health* (ed. G. Ziant), pp. 39–46, Excerpta Medica, Amsterdam.

Howson, C. P., Hiyama, T., and Wynder, E. L. (1986). The decline in gastric cancer: epidemiology of an unplanned triumph. *Epidemiol. Rev.,* **8,** 1–27.

Ikeda, M., Kasahara, M., Koizumi, A., and Watanabe, T. (1986). Correlation of cerebrovascular disease standardized mortality ratios with dietary sodium and the sodium/potassium ratio among the Japanese population. *Prev. Med.,* **15,** 46–59.

INTERSALT Co-operative Research Group (1988). INTERSALT: an international study of electrolyte excretion and blood pressure. Results for 24 hour urinary sodium and potassium excretion. *Br. Med. J.,* **297,** 319–28.

Joossens, J. V. and Geboers, J. (1981). Nutrition and gastric cancer. *Nutr. Cancer,* **2,** 250–61.

Joossens, J. V. and Kesteloot, H. (1988). Salt and stomach cancer. In *Gastric Carcinogenesis* (eds P. I. Reed and M. J. Hill), pp. 105–26, Excerpta Medica, Amsterdam.

Joossens, J. V. and Kesteloot, H. (1989). The value of ischaemic heart disease vital statistics since 1968. *Acta Cardiol.,* **44,** 389–405.

Joossens, J. V. and Kesteloot, H. (1990). Fats, cancer and cardiovascular disease. In *Lipids and health* (ed. G. Ziant), pp. 93–157, Excerpta Medica, Amsterdam.

Joossens, J. V. and Kesteloot, H. (1991). Trends in systolic blood pressure, 24-hour sodium excretion, and stroke mortality in the elderly in Belgium. *Am. J. Med.*, **90** (Suppl. 3A), 5S–11S.

Joossens, J. V., Verdonk, G., and Pannier, R. (1966). 'Normal' serum cholesterol values in Belgium as related to age and diet. A comparison with other countries. *Acta Cardiol.*, **21**, 431–45.

Joossens, J. V., Willems, J., Claessens, J., Claes, J. H., and Lissens, W. (1971). Sodium and hypertension. In *Nutrition and cardiovascular diseases* (eds F. Fidanza, A. Keys, G. Ricci, and J. C. Somogyi), pp. 91–110, Morgagni Edizioni Scientifiche, Rome.

Joossens, J. V., Geboers, J., and Kesteloot, H. (1989). Nutrition and cardiovascular mortality in Beligum. For the BIRNH Study Group. *Acta Cardiol.*, **44**, 157–82.

Kesteloot, H., Geboers, J., and Pietinen, P. (1987). On the within-population relationship between dietary habits and serum lipid levels in Belgium. *Eur. Heart J.*, **8**, 821–31.

Kesteloot, H., Geboers, J., and Joossens, J. V. (1989). On the within-population relationship between nutrition and serum lipids: the BIRNH study. *Eur. Heart J.*, **10**, 196–202.

Kesteloot, H., Lesaffre, E., and Joossens, J. V. (1991). Dairy fat, saturated animal fat, and cancer risk. *Prev. Med.*, **20**, 226–36.

Kono, S., Ikeda, M., and Ogata, M. (1983). Salt and geographical mortality of gastric cancer and stroke in Japan. *J. Epidemiol. Community Health*, **37**, 43–6.

Kromhout, D., de Lezenne Coulander, C., Obermann-de Boer, G. L., van Kampen-Donker M., Goddijn, E., and Bloemberg, B. P. M. (1990). Changes in food and nutrient intake in middle-aged men during the period 1960–1985 (the Zutphen Study). *Am. J. Clin. Nutr.*, **51**, 123–9.

Miguel, J. P. and de Pádua, F. (1980). Epidemiology of arterial blood pressure in Portugal. In *Epidemiology of Arterial Blood Pressure* (eds H. Kesteloot and J. V. Joossens), pp. 175–85, Martinus Nijhoff, The Hague.

National Research Council (1989). *Diet and health*, National Academy Press, Washington, D.C.

Perry, I. J. and Beevers, D. G. (1990). Is the relationship between salt intake and stroke independent of blood pressure? *J. Hypertension*, **8**, 1063.

Pietinen, P. (1982). *Studies on estimating sodium intake and sodium content of the Finnish diet*. Doctoral thesis, University of Helsinki.

Pietinen, P. (1990). Changing dietary habits in the population: the Finnish experience. In *Lipids and health* (ed. G. Ziant), pp. 243–64, Excerpta Medica, Amsterdam.

Puska, P., Iacono, J. M., Nissinen, A., Korhonen, H. J., Vartiainen, E., Pietinen, P., *et al.* (1983). Controlled, randomized trial of the effect of dietary fat on blood pressure. *Lancet*, **i**, 1–5.

Reddy, B. and Sugie, S. (1988). Effect of different levels of omega-3 and omega-6 fatty acids on azoxymethane-induced colon carcinogenesis in F344 rats. *Cancer Res.*, **48**, 6642–7.

Rose, D. P., Boyar, A. P., and Wynder, E. L. (1986). International comparisons of mortality rates for cancer of the breast, ovary, prostate, and colon, and per capita food consumption. *Cancer*, **58**, 2363–71.

Sasaki, N. (1964). The relationship of salt intake to hypertension in the Japanese. *Geriatrics,* **19,** 735–44.

Takamatsu, M. (1955). Figure of body fluid of farmers in the northeastern districts viewed from angle of water and salt metabolism. *Rodo Kagaku (J. Sci. Labour),* **31,** 349–70.

Tuyns, A. J., Kaaks, R., and Haelterman, M. (1988). Colorectal cancer and the consumption of foods: a case-control study in Belgium. *Nutr. Cancer,* **11,** 189–204.

Ueshima, H. (1989). Changes in dietary habits, cardiovascular risk factors and mortality in Japan. *Acta Cardiol.,* **44,** 475–7.

Weisburger, J. H. and Wynder, E. L. (1987). Etiology of colorectal cancer with emphasis on mechanism of action and prevention. In *Important advances in oncology 1987* (eds V. T. De Vita Jr, S. Hellman, and S. A. Rosenberg), pp. 197–220, J. B. Lippincott, Philadelphia, PA.

Yamori, Y. (1989). The salt balance in Asia. In *Salt and hypertension* (eds R. Rettig, D. Ganten, and F. Luft), pp. 319–28, Springer-Verlag, Berlin.

12

Design and analysis of multicentre epidemiological studies: the INTERSALT Study

P. Elliott

Large sample sizes are increasingly demanded of epidemiological studies and clinical trials (Peto 1987) in order to provide precise estimates of effect. Although statistical techniques are available to combine the results of different studies in formal meta-analyses (see Chapter 27 of this volume for discussion), there is also considerable interest in the multicentre study as a means of increasing sample size and enhancing statistical power. This approach offers other important and unique advantages over the more conventional single-centre study, but at the same time introduces a number of complexities into the study design, conduct, and analysis.

In this chapter, some of these theoretical and practical issues are discussed and illustrated with reference to the relation of systolic blood pressure (SBP) to sodium excretion in the INTERSALT study, an international co-operative study of electrolyte excretion and blood pressure (BP).

HIERARCHICAL DATA AND THE 'ECOLOGICAL FALLACY'

When data are collected at the individual as well as the group or population level (in contrast with a purely ecological design) they are said to have a *hierarchical structure* (Goldstein 1987). In educational research, for example, individual pupil performance may depend on peer grouping within classes, classes within schools, and other higher-level aggregates such as schools within education authorities (Aitken and Longford 1986).

Relatively little attention has been paid in the epidemiological literature to the implications of a hierarchical data structure. In one of the few epidemiological papers to address this issue, Feinleib and Leaverton (1984) reanalysed data from the first US National Health and Nutrition Survey (NHANES I) in which data collection took place in 100 examination centres across the USA based on a national probability sample of US residents (National Center for Health Statistics 1983). The data were originally presented as if from one large sample (ignoring centres), but in their reanalysis Feinleib and Leaverton retained the centre structure to examine relationships both within and across the centres. They found some striking differences between the within- and across-centre findings, for example in the relations of body weight to serum cholesterol. A similar analysis was carried out using data from the Second Health and Nutrition Survey (Piantadosi *et al.* 1988), and again some important within- and across-centre differences were found.

The danger of extrapolating from across-population findings to impute relations at the level of individuals is well known, and has been called the 'ecological fallacy' (Selvin 1958; Morgenstern 1982; Piantadosi *et al.* 1988). Piantadosi *et al.* suggest that it is usually only the individual-level relationships that are valid in making judgements as to causality. However, Blackburn and Jacobs (1984) argue that across-population findings can contribute importantly to the evidence, and cite as an example the relationship between saturated fat intake and serum cholesterol, which is strongly positive across populations (consistent with the experimental evidence) but weak or absent within populations.

Consider a hypothetical case where data are collected on individuals in a number of population *centres*. Figure 12.1 illustrates the hypothetical 'true' relationship between an outcome variable y and an 'explanatory' variable x measured in the different centres. The dots give the average x and y values of the centres, and the ellipses represent the cloud of observations on individuals in each centre.

Potentially, three different regression equations can be specified: an ecological (*across*-centre) regression of average y on average x, with true regression slope β_A; a *within*-centre regression of individual values of y on individual values of x, with true regression slope, β_W, and a regression of individual y on individual x *ignoring centre,* with true regression slope β_T. We shall assume that all three regression slopes coincide, i.e. the 'true' regression slope β of y on x, shown in the figure by the regression line, is such that $\beta = \beta_A = \beta_W = \beta_T$. In the discussion that follows, the convention is used that greek letters refer to 'true' values of the regression parameters (e.g. β) and their roman equivalents refer to the estimated values (e.g. b).

Now consider what might happen when the 'true' data illustrated in Fig. 12.1 are observed (measured) in practice, as shown in Fig. 12.2. Again, the full dots represent the 'true' across-centre relationship between y and x (as Fig. 12.1) and the open dots represent the observed relationship, with the difference being due to across-centre confounding by variables other than y and x and systematic differences in measurement between centres, resulting in positive 'cross-level' bias (Morgenstern 1982). The observed within-centre relationship of y on x is shown as circles around the open dots, again representing the cloud of individual observations within the centre; however,

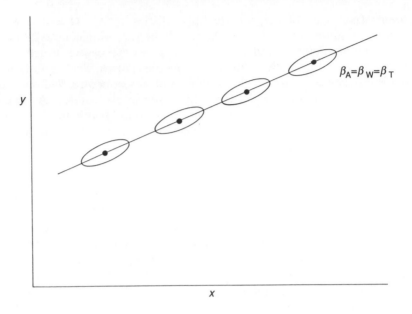

Fig. 12.1 Representation of the 'true' relationship between the response variable y and the independent variable x in different centres, with fitted regression lines: β_A, across-population slope; β_W, within-population slope; β_T, regression slope in individuals, ignoring centre.

in this example the relationship is considerably weakened by a combination of within-centre confounding, and intra-individual variability leading to so-called 'regression dilution' (MacMahon *et al.* 1990).

The observed across-centre regression of average y on average x is b_A, and the average observed within-centre regression slope is b_W. Whereas β_A, β_W, and β_T coincide (Fig. 12.1), in this example the observed regression slopes b_A and b_W are very different, with the regression being strongly positive across centres and essentially zero within centres. This situation is well known in epidemiology, for example the relation of dietary fat to serum cholesterol (Blackburn and Jacobs 1984) or salt to BP (Elliott 1991).

The regression b_T of y on x in individuals ignoring centre lies between b_W and b_A; in general, in simple regression, it can be shown to be the *weighted average* of b_W and b_A, with b_A given weight R_{XX} and b_W weight $1 - R_{XX}$, where R_{XX} is the proportion of the total sum of squares of x that is across centre (Aitken and Longford 1986; Piantadosi *et al.* 1988). Thus b_T, being a combination of b_W and b_A, is not in itself of interest; nevertheless, the data in most multicentre studies are combined and reported in this

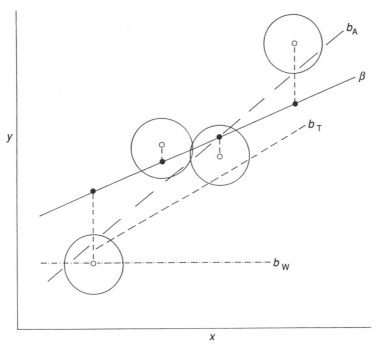

Fig. 12.2 Representation of 'observed' relationship between response variable y and independent variable x in different centres. The data in Fig. 12.1 have been subjected to positive ecological confounding across centres, and 'regression–dilution' bias within centres: β, 'true' regression slope (as in Fig. 12.1); b_A, observed across-population slope; b_W, observed within-population slope; b_T, observed slope in individuals, ignoring centre.

way without regard to the inherent hierarchical structure. This has been called 'lumping' or 'collapsing' of the data (Demets 1987).

Thus only two *independent* regression estimates are available: b_A and b_W. The approach adopted in INTERSALT is to obtain these empirically as follows.

1. Obtain an estimate b_A of the ecological regression coefficient by regressing average y on average x across the centres.

2. Obtain the average individual-level regression coefficient (within centres) b_W by *pooling* the separate within-centre regression coefficients b_i over all centres using $\mathrm{var}(b_i)^{-1}$ as weights, where b_i is the estimated regression coefficient in the ith centre.

Procedure 2 minimizes the variance of the pooled estimate b_W and gives the most powerful test of the null hypothesis that β_W (*and* all β_i) $= 0$. This is equivalent to a meta-analysis (overview) of clinical trials (Demets 1987), except that in the case of a well-conducted multicentre epidemiological study all data are obtained in a *single* study using common protocol, standardized field methods, etc., and there are no problems of publication bias or data missing from unknown or unavailable studies.

If the null hypothesis is rejected, there is good evidence for a *qualitative* relationship between y and x in individuals within centres. But what is the best *quantitative* estimate of that relationship? What is the distribution of the within-centre regression coefficients b_i, and do they appear to be measuring the same underlying quantity? Can the summary within-centre regression coefficient b_W be reconciled with the across-centre coefficient b_A?

THE INTERSALT STUDY

Some of the questions above are illustrated with reference to the relation between sodium excretion and SBP in the INTERSALT Study. Further discussion of the INTERSALT results can be found in Chapter 29 of this volume.

Details of the INTERSALT Study design and field methods are available in the literature (INTERSALT 1986, 1988, 1989; Elliott and Stamler 1988). Briefly, each centre was asked to recruit 200 men and women aged 20–59 years, stratified by age and sex into eight 10 year groups (i.e. men 20–29, men 30–39, etc.). Samples were selected by random sampling of population lists or chunk sampling of defined populations (e.g. whole island or village communities). BP was measured twice on a single occasion by trained observers using a random-zero sphygmomanometer, after participants had emptied their bladders and sat quietly for 5 min. Each participant provided a 24 hour urine collection, the start and end of which were supervised by clinic staff. Urine collections were rejected if found to be incomplete on interview, or if the urinary volume was less than 250 ml in 24 hours. A random 8 per cent of participants completed a second urine collection for the estimation of within-individual variability in electrolyte excretion, enabling a correction to be made (detailed below) for regression dilution bias in BP–electrolyte regression coefficients (INTERSALT 1988). Height and weight were measured in standard fashion, using a stadiometer and beam balance where possible. Seven day alcohol intake was assessed by questionnaire, using local data to convert consumption into millilitres of absolute alcohol per week.

Urine aliquots were kept locally at $-20\,^\circ\mathrm{C}$ and sent frozen to the Central Laboratory, Leuven, Belgium, for measurements of electrolyte concentration. Sodium and potassium were analysed by emission flame photometry. Duplicate samples were sent blind to the Central Laboratory for the estimation of technical error: the percentage technical error was 1.4 per cent (sodium) and 1.9 per cent (potassium).

Data analysis

Values of sodium and potassium excretion were the product of urinary concentration and volume corrected to 24 hours. Body mass index (BMI) was the ratio of weight (kg) to (height)^2 (m^2). Analyses are reported here for the 10 079 men and women with complete data, and for the relations of SBP to 24 hour sodium excretion both across and within the 52 centres of the study.

Across the centres, median sodium excretion was correlated with median slope of SBP with age (estimated by linear regression of SBP on age within each centre), and median SBP standardized for sex and age (20–39 years and 40–59 years). Medians were preferred to means because they are less affected by extreme values and, for BP, they reduce bias due to antihypertensive treatment (by assuming that all participants on treatment had BPs in the upper half of the distribution). Analyses were also carried out after adjustment for median BMI and alcohol intake entered as two centre-level variables: prevalence of drinkers and median alcohol intake in drinkers.

Four centres with low sodium excretion (less than 50 mmol/day), low BPs, and little or no rise of BP with age were found to have a strong influence on across-centre associations. The across-centre analyses were therefore carried out with and without these four centres (INTERSALT 1988).

Within centres, multiple linear regression of SBP on 24 hour urinary sodium excretion was carried out in each of the 52 centres of the study. Centre-specific regression coefficients adjusted for age and sex were then pooled, weighting by the inverse of the variance. Adjustments were also made for BMI, alcohol intake, and potassium excretion. Alcohol intake was entered as two (0,1) variables, i.e. zero versus 1–299 ml/week (0,1) and zero versus 300+ ml/week (0,1).

For each analysis, a test of significance (two-sided) was obtained by comparing the pooled regression coefficient with its pooled standard error, giving a z score. Within-centre regression estimates are seriously biased towards zero by intra-individual variability of electrolyte excretion (Liu *et al.* 1979). Regression coefficients were therefore corrected by dividing each coefficient by a study-wide estimate of the degree of 'regression dilution', which was obtained by correlating the first and second measures of sodium excretion in the 8 per cent of participants with repeated measurements (INTERSALT 1988).

Results

One unique feature of the INTERSALT study was its ability to examine the relationships across the centres between slope of BP with age and electrolyte excretion. The scatter plot for the median SBP slope with age

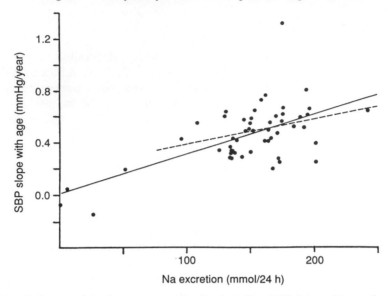

Fig. 12.3 Scatter plot of age–sex standardized median SBP slope with age (mmHg/year) against median 24 hour sodium excretion (mmol) and fitted regression lines: INTERSALT, 52 centres (full line) and 48 centres (broken line). Regression coefficients: 52 centres, $b = 0.030$ (SE 0.006) mmHg/year/10 mmol; 48 centres, $b = 0.019$ (SE 0.010) mmHg/year/10 mmol.

and median sodium excretion is shown in Fig. 12.3, together with fitted regression lines across the 52 and 48 centres (excluding the four low sodium centres). As can be seen, these four centres either had lower BPs with increasing age or only a small rise of BP with age. After adjustment for confounding variables, the 48 centre regression equation gave the estimate that the rise in SBP over a 30 year period (e.g. age 25 to age 55) would be less by 0.9 mmHg for daily sodium excretion lower by 10 mmol.

Results were less stable when the across-centre regression coefficients b_A relating median SBP and sodium excretion were examined (Table 12.1). Across the 52 centres, these coefficients were positive and significant in both the age–sex standardized analysis and in the analysis adjusted for other confounders, but across the 48 centres (excluding the four low sodium centres) the regression coefficient was negative in the age-standardized analysis and positive in the multiple-adjusted analysis, with neither result being statistically significant at the 5 per cent level.

In the first of the within-centre analyses, the number of positive SBP–sodium regression coefficients, the number of negative coefficients, and the number of coefficients nominally significant at $p < 0.05$ were calculated for each of the regression models as shown in Table 12.2. Under the null hypothesis of no relationship, one would expect that half the coefficients would be positive and half negative, with few if any statistically significant.

Table 12.1 Regression coefficients relating median SBP and 24 hour sodium excretion across 52 and 48 centres in INTER-SALT, standardized for age and sex, and multiple-adjusted[a]

	52 centres	48 centres[b]
Standardized age, sex (mmHg/10 mmol)	0.709**	−0.283
	(0.187)	(0.286)
Multiple-adjusted[a] (mmHg/10 mmol)	0.446*	0.251
	(0.152)	(0.259)

Standard error (SE) in parentheses.
[a] Standardized for age and sex, and adjusted for BMI and alcohol intake.
[b] Excluding four low sodium centres.
* $p < 0.01$; ** $p < 0.001$.

Table 12.2 Summary of within-centre regressions relating SBP and 24 hour sodium excretion in the 10 079 individuals in INTERSALT, adjusted for age and sex, and multiple-adjusted[a]

	Adjustment	
	Age, sex	Multiple[a]
No. of positive coefficients	39	33
No. significant ($p<0.05$)	15	8
No. of negative coefficients	13	19
No. significant ($p<0.05$)	2	2
Pooled regression coefficient		
(mmHg/10 mmol)	0.163	0.100
SE	0.023	0.026
z score	6.97*	3.79*
Pooled regression coefficient corrected		
for regression dilution bias[b]	0.354	0.217

[a] Adjusted for age, sex, BMI, potassium excretion, and alcohol intake.
[b] Correction for regression dilution estimated from data on repeat urine collections (INTERSALT 1988).
* $p < 0.001$.

In fact, in the age–sex model there were 39 positive coefficients, 15 of which were statistically significant at $p < 0.05$, and 13 negative coefficients, only two of which were statistically significant. With multiple adjustment, there were 33 positive coefficients, eight of which were statistically significant (Table 12.2 and Fig. 12.4).

The frequency distribution of the fully adjusted coefficients uncorrected for regression dilution is shown in Fig. 12.5, grouped into class sizes of width 0.1 mmHg/10 mmol; the modal value is 0.1 mmHg/10 mmol. As can be seen in Figs 12.4 and 12.5, there are two centres in the 'tails' of the

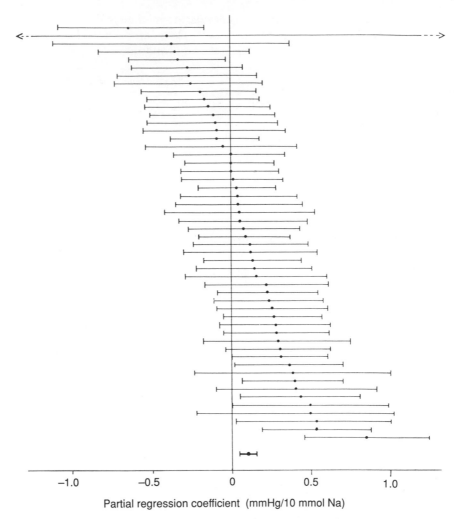

Fig. 12.4 Diagrammatic representation of the multiple-adjusted regression co-efficients and 95 per cent confidence intervals relating SBP (mmHg) and 24 hour sodium excretion (per 10 mmol) in the 10 079 persons in 52 INTERSALT centres. The bold point and line at the bottom of the figure give the pooled regression coefficient, and its 95 per cent confidence interval. The coefficients have not been corrected for regression dilution bias (see text).

distribution, one with a highly significant positive coefficient (Nanning, People's Republic of China) and one with a significant negative coefficient (Osaka, Japan).

For each regression model, the pooled within-centre regression coefficient b_{W} was obtained by weighting each centre's coefficient by the inverse of its

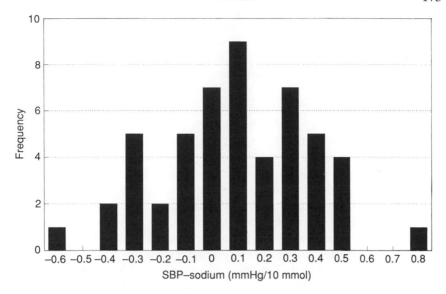

Fig. 12.5 Frequency distribution of the multiple-adjusted regression coefficients relating SBP (mmHg) and 24 hours sodium excretion (per 10 mmol) in the 10 079 persons in 52 INTERSALT centres. The coefficients have not been corrected for regression dilution bias (see text).

variance. As shown in Table 12.2, these pooled coefficients were positive and highly significant; with correction for regression dilution bias (as described above) the fully adjusted model gave the estimate of SBP lower by 0.22 mmHg/10 mmol sodium.

DISCUSSION

The INTERSALT analysis outlined above illustrates some important features of the multicentre design.

1. The design uniquely allowed the relationship with sodium of the slope of BP with age (a variable estimated *within* centres) to be examined across the centres.

2. The analysis across centres (based on 52 or 48 points) was much less stable than that within centres (based on 10 000+ individuals). In fact, the statistical power across centres was low once much of the variation in the *x* variable (sodium) was removed by excluding the four low sodium centres. The effect of these four centres on the size and direction of the across-centre regression coefficients (Table 12.1) illustrates the potential for ecological confounding and the danger of falling into the 'ecological fallacy'.

3. The analysis within centres gave a precise estimate of effect (based on a pooling of results in more than 10 000 individuals) and allowed the distribution of within-centre coefficients to be examined. This is a unique feature of the multicentre design. On the other hand, the size of the within-centre regression coefficients can be seriously attenuated towards zero by regression dilution bias, as was the case in INTERSALT.

4. In these analyses, the across- and within-centre findings could be reconciled. In the fully adjusted model, the analysis across 48 centres (i.e. after removing the ecological confounding introduced by the four low sodium centres) gave a regression estimate of 0.251 mmHg/10 mmol, similar to the pooled within-centre regression coefficient corrected for regression dilution bias, i.e. 0.217 mmHg/10 mmol. In general, the ecological regression coefficient b_A is estimated with less precision than the average within-centre regression coefficient b_W, unless there are large across-centre differences in average values of x, and b_A is particularly liable to unmeasured ecological confounding. However, b_A is much less sensitive than b_W to intra-individual variability (and regression dilution) provided that sample sizes within centres are adequate.

5. Examination of the distribution of regression coefficients (Fig. 12.5) revealed two coefficients in the 'tails' of the distribution, one significantly high (Nanning, People's Republic of China) and one significantly low (Osaka, Japan). In each case, the pooled coefficient was more than 3 standard deviations away from the mean coefficient in these centres (Fig. 12.4).

Further scrutiny of the data may indicate why results in some centres may have differed from the rest and could suggest useful clues as to aetiology. For example, in the Osaka sample (comprised of insurance company employees and their wives) the average daily sodium excretion was relatively low for Japan (168 mmol). More than 40 per cent of the hypertensive individuals reported having reduced their sodium intakes compared with only 12 per cent of the normotensive individuals ($p < 0.001$) (Hashimoto *et al.* 1989); it is conceivable that such differential changes in sodium intakes could have seriously biased the regression estimates towards negative values in the Osaka sample.

In contrast, the significantly positive results for the Nanning sample are broadly consistent with the similarly positive and significant results for the other Chinese centres in INTERSALT, although quantitatively larger (INTERSALT 1988); they are also consistent with results reported from other Chinese populations (Liu *et al.* 1984, 1988; Hsiao *et al.* 1986; Kesteloot *et al.* 1987; Pan *et al.* 1990). It is not clear whether these findings reflect truly stronger BP–sodium relationships in Chinese populations, or merely greater reliability of measurement (and hence less regression dilution bias) because of a more constant diet (Hsiao *et al.* 1986).

In conclusion, recent advances in techniques of meta-analysis and the understanding of hierarchical models make the multicentre approach an attractive design under certain circumstances. Not only can relationships at the level of individuals be examined with only trivial loss of statistical power, but across-centre relationships can also be investigated. In addition, the ability to examine within-centre relationships *across* the centres is gained, and some evidence for or against generalizability of results can be obtained from within a single study. These benefits have to be set against the many organizational difficulties of conducting studies in more than one centre, including the need for centralized training, co-ordination, standardization, and quality control.

ACKNOWLEDGEMENTS

I am pleased to acknowledge the collaborative effort of the INTERSALT Co-operative Research Group—a list of investigators, participating centres, and sponsors is published elsewhere (INTERSALT 1988). I am grateful to Martin Shipley, London School of Hygiene and Tropical Medicine, for carrying out the statistical analyses.

REFERENCES

Aitken, M. and Longford, N. (1986). Statistical modelling issues in school effectiveness studies (with discussion). *J. R. Statist. Soc. Ser. A,* **149,** 1–43.

Blackburn, H. and Jacobs, D. (1984). Sources of the diet–heart controversy: confusion over population versus individual correlations. *Circulation,* **70,** 755–80.

Demets, D. L. (1987). Methods for combining randomized clinical trials: strengths and limitations. *Statist. Med.,* **6,** 341–8.

Elliott, P. (1991). Observational studies of salt and blood pressure. *Hypertension,* **17** (Suppl. I), I-3–8.

Elliott, P. and Stamler, R. (1988). Manual of operations for 'INTERSALT', an international cooperative study of the relation of sodium and potassium to blood pressure. *Controll. Clin. Trials,* **9** (Suppl.), 1–118S.

Feinleib, M. and Leaverton, P. E. (1984). Ecological fallacies in epidemiology. In *Health information systems* (eds P. E. Leaverton and L. Massé), pp. 33–61, Praeger, New York.

Goldstein, H. (1987). *Multilevel models in educational and social research,* Charles Griffin, London.

Hashimoto, T., Fujita, Y., Ueshima, H., Kagamimori, S., Kasamatsu, T., Morioka, S., Mikawa, K., Naruse, Y., Nakagawa, H., Hara, N., Yanagawa, H., and Elliott, P. (1989). Urinary sodium and potassium excretion, body mass, alcohol intake and blood pressure in three Japanese populations. *J. Hum. Hypertension,* **3,** 315–21.

Hsiao, Z.-K., Wang, S. Y., Hong, Z. G., Liu, K., Cheng, T. Y., Stamler, J., and Tao, S.-C. (1986). Timed overnight sodium and potassium excretion and blood pressure in steel workers in north China. *J. Hypertension*, **4**, 345–50.

INTERSALT Co-operative Research Group (1986). INTERSALT Study, An international co-operative study on the relation of blood pressure to electrolyte excretion in populations. 1. Design and Methods. *J. Hypertension*, **4**, 781–7.

INTERSALT Co-operative Research Group (1988). INTERSALT: an international study of electrolyte excretion and blood pressure. Results for 24-hour urinary sodium and potassium excretion. *Br. Med. J.*, **297**, 319–28.

INTERSALT Co-operative Research Group (1989). The INTERSALT study: further results (ed. P. Elliott). *J. Hum. Hypertension*, **3**, 279–408.

Kesteloot, H., Huang, D. X., Li, Y.-L., Geboers, J., and Joossens, J. V. (1987). The relationship between cations and blood pressure in the People's Republic of China. *Hypertension*, **9**, 654–9.

Liu, K., Cooper, R., McKeever, J., McKeever, P., Byington, R., Soltero, I., Stamler, R., Gosch, F., Stevens, E. and Stamler, J. (1979). Assessment of the association between habitual salt intake and high blood pressure: methodological problems. *Am. J. Epidemiol.*, **110**, 219–24.

Liu, L. S., Tao, S. C., and Lai, S. H. (1984). Relationship between salt excretion and blood pressure in various regions of China. *Bull. WHO*, **62**, 255–60.

Liu, L., Xie, J., and Fang, W. (1988). Urinary cations and blood pressure: a collaborative study of 16 districts in China. *J. Hypertension*, **6** (Suppl. 4), S587–90.

MacMahon, S., Peto, R., Cutler, J., Collins, R., Sorlie, P., Neaton, J., Abbott, R., Godwin, J., Dyer, A., and Stamler, J. (1990). Blood pressure, stroke, and coronary heart disease. Part I, Prolonged differences in blood pressure: Prospective observational studies corrected for the regression dilution bias. *Lancet*, **335**, 765–74.

Morgenstern, H. (1982). Uses of ecological analysis in epidemiologic research. *Am. J. Publ. Health*, **72**, 1336–44.

National Center for Health Statistics (1983). Dietary intake and cardiovascular risk factors, Part 1, Blood pressure correlates. *Vital and Health Statistics* Series 11, No. 226. DHHS Pub. No. (PHS) 83–1676. Public Health Service. US Government Printing Office, Washington, DC.

Pan, W. H., Tseng, W. P., You, F.-Jr., Tai, Y., and Chou, J. (1990). Positive relationship between urinary sodium chloride and blood pressure in Chinese health examinees and its association with calcium excretion. *J. Hypertension*, **8**, 873–8.

Peto, R. (1987). Why do we need systematic overviews of randomised trials? (With discussion.) Transcript of oral presentation. *Statist. Med.*, **6**, 233–44.

Piantadosi, S., Byar, D. P., and Green, S. B. (1988). The ecological fallacy. *Am. J. Epidemiol.*, **127**, 893–904.

Selvin, H. C. (1958). Durkheim's 'suicide' and problems of empirical research. *Am. J. Sociol.*, **63**, 607–19.

13

Linoleic acid, antioxidant vitamins, and coronary heart disease

D. A. Wood and M. F. Oliver

INTRODUCTION

In our review of linoleic acid, antioxidant vitamins, and coronary heart disease (CHD) the scientific evidence from clinical, epidemiological, and experimental studies in man is examined. Most of the evidence presented comes from laboratory analyses of fatty acid composition of various tissues, particularly depot fat, and antioxidant vitamin levels in blood, all primarily used as surrogates for dietary intake. This review is divided into three main sections.

1. Clinical studies of patients with various manifestations of atherosclerosis (CHD, stroke, and peripheral arterial disease).
2. Epidemiological studies between and within populations:
   (a) cross-cultural comparisons of populations with different CHD mortality rates;
   (b) within-population studies of individuals, both retrospective and prospective, in relation to clinical manifestations of CHD (angina, myocardial infarction, and death).
3. Randomized experiments of dietary modifications of fatty acid intake in individuals (there are no prevention trials of antioxidant vitamins) in the primary prevention of CHD.

Burr and Burr (1929) first described the essentiality of dietary fat for animals and, by experiment, identified a deficiency of linoleic acid (C18: $2n-6$) as the essential fatty acid. Linoleic acid is termed essential because, for many animals and man, the only source is the diet (Sanders 1988); such species are unable to synthesize linoleic acid. When man is fed a fat-free diet, plasma linoleic acid rapidly decreases, and eicosatrienoic acid, normally only present in trace quantities, increases (Weir *et al.* 1975). These changes in fatty acids are identical with those reported in other species with essential fatty acid deficiency (Holman 1968).

Sinclair (1956) postulated a chronic relative deficiency of polyenoic essential fatty acids as a cause of coronary thrombosis. He proposed two mechanisms whereby 'a dietary high in saturated fats and unnatural fats, and relatively low linoleic and arachadonic acids' caused atheroma and thrombosis. Cholesterol becomes esterified with abnormal or unusually saturated fatty acids, he suggested, and these abnormal esters are less readily disposed of and so cause atheroma. He also proposed that phospholipids containing abnormal or unusually saturated fatty acids increase the coagulability of blood, thereby contributing to coronary thrombosis. Sinclair rejected Keys' (1952) initial hypothesis that total dietary fat, of whatever kind, was related to atheroma. In fact Keys' Seven Countries Study (Keys 1970), comprising 11 579 men agd 40–59 years, reported a positive correlation between percentage diet calories from total fat ($r = 0.50$), but a stronger correlation with saturated fat ($r = 0.84$) and CHD mortality. No association was found with polyunsaturated fatty acid intake and CHD even at the 15 year mortality follow-up (Keys *et al.* 1986). As the averages for calories from linoleic acid in these populations ranged from 3 to 7 per cent, with only trivial contributions from other polyenes, Keys concluded that 'such small variations in dietary polyunsaturated fat would have, at most, only a trivial effect on the concentration of cholesterol in the blood, or risk associated with it'. In contrast, no within-population dietary studies have shown any relationship between saturated fat and risk of CHD, although Shekelle *et al.* (1981) and Morris *et al.* (1977) found an inverse relationship between polyunsaturated fats and CHD. Yet saturated fat and CHD, mediated via blood cholesterol, has dominated research, and the influence of other types of fats has received less attention. As fat and vitamin consumption takes many days to measure accurately (Thomson *et al.* 1988) investigators have used dietary surrogates, usually tissue fatty acids and blood vitamin levels. Adipose tissue fatty acid composition is the most reliable reflection of long-term dietary intake of linoleic acid, with a slow turnover (50 per cent at 12 months) in the adipocyte triglyceride pool (Beynen *et al.* 1980), and this relationship has been confirmed in feeding experiments (Dayton *et al.* 1967). Fatty acid composition of blood lipid fractions in fasting man, particularly cholesterol esters, can also reflect medium-term dietary intake of linoleic acid. Antioxidant vitamin levels usually reflect recent, rather than long-term, consumption.

CLINICAL STUDIES OF PATIENTS WITH ATHEROSCLEROSIS

Retrospective studies

Fatty acids

Following Sinclair's letter, James *et al.* (1957) reported the fatty acid composition of blood lipids in 12 CHD patients and found no differences compared with healthy volunteers, but most subsequent investigators (Lewis 1958; Antonis and Bersohn 1960; Schrade *et al.* 1960; Lawrie *et al.* 1961; Böttcher and Woodford 1961; Bang *et al.* 1968; Allard *et al.* 1973) found lower linoleic acid in lipid fractions of patients with atherosclerosis (Table 13.1). Kingsbury *et al.* (1962) and others (Heffernen 1964; Antonini *et al.* 1970) extended these studies of plasma fatty acids to include adipose tissue composition and, although adipose linoleic acid was consistently lower in patients with atherosclerosis, this difference was not statistically significant. In the largest clinical study, comprising 79 men with acute myocardial infarction, Kirkeby *et al.* (1972*a,b*) found significantly lower adipose linoleic acid compared with surgical control patients only in those patients with no previous history of CHD.

Fatty acid composition of other blood components—platelets and erythrocytes—has also been examined and, with the exception of Nordøy and Rødset (1970), all subsequent investigators (Renaud *et al.* 1970; Lang *et al.* 1977; Valles *et al.* 1979; Lea *et al.* 1982; Simpson *et al.* 1982) found lower levels of linoleic acid and other long-chain polyunsaturated fatty acids in patients following acute myocardial infarction.

Antioxidant vitamins

Fewer clinical studies of antioxidant vitamins in CHD patients have been reported (Table 13.1). Ramirez and Flowers (1980) found that men with significant coronary artery obstructions and regional wall kinetic abnormalities had lower leucocyte ascorbic acid levels than those with normal arteriograms, irrespective of smoking status, whereas other workers (Mayet *et al.* 1986; Labadarios *et al.* 1987) found no difference in vitamin C levels in patients with a history of myocardial infarction compared with hospital controls. When studied at the time of myocardial infarction patients had significantly lower vitamin B6 (Serfontein *et al.* 1985; Vermaak *et al.* 1986), and in one study (Labadarios *et al.* 1987) significantly higher vitamins A and E, both reflecting higher lipid levels in those with CHD compared with controls.

Prospective studies

Fatty acids

A prospective relationship between polyunsaturated fatty acids and myocardial infarction was first reported by Kingsbury *et al.* (1969). A significant inverse relationship was found between the percentage of dienoic acids (reflecting alkaline isomerization of linoleic acid) in plasma cholesterol esters and incidence of myocardial infarction and vascular death (Table 13.1). In the lowest dienoic acid concentration, nearly all patients had a non-fatal myocardial infarction or died, whereas for those with the highest concentrations none developed a myocardial infarction

Table 13.1 Clinical studies of fatty acids and antioxidant vitamins in atherosclerotic patients

Reference	Cases	Controls	Measurements	Results
Retrospective: fatty acids				
James *et al.* 1957	12 CHD patients (40–51 years) of both sexes	Age- and sex-matched healthy volunteers	Red blood cells, plasma phospholipids, and acetone soluble fraction of plasma lipids	No differences in fatty acid composition
Lewis 1958	12 patients with cardiac infarction	8 control subjects	Plasma CE	Linoleic acid significantly lower in cases: 40.6% vs. 53.2%
Antonis and Bersohn 1960	23 patients (33–67 years) of both sexes with AMI	69 healthy subjects (18–62 years) of both sexes drawn from technical staff	Triglycerides within 1 week of admission	Dienoic (linoleic) and other polyenoic acids lower in cases
Schrade *et al.* 1960	31 atherosclerotic (angina MI, stroke or sclerosis of peripheral arteries) patients (41–76 years) of both sexes	21 controls: male patients (18–71 years) under observation, or members of hospital staff	Serum CE, phospholipids, glycerides, and unesterified fatty acids	Linoleic acid in serum (20.9% vs. 23.5%), CE (38.0% vs. 47.1%), and phospholipids (19.6% vs. 22.2%) was significantly lower in cases
Lawrie *et al.* 1961	16 CHD patients (47–77 years) of both sexes	16 apparently normal subjects	CE, triglycerides, and phospholipids	No differences in linoleic acid
Böttcher and Woodford 1961	4 men (41–57 years) following surgery for renal artery stenosis	4 healthy men (18–24 years)	CE, phospholipids, glycerides, and free fatty acids	Linoleic acid in CE significantly lower in cases: 48% vs. 55.5%
Kingsbury *et al.* 1962	9 atherosclerotic (angina or coronary thrombosis with peripheral arterial disease or aortic aneurysm) patients (51–74 years)	9 hospital controls (48–73 years) matched for age and other CHD risk factors	Plasma CE and AT	Significantly lower proportion of dienes (linoleic acid) and tetraenes, and higher hexaenes and triene/ tetraene and hexaene/ tetraene ratios in cases; adipose dienes and tetraenes also significantly lower in cases
Heffernen 1964	7 men (44–68 years) with MI	8 apparently healthy men (17–53 years)	AT	No difference in linoleic acid

Reference	Cases	Controls	Lipid fraction	Results
Bang et al. 1968	32 patients (40–91 years) of both sexes with AMI	28 subjects (23–69 years) of both sexes without any known coronary or atherosclerotic disease	CE, triglycerides, and phospholipids within 72 hours of onset of symptoms	No differences in fatty acid composition
Antonini et al. 1970	18 male (average age 68 years) and 15 female (average age 70 years) patients with cerebrovascular disease	22 apparently healthy subjects (average age 28 years) of both sexes	AT	Linoleic acid significantly lower (for males only) in cases: 8.2% vs. 10.6%
Nordøy and Rødset 1970	15 male CHD (angina pectoris or MI) patients (42–69 years)	20 healthy male controls (30–60 years)	Platelet phospholipids	No differences in linoleic acid for any of the platelet phospholipids
Renaud et al. 1970	10 male patients (mean age 43 years) 10 days after AMI	12 physicians or hospital employees (mean age 39 years) with no CHD risk factors	Platelet fatty acids	Platelet linoleic acid significantly lower in cases
Kirkeby et al. (1972a,b)	79 men (40–70 years) with AMI: 43 AMI cases with no previous history of CHD; 36 AMI cases with a previous history of CHD	25 surgical control patients matched for age	CE (within 24 hours) and AT (within 5 days of admission)	Linoleic acid in CE and AT lower in cases with no previous history: CE, 47.1% vs. 54.9%; AT, 8.0% vs. 9.5% compared with controls. Cases with a history of CHD had significantly *higher* adipose linoleic acid: AT, 11.5% vs. 9.5%
Allard et al. 1973	27 CHD patients (average age 54 years) including one woman, investigated by coronary arteriography	28 healthy subjects (average age 42 years) of both sexes free of CHD on coronary arteriography	CE, triglycerides, and phospholipids	No differences in linoleic acid in any of the lipid fractions
Lang et al. 1977	34 consecutive male (mean age 65 years) AMI patients	33 hospitalized male patients (mean age 33 years) free of CHD with normal resting ECGs	AT	Linoleic acid lower, although not significantly so, in cases

Table 13.1 (*contd.*)

Reference	Cases	Controls	Measurements	Results
Valles *et al.* 1979	24 AMI cases	24 age-matched controls	Platelet fatty acids within 24 hours of admission	Linoleic acid in the triglyceride fraction of platelets significantly lower in cases: 6.3% vs. 9.7%
Lea *et al.* 1982	20 MI patients	17 healthy age-matched controls	Erythrocyte fatty acid composition	Linoleic acid significantly lower in cases: 7.9% vs. 8.8%
Simpson *et al.* 1982	32 men (<60 years) with MI	Age- and social-class-matched occupational controls	Erythrocyte fatty acid composition	Linoleic acid in red cell membrane phospholipid choline was significantly lower in cases: 11.9% vs. 18.5%
Retrospective: vitamins				
Ramirez and Flowers 1980	150 patients (19–78 years) of both sexes who had cardiac catheterization		Leucocyte ascorbic acid levels	Ascorbic acid levels significantly lower in patients with significant coronary artery obstructions and wall motion abnormalities compared with patients with normal arteriograms
Serfontein *et al.* 1985	15 male patients (average age 56 years) with AMI	28 healthy male (average age 46 years) business executives	Plasma vitamin B6 measured within 24 hours of symptoms	Vitamin B6 significantly lower in cases: 5.4% vs. 11.4%
Vermaak *et al.* 1986	34 patients (average age 58 years) with AMI and 16 patients (average age 53 years) with chronic CHD	30 age- and sex-matched healthy volunteers (average age 55 years)	Plasma vitamin B6 measured within 48 hours of admission in AMI cases	Vitamin B6 significantly lower in AMI cases (5.2 vs. 11.5 mg/ml) but no difference found between chronic CHD cases and controls

Reference	Patients	Controls	Measurement	Results
Mayet et al. 1986	73 Indian patients (mean age 49 years) of both sexes with a diagnosis of MI	77 Indian control patients (mean age 36 years) of both sexes drawn from the medical wards of the same hospital	Leucocyte ascorbic acid levels	No difference in leucocyte ascorbic acid level
Labadarios et al. 1987	30 consecutive patients (27–73 years) with AMI	19 age-matched (30–75 years) and sex-matched surgical controls	Vitamins A, E, C, B6	Vitamin C lower and vitamins A, E, and total lipids all significantly higher in cases; no difference for vitamin B6
Prospective: fatty acids				
Kingsbury et al. 1969	146 consecutive male (35–75 years) patients with peripheral arterial disease of whom 18 had a non-fatal MI and 24 had a sudden death (21 MIs and 3 strokes) over a 4 year follow-up		Plasma CE	Significant inverse relationship between percentage dienoic (linoleic) acid and MI and vascular death
Kingsbury et al. 1974	80 male patients (average age 59 years) with peripheral arterial disease of whom 14 had a non-fatal vascular death (MI) and 13 had a vascular death (12 MIs and 1 stroke) over a 5 year follow-up		Plasma CE	Significant inverse relationship between linoleic acid and incidence of AMI and vascular death
Valek et al. 1985	107 male (<65 years) patients with MI who survived for 3 months and of whom 23 died of cardiac disease over a 5 year follow-up		Total serum lipids	Linoleic acid together with previous MI, heart volume index, and hyperlipoproteinaemia all significantly and independently related to risk of cardiovascular death

MI, myocardial infarction; AMI, acute myocardial infarction; CE, cholesterol esters; AT, adipose tissue; ECG, electrocardiogram.

and only one died. Kingsbury *et al.* (1974) later reported that only linoleate distinguished patients with non-fatal or fatal myocardial infarcts from those without symptoms of heart disease. One other study (Valek *et al.* 1985) has confirmed this prospective inverse relationship between linoleic acid, measured on this occasion in total serum lipids, and risk of cardiovascular death over 5 years in men following a myocardial infarction.

EPIDEMIOLOGICAL STUDIES OF POPULATIONS

Cross-cultural studies

In contrast with Keys' Seven Countries Study, all cross-cultural comparisons of tissue fatty acids and blood antioxidant vitamins have been retrospective and small in size.

Fatty acids

All early studies comparing adipose fatty acid composition between cultures found no significant differences in linoleic acid (Table 13.2), but subjects were highly selected, for example from out-patient clinics and hospital wards, and few in number (Antonis and Bersohn 1960; Hegsted *et al.* 1962; Lee *et al.* 1962; McLaren and Read 1962; Scott *et al.* 1962*a*; Shorland *et al.* 1969). A comparison of Korean soldiers on Korean and American diets with American soldiers found the highest adipose linoleic acid in Korean soldiers eating their own diet and the lowest in Americans, with Korean soldiers on an American diet in an intermediate position (Scott *et al.* 1962*b*). One autopsy study of adipose fatty acid composition found that Americans had higher proportions of saturated fatty acids, but less linoleic and longer-chain polyunsaturated fatty acids, compared with Japanese men who died suddenly and unexpectedly from CHD and other unrelated causes (Insull *et al.* 1969).

Unlike these earlier surveys, Logan *et al.* (1978) studied a representative sample of healthy people. Men aged 40 years living in two cities, Edinburgh and Stockholm, with a three-fold difference in CHD mortality for this age group were randomly selected. Numerous measurements were made, including lipoproteins, blood pressure, glucose tolerance, and insulin, but the proportionate storage of linoleic acid in adipose tissue was the most significant difference between the cities. Linoleic acid was lower in Edinburgh men with the higher CHD mortality, and a weighed dietary survey (Thomson *et al.* 1982) confirmed a lower consumption of linoleic acid in these men. Another cross-cultural comparison, based on random samples of healthy middle-aged men from three countries, found the lowest proportion of adipose linoleic acid in men from North Karelia, Finland, where CHD mortality was highest, and the highest proportion in

Italy where mortality was lowest, with intermediate proportions in Scotland and Southwest Finland (Riemersma *et al.* 1986). These regional differences in adipose linoleic acid remained highly significant in multivariate analysis when CHD risk factors—smoking, blood pressure, lipids, and obesity—were taken into account.

Antioxidant vitamins

Plasma antioxidant vitamins measured in the same cross-cultural study (Riemersma *et al.* 1986) of Finnish, Scottish, and Italian men (Table 13.2) showed no consistent relationship with CHD (Riemersma *et al.* 1990). Vitamin A did not differ between the three groups of men. β-carotene was lowest in Scotland but did not differ between Italian and Finnish men, and vitamin C showed the same pattern. Vitamin E cholesterol was lowest in Scotland, although not very different from Finnish men, and both these groups of men had lower levels compared with the Italians. Thus vitamin E cholesterol was the only naturally occurring antioxidant to be low in those populations with high CHD mortality, as might be expected from dietary differences between northern and southern Europe.

Gey *et al.* (1991) expanded this study of plasma antioxidant vitamins to 16 European study populations, including the four populations reported by Riemersma *et al.* (1990), in relation to CHD mortality. Healthy middle-aged men were selected at random from each country, except for the large cohort of Swiss industry employees in Thun. Vitamin E cholesterol ($r = 0.62$), and vitamin A cholesterol ($r = 0.24$) were both inversely related to CHD mortality, but there was no relationship with vitamin C or carotene. When other CHD risk factors in these populations—total cholesterol, diastolic blood pressure, and smoking—were examined in multivariate analysis, vitamin E cholesterol was more strongly associated with CHD mortality than any other factor.

Studies within populations

Retrospective studies

Fatty acids   Only a small number of retrospective population studies of fatty acids and CHD have been undertaken (Table 13.3).

Two population autopsy surveys, which examined the relationship between adipose fatty acid composition and CHD death, found no association with linoleic acid. Thomas and Scott (1981) studied autopsies from 10 areas in England and Wales and found that adipose linoleic acid was almost identical in CHD deaths compared with deaths from other causes. Strong *et al.* (1984) compared adipose fatty acid composition in black and white men who died from CHD with that of men who had died from external violence (accident, suicide, or homicide) or any natural cause other than atherosclerotic disease. Again, there was no difference in adipose linoleic

Table 13.2 Cross-cultural studies of fatty acids and antioxidant vitamins

Author	Populations	Results
Fatty acids		
Antonis and Bersohn 1960	57 healthy Bantu males (20–60 years) and 46 healthy European males (18–62), the latter drawn from the technical staff of a Research Institute	Dienoic (linoleic) acids in triglycerides higher in Bantu males
McLaren and Read 1962	26 Africans, 11 Asians, and 10 Europeans; AT samples taken at surgery	No differences in total unsaturated fatty acids
Lee et al. 1962	33 East African, 55 USA white, and 55 USA negro patients of both sexes (20–89 years) selected from hospital wards and clinics	No difference in adipose linoleic acid
Scott et al. 1962a	32 Guatemalans and 32 white North American patients of both sexes (30–70 years) selected from hospital wards and a church congregation	No difference in adipose linoleic acid
Hegsted et al. 1962	17 Bostonians (USA), 42 Nigerians from three tribal groups, 27 Japanese, 3 Colombians, and 12 Jamaican adults of both sexes; AT samples taken at surgery or autopsy	No difference in adipose linoleic acid
Scott et al. 1962b	21 Korean monks, 10 farmers, and 15 city dwellers, 20 Korean soldiers on Korean diet and 21 on an American diet, and 19 American soldiers with ages averaging between 23 and 44 years	Adipose linoleic acid significantly lower (8.9%) in American soldiers compared with Korean soldiers (17%), with Korean soldiers on an American diet in an intermediate position (12%)
Insull et al. 1969	Autopsies of 50 Americans and 56 Japanese men (15–65 years) with sudden unexpected deaths, mainly attributed to atherosclerotic diseases	Japanese had significantly higher adipose linoleic acid: 16.5% vs. 10.2%

Shorland et al. 1969	22 randomly selected male and female (18–77 years) Polynesians, and 15 Maori and 14 Europeans patients selected at random from hospital wards and clinics	No difference in adipose linoleic acid
Logan et al. 1978	Random population samples of 107 healthy men (40 years) in Edinburgh (Scotland) and 82 in Stockholm (Sweden)	Adipose linoleic acid significantly lower in Edinburgh men: 7.3% vs. 11.8%
Riemersma et al. 1986	Random population samples of men (40–49 years) from North Karelia and Southwest Finland, Scotland (Edinburgh), and Italy (Sapri)	Adipose linoleic acid lowest in North Karelia, Finland (7.4%), intermediate in Edinburgh, Scotland (8.8%) and Southwest Finland (8.1%), and highest in Sapri, Italy (13.5%)
Antioxidant vitamins		
Riemersma et al. 1990	Random population samples of men (40–49 years) from North Karelia and Southwest Finland, Scotland (Edinburgh), and Italy (Sapri)	Vitamin E cholesterol in Edinburgh, Scotland (3.4 µmol/mmol) and Finland (3.5 µmol/mmol) both significantly lower than in Sapri, Italy (4.8 µmol/mmol)
Gey et al. 1991	16 random population samples (with exception of employees in Thun, Switzerland) of men (40–49 years) from 10 countries: Denmark, Finland, France, German Democratic Republic, Israel, Italy, Northern Ireland, Scotland, Spain, and Switzerland	Vitamin E cholesterol ($r = -0.62$) and vitamin A cholesterol ($r = -0.24$) were independently related to CHD mortality

AT, adipose tissue.

Table 13.3 Population studies of fatty acids, antioxidant vitamins, and CHD

Author	Cases	Controls	Measurements	Results
Retrospective: fatty acids				
Thomas et al. 1981	Autopsy survey of 136 male CHD deaths from 10 geographic areas	95 deaths from other causes drawn from the same areas	AT	No difference in linoleic acid between cases and controls
Strong et al. 1984	New Orleans Community Pathology Survey of 66 black and white male (25–44 years) CHD deaths	988 black and white male (25–44 years) deaths from other causes	AT	No difference in linoleic acid
Wood et al. 1984	Edinburgh Fife Community (Prevalence) survey of 28 men (45–54 years) with newly diagnosed CHD	343 men (45–54 years) with no CHD	AT and P	Linoleic acid significantly lower in new CHD cases: 7.8% vs. 8.9%. No difference in P linoleic acid
Wood et al. 1987	Population case control study of 110 men (35–54 years) with newly diagnosed angina and 80 incident cases of AMI	408 healthy age- and sex-matched controls drawn from the same population	AT and P	Linoleic acid in both AT and P significantly lower for both cases of angina (AT, 8.6% vs. 9.8%; P, 5.6% vs. 5.9%) and AMI (AT, 8.8% vs. 9.8%; P, 5.3% vs. 5.9%)
Retrospective: antioxidant vitamins				
Roussow et al. 1985	71 men (45–54 years) with probable and possible CHD identified from a population survey	110 randomly selected controls with no evidence of CHD drawn from the same population	Plasma vitamin B6	No difference in vitamin B6 between either probable or possible CHD cases and controls
Saha et al. 1988	Autopsy survey of CHD deaths in Singapore ethnic groups (Chinese, Indian, Malay, Caucasian, and Eurasian) of both sexes	181 accidental deaths from the same populations	Liver	Vitamin A levels significantly higher in CHD deaths (209 vs. 200 mg/kg liver) compared with accidental deaths

Salonen *et al.* 1988	Kuopio Ischaemic Heart Disease Risk Factor (Prevalence) Survey of 175 men aged 54 years with chest pain, or history of CHD or ischaemic exercise ECG	449 men aged 54 years with no CHD	Plasma vitamins	No differences in vitamin C or vitamin E
Riemersma *et al.* 1991	Population case control study of 110 men (35–54 years) with newly diagnosed angina	394 healthy age and sex matched controls drawn from the same population	Plasma vitamins	Carotene (0.30 vs. 0.49 µmol/l), vitamin C (28.1 vs. 35.3 µmol/l), and vitamin E cholesterol (3.66 vs. 3.86 µmol/l) levels all significantly lower in cases
Prospective: fatty acids			
Miettinen *et al.* 1982	Prospective case control study of 33 men (40–55 years) with fatal or non-fatal MI or sudden death over 5–7 years from a population of 1222 men	64 controls matched for age, sex, and CHD risk factor (blood pressure, lipids, smoking, obesity, and glucose tolerance)	Fatty acids of CE, triglycerides, and phospholipids	Linoleic acid (phospholipids) was significantly lower in cases: 23.4% vs. 26.1%
Prospective: antioxidant vitamins			
Salonen *et al.* 1985	Eastern Finland Heart Study (prospective case control) of 92 CHD deaths in men and women (30–64 years) over 5 years from a population of 12155	92 controls matched for age, sex, and CHD risk factor (smoking, cholesterol, blood pressure, and history of cardiovascular disease)	Serum vitamins A and E	No relationship between vitamins A and E and CHD mortality

Table 13.3 (*contd.*)

Author	Cases	Controls	Measurements	Results
Lapidus *et al.* 1986	Prospective population study of 28 fatal and non-fatal AMIs, 13 strokes, and 75 deaths from all causes in women (38–60 years) over 12 years from a population of 1462 women in Gothenburg, Sweden	1424 women initially free of CHD	24 hour recall dietary interviews	No relationship between dietary vitamin C and cardiovascular disease (MI, stroke, and death)
Gey *et al.* 1987	Basel Prospective Occupational Study of 67 CHD deaths over 7 years from a population of 3000 male pharmaceutical employees	2707 healthy survivors	Plasma vitamins	No relationship between vitamins C or E cholesterol and CHD mortality
Kok *et al.* 1987	Prospective case control study of 84 cardiovascular (56 CHD, 15 cerebrovascular, 13 other) deaths in men and women aged 37–87 years at baseline over 6–9 years from a population of 10532 inhabitants of Zoetermeer, The Netherlands	168 age- and sex-matched healthy controls drawn from surviving population	Serum vitamins A and E	No relationship between vitamins A or E and cardiovascular, coronary, and stroke mortality

AMI, acute myocardial infarction; MI, myocardial infarction; AT, adipose tissue; P, platelets; CE, cholesterol esters; ECG, electrocardiogram.

acid, either in blacks or Caucasians dying from CHD, compared with other deaths. Whilst these findings may be true, autopsy studies are difficult to interpret because adipose fatty acid composition could change as a consequence of the development of diseases other than CHD.

Quantifying the risk of non-fatal CHD in relation to tissue fatty acids was first undertaken in a population survey of a random sample of 448 middle-aged men drawn from two areas, North Edinburgh and West Fife, on the east coast of Scotland (Wood *et al.* 1984). As a change of diet following a diagnosis of CHD may bias results, an observation originally made by Kirkeby *et al.* (1972*a*), the main analysis in this study was restricted to cases diagnosed at the time of the survey. Twenty-eight men were found to have CHD (either a positive response to the World Health Organization (WHO) Chest Pain Questionnaire, or Q waves (Minnesota Codes 1.1, 1.2) on their resting electrocardiogram (ECG)) without a history of myocardial infarction or angina pectoris.

Adipose linoleic acid was lower in the new cases compared with men with no CHD. As the proportionate storage of linoleic acid fell in this population, so the prevalence of new CHD increased, with nearly a quarter of all cases occurring in the bottom decile of linoleic acid distribution. Men with a history of CHD, either myocardial infarction or angina pectoris, had higher linoleic acid levels than newly diagnosed cases, and also higher levels compared with the healthy population, reflecting an increased consumption of polyunsaturated fats amongst survivors who knew their diagnosis. The ratio of polyunsaturated to saturated fats (P/S) was lower (0.28 versus 0.32) in the new CHD cases. Logistic regression found that adipose linoleic acid, age, total cholesterol, and weight/height index each made a significant and independent contribution to the explanation of new CHD in this population. A 7 day weighed dietary survey, undertaken in a random subsample of 164 men from this study, confirmed that new CHD cases had a significantly lower dietary linoleic acid intake and a lower P/S ratio compared with the healthy population.

A population case control study was then undertaken in Edinburgh to estimate the relative risk of CHD—separately for angina pectoris and acute myocardial infarction—in relation to adipose and platelet fatty acid composition (Wood *et al.* 1987). In a postal questionnaire survey of a systematic sample of 6000 men (35–54 years), angina pectoris cases were identified using the WHO Chest Pain Questionnaire: 125 new cases were found in men who reported no medical diagnosis of angina or myocardial infarction, and 80 new cases of acute myocardial infarction, also with no history of CHD, were identified from coronary care units in the city over 1 year. Healthy controls were drawn at random from the systematic sample of 6000 men with no history of CHD.

Adipose linoleic acid was lower in cases of angina pectoris and acute myocardial infarction, and the P/S ratio was also lower in both groups of cases. Unlike the earlier cross-sectional survey (Wood *et al.* 1984), platelet linoleic acid was also lower in both groups of cases and platelet eicosapentaenoic acid was lower in angina cases, although not in acute myocardial infarction cases. An inverse relation between adipose linoleic acid and both angina and acute myocardial infarction was found, with the highest unadjusted relative risk (95 per cent confidence intervals) for angina of 3.2 (1.5–7.0) and for acute myocardial infarction of 3.0 (1.3–7.2) occurring in the lowest quintile of adipose linoleic acid. In logistic regression low adipose linoleic acid made an independent contribution to the explanation of angina, together with low platelet eicosapentaenoic acid and smoking habit, whereas for acute myocardial infarction linoleic acid in adipose tissue and platelets was phased out by smoking habit, the only risk factor common to angina and acute myocardial infarction in this study.

Antioxidant vitamins   With one exception all retrospective population studies of antioxidant vitamins and CHD have found no associations (Table 13.3). Roussow *et al.* (1985) reported no difference in vitamin B6 between possible and probable CHD cases compared with controls. Salonen *et al.* (1988) also found no difference in plasma vitamin C or E cholesterol between those with and without CHD defined on the basis of symptoms, or a history of CHD, or objective evidence of ischaemia on a bicycle ergometer exercise test in the Kuopio Risk Factor Study. The vitamin A content of liver, the body's major store, did not differ between those dying from CHD and from accidental deaths (Saha *et al.* 1988) in a survey of ethnic groups in Singapore.

In a population case-control study already described (Wood *et al.* 1987) the relation between risk of angina pectoris and plasma concentrations of vitamins A, C, and E, and carotene was examined (Riemersma *et al.* 1991). Vitamins C and E and carotene were each inversely related to the risk of angina. The highest unadjusted relative risk (95 per cent confidence intervals) for angina occurred in the lowest quintile: vitamin C, 2.4 (1.2–4.8); vitamin E, 2.5 (1.2–5.1); carotene, 2.6 (1.3–5.3). After adjustment for CHD risk factors and season, only vitamin E cholesterol made a significant and independent contribution to the risk of angina.

Prospective studies

Fatty acids   A prospective relationship between CHD and fatty acid composition of plasma cholesterol esters was first reported by Miettinen *et al.* (1982) (Table 13.3). From a sample of 1222 middle-aged men who had one or more CHD risk factors, but were free of CHD at the start of the study, 33 experienced fatal or non-fatal myocardial infarction or sudden death during a follow-up of 7 years. For these, cases controls were selected from the remaining 1189 men to match for age, blood pressure, cholesterol and triglyceride concentrations, smoking, obesity, and glucose tolerance at the start of the follow-up. The fatty acid composition of phospholipids, cholesterol esters, and triglycerides was determined from fasting serum obtained at entry, and for serum phospholipids the cases had a significantly lower level of linoleic acid and lower total polyunsaturated fatty acids. As cases and controls were matched for CHD risk factors, this fatty acid pattern of serum lipids was considered an independent risk factor for CHD.

Antioxidant vitamins Vitamins A and E did not differ between cases dying from CHD and matched healthy controls in the Eastern Finland Heart Study (Salonen *et al*. 1985), and Kok *et al*. (1987) found a similar result for CHD and stroke deaths. Stähelin *et al*. (1982) also found no association between serum vitamin A and death from heart disease and stroke in the Basel Study of male pharmaceutical employees, and Gey *et al*. (1987) later reported no relationship between vitamin C and E cholesterol and subsequent death from CHD in the same population. Vitamin C intake in women, estimated from 24 hour diet recall interviews, was not related to non-fatal myocardial infarction and stroke or to death from cardiovascular disease (Lapidus *et al*. 1986).

DIETARY TRIALS

A dietary experiment can only test the converse of aetiological associations between fatty acids, antioxidant vitamins, and CHD by determining whether a change in diet can *reduce* the risk of this disease. All randomized dietary trials in the primary prevention of CHD have used experimental diets low in saturates and high in polyunsaturates, and therefore the effect of varying dietary intake of only one kind of fat at a time has never been tested in relation to CHD. Three randomized dietary trials of primary CHD prevention—Los Angeles Veterans Administration, Helsinki Mental Hospital, and the Oslo Study—have been reported.

In the Los Angeles trial of elderly institutionalized men (Dayton *et al*. 1969) vegetable oils were substituted for two-thirds of animal fat in the experimental diet, with linoleic acid accounting for 38 per cent of total fat compared with 12 per cent in the control diet. After 2 years adipose linoleic acid had risen to 24 per cent in the experimental group compared with 9 per cent in the control group. In the Finnish Mental Hospital Study (Turpeinen *et al*. 1979), which intervened in middle-aged male and female patients in two hospital populations, the experimental diet almost totally replaced dairy fats with vegetable oils, mainly soya bean. Whilst total fat intake remained the same in these two groups, there was a substantial reduction in saturated fat, no significant change in mono-unsaturates, and an increase in total polyunsaturates in the experimental group with a P/S ratio of 1.48 compared with 0.25 in controls. After 5 years adipose linoleic acid was 27 per cent in the experimental group compared with 10.3 per cent in the control group. In contrast with these earlier studies, the Oslo Diet Heart Study (Hjermann *et al.* 1981) intervened in high risk middle-aged men with hypercholesterolaemia and coronary risk score in the upper quintile of the distribution. A substantial reduction in saturated fat intake was the major dietary change with only a slight increase in polyunsaturated fats. A weighed dietary survey confirmed a lower total fat intake in the experimental group, largely due to a reduction in saturated fats, resulting in a P/S ratio greater than 1 in the intervention group compared with 0.39 in the control group.

All these experimental studies achieved substantial changes in dietary fat intake, both reduced saturated fats and increased polyunsaturates, with a corresponding rise in adipose linoleic acid over several years. Coronary incidence was lower in the experimental groups of each trial compared with the control groups, but there was no difference in CHD or total mortality.

DISCUSSION

From our review of linoleic acid, antioxidant vitamins, and CHD it is appropriate to consider some biological implications of this scientific evidence and make some recommendations for public health.

Whilst discussion of the mechanisms through which a low intake of linoleic acid and of antioxidant vitamins, and low tissue levels of these nutrients, might lead to CHD is beyond the scope of this epidemiological review, a brief comment is necessary. Linoleic acid, like other long-chain unsaturated fatty acids, is potentially unstable and prone to peroxidation. When this occurs, its biological availability is even further reduced. Peroxidation is potentiated when tissue antioxidant levels are low. It is probable that this situation would favour the incorporation of oxidized low density lipoprotein (LDL) into arterial walls. An increased tendency to peroxidation would also favour thrombosis by allowing saturated fatty acids to have an unbalanced influence on clotting mechanisms. Furthermore, platelet adhesiveness is increased when vitamin E levels are low. The myocardium may also be adversely affected after periods of ischaemia if tissue concentrations of free-radical scavengers, such as the antioxidant vitamins, are low. The importance of oxidative modification of LDL and increased atherosclerosis, thrombosis, and myocardial ischaemic damage, all leading to CHD, may therefore depend to some extent on the fatty acid composition and antioxidant vitamin content of the diet.

The inverse relationship between linoleic acid and CHD within coronary-prone populations appears to be as strong as the direct relationship of the classical CHD risk factors and is independent of them, apart from a close interrelationship with smoking. Whilst these findings for linoleic acid probably have a dietary explanation, because food is the only source of this essential faty acid, it is possible that CHD patients may absorb less of this nutrient—some will have relative mesenteric ischaemia on the basis of arterial disease—or may catabolize or store it differently from healthy people. Dietary surveys have actually confirmed a lower consumption of polyunsaturated fatty acids, particularly linoleic acid, in populations with a high CHD mortality (Thomson *et al.* 1982). Cigarette smokers in particular consume less food containing linoleic acid compared with non-smokers (Thomson *et al.* 1988), and consequently have a lower P/S ratio and a lower proportion of adipose linoleic acid. Furthermore, the more cigarettes that are smoked the lower is the percentage of adipose linoleate (Wood *et al.* 1987). Cigarette smokers also have a lower percentage of eicosapentaenoic acid in platelets than observed in non-smokers. However, the total energy, fat, carbohydrate, and protein intakes of smokers are the same as those of non-smokers. The reasons why smokers eat less linoleic acid is not clear. While the comparison with non-smokers may be fallacious, in so far as non-smokers may be more health conscious, it is also possible that cigarette smoking has altered palatability to such an extent, for example smokers add nearly twice as much salt to their food, that there is an unconscious rejection of foods rich in polyunsaturated oils, and this may be one reason why smokers are at higher risk of CHD in coronary-prone populations.

Therefore in summary dietary saturated fat is directly associated with CHD mortality across countries, whereas in some high mortality populations polyunsaturated fat, and in particular the essential fatty acid linoleic acid, is inversely related to an individual's risk of this disease. Clinical studies of patients with atherosclerosis have shown a lower proportionate storage of linoleic acid in several tissues compared with controls, and epidemiological studies, both retrospective and prospective, have quantified an inverse risk relationship between linoleic acid and CHD, separately for angina, acute myocardial infarction, and CHD death. Antioxidant vitamins, and in particular vitamin E, have a strong inverse relationship with CHD mortality in cross-cultural comparisons. In one case-control study a similar inverse relationship was found between vitamin E and angina, but three other retrospective studies and four prospective epidemiological studies have all found no association between antioxidant vitamins and CHD.

The inverse relationship between linoleic acid, and other polyunsaturated fatty acids, and CHD needs to be confirmed prospectively in other coronary-prone populations by measurement of dietary intake as well as by proportionate storage in tissues, so that interrelationships with other fatty acids—saturated, mono-unsaturated, and other long-chain polyunsaturated fatty acids—and other dietary nutrients, including antioxidant vitamins, can be examined.

PUBLIC HEALTH RECOMMENDATIONS

The epidemiological, clinical, and experimental evidence of an inverse relationship between linoleic acid and CHD is sufficiently strong to recommend that populations with a high CHD mortality should supplement their eating habits with more polyunsaturated oil, principally from cereals and vegetables, aiming at a P/S ratio in the region of 0.8. In particular, cigarette smokers who are unable to quit should follow this advice. Whilst the relationship between antioxidant vitamins and CHD is not yet sufficiently strong to justify dietary supplementation, a higher intake of foods rich in linoleic acid will naturally result in a greater consumption of the principal antioxidant vitamin E.

REFERENCES

Allard, C., Davignon, J., Marcel, Y. L., Goulet, C., Kuba, K., Alteresco, M., *et al.* (1973). Fatty acid profile of plasma lipid classes in coronary heart disease, in primary hyperlipoproteinaemias, and in healthy subjects. *Can. J. Biochem.,* **51,** 1509–14.

Antonini, F. M., Bucalossi, A., Petruzzi, E., Simoni, R., Morini, P. L., and D'Allessandro, A. (1970). Fatty acid composition of adipose tissue in normal, atherosclerotic and diabetic subjects. *Atherosclerosis,* **11,** 279–89.

Antonis, A. and Bersohn, I. (1960). Serum-triglycerides levels in South African Europeans and Bantu and ischaemic heart-disease. *Lancet,* **i,** 998–1002.

Bang, H. O., Hess Thaysen, E., and Thygsen, J. (1968). The plasma lipids and their fatty acid pattern in myocardial infarction. *Acta Med. Scand.,* **184,** 241–6.

Beynen, A. C., Hermus, R. J. J., and Hautvast, J. G. A. J. (1980). A mathematical relationship between the fatty acid composition of the diet and that of the adipose tissue in man. *Am. J. Clin. Nutr.,* **33,** 81–5.

Böttcher, C. J. F. and Woodford, F. P. (1961). Lipid and fatty-acid composition of plasma lipoproteins in cases of aortic atherosclerosis. *J. Atherosclerosis Res.,* **1,** 434–43.

Burr, G. O. and Burr, M. M. (1929). A new deficiency disease produced by the rigid exclusion of fat from the diet. *J. Biol. Chem.,* **82,** 345–67.

Dayton, S., Hashimoto, S., and Pearce, M. L. (1967). Adipose tissue linoleic acid as a criterion of adherence to a modified diet. *J. Lipid Res.,* **8,** 508–10.

Dayton, S., Pearce, M. L., Hashimoto, S., Dixon, W. J., and Tomiyasu, U. (1969). A controlled trial of a diet high in unsaturated fat in preventing complications of atherosclerosis. *Circulation,* **40** (Suppl. II), 1–63.

Gey, K. F., Stähelin, H. B., Puska, P., and Evans, A. (1987). Relationship of plasma level of vitamin C to mortality from ischemic heart disease. *Ann. N.Y. Acad. Sci.,* **498,** 110–23.

Gey, K. F., Pusha, P., Jordan, P., and Moser, U. K. (1991). Inverse correlation between plasma vitamin E and mortality from ischaemic heart disease in cross cultural epidemiology. *Am. J. Clin. Nutr.,* **53,** 3265–345.

Heffernen, A. G. A. (1964). Fatty acid composition of adipose tissue in normal and abnormal subjects. *Am. J. Clin. Nutr.,* **15,** 5–10.

Hegsted, D. M., Jack, C. W., and Stare, F. J. (1962). The composition of human adipose tissue from several parts of the world. *Am. J. Clin. Nutr.,* **10,** 11–18.

Hjermann, I., Velve Byre, K., Holme, I., and Leren, P. (1981). Effect of diet and smoking intervention on the incidence of coronary heart disease. *Lancet,* **ii,** 1303–9.

Holman, R. T. (1968). Essential fatty acid deficiency. In *Progress in the chemistry of fats and other lipids,* Vol. IX, Part 2, p. 275, Pergamon Press, Oxford.

Insull, W., Lang, P. D., Bartholomew, P., and Yoshimura, S. (1969). Studies of arteriosclerosis in Japanese and American men. *J. Clin. Invest.,* **48,** 1313–27.

James, A. T., Lovelock, J. E., Webb, J., and Trotter, W. R. (1957). The fatty acids of the blood in coronary-artery disease. *Lancet,* **i,** 705–8.

Keys, A. (1952). The cholesterol problem. *Verding,* **13,** 539–55.

Keys, A. (1970). *Coronary heart disease in seven countries.* Monogr. 29, American Heart Association.

Keys, A., Menotti, A., Karvonenn, M., Aravanis, C., Blackburn, H., Buzina, R., *et al.* (1986). The diet and 15-year death rate in the Seven Countries Study. *Am. J. Epidemiol.,* **124,** 903–15.

Kingsbury, K. J., Morgan, D. M., Aylott, C., Burton, P., Emmerson, R., and Robinson, P. J. (1962). A comparison of the polyunsaturated fatty acids of the plasma cholesterol esters and subcutaneous depot fats of atheromatous and normal people. *Clin. Sci.,* **22,** 161–70.

Kingsbury, K. J., Morgan, D. M., Stovold, R., Brett, C. G., and Anderson, J. (1969). Polyunsaturated fatty acids and myocardial infarction. Follow up of patients with aortoiliac and femoropopliteal atherosclerosis. *Lancet,* **ii,** 1325–9.

Kingsbury, K. J., Brett, C., Stovold, R., Chapman, A., Anderson, J., and Morgan, D. M. (1974). Abnormal fatty acid composition and human atherosclerosis. *Postgrad. Med. J.,* **50,** 425–40.

Kirkeby, K., Nitter-Hauge, S., and Bjerkedal, I. (1972a). Fatty acid composition of adipose tissue in male Norwegians with myocardial infarction. *Acta Med. Scand.,* **191,** 321–4.

Kirkeby, K., Ingvaldsen, P., and Bjerkedal, I. (1972b). Fatty acid composition of serum lipids in men with myocardial infarction. *Acta Med. Scand.,* **192,** 513–19.

Kok, F. J., de Bruijn, A. M., Vermeeren, R., Hofman, A., van Laar, A., de Bruin, M., *et al.* (1987). Serum selenium, vitamin antioxidants, and cardiovascular mortality: a 9-year follow-up study in the Netherlands. *Am. J. Clin. Nutr.,* **45,** 462–8.

Labadarios, D., Brink, P. A., Weich, H. S. H., Visser, L., Louw, M. E. J., Shephard, G. S., *et al.* (1987). Plasma vitamins A, E, C and B_6 levels in myocardial infarction. *S. Afr. Med. J.,* **71,** 561–3.

Lang, P. D., Degott, M., and Vollmar, J. (1977). Fatty acid composition of adipose tissue in patients with coronary heart disease. *Atherosclerosis,* **26,** 29–39.

Lapidus, L., Andersson, H., Bengtsson, C., and Bosaeus, I. (1986). Dietary habits in relation to incidence of cardiovascular disease and death in women: 12-year follow-up of participants in the population study of women in Gothenburg, Sweden. *Am. J. Clin. Nutr.,* **44,** 444–8.

Lawrie, T. D. V., McAlpine, S. G., Rifkind, B. M., and Robinson, J. F. (1961). Serum fatty acid patterns in coronary artery disease. *Lancet,* **i,** 421–4.

Lea, E. J. A., Jones, S. P., and Hamilton, D. V. (1982). The fatty acids of erythrocytes of myocardial infarction patients. *Atherosclerosis*, **41**, 363–9.

Lee, K. T., Shaper, A. G., Scott, R. F., Goodale, F., and Thomas, W. A. (1962). Geographic studies pertaining to arteriosclerosis. Comparison of fatty acid patterns of adipose tissue and plasma lipids in East Africans with those of North American white and negro groups. *Arch. Pathol.*, **74**, 481–8.

Lewis, B. (1958). Composition of plasma cholesterol ester in relation to coronary-artery disease and dietary fat. *Lancet*, **ii**, 71–3.

Logan, R. L., Riemersma, R. A., Thomson, M., Oliver, M. F., Olsson, A. G., Walldius, G., *et al.* (1978). Risk factors for ischaemic heart-disease in normal men aged 40. Edinburgh–Stockholm Study. *Lancet*, **i**, 949–55.

Mayet, F. H. G., Swedarsen, M., and Reinach, S. G. (1986). Ascorbic acid and cholesterol levels in patients with diabetes mellitus and coronary artery disease. *S. Afr. Med. J.*, **70**, 661–4.

McLaren, D. S. and Read, W. W. C. (1962). Fatty acid composition of adipose tissue. A study in three races in East Africa. *Clin. Sci.*, **23**, 247–50.

Miettinen, T. A., Naukkarinen, V., Huttenen, J. K., Mattila, S., and Kumlin, T. (1982). Fatty-acid composition of serum lipids predicts myocardial infarction. *Br. Med. J.*, **285**, 993–6.

Morris, J. N., Marr, J. W., and Clayton, D. G. (1977). Diet and heart: a postscript. *Br. Med. J.*, **2**, 1307–14.

Nordøy, A. and Rødset, J. M. (1970). Platelet phospholipids and their function in patients with ischemic heart disease. *Acta Med. Scand.*, **188**, 133–7.

Ramirez, J. and Flowers, N. C. (1980). Leukocyte ascorbic acid and its relationship to coronary heart disease in man. *Am. J. Clin. Nutr.*, **33**, 2079–87.

Renaud, S., Kuba, K., Goulet, C., Lemire, Y., and Allard, C. (1970). Relationship between fatty acid composition of platelets and platelet aggregation in rat and man. *Circul. Res.*, **26**, 553–64.

Riemersma, R. A., Wood, D. A., Butler, S., Elton, R. A., Oliver, M. F., Salo, M., *et al.* (1986). Linoleic acid content in adipose tissue and coronary heart disease. *Br. Med. J.*, **292**, 1423–7.

Riemersma, R. A., Oliver, M., Elton, R. A., Alfthan, G., Vartiainen, A., Salo, M., *et al.* (1990). Plasma antioxidants and coronary heart disease: vitamins C and E, and selenium. *Eur. J. Clin. Nutr.*, **44**, 143–50.

Riemersma, R. A., Wood, D. A., MacIntyre, C. C. A., Elton, R. A., Gey, K. F., and Oliver, M. F. (1991). Risk of angina pectoris and concentrations of vitamins A, C and E and carotene. *Lancet*, **i**, 1–5.

Roussouw, J. E., Labadarios, D., Jooste, P. L., and Shephard, G. S. (1985). Lack of a relationship between plasma pyridoxal phosphate levels and ischaemic heart disease. *S. Afr. Med. J.*, **67**, 539–41.

Saha, N., Ng, T. B., Tan, P. Y., and Wee, K. P. (1988). Vitamin A reserve of liver in health and coronary heart disease among ethnic groups in Singapore. *Br. J. Nutr.*, **60**, 407–12.

Salonen, J. T., Salonen, R., Penttila, I., Herranen, J., Jauhiainen, M., Kantola, M., *et al.* (1985). Serum fatty acids, apolipoproteins, selenium and vitamin antioxidants and the risk of death from coronary artery disease. *Am. J. Cardiol.*, **56**, 226–31.

Salonen, J. T., Salonen, R., Seppanen, K., Kantola, M., Parviainen, M., Alfthan,

G., *et al.* (1988). Relationship of serum selenium and antioxidants to plasma lipoproteins, platelet aggregability and prevalent ischaemic heart disease in Eastern Finnish men. *Atherosclerosis, 70,* 155–60.

Sanders, T. A. B. (1988). Essential and trans-fatty acids in nutrition. *Nutr. Res. Rev., 1,* 57–78.

Schrade, W., Boehle, E., and Biegler, R. (1960). Humoral changes in arteriosclerosis. Investigations on lipids, fatty acids, ketone bodies, pyruvic acid, lactic acid and glucose in the blood. *Lancet,* ii, 1409–16.

Scott, R. F., Hale, C., Hale, T., Goodale, F., and Tejada, C. (1962*a*). Chemicoanatomic studies in the geographic pathology of arteriosclerosis: a comparison of fatty acids of adipose tissue and plasma lipids in nondiabetics and diabetics from Guatemala and the United Staes. *Exp. Mol. Pathol., 1,* 44–56.

Scott, R. F., Daoud, A. S., Gittelsohn, A., Opalka, E., Florentin, R., and Goodale, F. (1962*b*). Lack of correlation between fatty acid patterns in adipose tissue and amount of coronary arteriosclerosis. *Am. J. Clin. Nutr., 10,* 250–6.

Serfontein, W. J., Ubink, J. B., De Violiers, L. S., Rapley, C. H., and Becker, P. J. (1985). Plasma pyridoxal-5-phosphate level as a risk index for coronary artery disease. *Atherosclerosis, 55,* 357–61.

Shekelle, R. B., Shryock, A. M., Paul, O., Lepper, M., Stamler, J., Liu, S., *et al.* (1981). Diet, serum cholesterol, and death from coronary heart disease: the Western Electric Study. *New Engl. J. Med., 304,* 65–70.

Shorland, F. B., Czochanska, Z., and Prior, I. A. M. (1969). Studies on fatty acid composition of adipose tissue and blood lipids of Polynesians. *Am. J. Clin. Nutr.,* 22(3), 594–605.

Simpson, H. C. R., Barker, K., Carter, R. D., Cassels, E., and Mann, J. I. (1982). Low dietary intake of linoleic acid predisposes to myocardial infarction. *Br. Med. J., 285,* 683–4.

Sinclair, H. M. (1956). Deficiency of essential fatty acids and atherosclerosis, ecetera. *Lancet,* i, 381–3.

Stähelin, H. B., Buess, E., Rösel, F., Widmer, L. K., and Brubacher, G. (1982). Vitamin A, cardiovascular risk factors, and mortality. *Lancet,* i, 394–5.

Strong, J. P., Oalmann, M. C., William, P. H., Newman, W. P., Tracy, R. E., Malcolm, G. T. *et al.* (1984). Coronary heart disease in young black and white males in New Orleans: Community Pathology Study. *Am. Heart J., 108,* 747–59.

Thomas, L. H. and Scott, R. G. (1981). Ischaemic heart disease and the proportions of hydrogenated fat and ruminant-animal fat in adipose tissue at post mortem examination: a case control study. *J. Epidemiol. Community Health, 35,* 251–5.

Thomson, M., Logan, R. L., Sharman, M., Lockerbie, L., Riemersma, R. A., and Oliver, M. F. (1982). Dietary survey in 40 year-old Edinburgh men. *Hum. Nutr. Appl. Nutr., 36A,* 272–89.

Thomson, M., Elton, R. A., Fulton, M., Brown, S., Wood, C. A., and Oliver, M. F. (1988). Individual variation in the dietary intake of a group of Scottish men. *J. Hum. Nutr. Dietet., 1,* 47–57.

Turpeinen, O., Karvonen, M. J., Pekkarinen, M., Miettinen, M., Elosuo, R., and Paavilainen, E. (1979). Dietary prevention of coronary heart disease: the Finnish Mental Hospital Study. *Int. J. Epidemiol., 8* (2), 99–118.

Valek, J., Hammer, J., Kohort, M., Grafnetter, D., Vondra, K., and Topinha, V. (1985). *Atherosclerosis, 54,* 111–18.

Valles, J., Aznar, J., and Santos, M. T. (1979). Platelet fatty acids in acute myocardial infarction. *Thromb. Res.,* **14,** 231–4.

Vermaak, W. J. H., Barnard, H. C., Potgeiter, E. M., and Marx, J. D. (1986). Plasma pyridoxal-5-phosphate levels in myocardial infarction. *S. Afr. Med. J.,* **70,** 195–6.

Weir, J. D., Connor, W. E., and Den Bester, L. (1975). The development of essential fatty acid deficiency in healthy men fed fat-free diets intravenously and orally. *J. Clin. Invest.,* **56,** 127–34.

Wood, D. A., Butler, S., Riemersma, R. A., Thomson, M., and Oliver, M. F. (1984). Adipose tissue and platelet fatty acids and coronary heart disease in Scottish men. *Lancet,* **ii,** 117–21.

Wood, D. A., Riemersma, R. A., Butler, S., Thomson, M., MacIntyre, C., Elton, R. A., *et al.* (1987). Linoleic acid eicosapentaenoic acids in adipose tissue and platelets and risk of coronary heart disease. *Lancet,* **i,** 177–83.

14

Fish, fibre, and heart disease

P. C. Elwood, M. L. Burr, and P. M. Sweetnam

FISH

Interest in fish and cardiovascular disease seems to have commenced with the observation, made around 1927, that heart disease is rare in Eskimos in Greenland. An early report refers to 'only three deaths from atherosclerotic heart disease from 1963–1967', and in 1978 the Annual Report of the Chief Medical Officer stated that deaths from coronary heart disease (CHD) accounted for only 3.5 per cent of all deaths in Greenland Eskimos.

Early interest in the Eskimos focused on their serum lipid levels, and in 1970 Bang and Dyerberg conducted an expedition to the northwest coast of Greenland. They obtained blood samples from 61 male and 69 female Eskimos, drawn from a total population of around 1350. The levels of total serum lipids were around 15 per cent lower than in adult Danes, cholesterol levels were around 20 per cent lower, and triglyceride levels were almost 60 per cent lower. High density lipoprotein levels were 45 per cent higher in the male Eskimos, but only marginally higher in the females. Bang *et al.* (1971) considered the possibility that these differences might be genetic in origin, and so they went on to compare the lipid levels of the Greenland Eskimos with those of Eskimos living in Denmark, who presumably had a dietary pattern more like that of the Danes. The differences between these Eskimo groups were similar in direction and in magnitude to those between the Greenland Eskimos and the Danes.

Hugh Sinclair seems to have been one of the first to go on to investigate the diets of Greenlanders, and in 1976 he joined Bang and Dyerberg in a study of the diets of 50 Eskimos using a 'double-portion' technique (Bang *et al.* 1980). They showed that, in comparison with an average Danish diet, the Eskimo diet was rich in polyunsaturated fatty acids of the linolenic class ($n-3$). This led them to suggest that the rarity of CHD in the Greenland Eskimos could be due not only to an effect of the fish oils on serum lipid levels, but also to an antithrombotic effect. In relation to the latter, they made particular reference to eicosapentaenoic acid (EPA) which comes mainly from fatty or oily fish.

Meanwhile, investigations in other communities were confirming a low mortality from CHD where there was a high dietary intake of fish. In

Japan, the incidence and mortality rates of cardiovascular diseases were shown to be lowest in an island community where fish consumption was about double that on the mainland (Kagawa *et al.* 1982). Another study of residents in a fishing village, where intakes of fish were around 250 g/day, showed lower CHD and cerebrovascular mortality than in an inland area where fish intake averaged around 90 g/day (Hirai *et al.* 1989).

Differences between communities are always difficult to interpret because factors such as fish eating could be no more than markers for a host of differences in life-style and environmental factors. Changes over time within the same community can yield evidence which has a rather different set of uncertainties. Therefore it is of interest that in Norway, where fish intakes fell during the Second World War and rose again at the end of hostilities, the incidence of myocardial infarction (MI) treated in Oslo hospitals showed a pattern inverse to this (Bang and Dyerberg 1981).

Prospective studies

Geographical evidence and trends over time are of interest to the eidemiologist, just as knowledge of metabolic pathways and biochemical mechanisms are of interest to biologists. However, none of the evidence on these aspects can be accepted as conclusive, or used as a basis for any therapeutic or prophylactic measure.

Therefore we turn to prospective studies and intervention trials. While evidence from randomized controlled trials can be as near to proof as scientific evidence can ever be, trials are very difficult to conduct in free-living human populations, and they always have the limitation that the extent to which subjects can be persuaded to modify their diets is limited, as is the time for which one can expect the changes to be maintained.

Evidence from prospective studies is therefore valuable, though these too have limitations. The major uncertainties arise because dietary differences within a community are undoubtedly confounded with numerous other differences, and in fact diet might again be no more than a marker for a particular life-style.

One of the first prospective studies relevant to fish and CHD was conducted retrospectively, in that serum samples which had been frozen and stored for 5–7 years were analysed for their phospholipid fatty acid content (Miettinen *et al.* 1982). The levels of EPA, which in the diet comes from fish alone, were found to be significantly lower in 33 men who had been free of CHD when the samples had been taken, but had had a cardiovascular event subsequently, compared with men who had remained free of CHD.

A cohort of 852 men in Zutphen, who had originally been enrolled in the Seven Countries Study, yielded similar results, but on this occasion the predictive data related to the consumption of fish of all kinds (Kromhout *et al.* 1985). During a 20 year period the CHD mortality of men who had regularly eaten a small amount of fish was less than half that of the men who had stated that they ate no fish. This study is of particular interest in that the amounts of fish eaten had been on the whole small, yet the protection against heart disease was substantial. Furthermore, the results related to fish of all kinds, and the authors estimated that only about one-third of this was fatty fish.

Since these studies were reported, the records of a number of other cohorts have been re-examined in relation to fish consumption. In the Western Electric Study there was evidence of a weak protective effect of fish in 1931 men who had been followed for 25 years (Shekelle *et al.* 1985). A study of almost 11 000 twins in Sweden showed a significant beneficial effect; those with the highest consumption of fish had a risk of MI which was about one-third lower than those with the lowest intakes of fish (Norell *et al.* 1986). More recently, the Multiple Risk Factor Intervention Trial (MRFIT) Research Group examined their data retrospectively and found evidence of a protective effect equivalent to a reduction of about one-third in CHD mortality in the regular fish eaters (Furburg 1989). The most recent prospective data come from the Caerphilly Prospective Study in South Wales (Fehily *et al.* 1991). Over 1000 men in this cohort ate fatty fish at least once every 2–3 weeks and their incidence of major CHD events was 1.04 per annum, while 811 men who never or rarely ate fatty fish had an incidence which was about 30 per cent higher ($p > 0.05$).

However, not all the results from cohort studies have been consistent with protection. A very large cohort in Norway showed no evidence of benefit from fish eating during a 13 year follow-up (Vollset *et al.* 1985), nor did the large cohort followed in the Honolulu Heart Programme give evidence of benefit from fish (Curb and Reed 1985).

Biochemical and metabolic studies

Numerous studies have been reported in which the effect of fish, or more usually fish oil, has been tested on a mechanism believed to be relevant to CHD. Many of these studies were reviewed by Herold and Kinsella (1986), and there is neither space nor reason to review them in detail in an epidemiological paper such as this. However, the two lines of investigation suggested earlier by Bang *et al.* (1980) are evident in all this work.

1. The effect on serum lipids. The greatest change appears to be on triglyceride levels, which are markedly lowered. Changes in other lipids are smaller, and are not consistent in the various studies (Kinsell *et al.* 1981).

2. The effect on thrombosis-related mechanisms. Here the action appears to be mainly through a reduction in platelet aggregation. This seems likely

to be due to the $n-3$ acids, in particular EPA, displacing arachidonic acid in the platelets and thereby reducing thromboxane synthesis (Galli *et al.* 1981).

Fish oils probably have other actions relevant to heart disease. These may include a reduction in blood pressure, though this has not been found consistently. An increase in red cell deformability may also be caused through incorporation of the $n-3$ acids in fish oil into the cell membranes (VonShacky *et al.* 1985). This last may lead to a reduction in whole-blood viscosity and possibly to a reduction of red-cell-generated adenosine diphosphate (ADP).

Although many of the $n-3$ fatty acids may be relevant to blood lipid levels, EPA (20:5 $n-3$) is particularly active in antithrombotic activity, both through PGI_3 and through the enhancement of the weak platelet agonist thromboxane A_3 rather than TXA_2. Interest has therefore focused mainly on fatty or oily fish, as the content of EPA is much higher in these than in white fish.

Fatty fish are pelagic, and include herring, mackerel, sardines, pilchards, trout, and salmon. The demersal, or bottom-feeding, fish have very much lower contents of EPA. At the same time it has to be pointed out that the focusing of interest on fatty fish is to a large extent based on the assumption that EPA is the relevant factor. However, present epidemiological evidence does not clearly indicate whether white fish is protective, and, as has been mentioned already, the reduced incidence of heart disease in the Zutphen Study was associated with the consumption of mostly white fish (Kromhout *et al.* 1985).

Randomized controlled trials

Although it has limitations, the randomized controlled trial is undoubtedly the most powerful tool available for the testing of a prophylactic measure. A number of trials have reported on the benefit of fish consumption, but before these are reviewed several general aspects of clinical trials need to be considered.

First, the ultimate test of a possible prophylactic measure must be against disease incidence. Trials which examine an effect on some biochemical or haematological measure are of value and may give a lead to further research. But benefit to health must not be assumed; it must be tested directly.

The adequate testing of a prophylactic measure in heart disease can be in relation to a number of outcomes. The best outcome is undoubtedly death or survival, and this will be argued shortly. However, the recent development of techniques by which atherosclerosis in the coronary arteries can be visualized and measured gives another most valuable measure and enables the progress of the underlying vascular disease to be monitored. Trials which evaluate the benefit of a prophylactic measure on the reduction of atheroma or the prevention of restenosis after angioplasty can therefore be informative. Thus it is of interest that in a number of trials of fish oil after angioplasty there has been angiographic evidence of a reduction in restenosis (Ilsley *et al.* 1987; Dehmer *et al.* 1988; Milner *et al.* 1988), though in two other trials no benefit of fish oil was detected (Grigg *et al.* 1989; Reis *et al.* 1989). At the same time, it must be recognized that the present techniques by which coronary arteries can be visualized are only acceptable in a small proportion of patients, selected on clinical grounds, and therefore trials with repeated measurements of coronary atheroma are likely to be possible only in patients with advanced disease. Furthermore, the relevance of atherosclerosis to death and MI is not fully understood, and while it is reasonable to assume that any measure which reduces atherosclerosis is likely to be beneficial, measures which protect against death and MI may do nothing to atherosclerosis.

This last seems likely to be a most important point in view of the evidence that tests relating to haemostatic mechanisms have a far greater predictive power than any lipid level (Elwood *et al.* 1991). The point is further emphasized by the success of aspirin in reducing mortality, a drug for which no one has postulated an effect on atherogenesis.

At first sight it seems attractive to evaluate measures of possible value against heart disease by their ability to reduce heart disease—fatal, non-fatal, or both. However, the dangers of drawing conclusions from indices other than total deaths has been well illustrated in the reports of trials of dietary fat reduction. In these, conclusions were based on either evidence of a reduction in deaths which had been attributed to CHD or total CHD incidence comprising both fatal and non-fatal CHD. However, overviews of these trials have shown that all-cause mortality is not affected (McCormick and Skrabanek 1988; Elwood 1990*a*; Muldoon *et al.* 1990). Heart disease is a major cause of death and therefore it is not unreasonable to expect that if a prophylactic measure does affect CHD, a reduction in total mortality will be apparent. Whatever steps are taken to avoid misclassification, bias in the certification of the cause of death and in the diagnosis of a non-fatal MI cannot be eliminated with certainty.

Second, there is a place for testing a prophylactic measure in subjects who have already had a non-fatal CHD event. Of course, trials of secondary prevention do raise questions as to whether or not the underlying disease has progressed too far for an event to be prevented. On the other hand, it does seem likely that mechanisms relevant to thrombosis may be of greater importance to cardiovascular mortality than are mechanisms of relevance to atherosclerosis. If this is true, then it is certainly not unreasonable to test protective measures which may affect thrombosis in secondary prevention. In any case it should be remembered that most clinical practice relates to patients, rather than the community, and it is therefore important to know whether or not it is worthwhile to recommend a prophylactic measure to patients who have already experienced a CHD event.

It has been said that attempts should be made to persuade every epidemiologist to set up one (if only one!) major prospective study or trial (Rose *c.* 1980). Secondary prevention trials are not easy, but unlike trials of primary prevention they are within the competence and resources of most epidemiologists. Suitable patients are common, they are usually well motivated to agree to enter a trial, and they are likely to comply with dietary changes for prolonged periods. In fact one could go further and plead that some of the effort and resources that are put into studies of biological mechanisms, and especially when the resources are put into animal studies, should be put into prophylactic trials on *Homo sapiens*, and in particular into secondary preventive trials.

In this connection it is intriguing to note that in one review of feeding trials of fish oils, evidence from 18 animal trials and 47 studies of human subjects were summarized. The conclusion calls for further research to give greater knowledge of the mechanisms by which $n-3$ polyunsaturated fats may act, but no need is expressed for trials to test benefit on health or survival (Herold and Kinsella 1986).

Having said all that, it has to be stated that to date only one randomized controlled trial of fish eating and mortality has been completed—but perhaps this demonstrates the appropriateness of the point just made. However, a further point can be made here. There have been a number of trials of diet and secondary prevention of death and/or reinfarction, most of which have tested a low fat diet with a high P/S ratio. All these trials have been totally unrealistic in size, ranging from 80 to 458, and a number of these have had serious design faults (Elwood 1990*a, b*).

The only trial of fish has been fully described elsewhere (Burr *et al.* 1989*a, b*; Fehily *et al.* 1989). However, before it is described, a further point of general relevance to trials should be made. This trial tested three prophylactic measures simultaneously. This was achieved by a factorial design in which each treatment is separately randomized. The effect of each intervention factor can therefore be tested in the full trial population, giving no limitation of power. The use of this design should be encouraged.

The three factors tested in the trial performed by Burr and his colleagues were fish, fat, and cereal fibre, but only the results for fish will be given in this section of the chapter. The advice given to the men was 'to have a main portion of fatty fish at two meals or more each week', giving at least 300 g per week. To ensure that the trial would have an 80 per cent likelihood of detecting (at $p < 0.05$) a true beneficial effect of the dietary change, equivalent to a reduction in mortality of 25 per cent or more, it was estimated that around 2000 men would be required, i.e. the advice would be given to around 1000 men and mortality in these compared with that in the 1000 men who had been given no such advice.

Subjects were men under 70 years of age who had recently suffered an MI, diagnosed according to World Health Organization (WHO) criteria. They were identified in 21 hospitals in South Wales and Southwest England. Men were eligible for the trial if they were non-diabetic, they had not had a serious illness such as malignant disease or renal failure, they were not being considered for a coronary artery bypass graft or heart transplant, and their diet did not already conform to any of the regimens being tested.

Men were visited at home by a doctor shortly after discharge from hospital and then each was then seen, together with his wife, by a Medical Research Council dietitian. A brief dietary history was taken, height and weight were measured, and a final decision was taken on the subjects' suitability for the trial. Subjects were then randomly allocated to receive or not to receive advice on each of the three factors. They were given a detailed explanation of the appropriate diet, together with a diet sheet and a specially prepared booklet with suitable recipes. Men allocated to 'no advice' were given a 'sensible eating' sheet which did not include advice on any of the intervention components. Smokers were advised to quit and each dietary regimen was modified to allow the inclusion of weight-reducing advice if appropriate.

At intervals during the trial subjects were revisited by a dietitian to reinforce the advice. Men who had been randomized to fatty fish advice but who were not able to eat two portions of these fish per week were given MaxEPA fish oil capsules as an alternative or partial replacement. At 6 months, 14 per cent of those given fish advice were taking fish oil capsules as a total or partial substitute and at 2 years the proportion was 22 per cent.

Compliance was monitored throughout the trial, primarily by means of detailed semi-quantitative food frequency questionnaires. These were supplemented by information from 7 day weighed intake records completed by a random subsample of men at 6 months and 2 years, and by food frequency charts completed for 1 month at 3 monthly intervals throughout the trial. More objective evidence on compliance was obtained by the determination of plasma fatty acid composition, including EPA, on random subsamples of men at 6 months and 2 years. Data from questionnaires completed at 6 months and 2 years were encouraging and showed that the effect of advice on consumption was just about that which had been hoped for. The EPA intake was 2.3 g/week at 6 months (controls 0.7 g/week) and 2.4 g/week at 2 years (controls 0.6 g/week).

The original plan for the trial was to examine mortality after every man had completed 2 years in the trial, and then, if no significant benefit had occurred, to continue the trial and make appropriate statistical allowances in the interpretation of any effects which occurred later. The first examination of the results gave evidence on fatty fish which was so convincing

Fish, fibre, and heart disease

Table 14.1

	Men advised to eat fatty fish	Men given no advice about fish
Number of men	1015	1018
Total deaths	93 (9.3%)	130 (12.8%)
CHD deaths	78 (7.7%)	116 (11.4%)
Non-fatal MI	49 (4.8%)	33 (3.2%)
All CHD events	127 (12.5%)	149 (14.6%)

(Table 14.1) that we judged it imperative to conclude the trial. The difference in all-cause mortality indicates a reduction in mortality of 29 per cent, and this is unaffected when the effects of all possible confounding factors are allowed for.

To put this figure of 29 per cent into context it is useful to consider it in terms of the likely saving of lives. If 1000 post-MI men are given advice to eat two or more meals of fatty fish each week, about 35 more will survive the next 2 years. This is of course a crude estimate and carries a considerable uncertainty, particularly as it is derived from the results of a single trial. However, it is probably very similar to the savings from low dose aspirin given to post-MI patients (about 25 in the first year and somewhat less in the second and subsequent years). It is far greater than any reasonable estimate of the effect of a low fat diet. On this last, it has been estimated from the results of a number of trials of secondary prevention, none of which yielded results which were statistically significant, that the saving of lives from a low fat diet might be equivalent to about one life per year per 9000 men advised (Elwood 1990*b*). In this context it is also of interest that Naylor *et al.* (1990) have estimated that 10.3 tonnes of the cholesterol-lowering drug Cholestyramine would be required to save one life (again, this estimate is based on a trial with a non-significant effect on total mortality).

It is notable that the data reported above from the trial carried out by Burr *et al.* (1989*a*) give no evidence that non-fatal MIs were reduced by fish eating. Therefore it is possible that the effect of fish, and probably EPA, is to reduce the risk of death after MI rather than to reduce the incidence of MI.

Evidence consistent with this last comes from work on experimentally induced MI in dogs. In one study the effect of fish oil was tested with electrically induced MI. The animals given fish oil had much smaller infarcts than the control animals, and had a lower incidence of ventricular ectopic beats (30 per cent compared with 80 per cent of the control animals) (Culp *et al.* 1980). Another group used diets with different oils in rats and tested the vulnerability of the myocardium to arrhythmia on coronary artery occlusion and reperfusion. The $n-3$ oils from a fish diet led to a very marked reduction in ventricular fibrillation (6 per cent of the animals) compared with the effects of a diet rich in sunflower seed oil (21 per cent) and a diet with high saturated fat (68 per cent of animals (McLennan *et al.* 1989)).

It is inevitable that work will continue on metabolic pathways of EPA, and on biochemical and other effects of fish oil. However, there is now an urgent need for further trials of fish and CHD. Results from a single trial can never be accepted as conclusive. Moreover, it is important that evidence is collected as to whether or not deaths are sudden, so that the effect of fish on deaths can be examined more carefully. It would also be of great interest to conduct a factorial trial in which fish is tested together with a purely antithrombotic agent such as aspirin.

FIBRE

It has been claimed that William Beaumont was the first to claim health benefits for dietary fibre (Beaumont 1833). However, it was Burkitt and Trowell (1975) who formulated the 'fibre hypothesis' linking low fibre intakes to numerous 'Western diseases' including CHD. Their reports, based on crude fibre estimations and even cruder epidemiological observations, generated a series of hypotheses, and these in turn stimulated a very large number of investigations. These have been repeatedly reviewed, and again it is not seen as appropriate to attempt to summarize the results in this epidemiological paper. However, it is notable that most of these studies have been biochemical, and most have focused on a possible hypolipidaemic effect of fibre.

It is also notable that many of the studies on dietary fibre have been very small and have used amounts of fibre which are quite unphysiological. Furthermore, it is a sad reflection on medical research, and on the media publicity it generates, that, despite the absence of evidence from randomized controlled trials with disease or death as their outcome, Eastwood and Passmore (1983) could claim that 'In 1982 the best-selling book in the United Kingdom was a guide to high-fibre diets based on wholemeal cereals . . .'.

Prospective studies

In the Zutphen Study 871 middle-aged men were followed for 10 years. Mortality from CHD was about 5.2 per cent in the fifth of men with the lowest intakes of total dietary fibre, about 1.3 per cent in the fifth with the highest intakes, and about 3.5 per cent in the remainder. A similar gradient was shown for total mortality (Kromhout *et al.* 1982). The serendipitous prospective study by Morris and his colleagues gave similar results, with a five-fold difference in CHD incidence between the thirds of men with the highest and the lowest intakes of cereal fibre (Morris *et al.* 1977).

In fact, there have been at least five prospective studies in which fibre intake has been related to subsequent disease incidence, and in all of them the subjects with lower intakes had a raised incidence of CHD (Morris *et al.* 1977; Kromhout and De Lezenne Coulander 1984; Kushi *et al.* 1985; Khaw and Barrett-Connor 1987; Fehily *et al.* 1991). At the same time, dietary fibre is not independent of energy in that, usually, the more food that is eaten, the more fibre is consumed. Therefore, although fibre does not contribute to energy, it does seem reasonable to standardize fibre intake for energy (using energy as a surrogate for bulk). When this is done the predictive power of fibre for incident CHD is reduced and in two of these studies it is lost altogether (Kromhout and De Lezenne Coulander 1984; Fehily *et al.* 1991).

The danger in all this work is that, to an extent which is probably greater than for any other food item, fibre is likely to be a marker for a life-style. Many dietary and environmental factors may differ in subjects who choose high fibre foods—often recognized as 'health foods'. That this might be the case is suggested by a large cohort study of almost 11 000 subjects whom Burr and his colleagues identified through health food shops and health food magazines. The strength of this study is that the 6000 or so subjects who have a high consumption of fibre can be compared with the 5000 or so who do not, but who also shop at health food shops and read health food magazines, and who seem to have a fairly similar life-style with regard to smoking, alcohol intake, exercise level, etc. During the first 5 years of follow-up there was no evidence of any difference in the heart disease mortality of these two groups despite a marked difference in cereal fibre consumption (Burr and Sweetnam 1982).

Again, the best evidence can only come from randomized controlled trials but sadly, as with fish, it has to be stated that only one trial of fibre and CHD has yet been reported. Again, one would like to repeat the call for some of the effort and resources that are put into metabolic and biochemical studies to be put into trials of disease prevention. And again, one would see trials of secondary prevention to be fully appropriate.

The one randomized controlled trial of fibre and CHD has given no evidence of any benefit on any index of disease. This was the factorial randomized controlled trial performed by Burr and colleagues which has already been described (Burr *et al.* 1989*a*, *b*; Fehily *et al.* 1989).

The advice given to the men who had been randomized to cereal fibre was 'to increase consumption of wholemeal bread and other cereal foods, sufficient to give an intake of at least 18 g cereal fibre (approximately 30 g total fibre) per day'. Intakes were monitored during the trial by question-naires administered to every man at 6 months and 2 years. These gave evidence consistent with a high level of compliance: cereal fibre intake,

Table 14.2

	Men advised to increase cereal fibre	Men given no advice about fibre
Number of men	1017	1016
Total deaths	123 (12.1%)	101 (9.9%)
CHD deaths	109 (10.7%)	85 (8.4%)
Non-fatal MI	41 (4.0%)	41 (4.0%)
All CHD events	150 (14.7%)	126 (12.4%)

19 g/day at 6 months (controls, 9 g/day) and 17 g/day at 2 years (controls, 9 g/day). However, the results obtained after every man had completed 2 years in the trial gave no encouragement whatever (Table 14.2). Indeed, although non-fatal MIs appeared to have been unchanged, the men given advice about cereal fibre had a higher mortality than those given no such advice.

Interest in fibre has shifted yet again and attention is now focused on 'soluble' fibre, which is quite a change from the early ideas about 'roughage' and insoluble fibre (Trowell and Burkitt 1981). Interest in soluble fibre arises primarily because in numerous small feeding trials it has been shown to reduce serum cholesterol if eaten in sufficient quantities. Soluble fibre, which includes pectin from apples and citrus fruits and guar gum from the cluster bean, is widely distributed in fruits and pulses. Baked beans and rolled oats are probably the most readily available source in the UK at present. Whatever its biochemical effects, the ultimate need is for randomized controlled trials and, in the first instance, these could well be of secondary prevention.

CONCLUSION

The vast bulk of the current literature on diet and heart disease consists of reports of small feeding trials which have examined the effects of a nutrient, or a food item, on lipid levels or occasionally, as with fish oils, on factors of relevance to thrombosis. On the evidence of such work, fish, in particular fatty fish, has effects which are consistent with benefit to health. The evidence suggestive of benefit from fibre is much less convincing, but soluble fibre is probably worth further consideration.

The greatest need in research on diet and heart disease is for randomized controlled trials of the effect of nutrients and food items which have been identified as of possible value in the small feeding trials, using survival as the index of benefit. Epidemiologists could do much more to meet the need for randomized controlled trials as studies of secondary prevention in heart disease are within the competence and resources of most Departments of Epidemiology.

Ideally, clinical practice should be based on evidence from intervention trials. On this criterion the consumption of fatty fish should be encouraged, though only cautiously at present as only one randomized controlled trial has been reported. By the same criterion, dietary fibre cannot be promoted, though soluble fibre has yet to be tested. However, it is quite unreasonable for any preventive strategy directed to the general population to be based on evidence other than the results of randomized controlled trials with death or survival as the outcome.

REFERENCES

Bang, H. O. and Dyerberg, J. (1981). Personal reflections on the incidence of ischaemic heart disease in Oslo during the Second World War. *Acta Med. Scand.*, **210**, 245–8.

Bang, H. O., Dyerberg, J., and Nelson, A. B. (1971). Plasma lipid and lipoprotein pattern in Greenlandic west-coast Eskimos. *Lancet*, **i**, 1143–6.

Bang, H. O., Dyerberg, J., and Sinclair, H. (1980). The composition of Eskimo food in north western Greenland. *Am. J. Clin. Nutr.*, **33**, 2657–61.

Beaumont, W. (1833). *Experiments and observations on the gastric juice and the physiology of digestions*, Allen, Plattsburgh, NY.

Burkitt, D. P. and Trowell, H. C. (1975). *Refined carbohydrate foods and disease: the implications of dietary fibre*, Academic Press, London.

Burr, M. L. and Sweetnam, P. M. (1982). Vegetarianism, dietary fibre and mortality. *Am. J. Clin. Nutr.*, **36**, 873–7.

Burr, M. L., Fehily, A. M., Gilbert, J. F., Rogers, S., Holliday, R. M., Sweetnam, P. M., *et al.* (1989*a*). Effects of changes in fat, fish and fibre intakes on death and myocardial reinfarction: diet and reinfarction trial (DART). *Lancet*, **ii**, 757–61.

Burr, M. L., Fehily, A. M., Rogers, S., Welsby, E., King, S., and Sandham, S. (1989*b*). Diet and reinfarction trial (DART): design recruitment and compliance. *Eur. Heart J.*, **10**, 558–67.

Culp, B. R., Lands, W. E. M., Lucchesi, B. R., Litt, B., and Romson, J. (1980). The effect of dietary supplementation of fish oil on experimental myocardial infarction. *Prostaglandins*, **20**, 1021–31.

Curb, J. D. and Reed, D. M. (1985). Fish consumption and mortality from coronary heart disease. *New Engl. J. Med.*, **313**, 821.

Dehmer, G. J., Popma, J. J., van den Berg, E. K., Eichhorn, E. J., Prewitt, J. B., Campbell, W. B., *et al.* (1988). Reduction in the rate of early restenosis after coronary angioplasty by a diet supplemented with $n-3$ fatty acids. *New Engl. J. Med.*, **319**, 733–40.

Eastwood, M. A. and Passmore, R. (1983). Dietary fibre. *Lancet*, **ii**, 202–5.

Elwood, P. C. (1990*a*). The fat debate—time to move on. *Chem. Ind.*, **3**, 59–62.

Elwood, P. C. (1990*b*). Lowering cholesterol concentrations and mortality. *Br. Med. J.*, **301**, 930.

Elwood, P. C., Yarnell, J. W. G., Burr, M. L., Sweetnam, P., Fehily, A. M.,

Baker, I. A., *et al.* (1991). *Epidemiological studies of cardiovascular disease*, Prog. Rep. VII, MRC Epidemiology Unit.

Fehily, A. M., Vaughan-Williams, E., Shiels, K., Williams, A., Horner, M., Bingham, G., *et al.* (1989). The effect of dietary advice on nutrient intakes: evidence from the diet and reinfarction trial (DART). *J. Hum. Nutr. Dietet.*, **2**, 225–35.

Fehily, A. M., Yarnell, J. W. G., and Elwood, P. C. (1991). Diet and IHD in the Caerphilly Study, in preparation.

Furberg, C. D. (1989). Private communication.

Galli, C., Agradi, E., Petroni, A., and Tremoli, E. (1981). Differential effects of dietary fatty acids on the accumulation of arachidonic acid and its metabolic conversion in platelets and vascular tissue. *Lipids*, **16**, 165–9.

Grigg, L. E., Kay, T. W. H., Valentine, P. A., Larkins, R., Flower, D. J., Manolas, E. G., *et al.* (1989). Determinants of restenosis and lack of effect of dietary supplementation with eicosapentaenoic acid on the incidence of coronary artery restenosis after angioplasty. *J. Am. College Cardiol.*, **13**, 665–72.

Herold, P. M. and Kinsella, J. E. (1986). Fish oil consumption and decreased risk of cardiovascular disease: a comparison of findings from animal and human feeding trials. *Am. J. Clin. Nutr.*, **43**, 566–98.

Hirai, A., Terano, T., Tamura, Y., and Yoshida, S. (1989). Eicosapentaenoic acid and adult diseases in Japan: epidemiological and clinical aspects. *J. Intern. Med.*, **225** (Suppl. 1), 69–75.

Ilsley, C. D. J., Nye, E. R., Sutherland, W., Ram, J., and Ablett, M. B. (1987). Randomised placebo-controlled trial of Maxepa and Aspirin/Persantin after successful coronary angioplasty. *Aust. NZ J. Med.*, **17**, 559.

Kagawa, Y., Nishizawa, M., Suzuki, M., Miyatake, T., Hamamoto, T., Goto, K., *et al.* (1982). Eicosapolyenoic acids of serum lipids of Japanese Islanders with low incidence of cardiovascular diseases. *J. Nutr. Sci. Vitaminol.*, **28**, 441–53.

Khaw, K. T. and Barrett-Connor, E. (1987). Dietary fibre and reduced ischaemic heart disease mortality rates in men and women: a 12-year prospective study. *Am. J. Epidemiol.*, **126**, 1093–102.

Kinsell, L. W., Michaels, G. D., Walker, G., and Visintine, R. E. (1981). The effect of fish oil on plasma lipids. *Diabetes*, **10**, 316.

Kromhout, D. and De Lezenne Coulander, C. (1984). Diet, prevalence and 10 year mortality from coronary heart disease in 871 middle-aged men: the Zutphen Study. *Am. J. Epidemiol.*, **119**, 733–41.

Kromhout, D., Bosscheiter, E. D., and De Lezenne Coulander, C. (1982). Dietary fibre and 10 year mortality from coronary heart disease, cancer and all causes. *Lancet*, **5**, 519–21.

Kromhout, D., Bosscheiter, E. D., and De Lezenne Coulander, C. (1985). The inverse relation between fish consumption and 20-year mortality from coronary heart disease. *New Engl. J. Med.*, **312**, 1205–9.

Kushi, L. H., Lew, R. A., Stare, F. J., Ellison, C. R., El Lozy, M., Bourke, G., *et al.* (1985). Diet and 20-year mortality from coronary heart disease: the Ireland–Boston diet-heart study. *New Engl. J. Med.*, **312**, 811–18.

McCormick, J. and Skrabanek, P. (1988). Coronary heart disease is not preventable by population interventions. *Lancet*, **ii**, 839–41.

McLennan, P. L., Abeywardena, M. Y., and Charnock, J. S. (1989). The influence of age and dietary fat in an animal model of sudden cardiac death. *Aust. NZ J. Med.*, **19**, 1–5.

Miettinen, T. A., Naukkarinen, V., Huttunen, J. K., Mattila, S., and Kumlin, T. (1982). Fatty-acid composition of serum lipids predicts myocardial infarction. *Br. Med. J.*, **285**, 993–6.

Milner, M. R., Gallino, R. A., Leffingwell, A., Packard, A. D., Rosenberg, J., and Lindsay, J. (1988). High dose omega-3 fatty acid supplementation reduces clinical restenosis after coronary angioplasty. *Circulation*, **78** (Suppl. III), 634.

Morris, J. N., Marr, J. W., and Clayton, D. G. (1977). Diet and heart: a postscript. *Br. Med. J.*, **2**, 1307–14.

Muldoon, M. F., Manuck, S. B., and Matthews, K. A. (1990). Lowering cholesterol concentrations and mortality: a quantitative review of primary prevention trials. *Br. Med. J.*, **301**, 309–12.

Naylor, C. D., Basinski, A., Frank, J. W., and Rachlis, M. M. (1990). Asymptomatic hypercholesterolemia: a clinical policy review. The Toronto Working Group on Cholesterol Policy. *J. Clin. Epidemiol.*, **43**, 1021–117.

Norell, S. E., Ahlbom, A., Feychting, M., and Pedersen, N. L. (1986). Fish consumption and mortality from coronary heart disease. *Br. Med. J.*, **2**, 426.

Reis, G. J., Boucher, T. M., Sipperly, M. E., Silverman, D. I., McCabe, C. H., Baim, D. S., *et al.* (1989). Randomised trial of fish oil for prevention of restenosis after coronary angioplasty. *Lancet*, **ii**, 177–81.

Rose, G. (*c.* 1980). Private communication.

Shekelle, R. B., Missell, L., Paul, O., Shryock, A. M., and Stamler, J. (1985). Fish consumption and mortality from coronary heart disease. *New Engl. J. Med.*, **313**, 820.

Trowell, H. C. and Burkitt, D. P. (eds) (1981). *Western diseases: their emergence and prevention*, Edward Arnold, London.

Vollset, S. E., Heuch, I., and Bjelke, E. (1985). Fish consumption and mortality from coronary heart disease. *New Engl. J. Med.*, **313**, 820–1.

VonShacky, C., Fischer, S., and Webber, P. C. (1985). Long term effects of dietary marine $n-3$ fatty acids upon plasma and cellular lipids, platelet function and eicosanoid formation in humans. *J. Clin. Invest.*, **76**, 1626.

15

Diabetes, insulin, ethnicity, and coronary heart disease

P. M. McKeigue and H. Keen

DIABETES AND CHD RISK

A striking feature of the association between diabetes and coronary heart disease (CHD) risk is that the relative risk is higher in women than in men, so that the sex difference in CHD risk is attenuated or even abolished in diabetic individuals. In the Framingham Study at 18 year follow-up the relative risk for incident CHD in diabetic subjects compared with non-diabetic subjects was 2.4 in men and 5.1 in women (Kannel 1985). This was confirmed in Rancho Bernardo where at 14 year follow-up the relative risk of CHD mortality was 1.8 in diabetic men and 3.3 in diabetic women (Barrett-Connor et al. 1991). Insulin-dependent diabetes is associated with an even higher relative risk of developing CHD than is non-insulin-dependent diabetes, and a similar attenuation of the sex differences in CHD risk is seen. In a cohort of 292 insulin-dependent patients from the Joslin Clinic in Boston the cumulative mortality from CHD by age 55 years was 35 per cent in both men and women (Krolewski et al. 1987). The relative risk of CHD mortality in this group compared with the Framingham population was 4.4 in men and 8.8 in women. The higher risk associated with insulin-dependent diabetes than with non-insulin-dependent diabetes may be because the metabolic disturbances of insulin-dependent diabetes are more severe, or simply because the onset of insulin-dependent diabetes is earlier and exposure to atherogenic disturbances of metabolism is consequently longer.

Early studies suggested that asymptomatic hyperglycaemia might be associated with increased cardiovascular risk even at lower degrees of glucose intolerance than those considered diabetic (Keen et al. 1965; Ostrander et al. 1965). A review of 15 population studies in 1979 concluded that the association had not yet been unequivocally established (Stamler and Stamler 1979). Since then, long-term follow-up results have been reported from three large prospective studies (Fuller et al. 1983; Eschwege et al. 1985; Pyörälä et al. 1985) of glucose tolerance and CHD risk in European men; in each there is a non-linear relationship between glucose tolerance and CHD risk. In the Helsinki, Paris, and Whitehall Studies there was no relationship between 2 hour glucose and CHD risk up to a threshold level of 2 hour glucose, above which level the risk was doubled. With known diabetic subjects excluded, the threshold for increased risk was at the 80th centile of the 2 hour glucose distributions in the Helsinki and Paris studies (Pyörälä 1979; Ducimetiere *et al.* 1980) and at the 95th centile in the Whitehall study (Fuller *et al.* 1983). The glucose load used in Helsinki and Paris was at least 75 g; in Whitehall a 50 g load was used, which may have made the test less sensitive. In all three studies the threshold for increased CHD risk was at a 2 hour glucose level low enough to include men with impaired glucose tolerance as well as diabetic men in the group at high risk. This apparent non-linear relationship between 2 hour glucose and CHD risk contrasts with the linear relationship of other coronary risk factors like blood pressure and plasma cholesterol. Glucose tolerance, unlike blood pressure, does not vary biologically in a continuous manner: plasma glucose is normally controlled within narrow limits and failure to maintain homeostasis may lead to decompensation (DeFronzo 1988).

Urinary albumin excretion is commonly raised in diabetics, and even at levels not detected by ordinary clinical testing albuminuria is a strong predictor of mortality in diabetic subjects (Jarrett *et al.* 1984; Mogensen 1984): in non-insulin-dependent diabetic subjects the relative risk associated with albumin excretion rates exceeding 30 µg/min ranges from 1.5 to 4.8. Cardiovascular causes account for most of these excess deaths. Albuminuria is associated with higher prevalence of hypertension (Allawi and Jarrett 1990) and CHD (Mattock *et al.* 1988) in non-insulin-dependent diabetic individuals. Increased urinary albumin excretion may be an indicator of diffuse vascular vulnerability or damage, affecting the coronary circulation as well as the glomeruli.

THE INSULIN RESISTANCE SYNDROME

Compared with normoglycaemic individuals, non-insulin-dependent diabetic patients have more central obesity, higher blood pressures, higher immunoreactive insulin levels, higher triglyceride, and lower high density lipoprotein cholesterol (HDL-cholesterol). These disturbances occur to a similar extent in non-diabetic individuals with impaired glucose tolerance (Table 15.1) and are associated with each other even in normoglycaemic individuals (Table 15.2). The intercorrelations of obesity, blood pressure, glucose intolerance, hyperinsulinaemia, high plasma triglyceride, and low HDL-cholesterol in population surveys have led to the idea of a common underlying disturbance (Abrams *et al.* 1969; Orchard *et al.* 1983; Cambien *et al.* 1987; McKeigue *et al.* 1988). In this view non-insulin-dependent diabetes is but one manifestation of a more fundamental process which is

Table 15.1 Coronary risk factors by glucose tolerance category in European men in West London

| | Glucose tolerance category | | |
	Normal	Impaired glucose tolerance	Diabetic
No. of individuals	1393	41	72
Waist/hip ratio	0.93	0.98	0.99 $p<0.001$
2 hour insulin (mU/l)	19	63	37[a] $p<0.001$
SBP (mmHg)	121	134	134 $p<0.001$
Fasting triglyceride (mmol/l)	1.47	1.97	2.54[a] $p<0.001$
HDL-cholesterol (mmol/l)	1.27	1.17	1.12 $p<0.001$

Age-adjusted means:
SBP, median systolic blood pressure.
[a] Based on 33 untreated diabetic subjects only.
From McKeigue *et al.* 1991.

Table 15.2 Correlations between variables in European men in West London

	Waist/hip ratio	2 hour insulin	Fasting TG	HDL-cholesterol
2 hour insulin	0.33			
Fasting TG	0.38	0.31		
HDL-cholesterol	−0.26	−0.29	−0.48	
DBP[a]	0.32	0.23	0.21	−0.07

Subjects with diabetes or impaired glucose tolerance are excluded ($n=1393$).
TG, triglyceride; DBP, diastolic blood pressure.
[a] Spearman rank correlation coefficients; treated hypertensives assigned to highest quartile of distribution.
From McKeigue *et al.* 1991.

common even in normoglycaemic individuals and is associated with increased risk of CHD. We have compared this hypothetical underlying disturbance to a submerged iceberg whose peaks include glucose intolerance, hypertension, and CHD. When genetic background and environmental milieu favour its emergence, this iceberg becomes visible as a single entity.

In recent years the view has gained ground that resistance to insulin-stimulated glucose uptake plays a fundamental role in this maladaptive complex (Reaven 1988; DeFronzo and Ferrannini 1991). In this model non-insulin-dependent diabetes represents a late stage in a process in which increasing hyperglycaemia and hyperinsulinaemia lead to beta cell failure (DeFronzo 1988). Reaven has tentatively given the name 'syndrome

Table 15.3 The insulin resistance syndrome

Resistance to insulin-stimulated glucose uptake
Central obesity
Glucose intolerance
Hyperinsulinaemia
Hypertension
Increased VLDL-triglyceride
Decreased HDL-cholesterol
Increased IDL
Small dense particles in LDL fraction

X' to the association of glucose intolerance, hyperinsulinaemia, hypertension, hypertriglyceridaemia, low HDL-cholesterol, and insulin resistance
(Reaven 1988): we would include central obesity in this list (Table 15.3).
Insulin resistance is present in non-insulin-dependent diabetic individuals
and in individuals with impaired glucose tolerance, and is common in
normoglycaemic individuals in association with increasing age, physical
inactivity, and central obesity. Although the degree of insulin resistance is
defined by steady state measurements of glucose disposal, in normoglycaemic individuals these measurements correlate with insulin levels
measured after glucose challenge (Hollenbeck and Reaven 1987), which
are more practicable in population surveys.

Associations between insulin and blood pressure have been demonstrated in several population studies (Florey *et al.* 1976; Jarrett *et al.* 1978;
Cambien *et al.* 1987). Steady state infusion studies have confirmed that
hypertensive patients are more insulin-resistant than normotensive controls (Ferrannini *et al.* 1987; Shen *et al.* 1988). Experimental findings
support a cause and effect relationship, though the mechanism remains
unclear (Reaven 1988): insulin could raise blood pressure by causing renal
sodium retention or by affecting vascular response to sympathetic stimuli.

The association between hyperinsulinaemia and elevated levels of very
low density lipoprotein triglyceride (VLDL-triglyceride) is probably not
simply an effect of insulin upon triglyceride synthesis; in normal individuals
euglycaemic insulin infusions lower triglyceride levels (Yki-Jarvinen *et al.*
1984). The explanation may be that insulin-resistant individuals fail to
suppress release of non-esterified fatty acids from adipose tissue: the combination of hyperinsulinaemia and elevated non-esterified fatty acids leads
to increased hepatic synthesis of VLDL-triglyceride (Olefsky *et al.* 1974*a*;
Yki-Jarvinen and Taskinen 1988). The elevated VLDL-triglyceride levels
are accompanied by disturbances in the concentration and composition of
the intermediate density lipoprotein (IDL), low density lipoprotein (LDL)
and HDL fractions. These include increased levels of the IDL fraction, an
LDL subclass pattern characterized by a preponderance of small dense

LDL particles, and low HDL-cholesterol levels (Austin *et al*. 1988; Barakat *et al*. 1988, 1990). These effects are also seen in comparisons of diabetic and normoglycaemic subjects (Kasama *et al*. 1987; Barakat *et al*. 1990; Iwai *et al*. 1990).

Based on the pathophysiological relationships outlined above, the insulin resistance syndrome can be considered as a group of disturbances resulting from a single perturbation in a system. This model is summarized in Fig. 15.1. The relationship between central obesity and insulin resistance is the least well understood of the linkages in this model; otherwise there is evidence to support most of the relationships shown.

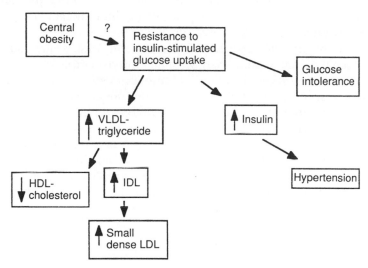

Fig. 15.1 The insulin resistance syndrome: possible pathways of association.

AETIOLOGY AND PREVENTION OF INSULIN RESISTANCE

The aetiology of insulin resistance and the mechanism of the association with central obesity are poorly understood. Skeletal muscle is the main site of insulin-mediated glucose disposal, and slow-twitch muscle fibres, which are specialized for endurance, are more insulin-sensitive than fast-twitch fibres which are specialized for short bursts of activity deriving energy from glycolysis (Holm and Krotkiewski 1988). Restriction of dietary energy intake and increased physical activity are the only known means of alleviating insulin resistance and the associated metabolic disturbances. In obese men, and also in women with central obesity, weight loss induced by either dietary restriction or exercise training reduces the insulin response to a glucose load (Olefsky *et al*. 1974*b*; Despres *et al*. 1988*a*; Andersson *et al*.

1991), lowers triglyceride (Olefsky *et al*. 1974*b*), and raises HDL-cholesterol (Wood *et al*. 1988). Even without loss of fat mass, exercise training increases insulin sensitivity, but this effect is lost within a few days of stopping exercise (LeBlanc *et al*. 1981; Heath *et al*. 1983). There is some evidence that, at least in men (Despres *et al*. 1985, 1988*a*) and in centrally obese women (Krotkiewski 1988; Wadden *et al*. 1988), dietary restriction or physical training causes loss of central rather than peripheral fat, and that the metabolic changes correlate with loss of central rather than peripheral fat (Despres *et al*. 1988*b*; Krotkiewski 1988).

A genetic predisposition to insulin resistance and central obesity may have been selected for under conditions of unreliable food supply and high physical activity levels. Central body fat, being more metabolically active than peripheral fat, could be stored quickly in time of surplus and mobilized quickly in time of need. Deposition of central fat would cause less interference with locomotion than accumulation of peripheral fat. Under conditions of starvation, resistance to insulin-mediated suppression of lipolysis and stimulation of glucose uptake by muscle would ensure that free fatty acids rather than glucose were used to fuel physical exertion: this would spare glucose for the brain, minimizing the need for ketogenesis or gluconeogenesis from protein. Urbanization and improved economic status are associated with reduction in physical activity and with higher energy intake in the form of fat and refined carbohydrates: in high risk populations diabetes and CHD would appear first in the most affluent, later spreading to other socio-economic groups.

INSULIN AS A CORONARY RISK FACTOR

The associations of triglyceride, HDL-cholesterol, and central obesity with CHD risk are reviewed elsewhere in this volume. It is of interest that, like diabetes, these risk factors appear to be stronger predictors of CHD in women than in men (Lapidus *et al*. 1984; Lerner and Kannel 1986). Since elevated serum insulin levels are associated with all these variables, it would be surprising if hyperinsulinaemia did not predict CHD risk. Two large prospective studies of the relationship between insulin and CHD in men have been reported: the Paris Prospective Study, with 126 CHD deaths at 10 year follow-up (Eschwege *et al*. 1985), and the Helsinki Policemen Study, with 63 new CHD cases at 9½ year follow-up (Pyörälä *et al*. 1985). In both studies fasting and 2 hour insulin levels were predictors of CHD and the association was non-linear, with most of the excess risk in the highest quintile of insulin levels. One possible explanation of the threshold relationship is that the highest quintile of the 2 hour insulin distribution identifies individuals who are at special risk from some underlying disturbance which has a more continuous distribution in the population.

Although there is some evidence from experimental studies that insulin may be directly atherogenic, there are also powerful objections to this as an explanation for the effects of the insulin resistance syndrome (Jarrett 1988). The absence of a dose–response relationship suggests that the association may not be directly causal. Insulin is one of the few putative cardiovascular risk factors to have been subjected (inadvertently) to a randomized controlled trial—the University Group Diabetes Program. In this study cardiovascular mortality was no higher in the groups treated with insulin than in the group treated with placebo (Knatterud et al. 1978). The interpretation of the observational studies has been complicated by the demonstration that standard commercial immuno-assays for insulin cross-react with intact pro-insulin and split pro-insulins (Temple et al. 1989); it is possible that CHD risk is associated with elevation of these insulin-like molecules rather than with insulin itself. A trial of treatment of diabetic patients with biosynthetic pro-insulin was terminated at 2 years when there were six myocardial infarctions in the pro-insulin-treated group and none in the control group (Galloway 1990); this has raised the possibility that pro-insulin itself may have atherogenic effects. Further population studies may help to elucidate these relationships.

HOW COULD THE INSULIN RESISTANCE SYNDROME CAUSE CHD?

A widely held view is that the presence in insulin-resistant individuals of a 'cluster' of coronary risk factors—hypertension, lipoprotein disturbances, and glucose intolerance—leads to cardiovascular disease (Reaven 1988). The assumption is that insulin resistance exerts effects on atherogenesis by several different mechanisms, including abnormal levels of insulin, glucose tolerance, blood pressure, triglyceride, and HDL-cholesterol. A more parsimonious explanation is that the effect of the insulin resistance syndrome upon atherogenesis is mediated principally through a single pathway, and that other features of the syndrome predict CHD because they are markers for this process. The standard approach to the problem of causation in cardiovascular epidemiology has been to attempt to identify 'independent' predictors of disease in multiple logistic regression analyses. The limitation of this approach is that the strongest predictive relationships are not necessarily with those factors that are causal but rather with those that can be most reliably characterized by a single measurement (Davey Smith and Phillips 1990). This argument applies especially to the labile and highly intercorrelated disturbances of body fat pattern, metabolism, and haemo-dynamics that comprise the insulin resistance syndrome. One approach to identifying causal relationships is to break some of the associations by studying differences between populations.

CHD IN POPULATIONS AT HIGH RISK FOR NON-INSULIN-DEPENDENT DIABETES

Several populations with a high prevalence of non-insulin-dependent diabetes have been described: the highest rates have been reported for Pima Native Americans (Knowler *et al*. 1978), Aboriginal Australians (Wise *et al*. 1976), and Nauruans (Zimmet *et al*. 1977). Common to most of these groups are a recent change towards urbanization, less physical activity, and the development of obesity. In some of these populations—urban South Asians (McKeigue *et al*. 1989) and Aboriginal Australians (Edwards *et al*. 1976; Bastian 1979)—CHD rates are also high. This association between population rates of diabetes and CHD would be expected if both high diabetes prevalence and high CHD risk were related to insulin resistance. In certain other populations of African and Native American origin prevalence of diabetes is high but CHD risk is relatively low.

South Asians

Mortality from CHD is higher in people of South Asian (Indian, Pakistani, and Bangladeshi) descent settled overseas than in other groups (McKeigue *et al*. 1989); the relative risk for CHD mortality ranges from 1.4 times higher than the national average for South Asian born migrants to England and Wales (OPCS 1990) to 3.6 for Indians compared with Chinese in Singapore (Hughes *et al*. 1990). The relative risk is highest in younger age groups; in Singapore, for instance, a relative risk of 10 has been reported for CHD mortality in Indians compared with Chinese before age 40 years (Hughes *et al*. 1990). In England and Wales the relative risk of CHD mortality associated with South Asian origin is higher for women than for men; in this respect the association with ethnicity resembles the association with diabetes. In England high CHD mortality is common to Gujarati Hindus, Punjabi Sikhs, and Muslims from Pakistan and Bangladesh (Balarajan *et al*. 1984; McKeigue and Marmot 1988), even though there are considerable differences between the dietary pattern and socio-economic status of these groups. The high risk is unexplained by established major risk factors including smoking, blood pressure, plasma cholesterol, and haemostatic activity. Although prevalence of non-insulin-dependent diabetes in South Asians in the UK is about four times higher than in the native British population (20 per cent versus 5 per cent in those aged over 40 years) (McKeigue *et al*. 1991), most South Asian patients with myocardial infarction are not diabetic and the high prevalence of diabetes cannot account for more than a small part of the excess CHD risk in this group. The most plausible explanation is that the high rates of both diabetes and CHD in this group are caused by insulin resistance. Mean fasting and post-load insulin levels are higher in South Asians than in Europeans, and the elevated insulin levels are generally associated with higher blood pressures, higher triglyceride, and lower HDL-cholesterol. South Asian men and women have a more central distribution of body fat than Europeans, with higher mean waist-to-hip girth ratios for a given level of body mass index (McKeigue *et al.* 1991). This tendency in South Asians to develop central obesity without overweight contrasts with American and Pacific populations in whom both the prevalence of non-insulin-dependent diabetes and the average weight-for-height are higher than in Europeans (Zimmet *et al.* 1977; Knowler *et al.* 1981; Stern *et al.* 1981).

Diabetes prevalence, waist-to-hip ratios, and serum insulin are higher in all main groups of South Asian migrants to the UK than in the native British population, but higher blood pressures, higher fasting triglyceride, and lower HDL-cholesterol are not present in all groups who share high CHD risk. Muslims from Pakistan and Bangladesh do not have higher blood pressures and Sikhs do not have lower HDL-cholesterol levels than the native British population (McKeigue *et al.* 1991). Since high CHD mortality is common to Hindus, Sikhs, and Muslims, it follows that this high risk is not mediated mainly through higher blood pressure or lower HDL-cholesterol. Triglyceride levels after a glucose load are higher in all groups originating from South Asia than in Europeans; this may be a marker for other disturbances of lipoprotein metabolism which are associated with insulin resistance.

Afro-Caribbeans and Afro-Americans

Non-insulin-dependent diabetes is commoner in Afro-Caribbeans and Afro-Americans than in Europeans. The ratio of diabetes prevalence in people of African descent to that in Europeans was 1.8 in the USA (Harris *et al.* 1987), 2.4 in Trinidad (Beckles *et al.* 1986), and 2.8 in the UK (McKeigue *et al.* 1991). In contrast with the high CHD mortality of South Asian people settled overseas, national data for the UK and the USA show lower CHD mortality in Afro-Caribbeans and Afro-Americans than in Europeans. The difference is greater for men than for women: in England and Wales in 1979–83 the standardized mortality ratio for CHD was 45 in Caribbean-born men and 76 in Caribbean-born women aged 20–69 (England and Wales = 100) (OPCS 1990). In the USA in 1986 the Black-to-White ratio for CHD mortality was 0.66 in men and 0.88 in women (Rothenberg and Aubert 1990). This relatively low mortality from CHD in Afro-Caribbeans and Afro-Americans contrasts with high mortality from stroke and hypertensive end-organ damage.

In our study in West London mean fasting and serum insulin levels were similar in Afro-Caribbean and European men aged 40–69 (McKeigue *et al.* 1991); in an American study fasting insulin levels were higher in Afro-

Americans than in Europeans aged 18–30 years and this difference was greater in women than in men (Folsom *et al*. 1989). It appears that the propensity to accumulate a high proportion of body fat intra-abdominally is not present in Afro-Americans and Afro-Caribbeans to the same extent as in South Asians; at any given body mass index mean waist-to-hip ratios are no higher in Afro-Caribbeans than in Europeans (Folsom *et al*. 1989; McKeigue *et al*. 1991). Plasma triglyceride levels are consistently lower and HDL-cholesterol levels consistently higher in Afro-Caribbean or Afro-American men than in men of European descent (Slack *et al*. 1977; Morrison *et al*. 1981). In women these differences in lipid pattern between Afro-Americans and Europeans are less evident, possibly because Afro-American women tend to be more obese (Ford *et al*. 1988). These findings suggest that the aetiology of non-insulin-dependent diabetes in Afro-Caribbeans differs from that in South Asians. In contrast with other groups, the high prevalence of diabetes and hypertension in Afro-Caribbeans is not accompanied by hyperinsulinaemia, intra-abdominal obesity, high triglyceride, and low HDL-cholesterol. Favourable body fat distribution and lipoprotein pattern in Afro-Caribbean and Afro-American men may partly explain the relatively low CHD rate in these groups.

Native Americans: Pimas and Mexican migrants

Some populations of Native American origin have a high prevalence of non-insulin-dependent diabetes but relatively low rates of CHD compared with the general population of the USA. In Pimas, an isolated Native American group living in Arizona, the prevalence of diabetes in men and women aged 35–64 was 42 per cent in 1975 (Knowler *et al*. 1978). Compared with Europeans, Pimas are resistant to insulin-mediated glucose uptake (Aronoff *et al*. 1977), are hyperinsulinaemic, and have higher triglyceride and lower HDL-cholesterol levels (Howard *et al*. 1983). Obesity is highly prevalent and the median body mass index in men and women aged 35–44 exceeds 30 kg/m^2. The interpretation of data on CHD rates in Pimas is complicated by the high all-cause mortality in this deprived population and by the small numbers of individuals surviving to middle age (Pettitt *et al*. 1982). CHD mortality rates are lower in Pimas than in the Framingham cohort, at least when diabetes is controlled for (Nelson *et al*. 1990). Plasma LDL-cholesterol levels are low in Pimas, despite levels of dietary fat intake which are similar to those of the general population of the USA (Reid *et al*. 1971); an ability to catabolize VLDL via the 'shunt' pathway, without conversion to LDL, may account for this (Howard *et al*. 1986).

Mexicans settled in the southern USA, who are of mixed European and Native American descent, also have high rates of non-insulin-dependent diabetes; prevalence in this group is about three times higher than in

Anglos (non-Hispanic Europeans) (Stern and Haffner 1988). In Texas in 1980 the ratio of CHD mortality in Mexicans to that in Anglos aged 35–64 was 0.81 in men and 1.06 in women (Stern *et al.* 1987). Mean body mass index, insulin, and triglyceride are higher and HDL-cholesterol is lower in Mexican-Americans than in Anglos, and the differences are larger in women than in men (Haffner 1987; Stern and Haffner 1988). Mean waist-to-hip ratios are no higher in Mexicans than in Anglos when the higher body mass index of Mexicans is taken into account. The relatively low CHD rates in Mexican-American men are unexplained: smoking and plasma cholesterol levels in this group are similar to the average for Anglos. Selection for fitness at migration and resistance to CHD conferred by mixed descent are possible explanations.

CONCLUSIONS

The insulin resistance syndrome may provide a unifying explanation for the relationship of CHD risk to obesity, hypertension, glucose intolerance, low HDL-cholesterol, and elevated triglyceride, and for the high risk in some ethnic groups. Risk factors associated with insulin resistance are stronger predictors of CHD in women than in men, and this suggests a close relationship with mechanisms underlying the sex difference in CHD risk. Some disturbance of lipoprotein metabolism, related to increased synthesis of VLDL-triglyceride, is the most likely mediator of the increased CHD risk. The basis of the association between CHD risk and microalbuminuria remain to be elucidated. The only known environmental influences on insulin resistance are energy intake and physical activity. Control of obesity and greater physical activity are likely to be the most effective means of preventing both diabetes and CHD in individuals and populations at risk of the adverse consequences of insulin resistance.

REFERENCES

Abrams, M. E., Jarrett, R. J., Keen, H., Boyns, D. R., and Crossley, J. N. (1969). Oral glucose tolerance and related factors in a normal population sample. II. Interrelationships of glycerides, cholesterol and other factors with the glucose and insulin response. *Br. Med. J.*, **1**, 599–602.

Allawi, J. and Jarrett, R. J. (1990). Microalbuminuria and cardiovascular risk factors in type 2 diabetes mellitus. *Diabet. Med.*, **7**, 115–18.

Andersson, B., Xu, X., Rebuffe-Scrive, M., Terning, K., Krotkiewski, M., and Bjorntorp, P. (1991). The effects of exercise training on body composition and metabolism in men and women. *Int. J. Obes.*, **15**, 75–81.

Aronoff, S. L., Bennett, P. H., Gorden, P., Rushforth, N., and Miller, M. (1977). Unexplained hyperinsulinaemia in normal and 'prediabetic' Pima Indians compared with normal Caucasians. An example of racial differences in insulin secretion. *Diabetes,* **26,** 827–40.

Austin, M. A., Breslow, J. L., Hennekens, C. H., Buring, J. E., Willett, W. C., and Kraus, R. M. (1988). Low density lipoprotein subclass patterns and risk of myocardial infarction. *J. Am. Med. Assoc.,* **260,** 1917–21.

Balarajan, R., Adelstein, A. M., Bulusu, L., and Shukla, V. (1984). Patterns of mortality among migrants to England and Wales from the Indian subcontinent. *Br. Med. J.,* **289,** 1185–7.

Barakat, H. A., Burton, D. S., Carpenter, J. W., Holbert, D., and Israel, R. G. (1988). Body fat distribution, plasma lipoproteins and the risk of coronary heart disease of male subjects. *Int. J. Obes.,* **12,** 473–80.

Barakat, H. A., Carpenter, J. W., McLendon, V. D., Khazanie, P., Leggett, N., Heath, J. *et al.* (1990). Influence of obesity, impaired glucose tolerance and NIDDM on LDL structure and composition: possible link between hyperinsulinacmia and atherosclerosis. *Diabetes,* **39,** 1527–33.

Barrett-Connor, E. L., Cohn, B. A., Wingard, D. L., and Edelstein, S. L. (1991). Why is diabetes mellitus a stronger risk factor for fatal ischemic heart disease in women than in men? The Rancho Bernardo Study. *J. Am. Med. Assoc.,* **265,** 627–31.

Bastian, P. (1979). Coronary heart disease in tribal Aborigines—the West Kimberley survey. *Aust. NZ J. Med.,* **9,** 284–92.

Beckles, G. L. A., Miller, G. J., Kirkwood, B. R., Alexis, S. D., Carson, D. C., and Byam, N. T. A. (1986). High total and cardiovascular disease mortality in adults of Indian descent in Trinidad, unexplained by major coronary risk factors. *Lancet,* **i,** 1298–301.

Cambien, F., Warnet, J-M., Eschwege, E., Jacqueson, A., Richard, J. L., and Rosselin, G. (1987). Body mass, blood pressure, glucose and lipids: does plasma insulin explain their relationships? *Arteriosclerosis,* **7,** 197–202.

Davey Smith, G. and Phillips, A. (1990). Declaring independence: why we should be cautious. *J. Epidemiol. Community Health,* **44,** 257–8.

DeFronzo, R. A. (1988). The triumvirate: beta cell, muscle, liver: a collusion responsible for NIDDM. *Diabetes,* **37,** 667–87.

DeFronzo, R. A. and Ferrannini, E. (1991). Insulin resistance: a multifaceted syndrome responsible for NIDDM, obesity, hypertension, dyslipidemia, and atherosclerotic cardiovascular disease. *Diabet. Care,* **14,** 173–94.

Despres, J-P., Bouchard, C., Tremblay, A., Savard, R., and Marcotte, M. (1985). Effect of aerobic training on fat distribution in male subjects. *Med. Sci. Sports Exerc.,* **17,** 113–18.

Despres, J-P., Tremblay, A., Nadeau, A., and Bouchard, C. (1988a). Physical training and changes in regional adipose tissue distribution. *Acta Med. Scand.,* Suppl. 723, 205–12.

Despres, J-P., Moorjani, S., Tremblay, A., Poehlman, E. T., Lupien, P., Nadeau, A., *et al.* (1988b). Heredity and changes in plasma lipids and lipoproteins after short-term exercise training in men. *Arteriosclerosis,* **8,** 402–9.

Ducimetiere, P., Eschwege, E., Papoz, L., Richard, J. L., Claude, J. R., and Rosselin, G. (1980). Relationship of plasma insulin levels to the incidence of myocardial infarction and coronary heart disease mortality in a middle-aged population. *Diabetologia,* **19,** 205–10.

Edwards, F. M., Wise, P. H., Thomas, D. W., Murchland, J. B., and Craig, R. J. (1976). Blood pressure and electrocardiographic findings in the South Australian Aborigines. *Aust. NZ J. Med.,* **6,** 197–205.

Eschwege, E., Richard, J. L., Thibult, N., Ducimetiere, P., Warnet, J. M., Claude, J. R., *et al.* (1985). Coronary heart disease mortality in relation with diabetes, blood glucose and plasma insulin levels: the Paris Prospective Study, ten years later. *Horm. Metab. Res.,* Suppl. 15, 41–6.

Ferrannini, E., Buzzigoli, G., Bonadona, R., Giorcio, M. A., Oleggini, M., Graziadei, L., *et al.* (1987). Insulin resistance in essential hypertension. *N. Engl. J. Med.,* **317,** 350–7.

Florey, C. du V., Uppal, S., and Lowy, C. (1976). Relationship between blood pressure, weight, and plasma sugar and serum insulin levels in schoolchildren aged 9–12 years in Westland, Holland. *Br. Med. J.,* **1,** 1368–71.

Folsom, A. R., Burke, G. L., Ballew, C., Jacobs, D. R. Jr, Haskell, W. L., Liu, K. A., *et al.* (1989). Relation of body fatness and its distribution to cardiovascular risk factors in young blacks and whites. The role of insulin. *Am. J. Epidemiol.,* **130,** 911–24.

Ford, E., Cooper, R., Simmons, B., Katz, S., and Patel, R. (1988). Sex differences in high density lipoprotein cholesterol in urban blacks. *Am. J. Epidemiol.,* **127,** 753–61.

Fuller, J. H., Shipley, M. J., Rose, G., Jarrett, R. J., and Keen, H. (1983). Mortality from coronary heart disease and stroke in relation to degree of glycaemia: the Whitehall Study. *Br. Med. J.,* **287,** 867–70.

Galloway, J. A. (1990). Treatment of NIDDM with insulin agonists or substitutes. *Diabet. Care,* **13,** 1209–39.

Haffner, S. M. (1987). Hyperinsulinemia as a possible etiology for the high prevalence of non insulin dependent diabetes in Mexican Americans. *Diabet. Metab.,* **13,** 337–44.

Harris, M. I., Hadden, W. C., Knowler, W. C., and Bennett, P. H. (1987). Prevalence of diabetes and impaired glucose tolerance and plasma glucose levels in U.S. population aged 20–74 yr. *Diabetes,* **36,** 523–34.

Heath, G. W., Gavin, J. R., III, Hinderliter, J. M., Hagberg, J. M., Bloomfield, S. A., and Holloszy, J. O. (1983). Effects of exercise and lack of exercise on glucose tolerance and insulin sensitivity. *J. Appl. Physiol. Resp. Environ. Exerc. Physiol.,* **55,** 512–17.

Hollenbeck, C. and Reaven, G. M. (1987). Variations in insulin-stimulated glucose uptake in individuals with normal glucose tolerance. *J. Clin. Endocrinol. Metab.,* **64,** 1169–73.

Holm, G. and Krotkiewski, M. (1988). Potential importance of the muscles for the development of insulin resistance in obesity. *Acta Med. Scand.,* Suppl. 723, 95–101.

Howard, B. V., Davis, M. P., Pettitt, D. J., Knowler, W. C., and Bennett, P. H. (1983). Plasma and lipoprotein cholesterol and triglyceride concentrations in the Pima Indians: distributions differing from those of Caucasians. *Circulation,* **68,** 714–24.

Howard, B. V., Egusa, G., Beltz, W. F., Kesaniemi, Y. A., and Grundy, S. M. (1986). Compensatory mechanisms governing the concentration of plasma low density lipoprotein. *J. Lipid Res.,* **27,** 11–20.

Hughes, K., Lun, K. C., and Yeo, P. P. B. (1990). Cardiovascular diseases in Chinese, Malays and Indians in Singapore. I. Differences in mortality. *J. Epidemiol. Community Health,* **44,** 24–8.

Iwai, M., Yoshino, G., Matsushita, M., Morita, M., Matsuba, K., Kazumi, T., *et al.* (1990). Abnormal lipoprotein composition in normolipidemic diabetic patients. *Diabet. Care,* **13,** 792–6.

Jarrett, R. J. (1988). Is insulin atherogenic? *Diabetologia,* **31,** 71–5.

Jarrett, R. J., Keen, H., McCartney, M., Fuller, J. H., Hamilton, P. J. S., Reid, D. D., *et al.* (1978). Glucose tolerance and blood pressure in two population samples: their relation to diabetes mellitus and hypertension. *Int. J. Epidemiol.,* **7,** 15–24.

Jarrett, R. J., Viberti, G. C., Argyropoulos, A., Hill, R. D., Mahmud, U., and Murrells, T. J. (1984). Microalbuminuria predicts mortality in non-insulin-dependent diabetes. *Diabet. Med.,* **1,** 17–19.

Kannel, W. B. (1985). Lipids, diabetes and coronary heart disease: insights from the Framingham Study. *Am. Heart J.,* **110,** 1100–7.

Kasama, T., Yoshino, G., Iwatani, I., Iwai, M., Hatanaka, H., Kazumi, T., *et al.* (1987). Increased cholesterol concentration in intermediate density lipoprotein fraction of normolipidemic non-insulin-dependent diabetics. *Atherosclerosis,* **63,** 263–6.

Keen, H., Rose, G., Pyke, D. A., Boyns, D., Chlouverakis, C., and Mistry, S. (1965). Blood sugar and arterial disease. *Lancet,* **ii,** 505–8.

Knatterud, G. L., Klimt, C. R., Levin, M. E., Jacobson, M. E., and Goldner, M. G. (1978). Effects of hypoglycemic agents on vascular complications in patients with adult-onset diabetes. VII. Mortality and selected nonfatal events with insulin treatment. *J. Am. Med. Assoc.,* **240,** 37–42.

Knowler, W. C., Bennett, P. H., Hamman, R. F., and Miller, M. (1978). Diabetes incidence and prevalence in Pima Indians: a 19-fold greater incidence than in Rochester, Minnesota. *Am. J. Epidemiol.,* **108,** 497–505.

Knowler, W. C., Pettitt, D. J., Savage, P. J., and Bennett, P. H. (1981). Diabetes incidence in Pima Indians: contributions of obesity and parental diabetes. *Am. J. Epidemiol.,* **113,** 144–56.

Krolewski, A. S., Kosinski, E. J., Warram, J. H., Leland, O. S., Busick, E. J., Asmal, A. C., *et al.* (1987). Magnitude and determinants of coronary artery disease in juvenile-onset, insulin-dependent diabetes mellitus. *Am. J. Cardiol.,* **59,** 750–5.

Krotkiewski, M. (1988). Can body fat patterning be changed? *Acta Med. Scand.,* Suppl. 723, 213–23.

Lapidus, L., Bengtsson, C., Larsson, B., Pennert, K., Rybo, E., and Sjostrom, L. (1984). Distribution of adipose tissue and risk of cardiovascular disease and death: a 12 year follow up of participants in the population study of women in Gothenburg, Sweden. *Br. Med. J.,* **289,** 1257–61.

LeBlanc, J., Nadeau, A., Richard, R., and Tremblay, A. (1981). Studies on the sparing effect of exercise on insulin requirements in human subjects. *Metabolism,* **30,** 1119–24.

Lerner, D. J. and Kannel, W. B. (1986). Patterns of coronary heart disease morbidity and mortality in the sexes: a 26-year follow-up of the Framingham population. *Am. Heart J.,* **111,** 383–90.

Mattock, M. B., Keen, H., Viberti, G. C., El-Gohari, M. R., Murrells, T. J., Scott, G. S., *et al.* (1988). Coronary heart disease and urinary albumin excretion rate in Type 2 (non-insulin-dependent) diabetic patients. *Diabetologia, 31,* 82–7.

McKeigue, P. M. and Marmot, M. G. (1988). Mortality from coronary heart disease in Asian communities in London. *Br. Med. J., 297,* 903.

McKeigue, P. M., Marmot, M. G., Syndercombe Court, Y. D., Cottier, D. E., Rahman, S., and Riemersma, R. A. (1988). Diabetes, hyperinsulinaemia and coronary risk factors in Bangladeshis in east London. *Br. Heart J., 60,* 390–6.

McKeigue, P. M., Miller, G. J., and Marmot, M. G. (1989). Coronary heart disease in South Asians overseas—a review. *J. Clin. Epidemiol., 42,* 597–609.

McKeigue, P. M., Shah, B., and Marmot, M. G. (1991). Relation of central obesity and insulin resistance with high diabetes prevalence and cardiovascular risk in South Asians. *Lancet, 337,* 382–6.

Mogensen, C. E. (1984). Microalbuminuria predicts clinical proteinuria and early mortality in maturity-onset diabetes. *N. Engl. J. Med., 310,* 356–60.

Morrison, J. A., Khoury, P., Mellies, M., Kelly, K., Horvitz, R., and Glueck, C. J. (1981). Lipid and lipoprotein distributions in black adults. The Cincinnati Lipid Research Clinic's Princeton School Study. *J. Am. Med. Assoc., 245,* 939–42.

Nelson, R. G., Sievers, M. L., Knowler, W. C., Swinburn, B. A., Pettitt, D. J., Saad, M. F., *et al.* (1990). Low incidence of fatal coronary heart disease in Pima Indians despite high prevalence of non-insulin-dependent diabetes. *Circulation, 81,* 987–95.

Olefsky, J. M., Farquhar, J. W., and Reaven, G. M. (1974a). Reappraisal of the role of insulin in hypertriglyceridemia. *Am. J. Med., 57,* 551–60.

Olefsky, J. M., Reaven, G. M., and Farquhar, J. W. (1974b). Effects of weight reduction on obesity: studies of carbohydrate and lipid metabolism. *J. Clin. Invest., 53,* 64–76.

Office of Population Censuses and Surveys (OPCS) (1990). *Mortality and geography: a review in the mid-1980s. The Registrar-General's decennial supplement for England and Wales, series DS no. 9,* HMSO, London.

Orchard, T. J., Becker, D. J., Bates, M., Kuller, L. H., and Drash, A. L. (1983). Plasma insulin and lipoprotein concentrations: an atherogenic association? *Am. J. Epidemiol., 118,* 326–37.

Ostrander, L. D., Francis, T., Hayner, N. S., Kjelsberg, M. O., and Epstein, F. H. (1965). The relationship of cardiovascular disease to hyperglycaemia. *Ann. Intern. Med., 62,* 1188–97.

Pettitt, D. J., Lisse, J. R., Knowler, W. C., and Bennett, P. H. (1982). Mortality as a function of obesity and diabetes mellitus. *Am. J. Epidemiol., 115,* 359–66.

Pyörälä, K. (1979). Relationship of glucose tolerance and plasma insulin to the incidence of coronary heart disease. Results from two population studies in Finland. *Diabet. Care, 2,* 131–41.

Pyörälä, K., Savolainen, E., Kaukola, S., and Haapakoski, J. (1985). Plasma insulin as coronary heart disease risk factor: relationship to other risk factors and predictive value during 9½-year follow-up of the Helsinki Policemen Study population. *Acta Med. Scand., 701,* 38–52.

Reaven, G. M. (1988). Role of insulin resistance in human disease. *Diabetes, 37,* 1595–607.

Reid, J. M., Fullmer, S. D., Pettigrew, K. D., Burch, T. A., Bennett, P. H., Miller, M., *et al.* (1971). Nutrient intake of Pima Indian women: relationships to diabetes mellitus and gallbladder disease. *Am. J. Clin. Nutr.,* **24,** 1281–9.

Rothenberg, R. B. and Aubert, R. E. (1990). Ischemic heart disease and hypertension: effect of disease coding on epidemiologic assessment. *Public Health Rep.,* **105,** 47–52.

Shen, D. C., Sheih, S. M., Fuh, M., Chen, Y. D., and Reaven, G. M. (1988). Resistance to insulin-stimulated glucose uptake in patients with hypertension. *J. Clin. Endocrinol. Metab.,* **66,** 580–3.

Slack, J., Noble, N., Meade, T. W., and North, W. R. S. (1977). Lipid and lipoprotein concentrations in 1604 men and women in working populations in north-west London. *Br. Med. J.,* **2,** 353–6.

Stamler, R. and Stamler, J. (1979). Asymptomatic hyperglycemia and coronary heart disease: a series of papers by the International Collaborative Group, based on studies in fifteen populations. *J. Chron. Dis.,* **32,** 683–837.

Stern, M. P. and Haffner, S. M. (1988). Do anthropometric differences between Mexican-Americans and non-Hispanic Whites explain ethnic differences in metabolic variables? *Acta Med. Scand.,* Suppl. 723, 37–44.

Stern, M. P., Gaskill, S. P., Allen, C. R., Garza, V., Gonzales, J. L., and Waldrop, R. H. (1981). Cardiovascular risk factors in Mexican Americans in Laredo, Texas. I. Prevalence of overweight and diabetes and distributions of serum lipids. *Am. J. Epidemiol.,* **113,** 546–55.

Stern, M. P., Bradshaw, B. S., Eifler, C. W., Fong, D. S., and Hazuda, H. P. (1987). Secular decline in death rates due to ischemic heart disease in Mexican Americans and non-Hispanic whites in Texas, 1970–1980. *Circulation,* **76,** 1245–50.

Temple, R. C., Carrington, C. A., Luzio, S. D., Owens, D. R., Schneider, A. E., Sobey, W. J., *et al.* (1989). Insulin deficiency in non-insulin-dependent diabetes. *Lancet,* **i,** 293–5.

Wadden, T. A., Stunkard, A. J., Johnston, F. E., Wang, J., Pierson, R. N., Van Italie, T. B., *et al.* (1988). Body fat distribution in adult obese women. II. Changes in fat distribution accompanying weight reduction. *Am. J. Clin. Nutr.,* **47,** 229–34.

Wise, P. H., Edwards, F. M., Craig, R. J., Evans, B., Marchland, J. B., Sutherland, B., *et al.* (1976). Diabetes and associated variables in the South Australian Aboriginal. *Aust. NZ J. Med.,* **6,** 191–6.

Wood, P. D., Stefanick, M. L., Dreon, D. M., Frey-Hewitt, B., Garay, S. C., Williams, P. T., *et al.* (1988). Change in plasma lipids and lipoproteins in overweight men during weight loss through dieting as compared with exercise. *N. Engl. J. Med.,* **319,** 1173–9.

Yki-Jarvinen, H. and Taskinen, M-R. (1988). Interrelationships among insulin's antilipolytic and glucoregulatory effects and plasma triglycerides in nondiabetic and diabetic patients with endogenous hypertriglyceridemia. *Diabetes,* **37,** 1271–8.

Yki-Jarvinen, H. Taskinen, M-R., Koivisto, V. A., and Nikkila, E. A. (1984). Response of adipose tissue lipoprotein lipase activity and serum lipoproteins to acute hyperinsulinaemia in man. *Diabetologia,* **27,** 364–9.

Zimmet, P., Taft, P., Guinea, A., Guthrie, W., and Thoma, K. (1977). The high prevalence of diabetes on a Central Pacific island. *Diabetologia,* **13,** 111–15.

16

Obesity and body fat distribution as predictors of coronary heart disease

B. Larsson

Obesity can be defined a 'an excess of body fat, frequently resulting in a significant impairment of health' (NIH 1985). Simple measurements of body fat, based on height and weight, are generally used as surrogate indices of obesity in epidemiological studies. The currently most widely used index is the body mass index (BMI), which is also known as Quetelet's index (weight (kg)/square of height(m)). Although BMI is strongly correlated with more direct estimates of body fatness, as determined by total body potassium (Larsson *et al.* 1981) or body density (Keys *et al.* 1972), it leaves 25–45 per cent of the variance in fatness unexplained.

OVERALL OBESITY AND MORTALITY

Epidemiological studies in large cohorts, with long follow-up periods, often report a J- or U-shaped association between obesity and all-cause mortality (Lew and Garfinkel 1979; Waaler 1983; Hoffmans *et al.* 1988; Rissanen *et al.* 1989; Manson *et al.* 1990). In the largest study to date, 1.8 million Norwegians have been followed for 10 years (Waaler 1983). In that study the U-shaped association of BMI with mortality, unadjusted for factors other than age and sex, was clear for both sexes. The optimum BMI in terms of survival was difficult to define since the U had a broad flat bottom from BMI around 22 to BMI about 29 in middle-aged subjects. Several studies suggest that the association of obesity with mortality after the sixth decade is weaker than in younger ages (Waaler 1983; Andres *et al.* 1985; Mattila *et al.* 1986; Tayback *et al.* 1990), and is weaker in women than in men (Waaler 1983; Tuomelehto 1987; Wienpahl *et al.* 1990). Both leanness and obesity seem to be detrimental to longevity, but via quite different mechanisms and disease patterns. Relative thinness is often associated with increased mortality from obstructive lung disease, tuberculosis, and stomach and lung cancer, and obesity-related causes of death are cardiovascular disease (CVD), cerebrovascular disease, and diabetes (Waaler 1983).

However, conflicting results have been reported on the association between obesity and longevity, as reviewed by Andres (1980), Ernsberger and Haskew (1987), Manson *et al.* (1987), and Keys (1989). Some of the inconsistencies can be explained by lack of statistical power in small studies and by biases (Manson *et al.* 1987).

OVERALL OBESITY AND CHD

The mortality curves for CVD versus initial BMI in the Norwegian study (smoking was not taken into account) were approximately J-shaped, with the lowest risk around BMI 23. From this point, the risk for death from cardiovascular disease increased by about 2 per cent for each kilogram of body weight (Waaler 1983). However, studies of overall obesity and risk for coronary heart disease (CHD) have been inconsistent, as reviewed by Keys (1980), Larsson *et al.* (1981), Simopoulos and van Itallie (1984), Barrett-Connor (1985), and Hubert (1986).

Contradictory findings between epidemiological studies are not uncommon, but in this field differences between results and conclusions have been greater than is usually the case. To be able to reach a conclusion based on all the evidence, we cannot simply count studies for or against an association; we have to understand the reasons for the different results.

There are a number of possible factors that could help to explain the inconsistent findings, as discussed by Barrett-Connor (1985), Stallones (1985), Manson *et al.* (1987), and Kissebah *et al.* (1989). Since the risk function between obesity and CHD in most large studies is rather flat and curvilinear, studies with few observations will have difficulty in demonstrating any correlation at all. Many studies have been too small, with too short a follow-up time, to have enough statistical power. In some studies the true effect of obesity has been underestimated because of lack of control of potential confounders such as smoking status (Garrison *et al.* 1983) or antecedent illness. Other possible confounders often not accounted for are physical inactivity, social group, dietary factors, or other behavioural risk factors for CHD (Stallones 1985). Control for potential intermediates (e.g. hypertension, hyperglycaemia, hyperlipidaemia) in a causal association between obesity and morbidity can also lead to underestimation of the true effect of obesity. Misclassification of both the degree of obesity and the outcome could obscure a true relationship. In a critical review considering these possible explanations for inconsistencies, it was concluded that 'inconsistent results with regard to the nature, strength and linearity of the association between obesity and atherosclerosis do not support the hypothesis that obesity causes atherosclerosis, despite its biologic plausibility' (Barret-Connor 1985). This conclusion was mainly based on results from smaller American cohorts. In most larger studies, however, general obesity is a risk factor for CVD in both men and women, as exemplified by two recent studies that are well designed and well analysed (Rissanen 1989; Manson *et al*. 1990). However, obesity is weaker than the major CHD risk factors. In all categories of BMI, smokers, for instance, have higher CHD incidence than non-smokers (Larsson *et al*. 1981; Royal College of Physicians 1983; Tuomilehto *et al*. 1987; Wannamethee and Shaper 1989).

Control for hypertension, hyperglycaemia, and hyperlipidaemia in most studies attenuates the strength of association between general obesity and CHD (Manson *et al*. 1987; Rissanen *et al*. 1989). This implies that, to a large extent, the excess risk associated with obesity is mediated by these risk factors. In some studies, obesity is shown to be a risk factor for CHD independently of these factors (Hubert *et al*. 1983), indicating a possible role of other mediating factors.

ABDOMINAL FAT DISTRIBUTION—A RISK FACTOR FOR CHD

Not all obese individuals are at high risk for CHD. Attempts have been made to find subgroups of obese individuals with a high CHD risk. Recent studies have indicated that subjects with a certain fat tissue distribution might be one such group (Seidell *et al*. 1987). More than 40 years ago, Vague used an index, adipomuscular ratio, derived from skinfold thicknesses and arm and thigh circumferences for differentiation of obesity into a masculine (android) and a feminine (gynoid) type. From cross-sectional findings, he concluded that android obesity was both diabetogenic and atherogenic (Vague 1956). More recent cross-sectional findings tend to support his conclusion. In a study of second-generation Japanese-American men, intra-abdominal cross-sectional fat area, determined by computer tomography (CT) scanning, was significantly elevated in men with signs of CHD compared with normal men, even after adjustment for glucose tolerance and BMI (Bergström *et al*. 1990).

Cross-sectional evidence for the possible importance of abdominal obesity has come from studies of another immigrant population—Asians living in England. Mortality from CHD is 50 per cent higher in men and women born in South Asia than in the general population (McKeigue and Marmot 1988). Factors such as smoking habits, diet, cholesterol, or blood pressure could not explain the difference in CHD incidence. However, Asians had diabetes three times more often, their plasma concentrations of insulin and triglycerides were high, and their high density lipoprotein (HDL) concentration was low. South Asians living in London also had a striking tendency to central adipose tissue distribution in the absence of obesity. It was concluded that abdominal adipose tissue distribution might account for the high CHD incidence in this population via insulin-resistance-related CHD risk factors (McKeigue *et al.* 1989).

The association between abdominal obesity and angiographically verified CHD has been studied, and the results suggest that in older women the risk increases with greater percentage of body fat in the abdomen (Hartz *et al.* 1990). A number of cross-sectional studies have shown that abdominal obesity *per se*, and especially the volume of the intra-abdominal fat depot, is associated with possible CHD risk factors such as insulin resistance, hyperinsulinaemia, impaired glucose tolerance, diabetes mellitus, atherogenic plasma lipid profile, and elevated blood pressure (Kissebah *et al.* 1982; Krotkiewski *et al.* 1983), and with haemostatic factors such as elevated fibrinogen levels and plasmin activator inhibitor (Sundell *et al.* 1989).

Limitations of inferences derived from cross-sectional studies make it desirable to confirm the associations in prospective studies. Abdominal obesity, assessed by circumferences or skinfolds, has been identified as a significant risk factor for CHD, independent of general obesity, in several prospective studies in both men and women (see Lapidus and Bengtsson (1988) and Larsson (1988 for reviews)): the Framingham Heart Study (Higgins *et al.* 1988), the Honolulu Heart Program (Donahue *et al.* 1987), the Paris Prospective Study (Ducemitiere *et al.* 1986), the Study of Men Born in 1913 (Larsson *et al.* 1984), and the Study of Women in Gothenburg (Lapidus *et al.* 1984). Indices of abdominal obesity are more predictive of CHD than are indices of general obesity, and, judging from a comparison of relative risks, abdominal obesity seems to be almost as strong a risk factor as the major CHD risk factors. Since obesity and abdominal adipose tissue distribution are common in most societies, they are also important risk factors from a public health point of view (Rose 1985).

CAUSAL ASSOCIATION?

Several possible mechanisms relating fat distribution, metabolism, and CHD risk have been discussed (Björntorp 1988; Kissebah *et al.* 1989). The intra-abdominal fat mass, and especially the 'portal' adipose tissue mass, has been suggested as a generator of risk factors for cardiovascular disease (see Björntorp 1990 for a review).

The portal adipose tissue mass has a very sensitive system for the mobilization of free fatty acids (FFA). When this mass is enlarged, the liver will therefore be exposed to elevated concentrations of portal FFA with important consequences for this organ. High FFA flux via the liver will stimulate hepatic production and secretion of very low density lipoprotein, activate gluconeogenesis, and, probably even more importantly, inhibit the hepatic uptake of insulin which will lead to peripheral hyperinsulinaemia (Björntorp 1990). Even in the absence of obesity, enlarged intra-abdominal adipose tissue mass might be an important underlying factor for the metabolic syndrome X (Reaven 1988) by altering the metabolic set-point of the liver.

Current data suggest that the regional distribution of body fat, rather than total fat, is a predictor of a number of CHD risk factors including HDL2 level. Fat distribution measured as waist-to-hip ratio explained much of the sex difference in HDL levels (Ostlund *et al.* 1990), and in another study adjustment for this ratio reduced the sex differences in levels of apolipoprotein B, triglycerides, and apolipoprotein A-I as well as HDL-cholesterol (Freedman *et al.* 1990). In a collaborative study in Gothenburg, Sweden, the sex difference in CHD incidence disappeared after controlling for the waist-to-hip ratio (Larsson *et al.* 1991).

Abdominal obesity might not only act via a number of CHD risk factors, but also to some extent be non-causally associated with CHD risk by acting as a marker for high CHD risk. Increased CHD risk in subjects with abdominal obesity could, at least in part, be a parallel phenomenon to increased genetically determined risk (Iverius and Brunzell 1985) or act as a surrogate for a cluster of unfavourable health habits associated with abdominal obesity such as high consumption of alcohol, smoking, physical inactivity, low education, etc. (Lapidus *et al.* 1989; Larsson *et al.* 1989). These factors need to be controlled for in future studies. Studies of determinants of abdominal obesity are urgently needed (Selby *et al.* 1990), as are intervention studies, to find out if the adverse consequences of abdominal obesity are reversible.

SUMMARY AND CONCLUSION

In summary, a quadratic association between obesity and all-cause mortality reflects several individual causes of death that have positive, negative, or quadratic associations with overall obesity. The optimal weight as regards mortality remains a subject of controversy. Optimal weight depends on personal characteristics such as age, sex, individual susceptibility, and cultural context. Obesity with BMI ≤ 30 is, if not associated with abdominal fat patterning, often rather well tolerated. Morbid obesity (BMI > 30) often leads to an adverse health outcome irrespective of the adipose tissue distribution. Even in the absence of obesity, abdominal adipose tissue distribution is an important marker of a cluster of behavioural, physiological, and metabolic risk factors for CHD, and might be causally associated with increased risk for CHD. Intervention strategies should be directed toward this group with high CHD risk.

ACKNOWLEDGEMENTS

This study was supported by grants from the Swedish Medical Research Council (90-27X-06276-09A), King Gustav V and Queen Victoria's Foundation, the Swedish Association against Heart and Chest Diseases, the Gothenburg Medical Association, and Gothenburg University.

REFERENCES

Andres, R. (1980). Effects of obesity on total mortality. *Int. J. Obes.*, **4**, 381–6.

Andres, R., Elahi, D., Tobin, J. D., Muller, D. C., and Brant, L. (1985). Impact of age on weight goals. *Ann. Intern. Med.*, **103**, 1030–3.

Barrett-Connor, E. L. (1985). Obesity, atherosclerosis, and coronary artery disease. *Ann. Intern. Med.*, **103**, 1010–19.

Bergström, R. W., Leonetti, D. L., Newell-Morris, L. L., Shuman, W. P., Wahl, P. W., and Fujimoto, W. Y. (1990). Association of plasma triglyceride and C-peptide with coronary heart disease in Japanese-American men with a high prevalence of glucose tolerance. *Diabetologia*, **33**, 489–96.

Björntorp, P. (1988). Possible mechanisms relating fat distribution and metabolism. In *Fat distribution during growth and later health outcomes* (eds C. Bouchard and F. E. Johnston), pp. 175–91, Alan R. Liss, New York.

Björntorp, P. (1990). 'Portal' adipose tissue as a generator of risk factors for cardiovascular disease and diabetes. *Arteriosclerosis*, **10**, 493–6.

Donahue, R. P., Abbott, R. D., Bloom, E., Reed, D. M., and Yano, K. (1987). Central obesity and coronary heart disease in men. *Lancet*, **i**, 821–4.

Ducimetiere, P., Richard, J., and Cambien, F. (1986). The pattern of subcutaneous fat distribution in middle-aged men and the risk of coronary heart disease. The Paris Prospective Study. *Int. J. Obes.*, **10**, 229–40.

Ernsberger, P. and Haskew, P. (1987). Health implications of obesity: an alternative view. *J. Obes. Weight Regul.*, **6**, 58–137.

Freedman, D. S., Jacobsen, S. J., Barboriak, J. J., Sobocinski, K. A., Anderson, A. J., Kissebah, A. H., *et al.* (1990). Body fat distribution and male/female difference in lipids and lipoproteins. *Circulation*, **81**, 1498–506.

Garrison, R. J., Feinleib, M., Castelli, W. P., and McNamara, P. M. (1983). Cigarette smoking as a confounder of the relationship between relative weight and long-term mortality: the Framingham Heart Study. *J. Am. Med. Assoc.*, **249**, 2199–203.

Hartz, A., Grubb, B., Wild, R., van Nort, J., Kuhn, E., Freedman, D. S. *et al.* (1990). The association of waist hip ratio and angiographically determined coronary artery disease. *Int. J. Obes.*, **14**, 657–65.

Higgins, M., Kannel, W., Garrison, R., Pinsky, J., and Stokes III (1988). Hazards of obesity—the Framingham experience. *Acta Med. Scand.*, Suppl. 723, 23–36.

Hoffmans, M. D. A. F., Kromhout, D., and De Lezenne Coulander, C. (1988). The impact of body mass index of 78,612 18-year old Dutch men on 32-year mortality from all causes. *J. Clin. Epidemiol.*, **41**, 749–56.

Hubert, H. B. (1986). The importance of obesity in the development of coronary risk factors and disease: the epidemiologic evidence. *Annu. Rev. Publ. Health,* **7,** 493–502.

Hubert, H. B., Feinleib, M., McNamara, P. M., and Castelli, W. P. (1983). Obesity as an independent risk factor for cardiovascular disease: a 26-year follow-up of participants in the Framingham Heart Study. *Circulation,* **67,** 968–77.

Iverius, P. H. and Brunzel, I. D. (1985). Obesity and common genetic metabolic disorders. *Ann. Intern. Med.,* **103,** 1050–1.

Keys, A. (1980). Overweight, obesity, coronary heart disease, and mortality. *Nutr. Rev.,* **38,** 297–307.

Keys, A. (1989). Longevity in man. Relative weight and fatness in middle age. *Ann. Med.,* **21,** 163–8.

Keys, A., Fidanza, F., Karvonen, M. J., Kimua, N., and Taylor, H. L. (1972). Indices of relative weight and obesity. *J. Chron. Dis.,* **25,** 329–43.

Kissebah, A. H., Vydelingum, N., Murray, R., Evans, K. J., Hartz, A. J., Kalkhoff, R. K. *et al.* (1982). Relation of body fat distribution to metabolic complications of obesity. *J. Clin. Endocrinol. Metab.,* **54,** 254–60.

Kissebah, A. H., Freedman, D. S., and Peiris, A. N. (1989). Health risks of obesity. *Med. Clin. N. Am.,* **73,** 111–38.

Krotkiewski, M., Björntorp, P., Sjöström, L., and Smith, U. (1983). Impact of obesity on metabolism in men and women. Importance of regional a dipose tissue distribution. *J. Clin. Invest.,* **72,** 1150–62.

Lapidus, L. and Bengtsson, C. (1988). Regional obesity as a health hazard in women—a prospective study. *Acta Med. Scand.,* Suppl. 723, 53–9.

Lapidus, L., Bengtsson, C., Larsson, B., Pennert, K., Rybo, E., Sjöström, L. (1984). Distribution of adipose tissue and risk of cardiovascular disease and death: a 12-year follow-up of participants in the population study of women in Gothenburg, Sweden. *Br. Med. J.,* **289,** 1257–61.

Lapidus, L., Bengtsson, C., Hällström, T., and Björntorp, P. (1989). Obesity, adipose tissue distribution and health in women—results from a population study in Gothenburg, Sweden. *Appetite,* **13,** 25–35.

Larsson, B. (1988). Regional obesity as a health hazard in men—prospective studies. *Acta Med. Scand.,* Suppl. 723, 45–51.

Larsson, B., Björntorp, P., and Tibblin, G. (1981). The health consequences of moderate obesity. *Int. J. Obes.,* **5,** 97–116.

Larsson, B., Svärdsudd, K., Welin, L., Wilhelmsen, L., Björntorp, P., and Tibblin, G. (1984). Abdominal adipose tissue distribution, obesity, and risk of cardiovascular disease and death: a 13-year follow-up of participants in the Study of Men Born in 1913. *Br. Med. J.,* **288,** 1401–4.

Larsson, B., Seidell, I., Svärdsudd, K., Welin, L., Tibblin, G., Wilhelmsen, L., *et al.* (1989). Obesity, adipose tissue distribution and health in men—the Study of Men Born in 1913. *Appetite,* **13,** 37–44.

Larsson, B., Bengtsson, C., Björntorp, P., Lapidus, L., Sjöström, L., Svärdsudd, K., *et al.* (1991). Is abdominal body fat distribution a main explanation for the sex difference in the incidence of myocardial infarction? *Am. J. Epidem.,* in press.

Lew, E. A. and Garfinkel, L. (1979). Variations in mortality by weight among 750,000 men and women. *J. Chron. Dis.,* **32,** 563–76.

Manson, J. E., Stampfer, M. J., Hennekens, C. H., and Willet, W. C. (1987). Body weight and longevity. A reassessment. *J. Am. Med. Assoc.*, **257**(3), 353–8.

Manson, J. E., Colditz, G., Stampfer, M. J., Willett, W. C., Rosner, B., Monson, R. R., *et al.* (1990). A prospective study of obesity and risk of coronary heart disease in women. *New Engl. J. Med.*, **322**, 882–9.

Mattila, M., Haavist, M., and Rajala, S. (1986). Body mass index and mortality in the elderly. *Br. Med. J.*, **292**, 867–8.

McKeigue, P. M. and Marmot, M. G. (1988). Mortality from coronary heart disease in Asian communities in London. *Br. Med. J.*, **297**, 903.

McKeigue, P. M., Miller, G. J., and Marmot, M. (1989). Coronary heart disease in South Asians overseas: a review. *J. Clin. Epidemiol.*, **42**, 597–609.

NIH (National Institutes of Health) Consensus Development Panel on the Health Implications of Obesity (1985). Health implications of obesity. *Ann. Intern. Med.*, **103**, 147–51.

Ostlund, R. E., Staten, M., Kohrt, W. M., Schultz, J., and Malley, M. (1990). The ratio of waist-to-hip circumference, plasma insulin level, and glucose intolerance as independent predictors of the HDL 2 cholesterol level in older adults. *New Engl. J. Med.*, **322**, 229–34.

Reaven, G. M. (1988). Role of insulin resistance in human disease. *Diabetes*, **37**, 1595–607.

Rissanen, A., Heliövaara, M., Knekt, P., Aromaa, A., Reunanen, A., and Maatela, J. (1989). Weight and mortality in Finnish men. *J. Clin. Epidemiol.*, **42**, 781–9.

Rose, G. (1985). Sick individuals and sick populations. *Int. J. Epidemiol.*, **14**, 32–8.

Royal College of Physicians (1983). Obesity. *J. R. Coll. Physic. Lond.*, **17**, 5–65.

Seidell, J. C., Durenberg, P., and Hautvast, J. G. A. J. (1987). Obesity and fat distribution in relation to health—Current insights and recommendations. *World Rev. Nutr. Diet*, **50**, 57–91.

Selby, J. V., Newman, B., Quesenberry, Jr C. P., Fabsitz, R. R., Carmelli, D., Meaney, F. J., and Slemenda, C. (1990). Genetic and behavioural influences on body fat distribution. *Int. J. Obes.*, **14**, 593–602.

Simopoulos, A. P. and van Ittalie, T. B. (1984). Body weight, health, and longevity. *Ann. Intern. Med.*, **100**, 285–95.

Stallones, R. A. (1985). Epidemiologic studies of obesity. *Ann. Intern. Med.*, **103**, 1003–5.

Sundell, B. T., Nilsson, T. K., Rönby, M., Hallmans, G., and Hellsten, G. (1989). Fibrinolytic variables are related to age, sex, blood pressure, and body build measurements: a cross-sectional study in Nordsjö, Sweden. *J. Clin. Epidemiol.*, **42**, 719–23.

Tayback, M., Kumanyika, S., and Chee, E. (1990). Body weight is a risk factor in the elderly. *Arch. Intern. Med.*, **150**, 1065–72.

Tuomilehto, J., Salonen, J. T., Marti, B., Jalkanen, L., Puska, P., Nissinen, A., *et al.* (1987). Body weight as risk of myocardial infarction and death in the adult population of eastern Finland. *Br. Med. J.*, **295**, 623–7.

Vague, J. (1956). The degree of masculine differentiation of obesities: a factor determining predisposition to diabetes, atherosclerosis, gout, and uric calculous disease. *Am. J. Clin. Nutr.*, **4**, 20–34.

Waaler, H. T. (1983). Height, weight, and mortality: the Norwegian experience. *Acta Med. Scand.*, Suppl. 3, 679.

Wannamethee, G. and Shaper, A. G. (1989). Body weight and mortality in middle aged British men: impact of smoking. *Br. Med. J.*, **299**, 1497–502.

Wienpahl, J., Ragland, D. R., and Sidney, S. (1990). Body mass index and 15-year mortality in a cohort of black men and women. *J. Clin. Epidemiol.*, **43**, 949–60.

17

Exercise versus heart attack: history of a hypothesis

J. N. Morris

The observation that physical activity can protect against heart attack was first made in studies of men in a variety of occupations. Conductors on London's double-decker buses (up and down stairs 11 days a fortnight, 50 weeks a year, often for decades) experienced half or less the incidence of acute myocardial infarction and 'sudden death' ascribed to coronary heart disease (CHD) in the sedentary bus drivers. Postmen (70 per cent of their shift walking, cycling, and climbing stairs to deliver the mail) were similarly protected by comparison with postal clerks and miscellaneous other groups of sedentary government workers (Morris *et al.* 1953). The self-selection issue soon presented: conductors were manifestly more lightly built than drivers. Perhaps the conductors were generally healthier than the drivers (as manifest in their leanness) and so less likely to suffer heart attack—and also to choose more active jobs? However, prospective analysis of rates of sudden death in relation to uniform trouser-waist (central obesity?) in the bus population found that slim, average, or portly conductors suffered about half or less the incidence of the drivers (Heady *et al.* 1961). Subsequent occupational studies in the UK and elsewhere mostly confirmed the main observation and its 'independence' from a variety of other relevant, possibly confounding factors (Paffenbarger *et al.* 1970; Powell *et al.* 1987; Kristensen 1989).

By the 1960s it had already become evident that if physical activity was to contribute in the years ahead to prevention of CHD it would increasingly have to be the exercise taken off the job, in leisure time, by a population increasingly employed in physically undemanding work and otherwise physically inactive. Therefore a survey was mounted among a group of male sedentary/physically very light workers in the executive grade of the civil service to test the hypothesis drawn (not very perceptively) from these occupational studies that such men with high totals of physical activity in their leisure time would suffer less CHD than comparable men with low totals. There was no support for this in prospective study. Instead, it was found that only the men engaging in vigorous activity showed a reduced incidence of the disease (Fig. 17.1). Vigorous activity was defined as that

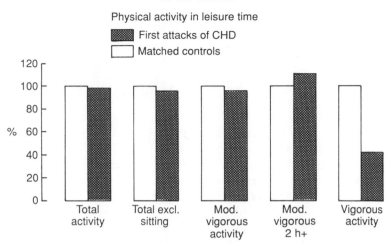

Fig. 17.1 Prospective survey (1968/70–78) of 16 882 British male executive grade civil servants, aged 40–64 at entry. First 214 fatal and non-fatal clinical attacks of coronary heart disease and 428 controls. Activity logged, 5 min × 5 min, on sample Friday and Saturday. (From Morris *et al.* 1973.)

liable to reach peaks of energy expenditure of 7.5 kcal/min (31.5 kJ/min), over six times basal oxygen uptake, say, and a gross oxygen uptake of 1.5 l/min or about 20 ml/kg/min. Furthermore, the men reporting dynamic vigorous aerobic exercise, in sports and getting about, showed much stronger and more consistent protection than those reporting heavy recreational 'work', the other form of vigorous activity (Morris *et al.* 1973, 1980).

Again, the benefits of such vigorous aerobic exercise were statistically independent of the other factors that were studied. For example, Table 17.1 shows the age-standardized percentage CHD incidence rates for men classified according to cigarette smoking and vigorous exercise at 8.5 years

Table 17.1 CHD incidence (per cent)

	VE	No. VE
Non-smokers		
Non-fatal first clinical attack	1.3	3.2
Fatal first clinical attack	0.85	1.7
Smokers		
Non-fatal	1.6	4.4
Fatal	3.3	5.2

VE, vigorous aerobic exercise.

follow-up. The reductions were substantially greater in men aged 50–64 than in the younger entrants.

VARIATIONS OF CHD

The advantage of men engaging in vigorous aerobic exercise was evident in the incidence of acute myocardial infarction (non-fatal and fatal), sudden death, angina pectoris, and coronary insufficiency.

In a cross-sectional approach a sample of 509 men was drawn from the cohort. Of these, 74 reported vigorous aerobic exercise. Their resting electrocardiograms (ECGs) were compared using the Minnesota Code (Rose and Blackburn 1968) with those of the 384 men reporting no vigorous exercise: 2.9 per cent of the former (age-standardized) showed definite or possible ischaemia against 10.4 per cent of the latter. Less expected were the differences in the frequency of ectopic beats (EBs). These were 2.9 per cent in the 74 men reporting exercise versus 7.1 per cent in the 384 others: 0 versus 10 instances of supraventricular EBs, 2 versus 17 instances of ventricular EBs, and 0 versus 14 instances of EBs comprising 10 per cent or more of recorded cycles. Electrical instability?

Exclusion of men with evidence of clinical or subclinical cardiovascular disease did not affect this contrast. The 51 men reporting heavy recreational work showed no such immunity (Epstein *et al.* 1976).

NEXT STEPS

The indication that a threshold of intensity of exercise has to be reached for protection against CHD, and the further suggestion that vigorous *aerobic* exercise is distinctively effectual, raised questions for theory (Fentem *et al.* 1988; Pollock and Wilmore 1990) and for public health. Thus we could be identifying a level of activity in this homogeneous population of middle-aged middle-class office workers whose health was average or above, sufficiently intense on average, i.e. entailing over 50–60 per cent of individual maximal aerobic power, and of sufficient quantity, to produce 'overload' and a training stimulus. And this could be improving cardio-respiratory fitness to moderately high levels. Plainly, health education messages would be affected if such a proposition superseded that of the benefits of high total physical activity levels (Morris 1975). Therefore a further survey was mounted in 1976 to test the new hypothesis directly.

Fresh hypothesis

The prospective survey of 1976–86, again in men of the executive grade in the civil service, was designed to test the following propositions.

1. Vigorous habitual frequent aerobic exercises in sports and in getting about would offer substantial protection against CHD.

2. More tentatively, heavy (vigorous) recreational work in jobs and hobbies in and about the house and garden and on the car (the other main form of physical activity in leisure time), which had shown an inconsistent and weaker association with incidence of CHD in the previous survey, would also confer some protection.

3. Other physical activity would not be protective.

4. High totals of energy expenditure *per se* would not be protective (Morris *et al*. 1990).

Exercise and incidence

Table 17.2 orders the data of this second survey in terms of the principal proposition 1. The total cohort consisted of 9375 men having no history or record of CHD. There were 474 first clinical events in a 9.3 year follow-up and 87 563 man-years' observation. Table 17.2 shows the data for men aged 55–64 at entry which relate to proposition 1.

Group 1 consists of the men (9 per cent of the cohort) reporting vigorous sports (swimming, jogging, hill-climbing, rowing, soccer and hockey (mostly refereeing), racket games, etc., at least twice a week), and/or rating the usual pace of their regular walking to and from work and in their leisure time as 'fast' (over 4 mph or 6.4 kmph), and/or recording considerable cycling. Group 2 comprises the next highest degree of such vigorous aerobic exercise, i.e. vigorous sports at least once but less than twice a week, and/or 'fairly brisk' walking for over 30 min per day, and/or other cycling. Group 3 includes residual vigorous aerobic exercise, i.e. very little, occasional sports, and/or shorter 'fairly brisk' walks. Group 4, the largest comprising just over half the men, is made up of those who reported no vigorous aerobic exercise. This category includes the very popular non-vigorous sports and games, the commoner regular walking at 'normal' pace or 'strolling', and a huge volume of recreational work in gardening and do-it-yourself, whether vigorous, moderate, or light.

Group 1 of the cohort had low CHD attack rates compared with the rest of the men ($p < 0.001$). This was evident in both non-fatal and fatal first clinical events. For younger men, aged 45–54, there were no differences in attack rates among groups 2–4. However, the attack rate in entrants aged 55–64 was significantly lower in group 2 than in groups 3 and 4 ($p \approx 0.01$). Moreover, keep-fit exercises five or more times a week, and climbing 500 plus stairs each day—dynamic aerobic activities, plausibly vigorous items from the previous survey—which were not associated with incidence in the younger entrants did show significantly lower CHD rates in these older men. Therefore they have been included in group 2. This makes sense in

Table 17.2 Vigorous aerobic exercise, other CHD factors, and the attack rate of CHD (1976–86) in male executive grade civil servants aged 55–64 at entry (rates per 1000 man-years)

	Group 1 (frequent vigorous aerobic exercise)	Group 2 (next lesser degree of this)	Group 3 (residual vigorous aerobic exercise)	Group 4 (no vigorous aerobic exercise)	p[a]
Vigorous aerobic exercise	2.3	3.3	4.5	5.9	<0.001
Standardized for other factors	2.4	3.6	4.8	5.6	<0.005

Non-fatal first events, 55–59 years; fatal, 55–73 years.

[a] Tests for trend; tested for heterogeneity, the results are similar.

[b] Other factors, from data reported at entry, were premature parental mortality from CVD, stature, cigarette smoking, body mass index, history of high blood pressure, history of diabetes, positive/negative on LSHTM angina questionnaire (Rose and Blackburn 1968).

From Morris et al. 1990.

terms of both the probable greater variability in intensity of these two activities on the one hand and the reduction with age of the oxygen utilization capacity of muscles on the other, so that less exercise is required for overload and a training stimulus (though of course it still has to be more intense than customary). The net result is that 30 per cent of the older entrants showed such exercise-related reduction of heart disease.

In group 3 there is a non-significant continuation of the favourable trend in the older men. Thus there was some indication of dose–response of CHD with frequency/intensity in vigorous aerobic exercise. A threshold effect of such exercise alone is seen in the younger men, at the highest level of intensity that was identified (group 1). High coronary incidence at all ages was recorded in group 4.

Table 17.3 further illustrates the failure of popular non-vigorous sports and games (dancing was reported by 14 per cent of the men and golf by 10 per cent) to affect CHD rates. The outcome is similar with the quantity of regular walking if pace is disregarded. The negative findings with the detailed and more representative record in this survey of recreational work are clear; the results are the same for gardening. The situation chosen in Table 17.3 is that most likely to elicit association with coronary disease: first clinical events in men over 60 and the harder mortality data. At ages under 60 the results are the same for both non-fatal and fatal events. Because of the popularity and appeal of the non-vigorous sports and games, they were subjected to an intensive study, searching for example for possible associations with CHD in vulnerable groups such as cigarette smokers, the overweight, those with subclinical CVD, and so on, which might be expected to show a response to such exercise of lower intensity. Again, none was found.

Table 17.3 Miscellaneous activities in leisure time and mortality from CHD in male executive grade civil servants (1976–86) aged 60–73 (rates per 1000 man-years)

Episodes in previous 4 weeks[a]	Ballroom dancing	Golf	Long walks[b]	Do-it-yourself		
				Heavy	Moderate	Light
0	4.2	4.2	4.4	4.3	4.2	4.0
1–3	4.3	4.0	3.8	3.9	3.9	3.6
4–7	5.5	5.1	4.1	4.7	5.4	5.1
≥8	(3.1)	6.2	4.2	6.5	3.4	4.6

Regular walking to and from work, and elsewhere, regardless of pace, per day: 0, 3.9 per 1000 man-years; ≤30 min, 4.2 per 1000 man-years; >30 min, 3.7 per 1000 man-years. (The 0 is an overstatement since episodes of activity <5 min were disregarded throughout.)
[a] Reported at entry in 1976. (Rates for less than 5 cases in brackets.)
[b] Walks of at least an hour, additional to 'regular' walking.

Multivariate analysis

The lower line of Table 17.2 controls for possible confounding by some CHD risk factors. The familiar dilemmas and limitations of such adjust-ment arise (Davey Smith and Phillips 1990), including circularity and double-counting of such factors as body mass, subclinical cardiovascular disease (and blood cholesterol levels). These factors themselves are likely to be lowered by exercise, and may indeed be mechanisms of the effect of exercise on CHD. Therefore their introduction into the multivariate analysis may misleadingly reduce the value of the exercise factor itself in the outcome. This can be illustrated by data on 'personal control'.

In these men, there is a significant association between confidence in the possibility of personal control of future health and future coronary inci-dence. When the psychological variable is 'adjusted' for vigorous aerobic exercise, the association is considerably weakened, and if cigarette smoking is then introduced it disappears altogether. It is possible that this belief/attitude/knowledge is effectual through or mediated by these (and other health-directed) behaviours. This is attractive, but for understanding of aetiology—and for public health and its need to understand motives—how much is being lost by such computation and the summary dismissal of antecedent by later stages in the long natural history of CHD? (The difference in the precision of classification of exercise and smoking com-pared with that of the attitude, and how far this is responsible for the result, need not detain us now.)

Be all this as it may, the striking feature of Table 17.2 is the similarity of before and after profiles, again pointing to statistical independence of the exercise factor and some freedom from its confounding by the other factors studied. Of course, multivariate analyses are now ritual in epidemiological research, and in the relation between physical activity and CHD they have included all the standard risk factors and show the same general picture (Powell *et al.* 1987).

OVERVIEW

A few points can be made about some recent reports. First, a remarkable variety of populations have shown lower CHD rates with high physical activity. Thus the two most detailed studies are of elite affluent Harvard alumni (Paffenbarger *et al.* 1978) and our own British civil servants (social class II in the national scale) on modest incomes and generally without tertiary educational qualifications. The Finnish general population sample is from an area with a notably high prevalence of CHD (Salonen *et al.* 1988). The Honolulu Study follows a cohort of men of Japanese ancestry (Donahue *et al.* 1988). The Multiple Risk Factor Intervention Trial

(MRFIT) is an experiment on American men selected for high risk of CHD by elevated lipid and blood pressure levels (Leon *et al.* 1987).

There are difficulties in interpreting discrepancies between the findings of these studies. Thus, in contrast with our findings, Paffenbarger *et al.* (1978) report substantial benefit from more than 2000 kcal per week of leisure time activity, however this is accomplished. On analysis, two-thirds of the men with such high totals engaged in vigorous sports, but those reporting other non-vigorous aerobic exercise also show some, albeit less, advantage. Could it be that the American cohort is basically less active and less fit than the British and thus capable of benefiting from less intense exercise? (The same point has previously been made on age.) Other obvious differences in the populations are that the British are subject to governmental medical recruitment and retirement policies, and that they are men actually in post and hence are a 'healthy worker' cohort. Comparative physiological studies on American and British men could be rewarding.

Another question arises with regard to the methods of assessment of physical activity that are being used and, in particular, on their probability of identifying training or conditioning exercise. Because of the frequency of do-it-yourself and gardening in our British study (90 per cent of the men gardened and 80 per cent reported moderate or heavy work), overall assessment of activity by totals of energy expenditure blur the picture: neither of these two classes of activity contain much of the sustained rhythmic contraction/relaxation of large muscle groups that is required for cardiorespiratory training. Again, as previously found, total physical activity estimates do not identify groups with different CHD risk in this population. Thus, in group 4, who reported no vigorous aerobic exercise, incidence rates per 1000 man-years by total physical activity in leisure time per week, summing all the forms previously considered, were as follows: <2000 kcal, 5.9; 2,000–2,999 kcal, 6.5; ≥3000 kcal, 7.0.

The other studies mentioned above are uniform and total in their assessments and do not seek to report predominantly aerobic exercise, vigorous or not, so that rival hypotheses can be tested. The fact that these studies produce positive results could mean that it is not training and fitness that matter but high total energy expenditure, thus refuting the British findings, or perhaps indicating that they apply only to a relatively healthy population. Alternatively, the overall profiles among those scoring high totals in these other studies may include enough vigorous aerobic exercise for benefit in their populations. It should be possible to disaggregate the data and extract such information. Highlighted by this discussion is the lack, exposed by the needs of epidemiological research, of physiological information on real-life everyday physical activities in leisure time (in people of disparate occupation): on caloric expenditures, dynamic/static components, vascular reactions, metabolic responses, and short-, medium-, and long-term risk factor relationships. (The contrast with the richness of data on athletes and athleticism (Reilly *et al*. 1990) is striking.) Clinical and psychological data are frequently equally sparse.

MECHANISMS OF PROTECTION

With little qualification it can be said that exercise improves all physiological function, and of course there are also psychological and social benefits. In that sense exercise is a 'general cause' of good health (Morris 1975). Therefore, not surprisingly, major risk factors for CHD are liable to be diminished: lipid profiles, blood pressure, insulin sensitivity, glucose levels, and body mass (Powell *et al*. 1987; Fentem *et al*. 1988). At the same time, exercise both counteracts these risk factors and is some defence against them, as seen in the data previously given on smoking. Thus it might be expected that coronary atherosclerosis will be retarded or reduced, but so far the evidence in man is not impressive.

The more interesting suggestion in our study is that in such a different body of data it confirms and amplifies the observation by Paffenbarger *et al*. (1978) that, for benefit, the exercise has to be current. A history of exercise in the past, which has been abandoned, confers no protection. For example, Table 17.4 reports the experience among men who reported no vigorous sports in the 1976 survey. By the same token, men who reported taking part in vigorous sports in 1976 had the same low incidence over the period 1976–86 whether or not they had been 'athletic' when young (as attested by a record of the most vigorous sports such as squash, rugby, athletics, and wrestling). The future rates in men reporting vigorous sports at least once a week in 1976 were 3.2 and 3.0 per 1000 man-years respectively in those with and without such a record.

These observations point to the acute phases of the heart disease rather than the slow build-up of chronic coronary atherosclerosis as the main locus of protection by exercise: to acute ischaemia, thrombosis, occlusion,

Table 17.4

	Cases 1976–86	Rate per 1000 man-years
Played no vigorous sports previously	128	5.7
Played up to 25 years of age	27	4.1
Played up to 30 years of age	54	6.4
Played up to 40 years of age	92	5.7
Played past 40 years of age	112	6.2

dysrhythmia and electrial instability. Evidence that exercise is related to improved haemostatic profile in particular is increasing (Davey Smith *et al.* 1989; Meade 1991). This is a field ripe for systematic study.

An alternative or complementary interpretation of the necessity for the exercise to be maintained is that the protection is related not so much to the exercise itself, for example the dynamic exercise that raises the level of high density lipoprotein cholesterol, as to the cardiorespiratory fitness and improved cardiac performance that is induced. It is well known that fitness cannot be stored; it depends on the maintenance of adequate aerobic exercise (Saltin *et al.* 1968). Studies of CHD incidence in relation to fitness are accumulating, mostly with positive results (Gyntelberg *et al.* 1980; Blair *et al.* 1989). A difficulty here is that endurance capacity or stamina, the manifestation of cardiorespiratory fitness likely to be most responsive to the exercise under consideration, cannot yet be readily measured in the field, and estimates of maximum aerobic power (VO_2 max) are not satisfactory substitutes. Interestingly, the association of cardiorespiratory fitness with CHD risk factors, as distinct from CHD incidence, is more controversial (Sedgwick *et al.* 1989, 1990; Bouchard *et al.* 1990*a*).

RESTATEMENT OF HYPOTHESIS

The initial hypothesis has undergone several transformations in the course of its 40 years. It can now be stated as follows.

Adequate aerobic exercise in leisure time, which is habitual and ongoing, and the training and improved cardiorespiratory fitness and performance this produces, confer substantial protection against the occurrence of CHD in middle-aged and elderly men. The total death rate is also lowered. This is the case whatever the risk status of the men with respect to other factors. Protection by exercise is effectual mainly in the acute phases of the disease, in particular against thrombosis, though there is also some benefit from reducing and counteracting standard risk factors and the build-up of chronic coronary atherosclerosis.

In this statement 'adequate' refers to both vigour (intensity) and quantity (frequency/duration) of exercise. The hypothesis refers to ordinary relatively healthy men engaged in sedentary and physically light occupations, and not to athletes.

FROM AETIOLOGY TO PUBLIC HEALTH

There is now good reason to believe that the decline of physical activity in work, recreation, transport, and daily living is an integral part of the modern epidemic of CHD in developed industrial societies. This decline may well have been greatest in adequate aerobic exercise, and hence in cardiorespiratory fitness. Moreover, the increase in CHD has entailed an increase in coronary thrombosis—perhaps the main pathological change (Morris 1951)—and again a link with physical activity/inactivity can be postulated.

The UK is underachieving in several aspects of health, particularly in its persistent high rates of CHD, and the need to address major possible causes is now, at last, widely recognized. Exercise is today's best buy in public health, not only because of the need and potential, but because it is positive and acceptable, has insignificant side-effects, and can be inexpensive. Also, the opposition to be overcome is feeble in comparison with the tobacco barons and the Common Agricultural Policy for instance.

In seminal papers, Rose (1981, 1985) has interpreted modern aetiological research for public health practice in the prevention of CHD. He describes two strategies: the individual high risk strategy involving case-finding and personal care, and the population strategy which, by attacking the causes of incidence, seeks to reduce the mean level of risk factors and 'to shift the whole distribution of exposure in a favourable direction'. Each has its advantages and its drawbacks, though there is no question about the importance of the population strategy for this mass scourge.

However, two points can be made in applying Rose's thesis to our present concern with exercise. Only a minority of the population takes anything worthy of the name of exercise, and only a small minority of the lower social classes that are most vulnerable to heart attack (*General Household Survey* 1989). Thus the majority, or the great majority, of the population is probably at high risk in these terms, and the approach to them and to the population at large must be much the same. Moreover, the 'prevention paradox' of the population strategy, that participating individuals will themselves derive little benefit from their contribution to the common good (for example by lowering their blood pressure), may not apply in the case of exercise. Altruistic participating individuals can be assured that by taking exercise, as encouraged, they will rapidly feel and function better as a result of the manifold benefits that exercise confers.

The evidence on CHD can be matched by that on the general benefits of exercise to physical capacity and mobility, mental and social function, and well-being, all perhaps most notably in the elderly; to the prevention of obesity, maturity onset diabetes, osteoporosis, and so on; and to the relief of anxiety and depression. Equally, benefits in the rehabilitation of chronic disease and in the life of people with disabilities could be included (Bouchard *et al.* 1990*b*). In the present chapter we have dealt with only one aspect.

Practical application

There are several practical messages for public health practice from the kind of positive and encouraging observations reported in the present chapter. The commitment to exercise manifestly has to be continuing and serious (Department of Health and Human Services 1980; American College of Sports Medicine 1986). Examples given here are vigorous aerobic exercise at least twice a week and the expenditure of more than 2000 kcal per week in leisure time activities. Therefore such a commitment has to be emphasized in health education. However, aetiological studies are urgently required in other social and occupational samples, particularly among the lower socio-economic groups, to aid the formulation of population strategy.

Congruent with the physiology that, with adequate exercise, training is possible at all ages, there is encouragement for middle-aged men to start exercising and for the elderly to continue. Direct evidence on the former will soon be available (Paffenbarger 1991), and there is already some evidence of protection against CHD in the elderly (Donahue *et al*. 1988) and our own data for individuals up to 73 years of age.

Individual and family, society and culture

The appeal must be seen to apply to the whole population. At the same time exercise typifies the individual–social, personal–environmental, and private–public interactions and parternships that health promotion and prevention of disease require today (Morris 1975). The individual takes exercise and can continue to do so. The individual alone can tell when he/she is taking enough exercise for 'overload' or too much for safety. We are slowly learning about individual and family motivations. However, culture and society have to reinforce motivation, help with education and research, and, above all, provide support with facilities. Among the civil servants in our study, swimming is the most popular and beneficial exercise: the provision of pools to generate and meet growing demand is under perennial threat from local government financial constraints. Similarly, both walking and cycling entail the partnership of individual and government; the latest British national plan to spend more than £12 billion on roads considers neither walking nor cycling.

The return of physical activity as the norm in everyone's everyday life— the 'restoration of biological normality' in Rose's words—will require cultural change on a scale similar to that which has occurred with smoking. Meanwhile, there is little advance among those who need it most. Hopefully, the findings of the National Fitness Survey (1990–1) may provide the impetus. The challenges to epidemiology are great: in a wide range of research, in information of the public, health service, and government, in teaching, in the example we set, and, as part of the wider public health movement, in our collective political message.

ACKNOWLEDGEMENTS

Readers of this account will know how much teamwork is required in these studies. I am deeply grateful to my colleagues for their contributions.

REFERENCES

American College of Sports Medicine (1986). *Guidelines for exercise testing and prescription* (3rd edn), Lea & Febiger, Philadelphia, PA.

Blair, S. N., Kohl, H. W., III, Paffenbarger, R. S., Jr, Clark, D. G., Cooper, K. H., and Gibbons, L. W. (1989). Physical fitness and all-cause mortality: a prospective study of healthy men and women. *J. Am. Med. Assoc.*, **262**, 2395–401.

Bouchard, C., Leon, A. S., Rao, D. C., Skinner, J. S., and Wilmore, J. H. (1990*a*). Cross-sectional and longitudinal relationships between physical fitness and risk factors for coronary heart disease in men and women: 'The Adelaide 1000'. *J. Clin. Epidemiol.*, **43**, 1005–7.

Bouchard, C., Shephard, R. J., Stephens, T., Sutton, J. R., and McPherson, B. M. (eds) (1990*b*). *Exercise, fitness and health: a consensus of current knowledge*, Human Kinetics, Champaign, IL.

Davey Smith, G. and Phillips, A. (1990). Declaring independence: why we should be cautious. *J. Epidemiol. Community Health*, **44**, 257–8.

Davey Smith, G., Marmot, M. G., Etherington, M., and O'Brien, J. (1989). A work stress-fibrinogen pathway as a potential mechanism for employment grade differences in coronary heart disease rates. Abstracts, 2nd Int. Conf. on Preventive Cardiology, Washington, DC.

Department of Health and Human Services (1980). *Promoting health/preventing disease: objectives for the nation*, US Government Printing Office, Washington DC.

Donahue, R. P., Abbott, R. D., Reed, D. M., and Yano, K. C. (1988). Physical activity and coronary heart disease in middle-aged and elderly men. *Am. J. Public Health*, **78**, 683–5.

Epstein, L., Miller, G. J., Stitt, F. W., and Morris, J. N. (1976). Vigorous exercise in leisure-time, coronary risk factors, and resting electrocardiogram in middle-aged male civil servants. *Br. Heart J.*, **38**, 403–9.

Fentem, P. H., Bassey, E. J., and Turnbull, N. B. (1988). *The new case for exercise*, Health Education Authority and Sports Council, London.

General Household Survey 1986 (1989). HMSO, London.

Gyntelberg, F., Lauridsen, L., and Schubell, K. (1980). *Scand. J. Work Environ. Health*, **6**, 170–8.

Heady, J. A., Morris, J. N., Kagan, A., and Raffle, P. A. B. (1961). Coronary heart disease in London busmen: a progress report with particular reference to physique. *Br. J. Prev. Social Med.*, **15**, 143–53.

Kristensen, T. S. (1989). Cardiovascular diseases and the work environment. *Scand. J. Work and Environ. Health*, **15**, 165–79.

Leon, A. S., Connett, J., Jacobs, D. R., Jr, and Rauramaa, R. (1987). Leisure-time physical activity levels and risk of coronary heart disease and death. *J. Am. Med. Assoc.*, **258**, 2388–95.

Meade, T. W. (1991). In preparation.

Morris, J. N. (1951). Recent history of coronary disease. *Lancet*, **i**, 1–7, 69–73.

Morris, J. N. (1975). *Uses of epidemiology* (3rd edn), Churchill Livingstone, London (reprinted 1983).

Morris, J. N., Heady, J. A., Raffle, P. A. B., and Parks, J. W. (1953). Coronary heart disease and physical activity of work. *Lancet,* **ii,** 1053–7, 1111–20.

Morris, J. N., Chave, S. P. W., Adam, C., Sirey, C., and Epstein, L. (1973). Vigorous exercise in leisure-time and the incidence of coronary heart disease. *Lancet,* **i,** 333–9.

Morris, J. N., Everitt, M. G., Pollard, R., Chave, S. P. W., and Semmence, A. M. (1980). Vigorous exercise in leisure-time: protection against coronary heart disease. *Lancet,* **ii,** 1207–10.

Morris, J. N., Clayton, D. G., Everitt, M. G., Semmence, A. M., and Burgess, E. H. (1990). Exercise in leisure-time: coronary attack and death rate. *Br. Heart J.,* **63,** 325–34.

Paffenbarger, R. S., Jr (1991). In preparation.

Paffenbarger, R. S., Jr, Laughlin, M. E., Gima, A. S., and Black, R. A. (1970). Work activity of longshoremen as related to death from coronary heart disease and stroke. *New Engl. J. Med.,* **282,** 1109–13.

Paffenbarger, R. S., Jr, Wing, A. L., and Hyde, R. T. (1978). Physical activity as an index of heart attack risk in college alumni. *Am. J. Epidemiol.,* **108,** 161–75.

Pollock, M. and Wilmore, J. H. (1990). *Exercise in health and disease* (2nd edn), W. B. Saunders, Philadelphia.

Powell, K. E., Thompson, P. D., Caspersen, C. J., and Kendrick, J. S. (1987). Physical activity and the incidence of coronary heart disease. *Ann. Rev. Publ. Health.,* **8,** 251–87.

Reilly, T., Secher, N., Snell, P., and Williams, C. (eds) (1990). *Physiology of sports.* Spon, London.

Rose, G. and Blackburn, H. (1968). *Cardiovascular survey methods.* World Health Organization, Geneva.

Rose, G. (1981). Strategy of prevention: lessons from cardiovascular disease. *Br. Med. J.,* **282,** 1847–51.

Rose, G. (1985). Sick individuals and sick populations. *Int. J. Epidemiol.,* **14,** 32–8.

Salonen, J. T., Slater, J. S., Tuomilehto, J., and Rauramaa, R. (1988). Leisure-time and occupational physical activity: risk of death from ischaemic heart disease. *Am. J. Epidemiol.,* **127,** 87–94.

Saltin, B., Blomquist, G., Mitchell, J. H., Johnson, R. L., Wildenthal, K., and Chapman, C. B. (1968). Response to exercise after bed rest and after training. *Circulation,* **38** (Suppl. VII), 1–77.

Sedgwick, A. W., Thomas, D. W., Davies, M., Baghurst, K., and Rouse, I. (1989). Cross-sectional and longitudinal relationships between physical fitness and risk factors for coronary heart disease in men and women: 'The Adelaide 1000'. *J. Clin. Epidemiol.,* **42,** 189–200.

Sedgwick, A. W., Thomas, D. W., Davies, M., Baghurst, K., and Rouse, I. (1990). Cross-sectional and longitudinal relationships between physical fitness and risk factors for coronary heart disease in men and women: 'The Adelaide 1000'. *J. Clin. Epidemiol.,* **43,** 1007–12.

18

The psycho-social environment, stress, and coronary heart disease

T. Theorell

The success of any scientific endeavour depends upon the rigour and relevance of its scientific concepts. The methods that are developed also depend upon these concepts and in addition determine the extent to which they can be used for scientific enquiry. The psycho-social sphere is no exception to these rules. This chapter focuses on the introduction and development of some of the most frequently used concepts and methods in the field.

INDIVIDUAL AND ENVIRONMENT

By definition, psycho-social research is a cross-disciplinary field. Input is mainly from three disciplines.

Epidemiology and social science The focus for the epidemiologist and social scientist is the way in which the environment influences individuals. In the discipline of psycho-social factors developed in the 1960s this corresponds to an interest in the social class correlates of cardiovascular disease risk. This era is interesting because it represents a turning-point. Previously, the most frequent opinion was that cardiovascular disease was restricted to the upper classes. However, Antonovsky (1968) and, later, Marmot (1982), among others, noted that in the USA and the UK this was not the case. The social class question is still one of the most important in cardiovascular epidemiology. However, the concept of social class is not ideal from the point of view of scientific enquiry. It originates in the Marxist theory of buying and selling labour in the production process. It could be regarded as puzzling that, despite historical changes in ownership and production systems and the crude categorizations that have been used, such a vague concept still forms the basis of one of the most powerful correlates of cardiovascular disease risk. It is even more puzzling that in some countries, for instance in Southern Europe, the pattern is opposite to that in Northern Europe and North America—a higher disease risk for higher social class in the former countries and a higher risk for lower social class in the latter countries. The observations on social class have generated a great deal of interest among cardiovascular epidemiologists. However, more precise concepts and methods have slowly developed, as we shall see below.

Psychology and behavioural science   The psychological scientific tradition focuses on individuals. Its explanations involve individual mechanisms, although mechanisms on a group level are often taken into account. Psychology has played an important role in psycho-social cardiovascular epidemiology. Some of the most fruitful concepts, such as the Sisyphus syndrome (Wolf 1969), type A behaviour (Friedman and Rosenman 1959), and social support (Henry and Cassell 1969; Cobb and Kasl 1977), have been initiated by physicians rather than psychologists, but they have been given a scientific formulation by psychologists. The starting point in the formation of concepts relevant to this area has always been the following questions. Is there a particular behaviour pattern or psychological trait that increases cardiovascular vulnerability? Can this be treated psychologically? However, the concepts have been loosely defined at the start, and this has created difficulty in later stages.

Medicine   The starting point for medical science in the psycho-social field has always been the question of whether there are medical prescriptions (e.g. drugs, operations, diet) that may decrease the effects of adverse psycho-social factors. Some of the most important advances in pharmacology since the 1960s, such as the beta blockers, have been in this field.

  Each of these approaches has contributed to the psycho-social field, and there has been collaboration between them. However, the underlying philosophies are quite different. The epidemiologist wants to change environmental conditions, whereas the psychologist wants to strengthen the individual's ability to resist and the physician considers that his main task is to change the bodily reactions themselves. Social class, type A behaviour, and beta blockade could represent the three traditions. Most of these have gone through a gradual process of improving the precision of concepts and refining methodology during the period covered in this chapter.

SOCIAL ENVIRONMENT

Social class

Social class has always been a vaguely defined concept from an epidemiological research perspective. In most countries systems of three or five classes have been used, all based on education and/or income. A few attempts have been made to operationalize social class in other ways, but they have never been widely used. The use of more than five social groups has never proved to provide additional precision. For instance, in Sweden a 10 grade scale has been tried (Lundberg 1990). Recently, it has been observed in both Sweden (Diderichsen and Lindberg 1989) and the UK (Marmot and McDowell 1986) that the differences in cardiovascular mortality between social classes have widened. This has enforced the need to investigate which aetiological factors may differ between the social classes.

During the period under review there have been attempts to determine whether differences in childhood conditions are associated with differences in the risk of cardiovascular illness. Explanations of such differences have been discussed extensively (Davey Smith *et al.* 1990). More recently, much attention has been paid to two areas which both can be related to social class and may be amenable to intervention, namely working conditions and social networks.

Demand and control

Working conditions were studied systematically in the 1960s. For instance, in a retrospective study of two cohorts of bank employees in Belgium, Kornitzer and his collaborators observed that the cohort drawn from private banks had a higher incidence of coronary heart disease (CHD) than the cohort drawn from state-owned banks (Kornitzer *et al.* 1982). This could not be explained by biomedical risk factors (Kittel *et al.* 1980). Kornitzer's group have also discussed the complex relationships between stress, biomedical risk factors, and cardiovascular risk (Kornitzer and Kittel 1986). This study was one of the first to indicate a possible relationship between certain types of working conditions, work demands (which were higher in the private banks), and risk of myocardial infarction. Other cross-sectional studies during this period (Biörck *et al.* 1958; Russek and Zohman 1958; Buell and Breslow 1960; Kasanen *et al.* 1963) indicated that there may be a relationship between excessive overtime work and cardiovascular illness risk. Hinkle's study of employees of the Bell Telephone Company was the first prospective indication in this direction (Hinkle *et al.* 1968). During the same period there were also studies which indicated a higher incidence of myocardial infarction among lower-level employees in large companies (Pell and d'Alonzo 1963). Of course, this is related to the social class observation discussed above and for the first time raised the suspicion that psycho-social stress may not primarily be a problem for people with a lot of responsibility, as researchers had tended to believe previously.

During this phase of confusion and lack of theoretical models sociologists entered the field. Karasek (1979) introduced his demand–control model which was an architect's synthesis of the demand (equivalent to 'stress') and the 'lack of control' (sociological) research traditions. In generating the concept 'lack of control', or 'lack of decision latitude' as Karasek labelled it, sociologists had been following Marxist traditions. The question was: Is the worker alienated from the work process? It was assumed that the absence of possibilities of utilizing and developing skills (*skill utilization*), a concept developed in work psychology, was closely related to *authority over decisions*. In factor analysis of responses to questions about work content these two factors mostly go together, and accordingly they have been added to one another to constitute *decision latitude* (Karasek and Theorell 1990). The other dimension, *psychological demands*, included qualitative as well as quantitative demands.

Karasek's original hypothesis, that excessive psychological demands interact with lack of decision latitude in generating increased risk of cardiovascular disease, was tested in a number of epidemiological studies in the 1980s (Karasek and Theorell 1990). Ten prospective or cross-sectional studies have been published. The methodology has varied considerably. The most important distinction is that in some studies the subjects' own descriptions of their work situations were used, whereas others relied on aggregated job descriptive data, based on representative workers in the occupations in the population. Both methods have advantages and disadvantages. However, individual traits can be associated with systematically distorted work descriptions, and this systematic distortion may be related to illness risk, with both overestimation and underestimation as a possible result. The use of aggregated data provides an opportunity of avoiding individual distortion (although collective distortion may still take place of course), but it does not allow for variations between work sites. This may lead to substantial underestimation of true associations (Alfredsson 1982). The underestimation problem in the use of aggregated data is probably more important in estimating the importance of psychological demands, since this variable shows relatively small variance between occupations. Decision latitude, however, shows considerable variance between occupations (Karasek and Theorell 1990). Even the aggregated methodology has varied across studies. In some studies, the classifications have been based on means for each of the dimensions from employees in the different occupations in the working population. In others, the dimensions have been represented by single questions, and several combinations (demand–skill utilization and skill–authority over decisions) have been tested.

True (multiplicative) interactions have only been observed in two studies (Alfredsson and Theorell 1983; Johnson and Hall 1988), whereas in the others additive interactions were seen. There is no doubt, however, that the use of the two dimensions together has provided better predictions than using either one of them alone.

The summary of relative risks indicates, as expected, that studies utilizing self-reported work descriptions have shown higher relative risks (2.0–4.0 versus 1.3–2.0). Demands have been shown to be relatively more important in studies utilzing self-reported data than in studies utilizing aggregated data. Some of the studies have covered other risk factors, and one has also included type A behaviour (La Croix 1984). In general, the adjustment for standard risk factors for cardiovascular disease does not eliminate the association between the high demand–low decision latitude combination and risk of cardiovascular disease (in most studies clinically verified myocardial infarction and in three studies CHD). In one case, the Framingham Study (La Croix 1984), the adjustment for other risk factors strengthened the association.

Only the Hawaii Cardiovascular Survey (Reed *et al.* 1989), showed no association at all between high demand–low decision latitude and risk of cardiovascular illness. Interestingly, the participants in this study were above 55 years of age at the start of the follow-up period. Studies of participants younger than 55 years of age have generally shown stronger associations than those including older subjects. Another observation is that the high demand–low decision latitude has provided to be a more powerful predictor of cardiovascular illness risk in blue-collar men than in white-collar men. For instance, a Finnish study (Hahn 1985) included mainly blue-collar workers and showed a strong association. The study by Johnson and Hall (1988) contains separate analyses of blue-collar and white-collar men which illustrate this point. For further discussion see Marmot and Theorell (1988).

A small clinical 5 year follow-up study of men in Stockholm below age 45 who had suffered a myocardial infarction indicated that returning to a job perceived as psychologically demanding and with a low decision latitude may be associated with increased risk of reinfarction death (Theorell *et al.* 1991). This was true even after adjustment for biomedical risk factors, degree of coronary atherosclerosis, type A behaviour, and education. This finding emphasized the potential importance of this research to cardio-vascular rehabilitation.

There are two recent developments in this field. First, Johnson and co-workers have included social support in the theoretical models. A study of the prevalence of cardiovascular disease in a large random sample of Swedish men and women indicated that the joint action of high demands and lack of control (decision latitude) is of particular importance to blue-collar men, whereas the joint action of lack of control and lack of support is more important for women and white-collar men. The multiplicative inter-action between all three of them (iso-strain) was tested in a 9 year prospec-tive study of 7000 randomly selected Swedish working men. Interestingly, for the most favoured 20 per cent of men (low demands, good support, good decision latitude) the progression of cardiovascular mortality with increasing age was equally slow in the three social classes. In blue-collar workers, however, the age progression was much steeper in the worst iso-strain group than it was in the corresponding iso-strain group in white-collar workers (Johnson *et al.* 1989) (see Fig. 18.1).

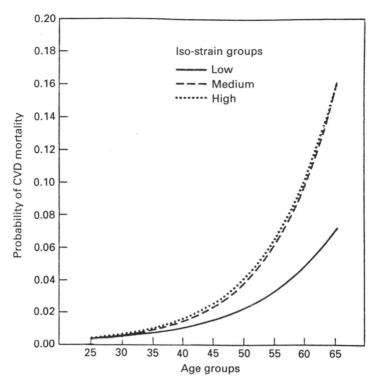

Fig. 18.1 The combined effects of job strain and social isolation on cardiovascular (CVD) mortality in randomly selected Swedish working men (*n* = 7219, 9 year follow-up). (From Johnson *et al.* 1989.)

Second, attempts are now being made to use the occupational classification systems in order to describe the 'psycho-social work career'. Researchers have pointed out that an estimate of work conditions at only one point of time may provide a very imprecise estimation of the total exposure to adverse conditions (House *et al.* 1986). Descriptions of all the occupations during the whole work career are obtained for the participants. Occupational scores are subsequently used for a calculation of the 'total lifetime exposure'. The 'total job control exposure' in relation to 9 age-adjusted cardiovascular mortality in working Swedish men was studied. It was observed for both men and women that the cardiovascular mortality difference between the lowest and highest quartiles was three-fold for both men and women (Johnson *et al.* 1991). It should be pointed out, however, that these age-specific differences are unadjusted for biomedical risk factors.

A model similar to the demand–control model has been developed and tested by Siegrist and co-workers (Siegrist *et al.* 1990). They use 'effort' and 'social reward' as the crucial dimensions, and the hypothesis to be tested is that a high level of effort without social reward is pathogenetic.

The social reward dimension has elements of both decision latitude and social support. In a recently published study of industrial workers (Siegrist *et al.* 1990) it was shown that combinations of high levels of effort and lack of reward predicted increased myocardial infarction risk independently of biomedical risk factors. The relative risk was of the order of 4.0.

Working hours

Although previously no relationship was believed to exist between exposure to shift work and risk of myocardial infarction, several new studies support the hypothesis that there is a relationship. For example, a study of a cohort of paper-pulp factory workers in Northern Sweden showed that there was such a relationship and that it became successively stronger with longer duration of exposure—up to 20 years of exposure at which time the relationship was attenuated or even reversed (Knutsson *et al.* 1986). The authors speculated that the attenuated effect after the longest exposure periods could be a 'selection' effect—only the most healthy workers remained till the end. 'Aggregated' studies of typical shift work occupations have also shown increased myocardial infarction risk compared with other occupations (Åkerstedt *et al.* 1987). There has been speculation regarding mechanisms underlying these relationships. Both direct (catecholamines) and indirect mechanisms–for instance, via unhealthy diet during night work—have been discussed (Knutsson 1989). There is also an indication that improved shift work schedules may be associated with improved cardiovascular risk profiles (Orth-Gomér 1983).

Long working hours have also been studied. The classical study by Hinkle and co-workers of employees of the Bell Telephone Company indicated that men who worked full time and also went to night school had an increased age-adjusted cardiovascular death risk (Hinkle *et al.* 1968). A study of working men and women in five counties in Sweden provided an analysis of the 1 year incidence of hospitalization for myocardial infarction (Pell and d'Alonzo 1963). The results indicated a pronounced difference between men and women. Men in occupations classified as 'overtime occupations' in the national surveys had a lower age-adjusted hospitalization incidence than other working men, even after adjustment for a number of possible social confounders. The opposite was true for women—'overtime work' occupations had higher hospitalization incidence than others. An 'overtime occupation' was defined as an occupation in which at least 10 hours of overtime work per week was reported 'frequently' (occupations with above median frequency). It should be emphasized that this is a relatively modest cut-off point. The level of overtime work in Hinkle's study, for instance, is much higher. The gender difference is most probably due to the double role of women. Since women, in Sweden as well as in other countries, have more responsibility for home and children, it is more difficult for them to handle overtime work. The interactive effects between home work and paid work on psychosomatic symptoms are more pronounced for women than for men (Hall *et al.* 1991). Another possible explanation may be associated with the fact that men perceive that they have a higher level of skill utilization and authority over decisions than do women (Hall 1989). Accordingly, overtime work could be less rewarding for women than for men. In addition, a modest level of overtime for a man is associated with stimulating work (Alfredsson 1983).

There has been considerable activity in the area of work organization and cardiovascular disease. The concepts and theoretical models that have been used are relatively simple, and it has turned out that they are also robust in the sense that they have been testable by means of widely differing methodologies. However, theoretical analysis of the concepts of demand, control, and support are still necessary since there is no universal agreement about definitions. As expected, the models are not universally applicable to all kinds of populations under study. The demand–control model, for instance, is very useful for blue-collar men below age 55, but less useful for other groups. The total demand–control–support model, however, may be more universally applicable.

Social network and social support

As mentioned earlier, social support at work has been shown to be of importance at least to the development of cardiovascular symptoms (House 1981; Marmot and Theorell 1988). It has also been shown recently that continuously monitored heart rate is associated with job social support—the poorer the support the higher the heart rate (Undén *et al.* 1991). In addition, our group has shown that spontaneous variations in social support at work are associated with variations in mean systolic blood pressure during a working day. During periods of poor support the systolic blood pressure is higher and vice versa. This observation was based upon working men and women in six occupations who were observed on four different days 3–4 months apart. Blood pressure was measured once every hour on each of these days (Theorell 1990).

Although social support at work has not been extensively explored in relation to cardiovascular disease, social support in general has been one of the main interests in the area of psycho-social factors and cardiovascular disease. At the beginning of the period covered in this chapter the idea that cultural cohesiveness may protect against cardiovascular disease was introduced (Marmot and Syme 1976; Bruhn and Wolf 1979; Matsumoto 1979). This idea was followed up in several prospective studies of random samples of communities (Berkman and Syme 1979; House *et al.* 1982; Welin *et al.* 1985; Orth-Gomér and Johnson 1987). In all these studies it was found that the more social contacts a person had, the more likely he/she was to survive the follow-up period. Several of these studies have included bio-medical risk factors and indicators of subjective health. The association between social network and mortality has remained significant even after adjustment for these factors. Predictions of cardiovascular mortality by means of social network information have been as successful as those of total mortality (House *et al.* 1988). Recently, a prospective study of middle-aged men in Gothenburg, Sweden, indicated that in multivariate statistics an index of number of social contacts ('availability of social integration') was a better predictor of myocardial infarction risk than any of the accepted biomedical cardiovascular risk factors (Orth-Gomér *et al.* 1990). In the studies of various indices of social support and social net-work, relatively simple indicators of number of social contacts have been more successful predictors than subjective estimations of the adequacy of support or measurements of emotional supportive ties. It has been sus-pected that this may be due to the difficulties of measuring deeper aspects of social support by means of self-administered questionnaires. There is intuitive reason to suspect that the emotional support available to a person should be more important than the superficially recorded number of social contacts. A question that has accompanied this research is how important the person's own individual characteristics are in this relationship. Is it the person himself/herself who repels social contacts or has the environment been deficient? One study that has illuminated this indirectly has recently been published by Orth-Gomér and Undén (1990): a follow-up of 150 Swedish men indicated that a combination of a poor social network and type A behaviour (according to a structured interview) was a powerful predictor of cardiovascular death risk during the follow-up period. The individual components in social support will be a future area of research. Methods which measure 'social competence', for instance, should be explored.

Social network and social support research has provided some of the strongest findings in psycho-social cardiovascular epidemiology. As in the case of work environment, it will be necessary for researchers to explore the theoretical constructs more thoroughly since definitions vary in a con-fusing way. This will have enormous importance for efforts to use this knowledge in future interventions. The most crucial question will be whether the main component is individual or environmental. Should we focus on strengthening individual competence or on improving networks?

LIFE EVENTS

The conceptual conflict between individual and environment has also been problematic in the area of life change research in relation to cardiovascular disease. This research area has been reviewed elsewhere (Theorell 1987). Two different lines of research have developed. In the first, the effect of specific life crises, for example bereavement, migration, and retirement, on cardiovascular risk has been examined. For instance, an association between bereavement and increased subsequent near-future cardiovascular death risk has been found (Parkes *et al*. 1969). In the other, change in general has been explored.

The study of change in general is a difficult field. One of the most prominent difficulties is that the incidence of myocardial infarction following the measurement of total life change indices should be recorded during a short period—otherwise new events may occur which will make interpretation difficult. This means that very large samples are required. A laborious design with repeated observations on relatively large samples could also be tried. The research is further complicated by conceptual problems. Is it the characteristics and the social circumstances around the life change that are important or is it the perception? Of course, in order to explore the former, the researcher has to interview the subject thoroughly and make judgements regarding the character of the event, deliberately disregarding the subject's perception of it. Such interview methodology has been introduced (Brown *et al*. 1973). However, interviews of this kind are time-consuming and require substantial resources if they are to be used on large samples. So far the technique has only been used in retrospective studies (Connolly 1976; Falger 1989). In exploring the perception of life changes, questionnaires could be used, and various techniques have been proposed such as 'daily hassles and uplifts' (de Longis *et al*. 1982) and ratings of controllability, possibility of anticipation, desirability, negative/positive, and loss/gain (Dohrenwend and Dohrenwend 1974). The more the psychological perception side dominates, the less the measures have anything to do with an environmental measure, and it would be argued that measures of psychological coping would probably measure the same dimension. Most of these techniques have not been used in the study of life changes in relation to the onset of myocardial infarction. Using standard weights of 'degree of upset' derived from a reference population on a list of life events explored according to Holmes and Rahe (1967) for the year preceding the study, our group was able to show that a high total life change score did not predict myocardial infarction risk during 1 year of follow-up in middle-aged building construction workers, although 'increased responsibility at work' did (Theorell *et al*. 1975). Episodes of cardiovascular illness could be predicted by means of a high life change score and a high 'chronic discord' score (Theorell 1976). Also, psychological work load was predictive of elevated myocardial infarction risk during 2 years of follow-up (Theorell and Flodérus-Myrhed 1977).

The most fruitful life change approach seems to have been the study of specific crisis situations. These can also easily be identified by the epidemiologist so that risk situations for support can be identified. Successful controlled psycho-social intervention trails have also been published in relation to bereavement (Parkes 1980) and to the case when a relative develops cancer (Häggmark *et al.* 1991). However, so far studies of this type have not been made in relation to cardiovascular disease.

INDIVIDUAL PSYCHOLOGICAL CHARACTERISTICS

Perception of life change brings us to the individual's way of handling challenges and difficulties. This has been a favourite subject among psychologists. The type A behaviour concept was introduced by Friedman and Rosenman (1959) and has subsequently stimulated enormous research interest. A somewhat similar concept, the Sisyphus syndrome, had been introduced earlier (Wolf 1969). It became apparent quite early that the behaviour pattern that the physicians Rosenman and Friedman described had several components, and different researchers have subsequently focused on these. Type A behaviour was originally formulated as being provoked by certain situations. Other researchers have subsquently treated the behaviour pattern as a stable trait. The structured interview designed for detecting type A behaviour contains some provocation. Not only the verbal content in the responses during the interview but also the *behaviour* is rated. The interview technique is accordingly more consistent with the original Friedman–Rosenman conceptualization. Studies utilizing the structured interview for classification of type A behaviour have been more successful in the prediction of cardiovascular disease than those utilizing questionnaires (Mathews and Haynes 1986). However, because the original concept had several components, the structured interview has been developed somewhat differently by different groups. Some critics have stated that this may be one reason why type A behaviour ratings failed to predict cardiovascular disease in the Multiple Risk Factor Intervention Trial (MRFIT 1982)—the interview technique was focusing on the wrong component. During later years several researchers have focused on one single aspect of type A behaviour—hostility—which has been easier to define and has been a successful predictor in several studies (MRFIT 1982).

Recently, great attention has been paid to the findings in the 20 year follow-up of the original prospective structured interview study of type A behaviour—the Western Collaborative Group Study. It was shown that those subjects who exhibited type A behaviour during the interview showed excess risk of myocardial infarction mainly during the first and, to some extent, the second year of follow-up, while no excess risk was shown subsequently. One interpretation of this is that the interview captures a hyper-responsive behaviour pattern caused by a stressful life situation. When the situation improves the behaviour disappears. The somewhat related concept of vital exhaustion—a feeling in the person that he is emptied and unable to recharge his energy—was used by Appels and co-workers for predicting risk of myocardial infarction (Appels and Mulder 1988). Initially, it was believed that vital exhaustion was caused by asymptomatic early stages of the heart disease itself. However, recent prospective studies taking account of biomedical risk factors (Appels 1990) have refuted this interpretation—a high score on the vital exhaustion questionnaire scale is associated with increased risk of near-future myocardial infarction regardless of biomedical risk factors. It is quite possible that the behaviour recorded by the structured type A interview is closely related to vital exhaustion.

The German sociologist Siegrist and his collaborators have developed a theory somewhat related to the vital exhaustion concept, with the main difference being that Siegrist's theory also takes the time dimension into account. According to this theory, a young person prone to myocardial infarction would typically start his working careeer with extreme vigour. The only observable phenomenon that is related to cardiovascular risk during this phase is enhanced cardiovascular reactivity to challenges. As the person grows older, vigour is replaced by immersion—the energy expended does not result in social reward despite 'immersed' efforts. This phase corresponds to increased prevalence of cardiovascular risk factors. The final phase corresponds to overt cardiovascular disease (Siegrist *et al.* 1986). Siegrist's theory incorporates the individual with his history as well as his environment. 'Chronic work stress', defined according to combined subjective and objective criteria, was associated with an elevated ratio of low density lipoprotein cholesterol to high density lipoprotein cholesterol (Siegrist *et al.* 1988).

A new line of research has focused on alexithymia—inability to differentiate emotions. Early results suggest that it may be related to hypertension (Knox *et al.* 1988).

PHYSIOLOGICAL BASIS

Type A behaviour (including hostility), Sisyphus syndrome, vital exhaustion, immersion, and alexithymia are all psychological concepts. Identification of them in individuals could lead to treatment licensed by the psychological profession. An individual trait that has a physiological basis, and would accordingly respond to medical or physiological treatments, is shown by the 'hot reactor'—a person who has strong physiological reactions to challenges. Such a person may or may not exhibit type A behaviour. The identification of the risk trait is made by means of physiological reactivity tests (Eliot 1986). This has turned out to be a fruitful approach in preventive work.

The physiological basis for the associations between psycho-social factors and CHD has been a lively research field during the period under review. Catecholamines have been suspected of mediating some of the relationship, and it has become possible to study not only urinary excretion of these compounds (which is still a good way of collecting data on sympatho-adrenal activity during integrated periods of time) but also the small concentrations that exist in venous plasma during rest. A study by our group of men aged 28 years has recently shown that poor social network and support as well as a job 'classified' as boring all contribute to an elevated venous plasma adrenaline at rest (Knox *et al.* 1985). However, the main endeavour has been the study of urinary catecholamine excretion. Recently, epidemiological studies have shown a correlation between poor social network and high urinary catecholamine excretion (Eide 1982) and also between poor decision latitude and high catecholamine excretion (Härenstam and Theorell 1988). However, it has also been found that sympatho-adrenal reactions in different organs may be specific, and accordingly generalizations should not be made in all instances (Hjemdahl *et al.* 1989).

The possibilities of monitoring physiological functions continuously have produced a revolution in this field. For instance, since we can now study heart rate and blood pressure during activity and sleep we have started to explore how psycho-social factors relate to the development of coronary atherosclerosis for instance. The lowest heart rate during sleep correlates with the degree and progression of coronary atherosclerosis (Perski *et al.* 1989 and Perski *et al.* 1991). It is possible that inability to relax is associated with a high heart rate during sleep as well as with progression of coronary atherosclerosis. Similarly, Undén *et al.* (1991) have shown that poor social support at work is associated with a high heart rate throughout the day and the night. The interpretations of these associations are not clear, but it is possible that feelings of loneliness may activate the sympatho-adrenal system.

A growing field that also relates to catecholamines is coagulation. For instance, in one study a boring job (or job strain) has been related to high plasma fibrinogen levels (Markowe *et al.* 1985). The question that arises could be formulated in the following way. To what extent do psycho-social clots and psycho-social atherosclerosis exist? Certainly, the common theme in the lack of social support in life in general and the lack of possibilities to learn and to influence decision-making at work may be boredom. Research in cardiovascular psycho-social epidemiology has not provided any final answers, but several very useful concepts have been developed and utilized, and many empirical results point to possible interventions in, for instance, work organization and social networks.

REFERENCES

Åkerstedt, T., Alfredsson, L., and Theorell, T. (1987). *Arbetstid och sjukdom—en studie med aggregerade data*. Stressforskningsrapporter 190.

Alfredsson, L. (1983). *Myocardial infarction and environment: use of registers in epidemiology*, Acad. thesis, Karolinska Institute, Stockholm.

Alfredsson, L. and Theorell, T. (1983). Job characteristics of occupations and myocardial infarction risk: effects of possible confounding factors. *Soc. Sci. Med.*, **17**, 1497–503.

Alfredsson, L., Spetz, C-L., and Theorell, T. (1985). Type of occupation and near-future hospitalization for myocardial infarction and some other diagnoses. *Int. J. Epidemiol.*, **14**, 378–88.

Antonovsky, A. (1968). Social class and the major cardiovascular diseases. *J. Chron. Dis.*, **21**, 65–106.

Appels, A. (1990). Mental precursors of myocardial infarction. *Abstract, 18th Eur. Conf. on Psychosomatic Research, Helsinki, Finland.*

Appels, A. and Mulder, P. (1988). Excess fatigue as a precursor of myocardial infarction. *Eur. Heart J.*, **9**, 758–64.

Berkman, L. and Syme, S. L. (1979). Social networks, host resistance and mortality: a nine-year study of Alameda county residents. *Am. J. Epidemiol.*, **109**, 186–204.

Biörck, G., Blomqvist, G., and Sievers, J. (1958). Studies on myocardial infarction in Malmö 1935–1954. II. infarction rate by occupational group. *Acta Med. Scand.*, **161**, 21.

Brown, G. W., Sklair, F., Harris, T. O., and Birley, J. L. T. (1973). Life events and psychiatric disorders: 1. Some methodological issues. *Psychol. Med.*, **3**, 74–87.

Bruhn, J. and Wolf, S. (1979). *An anatomy of health: the Roseto story*, University of Oklahoma Press, Oklahoma City, OK.

Buell, P. and Breslow, L. (1960). Mortality from coronary heart disease in California men who work long hours. *J. Chron. Dis.*, **11**, 615–26.

Cobb, S. and Kasl, S. (1977). *Termination: the consequences of job loss*, NIOSH Publ. 77–224, National Institute for Occupational Safety and Health, Cincinnati, OH.

Connolly, J. (1976). Life events before myocardial infarction. *J. Hum. Stress*, **2**, 3.

de Longis, A., Coyne, J. C., Dakof, G., Folkman, S., and Lazarus, R. S. (1982). Relationship of daily hassles, uplifts, and major life events to health status. *Health Psychol.*, **1**, 119–36.

Davey Smith, G., Shipley, M. J., and Rose, G. (1990). Magnitude and causes of socioeconomic differentials in mortality: further evidence from the Whitehall Study. *J. Epidemiol. Commun. Health*, **44**, 265–70.

Diderichsen, F. and Lindberg, G. (1989). Better health—but not for all. The Swedish public health report 1987. *Int. J. Health Serv.*, **19**, 221–55.

Dohrenwend, B. S. and Dohrenwend, B. P. (eds) (1974). *Stressful life events, their nature and effects*, Wiley, New York.

Eide, R. (1982). *Psychosocial factors and indices of health risks*, Acad. Thesis, University of Bergen.

Eliot, R. S. (1986). Stress and cardiovascular disease: mechanisms and measurement. *Ann. Clin. Res.*, **19**(2), 88–95.

Falger, P. R. J. (1989). *Life-span development and myocardial infarction: an epidemiological study*, Doctoral Thesis, University of Maastricht.

Friedman, M. and Rosenman, R. H. (1959). Association of specific overt behavior pattern with blood and cardiovascular findings. *J. Am. Med. Assoc.*, **169**, 1286–97.

Häggmark, C., Bachner, M., and Theorell, T. (1991). A follow-up of psychological state in relatives of cancer patients one year after the patient's death. *Acta Oncol.*, **30**, 677–84.

Hahn, M. (1985). Job strain and cardiovascular disease: a ten-year prospective study. *Am. J. Epidemiol.*, **122**, 532–40.

Härenstam, A. and Theorell, T. (1988). Work conditions and urinary excretion of catecholamines—a study of prison staff in Sweden. *Scand. J. Work Environ. Health*, **14**, 257–64.

Hall, E. M. (1989). Gender, work control, and stress: a theoretical discussion and an empirical test. *Int. J. Health Serv.*, **19**(4), 725–45.

Hall, E. M., Johnson, J. V., and Stewart, W. (1991). Double exposure: the combined impact of the home and work environments on mental strain and physical illness. *J. Health Soc. Behav.*, in press.

Henry, J. P. and Cassel, J. (1969). Psychological factors in essential hypertension: recent epidemiological and animal experimental evidence. *Am. J. Epidemiol.*, **90**, 171–200.

Hinkle, L. E., Whitney, L. H., Lehman, E. W., Dunn, J., Benjamin, B., King, R., et al. (1968). Occupation, education and coronary heart disease. *Science*, **161**, 238–48.

Hjemdahl, P., Fagius, J., Freyschuss, B., Wallin, B. G., Daleskog, M., Bohlin, G., et al. (1989). Muscle sympathetic activity and norepinephrine release during mental challenge in humans. *Am. Physiol. Soc.*, E654–64.

Holmes, T. H. and Rohe, R. H. (1967). The social readjustment scale. *J. Psychosom. Res.*, **11**, 213–18.

House, J. S. (1981). *Work, stress and social support*, Addison-Wesley, Reading, MA.

House, J., Robbins, C., and Metzner, H. (1982). The association of social relationships and activities with mortality: prospective evidence from the Tecumseh community health study. *Am. J. Epidemiol.*, **116**, 123–40.

House, J. S., Strecher, V., Metzner, H. L., and Robbins, C. (1986). Occupational stress and health among men and women in the Tecumseh Community Health Study. *J. Health Soc. Behav.*, **27**, 62–77.

House, J., Landis, N. R., and Umberson, D. (1988). Social relationships and health. *Science*, **241**, 540–5.

Johnson, J. V. and Hall, E. M. (1988). Job strain, workplace social support and cardiovascular disease: a cross-sectional study of a random sample of the Swedish working population. *Am. J. Publ. Health*, **78**, 1336–42.

Johnson, J. V., Hall, E. M., and Theorell, T. (1989). Combined effects of job strain and social isolation on cardiovascular disease morbidity and mortality in a random sample of the Swedish male working population. *Scand. J. Work Environ. Health*, **15**, 271–9.

Johnson, J. V., Hall, E. M., Stewart, W., Fredlund, P., and Theorell, T. (1991). Combined exposure to adverse work organization factors and cardiovascular disease: towards a life-course perspective. *Arch. Complex Environ. Stud.*, **3**, 117–22.

Karasek, R. A. (1979). Job demands, job decision latitude, and mental strain: implications for job redesign. *Administrative Science Quarterly,* **24,** 285–307.

Karasek, R. A. and Theorell, T. (1990). *Healthy work,* Basic Books, New York.

Karasek, R. A., Baker, D., Marxer, F., Ahlbom, A., and Theorell, T. (1981). Job decision latitude, job demands, and cardiovascular disease: a prospective study of Swedish men. *Am. J. Publ. Health,* **71,** 694–705.

Kasanen, A., Kallio, V., and Forsström, J. (1963). The significance of psychic and socio-economic stress and other modes of life in the etiology of myocardial infarction. *Ann. Med. Intern. Fenn.,* **52** (Suppl. 43).

Kittel, F., Kornitzer, M., and Dramaix, M. (1980). Coronary heart disease and job stress in two cohorts of bank clerks. *Psychother. Psychosom.,* **34,** 110–23.

Knox, S., Theorell, T., Svensson, J., and Waller, D. (1985). The relation of social support and working environment to medical variables associated with elevated blood pressure in young males: a structural model. *Soc. Sci. Med.,* **21,** 525–31.

Knox, S., Svensson, J., Theorell, T., and Waller, D. (1988). Emotional coping and elevated blood pressure. *Behav. Med.,* **14,** 52–8.

Knutsson, A. (1989). Shift work and coronary heart disease. *Scand. J. Soc. Med.,* **17,** Suppl. 44.

Knutsson, A., Åkerstedt, T., Jonsson, B. G., and Orth-Gomér, K. (1986). Increased risk of ischaemic heart disease in shift workers. *Lancet,* **ii,** 89–92.

Kornitzer, M. and Kittel, F. (1986). How does stress exert its effects—smoking, diet and obesity, physical activity. *Postgrad. Med. J.,* **62,** 695–6.

Kornitzer, M., Kittel, F., Dramaix, M., and de Backer, G. (1982). Job stress and coronary heart disease. *Adv. Cardiol.,* **19,** 56–61.

La Croix, A. Z. (1984). *Occupational exposure to high demand/low control work and coronary heart disease incidence in the Framingham cohort.* Ph.D. Dissertation, Department of Epidemiology, University of North Carolina.

Lundberg, O. (1990). *Den ojämlika hälsan,* Doctoral Thesis, Institute for Social Research, Stockholm's University.

Markowe, H. L., Marmot, M. G., Shipley, M. J., Bulpitt, C. J., Meade, T. W., Stirling, Y., *et al.* (1985). Fibrinogen: a possible link between social class and coronary heart disease. *Br. Med. J.,* **9,** 291.

Marmot, M. G. (1982). Socio-economic and cultural factors in ischemic heart disease. *Adv. Cardiol.,* **29,** 68–76.

Marmot, M. G. and McDowell, M. E. (1986). Mortality decline and widening social inequalities. *Lancet,* **ii,** 274–6.

Marmot, M. G. and Syme, S. L. (1976). Acculturation and coronary heart disease in Japanese-Americans. *Am. J. Epidemiol.,* **104,** 225–47.

Marmot, A. and Theorell, T. (1988). Social class and cardiovascular disease: the contribution of work. *Int. J. Health Serv.,* **18**(4), 659–74.

Mathews, K. A. and Haynes, S. G. (1986). Type A behavior pattern and coronary disease risk: up-date and critical evaluation. *Am. J. Epidemiol.,* **123,** 923–60.

Matsumoto, Y. S. (1979). Social stress and coronary heart disease in Japan: a hypothesis. *Milbank Mem. Fund. Q. Bull.,* **48,** 9–36.

MRFIT (Multiple Risk Factor Intervention Trial) Research Group (1982). Risk factor changes and mortality results. *J. Am. Med. Assoc.,* **248,** 1465–77.

Orth-Gomér, K. (1983). Intervention on coronary risk factors by adapting a shift work schedule to biologic rhythmicity. *Psychosom. Med.,* **45,** 407–15.

Orth-Gomér, K. and Johnson, J. V. (1987). Social network interaction and mortality: a six year follow-up of a random sample of the Swedish population. *J. Chron. Dis.*, **40**, 949–57.

Orth-Gomér, K. and Undén, A.-L. (1990). Type A behavior, social support, and coronary risk: interaction and significance for mortality in cardiac patients. *Psychosom. Med.*, **52**, 59–72.

Orth-Gomér, K., Rosengren, A., and Wilhelmsen, L. (1990). *Social support and coronary heart disease* (abstract), European Society of Cardiology, Stockholm.

Parkes, C. M. (1980). Bereavement counselling: does it work? *Br. Med. J.*, **3**, 281.

Parkes, C. M., Benjamin, B., and Fitzgerald, R. G. (1969). Broken heart: a statistical study of increased mortality among widowers. *Br. Med. J.*, **1**, 740–3.

Pell, S. and d'Alonzo, C. A. (1963). Acute myocardial infarction in a large employed population: report of six-year study of 1,356 cases. *J. Am. Med. Assoc.*, **185**, 831–41.

Perski, A., Hamsten, A., Lindvall, K., and Theorell, T. (1989). Heart rate correlates with severity of coronary atherosclerosis in young postinfarction patients. *Am. Heart J.*, **116**(5), part 1, 1369–73.

Perski, A., Olsson, G., Landou, C., de Faire, U., Theorell, T., and Hamsten, A. (1991). Minimum heart rate and coronary atherosclerosis: independent relations to global severity and rate of progression of angiographic lesions in men with myocardial infarction at young age. *Am. Heart J.* in press.

Reed, D. M., La Croix, A. Z., Karasek, R. A., Miller, D., and McLean, C. A. (1989). Occupational strain and the incidence of coronary heart disease. *Am. J. Epidemiol.*, **129**, 495–502.

Russek, H. I. and Zohman, B. L. (1958). Relative significance of heredity, diet and occupational stress in coronary heart disease among young adults. *Am. J. Med. Sci.*, **235**, 266.

Siegrist, J., Siegrist, K., and Weber, I. (1986). Sociological concepts in the etiology of chronic disease: the case of ischemic heart disease. *Soc. Sci. Med.*, **22**, 247–53.

Siegrist, J., Matschinger, M., Cremer, P., and Seidel, D. (1988). Atherogenic risk in men suffering from occupational stress. *Atherosclerosis*, **69**, 211–18.

Siegrist, J., Peter, R., Junge, A., Cremer, P., and Seidel, D. (1990). Low status control, high effort at work and ischemic heart disease: prospective evidence from blue-collar men. *Soc. Sci. Med.*, **31**(10), 1127–34.

Theorell, T. (1976). Selected illnesses and somatic risk factors in relation to two psychosocial stress indices—a prospective study of middle-aged building-construction workers. *J. Psychosom. Res.*, **20**, 7.

Theorell, T. (1987). Relationships between critical life events, job stress and cardiovascular illness. *Rev. Épidémiol. Santé Publ.*, **35**, 36–45.

Theorell, T. (1990). Socialt stöd i arbetet. *Socialmed. Tidskrft.*, **67**, 27–31.

Theorell, T. and Flodérus-Myrhed, B. (1977). 'Workload' and risk of myocardial infarction: a prospective psychosocial analysis. *Int. J. Epidemiol.*, **6**, 17–21.

Theorell, T., Flodérus, B., and Lind, E. (1975). The relationship of disturbing life-changes and emotions to the early development of myocardial infarction and other serious illnesses. *Int. J. Epidemiol.*, **4**, 281–96.

Theorell, T., Perski, A., Orth-Gomér, K., Hamstem, A., and de Faire, U. (1991). The effects of the strain of returning to work on the risk of cardiac death after a first myocardial infarction before age 45. *Int. J. Cardiol.*, **30**, 61–7.

Undén, A.-L., Orth-Gomér, K., and Elofsson, S. (1991). Cardiovascular effects of social support in the workplace: 24 hour ECG monitoring of men and women. *Psychosom. Med.*, **53**, 50–60.

Welin, L., Tibblin, G., Svärdsudd, K., Tibblin, B., Ander-Peciva, S., Larsson, B., and Wilhelmsen, L. (1985). Prospective study of social influences on mortality: the study of men born in 1913 and 1923. *Lancet,* **i,** 915–18.

Wolf, S. (1969). Psychosocial forces in myocardial infarction and sudden death. *Circulation*, **28,** (Suppl. 4), 74–82.

19

Sex differences, hormones, and coronary heart disease

K.-T. Khaw and E. Barrett-Connor

SEX DIFFERENCES IN CHD RATES

The male preponderance for coronary heart disease (CHD) is well recognized: the magnitude of this excess ranges from two- to six-fold, tending to be greater at younger ages. Table 19.1 shows age-adjusted CHD mortality rates for men and women aged 40–69 years in different countries; despite a ten-fold variation in CHD rates, there is a consistent three- to four-fold male excess in all countries. Table 19.2 shows age-specific rates in England and Wales; the male-to-female ratio decreases with increasing age but does not disappear, even in the oldest age groups. This observation also appears consistent in different countries, whether CHD rates are high or low. Both behavioural and biological explanations have been postulated for this sex difference. Men may have life-styles that are more likely to lead to adverse risk factor profiles and to CHD. Alternatively, women may be biologically less susceptible to CHD such that for a given level of exposure, such as a high saturated fat diet, or of risk factor, such as serum cholesterol, men may respond more adversely with atherosclerotic changes compared with women. These factors may well interact in that behavioural factors such as diet or physical activity might influence factors such as sex hormone levels which might determine biological susceptibility to CHD.

Are gender differences in CHD due to differences in levels of classical risk factors?

The simplest explanation for sex differences in CHD is that classical risk factors including high blood pressure, high blood cholesterol, and cigarette smoking are all more common in men, possibly because men are more likely to have life-styles leading to high levels of such risk factors. However, higher prevalence of these risk factors does not satisfactorily account for the sex differential. Cigarette smoking is usually, but not always, commoner in men. Women are more likely to have lower blood pressures and cholesterol levels prior to the menopause, but higher levels post-

Table 19.1 CHD (ICD 410–414) annual mortality rates per 100 000 by country and sex for ages 40–69 years (age-adjusted), 1987–8

Country	Men	Women	Sex ratio M:F
Northern Ireland	511.9	175.4	2.9
Scotland	507.3	183.2	2.8
Finland	469.1	114.9	4.1
Czechoslovakia	457.8	134.2	3.4
Ireland	456.5	144.1	3.2
Hungary	431.4	115.8	3.7
New Zealand	399.6	130.3	3.1
England and Wales	384.9	117.6	3.3
Norway	364.3	115.8	3.1
Denmark	306.7	89.2	3.4
Sweden	301.5	70.2	4.3
Israel	284.0	106.9	2.7
Australia	283.3	89.1	3.2
United States of America	282.6	101.7	2.8
Bulgaria	276.4	87.8	3.1
Netherlands	260.1	65.6	4.0
German Democratic Republic	251.2	72.4	3.5
Federal Republic of Germany	244.1	62.4	3.9
Austria	239.5	64.8	3.7
Belgium	202.1	52.0	3.9
Greece	186.1	48.0	3.8
Italy	176.0	41.4	4.3
Poland	140.3	44.9	3.1
Spain	139.1	30.7	4.5
France	109.4	22.9	4.8
Japan	44.0	15.2	2.9

Source: *WHO Statistics Annual*, World Health Organization, Geneva.

menopausally compared with men the same age, yet the sex differences still persist after the menopause well into the seventies. Moreover, adjusting for risk factor level including blood pressure, serum cholesterol, and cigarette smoking may reduce the male excess in CHD, but does not wholly explain or eliminate it (Wingard 1984). However, such adjustment may not be adequate because of measurement error, particularly if the crucial years for exposure for the development of atherosclerotic disease occur at earlier ages, for example 20–40 years rather than at the older ages at which risk factor levels have been documented in prospective studies. Sex differences in the prevalence of other documented risk factors for

Table 19.2 CHD (ICD 410–414) annual mortality rates by sex and age group, England and Wales 1986

Age	Men	Women	Sex ratio M:F
35–44	41.4	6.1	6.8
45–54	215.0	40.8	5.3
55–64	670.0	201.0	3.3
65–74	1561.1	672.8	2.3
75+	3343.7	2122.1	1.6

Source: *WHO Statistics Annual*, World Health Organization, Geneva, 1987.

CHD, including clotting factors such as fibrinogen and factor VII (Meade *et al.* 1977), and glucose intolerance (Wingard 1990), undoubtedly exist, but even fewer data are available to examine whether, and to what extent, these may account for the sex difference in CHD.

Nevertheless, of all the risk factors, serum lipid levels are the most closely associated with CHD risk, and at least some of the sex differential has been attributed to differences in specific lipid and lipoprotein components, extensively reviewed elsewhere (Hazzard 1986; Godsland *et al.* 1987). The most consistent difference has been the higher levels of high density lipoprotein cholesterol (HDL-cholesterol), a protective factor, in women compared with men (Rifkind *et al.* 1979).

It may also be that women are more resistant to the effects of a given risk factor. In those prospective population studies which have directly compared relative risks in men and women, the classical risk factors for CHD—cigarette smoking, raised serum cholesterol, and raised blood pressure—appear to confer increased risk for CHD in women as well as men (Kannel 1978; Barrett-Connor *et al.* 1984). Whilst the magnitude of the increased relative risks for a given risk factor may not be identical in men and women, gender differences in relative risks are not consistent in differing populations and may well be explained by selective mortality, differences in prevalences of various risk factors, and competing risks within the margins of measurement error. However, the Framingham Study reported that, while cholesterol level overall was associated with CHD mortality in both men and women, decreasing HDL and increasing low density lipoprotein cholesterol (LDL-cholesterol) level were stronger risk factors in men compared with women, suggesting that women might be more resistant (Gordon *et al.* 1977; Lerner and Kannel 1986). Thus, some of the sex differences might be partly explained by both higher levels and a stronger protective effect of HDL-cholesterol in women compared with men.

Are women less susceptible to the effects of a potentially atherogenic diet?

There may be both behavioural and biological reasons for higher HDL-cholesterol levels, and hence higher HDL/LDL ratios in women. Women might have diets more likely to result in higher HDL/LDL ratios, or women might be less likely than men to lower the HDL/LDL ratio in response to such a diet. Kesteloot (1987) reported that in Belgium, despite similar dietary saturated fat intake in men and women, and similar LDL levels, HDL levels were substantially higher in women compared with men. This, coupled with his observations that, in communities with low CHD prevalence and low dietary fat intake such as Korea or the People's Republic of China (Kesteloot *et al.* 1985), men and women had similar low LDL-cholesterol and HDL-cholesterol levels led him to suggest that HDL-cholesterol in females reacts in a different way to a high intake in saturated fat or other atherogenic diet. Metabolic and clinical studies as well as other observational data lend some support to this hypothesis. Crouse (1989) argued that, in intervention studies, changing from a Western diet to the American Heart Association step I diet (reduce fat intake from 40 to 30 per cent of calories, reduce saturated fat from 20 to 10 per cent of total calories) reduced LDL-cholesterol considerably in both men and women, but women showed much greater reductions than men in HDL-cholesterol. However, not all studies confirm this: Mensink and Katan (1989) showed no such differential effect in men and women when changing from a high saturated fat to a mono-unsaturated fat diet. However, levels of sex hormones, namely oestrogens, have been suggested as one possible explanation for the sex differences in HDL-cholesterol levels.

SEX HORMONE DIFFERENCES: A LINK WITH CHD?

The obvious differences in sex hormone levels between men and women have led to a common supposition that endogenous oestrogens in women may be protective against CHD or testicular androgens in men may be detrimental. Surprisingly, this supposition has rarely been formally tested. The notion that low levels of oestrogens or high levels of androgens confer adverse CHD risk has largely gained credence from studies in men and women using exogenous hormones.

Exogenous hormones and CHD

The major support for the hypothesis that women are protected from CHD because of high oestrogen levels comes from the numerous case–control and prospective studies, reviewed elsewhere (Bush and Barrett-Connor 1985), showing a striking decrease in CHD of the order of 0.3–0.5 relative risk in women taking post-menopausal exogenous oestrogens, coupled with the observation that women with a premature menopause due to oophorectomy are at increased risk of heart disease. This increased risk is abolished with oestrogen replacement therapy (Stampfer *et al.* 1985). Observational and trial data showing that oral unopposed exogenous oestrogen therapy post-menopausally is associated with increasing HDL-cholesterol levels and reducing LDL-cholesterol levels (Hirvonen *et al.* 1981; Matthews *et al.* 1989) provide a coherent and biologically plausible mechanism for a cardioprotective effect of exogenous oestrogens in post-menopausal women. However, giving oestrogens to men does not appear to be protective for CHD (Coronary Drug Project Research Group 1973); studies have in fact shown quite the converse, that exogenous oestrogens (admittedly in high doses) are associated with higher rates of CHD (Henriksson and Johansson 1987). Additionally, oral contraceptives in pre-menopausal women are associated with increased cardiovascular risk; one study which reported increased CHD risk in post-menopausal oestrogen users may have in fact included women who used oestrogens pre-menopausally (Wilson *et al.* 1985).

Data on the effects of exogenous androgen administration are mainly based on large doses given to sports participants. These are generally reported to have adverse effects on lipid profiles in both sexes (Solyom 1971; Barton *et al.* 1973; Reeves *et al.* 1976).

Hence, while the bulk of the evidence suggests that exogenous oestrogen use is cardioprotective for post-menopausal women, this is not the case for either men or pre-menopausal women; rather, the converse holds. Thus it is unlikely that lack of oestrogens in men confers susceptibility, though it is still possible that androgen excess in men might be related to CHD risk. One possible explanation for the variable findings is that other hormones such as androgens (in men) or progestogens (in oral contraceptive formulations) may interact with oestrogens to reduce or abolish any cardioprotective effect. Several studies suggest that progestogens with androgenic properties abolish the HDL-cholesterol-raising effect of oestrogen administration in women (Hirvonen *et al.* 1981; Wahl *et al.* 1983; Crook *et al.* 1988; La Rosa 1988).

Problems of interpretation of all these studies of exogenous hormone administration arise from the use of differing and non-physiological hormone doses in varying formulations including different oestrogens, androgens, and progestogens which have been shown to have very variable effects on risk factor profiles such as lipids, and in differing modes of administration including oral and parenteral routes which have variable effects on liver metabolism and on carrier protein and enzyme induction. The use of a variety of age-selected patient groups leading to different results make generalizability of findings difficult. The relevance of data based on administration of exogenous hormones to explaining sex differences in CHD is questionable without other supporting evidence.

Endogenous hormones and CHD risk

Is there any evidence that endogenous hormone levels relate to CHD in either men or women?

Consistent with the observed adverse effects of exogenous oestrogens on coronary risk in men, several case–control studies report higher levels of oestrogens in men who survived a heart attack compared with controls (Phillips 1978, 1984). The case–control design does not make it possible to tell if high oestrogen levels preceded CHD, or were simply a consequence of the disease or its treatment, or were associated with improved survival. In contrast, case–control studies using angiographic evidence of CHD to define cases did not have consistent results (Small *et al*. 1985), and prospective studies have found no significant associations between baseline oestrogen levels and subsequent CHD in men (Barrett-Connor and Khaw 1988*a*).

An inverse relationship of dehydroepiandrosterone sulphate, a weakly androgenic adrenal steroid, with CHD in men has been reported (Barrett-Connor *et al*. 1986), though again this finding has not been consistent in all studies. While prospective data in men also did not show any significant association of baseline testosterone levels with subsequent CHD (Barrett-Connor and Khaw 1988*a*), a positive relationship between total testosterone levels and HDL levels in men has been reported in several cross-sectional studies (Nordoy *et al*. 1979; Gutai *et al*. 1981; Heller *et al*. 1981; Dai *et al*. 1984). The observation that low plasma testosterone related to low lipoprotein lipase activity and low HDL-cholesterol, which in turn were related to the severity of coronary artery disease in men (Breier *et al*. 1985), provides some biological plausibility for this unexpected favourable association. However, the few studies that were also able to examine HDL-cholesterol levels with estimates of free testosterone levels reported findings in all directions: associations were no longer significant, were reversed, or still remained (Semmens *et al*. 1983). The role of sex hormone binding globulin (SHBG) may be of significance in this respect but has not been explored in detail.

The clinical observation that pre-menopausal women with polycystic ovaries have high levels of androgens which correlate with higher LDL-cholesterol and lower HDL-cholesterol levels (Wild *et al*. 1985; Wild and Bartholomew 1988) has led to the suggestion that androgens in women may confer adverse cardiovascular risk, though the relationship to CHD end-points has not been documented. Diabetes and cigarette smoking in women are both associated with a much greater relative risk of CHD (Barrett-Connor and Wingard 1983) and hence reduction of the sex differential; both raised plasma glucose levels and cigarette smoking have been associated with increased androgen levels in women (Khaw *et al.* 1988; Khaw and Barrett-Connor 1991). Though positive associations of oestradiol with HDL-cholesterol have been reported in post-menopausal women (Maserai *et al.* 1980), neither androgen nor oestrogen levels have been consistently related to HDL-cholesterol in most studies. There are no convincing prospective data for endogenous hormone levels with CHD in women: a preliminary finding from the Rancho Bernardo study reported a U-shaped relationship with dehydroepiandrosterone sulphate, an adrenal androgen (Barrett-Connor and Khaw 1988*b*).

Studies between populations at high and low risk of CHD may give some clues. Populations with low CHD rates, such as Japanese or Chinese women, have lower levels of both HDL-cholesterol (Kesteloot *et al.* 1985) and oestrogen (Goldin *et al.* 1986) compared with women in populations with high CHD rates. A vegetarian or low fat diet has been reported to be related to higher urinary oestrogen levels, lower serum oestrogen levels, and higher SHBG levels in women (Goldin *et al.* 1986). A Western-type diet has also been associated with higher androgen and lower SHBG levels in post-menopausal women (Adlercreutz *et al.* 1989). One possible hypothesis which attempts to reconcile some of the diverse observations is shown in Table 19.3. This postulates that some component of a 'Western' diet, most probably a high saturated fat intake, is associated with an increase in LDL-cholesterol levels which increase CHD risk in both men and women. A high saturated fat diet also results in increased oestrogen levels: the high oestrogen levels in women in the presence of a high fat diet result in high levels of HDL-cholesterol, which are protective. This HDL-cholesterol-raising effect of high oestrogen levels is abolished by high levels of androgens. This model might explain why men, who in fact have higher absolute oestrogen levels than post-menopausal women, are still at increased CHD risk, as well as why the sex differential is reduced in women with high levels of androgens, such as diabetic women who smoke. This model is unlikely to provide a complete explanation, since in communities with low CHD prevalence such as Japan and Korea, where HDL-cholesterol levels tend to be similar in men and women, a marked male excess in CHD mortality is still apparent; it also does not explain the observed inverse association of testosterone with HDL-cholesterol levels in men. However, Laskarzewski *et al.* (1983) observed variable relationships between lipoprotein profiles at different absolute and relative oestradiol and testosterone levels and ratios in adolescent boys, and suggested that the various hormones interact at different levels in as yet undefined ways.

The somewhat surprising paucity of information on endogenous hormone levels, risk factor levels, and CHD risk, and the lack of consistent findings, may reflect methodological limitations. Sex differences are greatest at

Table 19.3 A proposed model for sex differences in CHD

1. *Low incidence population (e.g. Japan)*

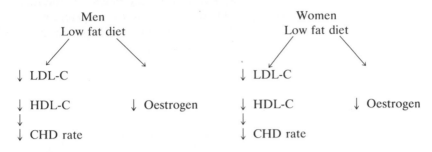

2. *High incidence population (e.g. USA)*

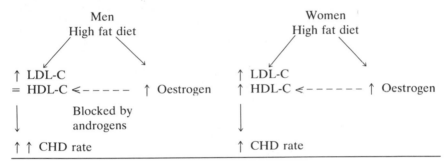

LDL-C, LDL-cholesterol; HDL-C, HDL cholesterol.

younger ages and the critical period of hormonal exposure may not be in middle age, when prospective studies with available data have commenced, but earlier in life. Sex hormone assay methods have been time-consuming and inaccurate. The advent of precise radio-immunoassay methods have made large-scale epidemiological studies, though still expensive, more feasible. Even so, in men and post-menopausal women, oestradiol levels are at the lower limit of sensitivity of assay methods. Additionally, single measures of hormones may inadequately characterize pre-menopausal women in whom hormone levels vary with menstrual cycle phase. Moreover, it has been suggested that over 90 per cent of the endogenous hormones are protein bound and only the free hormone is biologically active; most studies have measured only total hormone levels and we may well need to take into account other factors such as protein binding.

In summary, the role of sex hormones seems intuitively attractive, but there is little direct evidence that high endogenous oestrogens *per se* protect women, nor that high endogenous androgens *per se* are adverse for men, nor that differences in hormone levels *per se* explain the male excess.

Any explanation for the sex differences involving sex hormone levels, at least at older ages where absolute rates of CHD are greatest, would need to invoke other factors including possibly differential and sex-specific receptor sensitivity, sex hormone interactions or ratios, particularly oestrogen-to-androgen ratios, the role of SHBG or interactions with other, as yet unknown, environmental factors.

AREAS FOR FUTURE RESEARCH

There are several directions in which the sex difference in CHD could be usefully explored. The roles of other known and potential risk factors for CHD, such as clotting factors, hormones such as insulin, and their relationship to life-style factors, such as antioxidants (e.g. β-carotene, ascorbic acid, or α-tocopherol), intake of specific fatty acids (e.g. Ω-3 fatty acids), or physical activity, their interaction with classical factors such as blood pressure and lipids, and sex hormone profiles need be documented in both sexes. Clues may come from comparing different populations where sex ratios vary, for example different ethnic or age groups (Sempos *et al.* 1988), or from comparing conditions such as diabetes in which the sex difference for CHD is decreased or disappears. Studies in the past have mainly focused on men for practical reasons, including the accessibility of working populations and their higher frequency of CHD. However, CHD is also the leading cause of death in women. It is now apparent that data for women are badly needed, not just to obtain direct evidence in women for their own benefit, but also because a better understanding of why men are at so much greater risk of CHD may lead to better methods of prevention and treatment for both sexes.

CONCLUSION: IMPLICATIONS FOR PUBLIC HEALTH

While the role of sex hormones and the reasons for a sex differential in CHD are still not clear, there may still be important public health implications.

First, while the relative risk for CHD associated with risk factors such as blood pressure and cholesterol are similar in women and men, the lower absolute CHD rates in women associated with a given level of risk factor results in different potential risk–benefit balances from any interventions. The risk–benefit equation in women is hence more sensitive to any potential adverse effects of intervention, and this must be borne in mind when advocating any public health programme.

Second, some, but not all, the sex differences in CHD can be explained by higher prevalence of known risk factors in men, notably cigarette smoking and, at least in younger men, higher blood pressure and serum cholesterol levels, and lower HDL levels. These are all known to be amenable to life-style modification, such as reduction of dietary fat and sodium intake, and there is potential for reduction of gender differences as men adopt these life-style changes.

Most important, while men are clearly more susceptible to CHD, the ranking order of CHD between different countries for women is close to that for men, suggesting that whatever factors influence CHD occurrence in men also affect women, although to a lesser extent. Men in populations where CHD is lowest have lower rates than women in populations where CHD is high. The striking geographical and secular variation in CHD suggests that the role of environmental factors can outweigh the magnitude of any sex differences within each population.

REFERENCES

Adlercreutz, H., Hamalainen, E., Gorbach, S. L., Goldin, B. R., Woods, M. N., and Dwyer, J. T. (1989). Diet and plasma androgens in postmenopausal vegetarian and omnivorous women and postmenopausal women with breast cancer. *Am. J. Clin. Nutr.*, **49**, 433–42.

Barrett-Connor, E. and Khaw, K-T. (1988*a*). Endogenous sex hormones and cardiovascular disease in men. *Circulation*, **78**, 539–45.

Barrett-Connor, E. and Khaw, K.-T. (1988*b*). Absence of an inverse relationship of dehydroepiandrosterone sulfate with cardiovascular mortality in postmenopausal women. *New Engl. J. Med.*, **317**, 711.

Barrett-Connor, E. and Wingard, D. L. (1983). Sex differential in ischaemic heart disease mortality in diabetics: a prospective population-based study. *Am. J. Epidemiol.*, **118**, 489–96.

Barrett-Connor, E., Suarez, L., and Khaw, K-T. (1984). Ischemic heart disease risk factors over age 50. *J. Chron. Dis.*, **37**, 903–8.

Barrett-Connor, E., Khaw, K-T., and Yen, S. S. C. (1986). A prospective study of dehydroepiandrosterone sulphate, Mortality, and cardiovascular disease. *New Engl. J. Med.*, **315**, 1519–24.

Barton, G. M. G., Gillam, P. M. S., Longridge, R. G. M., and Freeman, P. R. (1973). Trial of an anabolic steroid (oxymetholone) in atherosclerosis with hyperlipoproteinemia. *Atherosclerosis*, **18**, 505.

Breier, C. H., Drexel, H., Lisch, H. J., Muhlberger, V., Herold, M., Knapp, E., *et al.* (1985). Essential role of post-heparin lipoprotein lipase activity and of plasma testosterone in coronary artery disease. *Lancet*, **ii**, 1242–4.

Bush, T. L. and Barrett-Connor, E. (1985). Non-contraceptive estrogen use and cardiovascular disease. *Epidemiol. Rev.*, **7**, 80.

Coronary Drug Project Research Group (1973). The Coronary Drug Project. Findings leading to discontinuation of the 2.5 mg/day estrogen group. *J. Am. Med. Assoc.*, **226**, 652.

Crook, D., Godsland, I. F., and Wynn, V. (1988). Oral contraceptives and coronary heart disease: modulation of glucose tolerance and plasma lipid risk factors by progestins. *Am. J. Obstet. Gynecol.,* **158,** 1612–20.

Crouse, J. R. (1989). Gender, lipoproteins, diet, and cardiovascular risk. *Lancet,* **i,** 318–20.

Dai, W. S., Gutai, J. P., Kuller, L. H., LaPorte, R. E., Falvo-Gerard, L., and Caggiula, A. (1984). Relation between plasma high density lipoprotein cholesterol and sex hormone concentrations in men. *Am. J. Cardiol.,* **53,** 1259–63.

Godsland, I. F., Wynn, V., Crook, D., and Miller, N. E. (1987). Sex, plasma lipoproteins, and atherosclerosis: prevailing assumptions and outstanding questions. *Am. Heart J.,* **114,** 1467–503.

Goldin, B. R., Adlercreutz, H., Gorbach, S. L., Woods, M. N., Dwyer, J. T., Conlon, T., *et al.* (1986). The relationship between estrogen levels and diets of Caucasian American and Oriental immigrant women. *Am. J. Clin. Nutr.,* **44,** 945–53.

Gordon, T., Castelli, W. P., Hjortland, M. C., Kannel, W. B., and Dawber, T. R. (1977). High density lipoprotein as a protective factor against coronary heart disease. The Framingham Study. *Am. J. Med.,* **62,** 707–14.

Gutai, J., LaPorte, R., Kuller, L., Dai, W., Falvo-Gerard, L., and Caggiula, A. (1981). Plasma testosterone, high density lipoprotein cholesterol and other lipoprotein fractions. *Am. J. Cardiol.,* **48,** 897–902.

Hazzard, W. R. (1986). Biological basis of the sex differential in longevity. *J. Am. Geriatr. Soc.,* **34,** 455–71.

Heller, R. F., Miller, N. E., Lewis, B., Vermeulen, A., Fairney, A., and James, V. H. T. (1981). Associations between sex hormones, thyroid hormones and lipoproteins. *Clin. Sci.,* **61,** 649–51.

Henriksson, P. and Johansson, S.-E. (1987). Prediction of cardiovascular complications in patients with prostatic cancer treated with estrogen. *Am. J. Epidemiol.,* **125,** 970–8.

Hirvonen, E., Malkonen, M., and Manninen, V. (1981). Effects of different progestogens on lipoproteins during postmenopausal replacement therapy. *New Engl. J. Med.,* **304,** 560–3.

Kannel, W. B. (1978). Hypertension, blood lipids and cigarette smoking as co-risk factors for coronary heart disease. *Ann. NY Acad. Sci.,* **304,** 128.

Kesteloot, H., Huang, D. X., Yang, X. S., Claes, J., Rosseneu, M., Geboers, J., *et al.* (1985). Serum lipids in the People's Republic of China. *Arterosclerosis,* **5,** 427–33.

Kesteloot, H. (1987). Cardiovascular risk factors and mortality in women. *Herz,* **12,** 248–54.

Khaw, K.-T. and Barrett-Connor, E. (1991). Fasting plasma glucose and endogenous androgens in non-diabetic postmenopausal women. *Clin. Sci.,* **80,** 199–203.

Khaw, K.-T., Tazuke, S., and Barrett-Connor, E. (1988). Cigarette smoking and raised adrenal androgens in postmenopausal women. *New Engl. J. Med.,* **318,** 1705–9.

La Rosa, J. C. (1988). The varying effects of progestins on lipid levels and cardiovascular disease. *Am. J. Obstet. Gynecol.,* **158,** 1621–9.

Laskarzewski, P. M., Morrison, J. A., Gutai, J., Orchard, T., Khoury, P. R., and Glueck, C. J. (1983). High and low density lipoprotein cholesterols in adolescent boys: relationships with endogenous testosterone, estradiol, and quetelet index. *Metabolism,* **32,** 262–71.

Lerner, D. J. and Kannel, W. B. (1986). Patterns of coronary heart disease morbidity and mortality in the sexes: a 26 year follow-up in the Framingham population. *Am. Heart J.,* **111,** 383–90.

Maserai, J. R. L., Armstrong, B. K., Skinner, M. W., Rataczjak, T., Hahnel, R., and Crooke, D. (1980). HDL-cholesterol and sex hormone status. *Lancet,* **i,** 208.

Matthews, K. A., Meilahn, E., Kuller, L. H., Kelsey, S. F., Caggiula, A. W., and Wing, R. R. (1989). Menopause and risk factors for coronary heart disease. *New Engl. J. Med.,* **321,** 641–6.

Meade, T. W., North, W. R. S., Chakrabarti, R., Haines, A. P., and Stirling, Y. (1977). Population-based distributions of haemostatic variables. *Br. Med. Bull.,* **33,** 283–8.

Mensink, R. P. and Katan, M. B. (1989). Effect of a diet enriched with monounsaturated or polyunsaturated fatty acids on levels of low-density and high-density lipoprotein cholesterol in healthy women and men. *New Engl. J. Med.,* **321,** 436–41.

Nordoy, A., Aakvaag, A., and Thelle, D. (1979). Sex hormones and high density lipoproteins in healthy males. *Atherosclerosis,* **34,** 431–6.

Phillips, G. B. (1978). Sex hormones, risk factors and cardiovascular disease. *Am. J. Med.,* **65,** 7–11.

Phillips, G. B. (1984). Evidence for hyperestrogenemia as the link between diabetcs mellitus and myocardial infarction. *Am. J. Med.,* **76,** 1041–8.

Reeves, R. D., Morris, M. D., and Barbour, G. L. K. (1976). Hyperlipidemia due to oxymetholone therapy. *J. Am. Med. Assoc.,* **236,** 469.

Rifkind, B. M., Tamir, I., Heiss, G., Wallace, R. B., and Tyroler, H. A. (1979). Distribution of high density and other lipoproteins in selected LRC Prevalence Study populations. *Lipids,* **14,** 105.

Semmens, J., Rouse, I., Beilin, L. J., and Masarei, J. R. L. (1983). Relationship of plasma HDL-cholesterol to testosterone, oestradiol, and sex-hormone-binding globulin levels in men and women. *Metabolism,* **32,** 428–32.

Sempos, C., Cooper, R., Kovar, M. G., and McMillen, M. (1988). Divergence of the recent trends in coronary mortality for the 4 major race-sex groups in the US. *Am. J. Publ. Health,* **78,** 1422–7.

Small, M., Lowe, G. D. O., Beastall, G. H., *et al.* (1985). Serum oestradiol and ischaemic heart disease—relationship with myocardial infarction but not coronary atheroma or haemostasis. *Q. J. Med.,* **57,** 775–82.

Solyom, A. (1971). Effects of androgens on serum lipids and lipoproteins. *Lipids,* **7,** 100.

Stampfer, M. J., Willett, W. C., Colditz, G. A., Rosner, B., Speizer, F. E., and Hennekens, C. H. (1985). A prospective study of postmenopausal estrogen therapy and coronary heart disease. *New Engl. J. Med.,* **313,** 1044–9.

Wahl, P., Walden, C., Knopp, R., Hoover, J., Wallace, R., Heiss, G., *et al.* (1983). Effect of oestrogen/progestin potency on lipid/lipoprotein cholesterol. *New Engl. J. Med.,* **308,** 862–7.

Wild, R. A. and Bartholomew, M. J. (1988). The influence of body weight on lipoprotein lipids in patients with polycystic ovary syndrome. *Am. J. Obstet. Gynecol.,* **159,** 423–7.

Wild, R. A., Painter, P. C., Coulson, P. B., Carruth, K. B., and Ranney, G. B. (1985). Lipoprotein lipid concentrations and cardiovascular risk in women with polycystic ovary syndrome. *J. Clin. Endocrinol. Metab.*, **61**, 946–51.

Wilson, P. W. F., Garrison, R. J., and Castelli, W. P. (1985). Postmenopausal oestrogen use, cigarette smoking, and cardiovascular morbidity in women over 50. *New Engl. J. Med.*, **313**, 1038–43.

Wingard, D. L. (1984). The sex differential in morbidity, mortality, and lifestyle. *Annu. Rev. Publ. Health*, **5**, 433–58.

Wingard, D. L., Sinsheimer, P., Barrett-Connor, E., and McPhillips, J. B. (1990). Community-based study of prevalence of NIDDM in older adults. *Diabet. Care*, **13**, 3–8.

20

Atheroma and thrombosis in cardiovascular disease: separate or complementary?

T. W. Meade

INTRODUCTION

There is now very general agreement about a central role for thrombosis in the onset of clinically manifest coronary heart disease (CHD) and in many cases of stroke also. However, this recognition is comparatively recent. Stimulated by an alarming increase in incidence and mortality, the growing research endeavour on CHD that started after the Second World War centred almost exclusively on atheroma and, because of its lipid content, the place of dietary fat and blood cholesterol levels. True, earlier work on the thrombogenic or encrustation theory of atheroma was not entirely overlooked and the term 'coronary thrombosis' (Herrick 1912) implied that at least some clinicians and pathologists had long ago recognized processes that we are now rediscovering. But until the late 1970s or early 1980s, almost no systematic attention has been paid to processes responsible for luminal occlusion.

THROMBOSIS, MYOCARDIAL INFARCTION, AND CORONARY DEATH

When the topic of thrombosis began to re-emerge in the mid-1970s, it was characterized by two major controversies. The first was whether thrombosis precedes or follows transmural myocardial infarction (MI). The issue was settled, as far as it then could be, by the unsatisfactory process of a consensus view of the evidence, which concluded that thrombosis does precede and probably causes transmural MI (Chandler *et al.* 1974). With the advent of thrombolytic therapy and the need to establish the rationale for its use and effects, angiography clearly demonstrated the high frequency of total coronary occlusion during MI (DeWood *et al.* 1980) and there is now no doubt about the significance of thrombosis in transmural MI

(Davies 1987). The place of thrombosis in subendocardial infarction is less clear (Davies 1987), though probably real. The second controversy, settled even more recently, was the place of thrombosis in sudden coronary death. In the mid-1970s, reports of platelet thrombi and microemboli in the coronary vessels of those dying sudden vascular deaths (Haerem 1974) were often viewed, wrongly, with scepticism. It was not until the results of a series of particularly careful autopsy studies became available in the 1980s (Davies and Thomas 1984; van Dantzig and Becker 1986; El Fawal *et al*. 1987; Frink *et al*. 1988) that the almost universal occurrence of thrombosis in sudden coronary death was recognized and accepted as directly contributing to these events. Most, though not all, sudden coronary deaths are the result of a ruptured atheromatous plaque in which thrombosis contributes to the intramural pathology or to luminal occlusion or to both. The minority of events in which thrombosis is not apparently associated with plaque rupture—between 2 per cent (Davies and Thomas 1984) and about 25 per cent (El Fawal *et al*. 1987)—are interesting in suggesting that characteristics of the circulating blood play a part in initiating some arterial thrombi. The observation that thrombi associated with sudden coronary death do not totally occlude the arterial lumen as often as those causing transmural MI may be due to the intense fibrinolytic activity accompanying sudden death, with the consequence that thrombi initially responsible for the episode are at least partially lysed by the time of autopsy (Meade *et al*. 1984; Davies 1987).

These crucial advances in the pathology of arterial disease are the basis for much of the work and many of the clinical and therapeutic advances of the last few years, and those likely during the next decade.

On the epidemiological side, it was Morris (1951) who first drew attention to the involvement of a major process other than atherogenesis through his analysis of post-mortem findings at the London Hospital. There was no increase—if anything a decrease—in the prevalence of advanced atheroma over a period of time during which mortality from CHD had increased several-fold. Morris pointed out that the main epidemic had started just after the First World War and that some environmental change that had occurred about then might provide at least a partial explanation. One such possibility was the widespread adoption of smoking by men. If this was involved, it suggested a relatively short-term acute effect rather than a longer-term influence.

PLATELETS AND FIBRIN

Coronary artery thrombi may vary from predominantly platelet bodies in the vessel wall to mainly fibrin accumulations in the lumen. As interest in thrombosis and CHD grew, most attention was initially directed towards the contribution of platelets. Their very rapid adhesion to damaged endo-thelium and then to each other is central to arterial thrombosis. The formation and incorporation of fibrin is a slower and therefore, for some, a less exciting event, but it is fibrin which gives many developing thrombi their ultimate stability and volume. A recent biochemical (as distinct from morphological) study concluded that fibrin formation and platelet activa-tion are probably equally important in the early hours of MI (Rapold *et al.* 1989). If so, this is an added reason for recognizing that the mechanical obstruction of the coronary artery is due to two main processes and that the most effective approach to antithrombotic therapy may involve platelet-active agents and anticoagulants simultaneously, a point considered in more detail later.

HAEMOSTATIC FUNCTION AND CHD

Is it possible to characterize those at risk of MI or sudden coronary death on account of a thrombotic tendency? The answer to this question mainly depends on prospective studies which include measures of haemostatic function. The first study specifically designed for this purpose was the Northwick Park Heart Study (NPHS) (Meade and North 1977). Its main objective has always been the epidemiological study of possible mechan-isms in the pathogenesis of CHD, as distinct from simply the prediction of those at high risk regardless of the underlying explanations.

When NPHS started in 1972, what limited interest there was in the contribution of thrombosis to CHD centred almost entirely on platelets. There is of course no doubt whatever about the central role of platelets in the process of thrombogenesis. However, there is still no generally accepted measure of platelet function that has been shown to be associated with the later onset of CHD in those so far free of clinical disease, though spontaneous platelet aggregation may well be associated with recurrence (Trip *et al.* 1990). Epidemiologically, the assessment of coagulability has been much more rewarding. Figure 20.1 is a simple representation of the coagulation system. Besides its well-known role in the conversion of fibrinogen to fibrin, thrombin is a potent platelet-aggregating agent. The assessment of coagulability may therefore provide one approach, albeit indirect, to platelet function. Furthermore, fibrinogen at levels within the physiological range is an important cofactor for platelet aggregability, so here too the coagulation system may exert a significant influence on platelet behaviour.

The main prospective findings of NPHS were of strong and independent associations between the levels of factor VII activity and plasma fibrinogen and the incidence of CHD (Meade *et al.* 1980, 1986). Since the first prospective results from NPHS (Meade *et al.* 1980), four other prospective

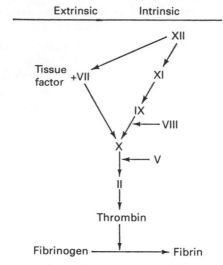

Fig. 20.1 An outline of the coagulation cascade.

studies have also reported strong relationships between the fibrinogen level and CHD (Wilhelmsen *et al.* 1984; Stone and Thorp 1985; Kannel *et al.* 1987; Yarnell *et al.* 1991). A number of cross-sectional studies support the likely involvement of fibrinogen and factor VII activity levels in CHD as well (Poller 1957; Meade 1987*a*). High fibrinogen levels increase viscosity, enhance platelet aggregability, contribute to the amount of fibrin formed in the rabbit, and probably contribute to the development of atheroma at least in its more advanced stages, so they may be of causal significance through one or a combination of pathways (Meade 1987*a*). Part of the evidence that high factor VII activity levels are of causal significance are the results of studies showing the influence of the extrinsic pathway on coagulability and thrombin production (Bauer and Rosenberg 1987; Bauer *et al.* 1989, 1990).

However, factor VII activity and the fibrinogen level are almost certainly not the only components of the coagulation system involved in the onset of CHD. Although much weaker than for factor VII and fibrinogen, in NPHS there were also suggestive associations of high factor VIII levels and poor fibrinolytic activity with CHD incidence (Meade *et al.* 1980, 1986), and impaired fibrinolytic activity may also influence the recurrence of MI (Hamsten *et al.* 1987). In the case of factor VIII, supporting evidence comes from interesting Dutch studies which show a much lower than expected incidence of CHD in haemophiliacs (Rosendaal *et al.* 1989).

The emphasis is now shifting from the *potential* of the coagulation system in contributing to CHD to indices of actual *activity*—for example, the activation peptide of factor X, fragment F 1.2 as an index of thrombin generation, and fibrinopeptide A (FPA) as an index of the action of thrombin on fibrinogen.

DETERMINANTS OF COAGULABILITY

The main environmental determinant of fibrinogen levels is smoking. All the large epidemiological studies have consistently found the highest levels in smokers, intermediate levels in ex-smokers, and the lowest levels in non-smokers (Meade 1987*b*). There is a dose–response relationship between the number of cigarettes smoked and the fibrinogen level (Wilkes *et al.* 1988). Finally, starting or resuming smoking is accompanied by an increase in fibrinogen, while stopping is accompanied by a decrease (Meade *et al.* 1987). Figure 20.2, from data at entry to NPHS, shows a rapid initial decline in fibrinogen on stopping smoking, but levels remain above those for non-smokers for up to 5 and perhaps 10 years after discontinuation—a time course that closely mirrors the decline in the risk of CHD itself after smoking cessation (Cook *et al.* 1986). In fact, given the very strong relationship between fibrinogen levels and the risk of CHD or stroke, the fall in fibrinogen in ex-smokers is enough to account for a large part of the decline in their risk of CHD. This strengthens the conclusion that much and perhaps most of the relationship between smoking and CHD is mediated through the fibrinogen level, though it is important to remember that high fibrinogen levels are associated with an increased risk of CHD in non-smokers as well (Meade *et al.* 1986).

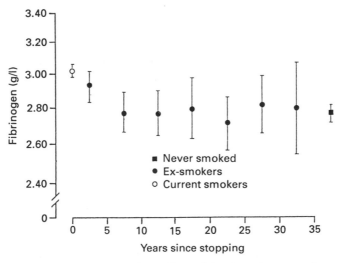

Fig. 20.2 Plasma fibrinogen level (age-adjusted) by time since stopping smoking in 518 ex-smokers and in current and non-smokers.

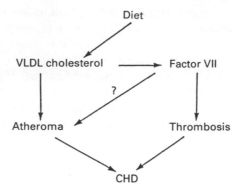

Fig. 20.3 Scheme of dietary contribution to pathogenesis of CHD. Fibrin, possibly due to coagulation initiated via the extrinsic system, contributes to atheroma as well as thrombosis (as does fibrinogen).

The leading environmental determinant of factor VII activity levels is dietary fat intake (Miller *et al*. 1986, 1989). Taken together, the evidence leaves little doubt that dietary fat influences the risk of CHD through both a long-term atherogenic pathway and an acute short-term thrombogenic pathway (Fig. 20.3). This emphasizes the complementary nature of athero-genesis and thrombosis in CHD and the need to avoid any further polarization of hypotheses for CHD as purely atherogenic or purely thrombogenic. Another consideration, perhaps with important practical implications, is that lipid-lowering regimes may reduce CHD risk at least as much by their effects on coagulability and thrombin production as through the more difficult process of reversing atheroma (if, indeed, this is feasible at all under any but exceptional conditions).

The probable benefit of fish oil in preventing CHD (Burr *et al*. 1989) is likely to be mediated through its effect on platelet activity.

PRACTICAL IMPLICATIONS

The risk of CHD can be modified either through changes in life-style or pharmacologically.

Life-style changes can be encouraged by central policies affecting dietary habits or tobacco advertising, for example, and directed at populations as a whole, or they can be adopted through individual choice. They have almost certainly been responsible for much of the decline in CHD incidence in many countries over the last 25 years. However, their acceptance and implementation take time. Many find the recommended changes difficult or impossible to adhere to, and they are ineffective in some of those who do take them up. Thus there is always likely to be a case for pharmacological intervention. Before considering this in further detail, however, there are some lessons for prevention through life-style changes that are emerging from the recognition of the thrombotic component in CHD and its characteristics. While this new information alters no general principles, it does in some respects enable their more efficient application. First, the independent relationship between high fibrinogen levels and the risk of CHD is sufficiently strong to warrant the addition of the fibrinogen level to the definition of the 'high risk profile'. Second, the similarity of the time course for the fall in fibrinogen and in the risk of CHD itself in ex-smokers emphasizes the importance of not overlooking the considerable period of time during which an ex-smoker remains at increased risk or the thrombotic contribution to this risk. Turning to diet, the very rapid effect of changes in fat intake on coagulability provides a sound basis for the adoption of dietary measures at any age and argues strongly against any remaining belief that these will only succeed if they are adopted in early life (though doing so then may well influence atherogenesis as well). The potential value of fish oils on platelet activity carries the same implication.

Where pharmacological measures for primary prevention are necessary, it is of course with the modification of platelet aggregation and fibrin formation that antithrombotic measures are concerned. The value of aspirin in primary prevention is still rather uncertain: the trial in American doctors (Physicians' Health Study Research Group 1989) suggested a reduction of 44 per cent in the incidence of MI but no effect on death from all vascular causes, while the trial in British doctors (Peto *et al.* 1988) showed no apparent benefit against MI. An overview of the two trials suggests a significant reduction of 32 per cent (Hennekens *et al.* 1989), although there is marginally significant heterogeneity between the two trials in this respect, and an increase of 18 per cent in non-fatal stroke, which is not significant, however, and contrasts with the obvious reduction in stroke ascribed to aspirin in the secondary prevention trials. Therefore there is a need for further information from primary prevention trials of aspirin, including the effects of aspirin doses in the range of 40–80 mg daily. A fairly consistent finding in secondary prevention trials so far has been a somewhat greater benefit due to oral anticoagulants than aspirin, though this conclusion is mainly based on indirect comparisons. Thus the reduction in mortality attributable to anticoagulants is, at between 20 and 25 per cent, somewhat more than the typical figures of between 15 and 20 per cent for aspirin. Similarly, anticoagulants reduce recurrent MI between a third and a half compared with a reduction of 25 or 30 per cent in the case of aspirin.

If there truly is a more than marginal advantage of anticoagulants over aspirin, the greater complexity of anticoagulant treatment should not automatically rule it out in what is, after all, a common condition in which even small differences in effectiveness may be reflected in many lives saved and events avoided. A second consideration for the potential value of anticoagulants is the growing conviction that their benefit may perhaps be achieved at much lower than conventional levels of anticoagulation. There would also be less bleeding and less need for monitoring. In addition, there is also the real possibility that the simultaneous modification of platelet function and fibrin formation may be more effective than the modification of either process on its own. The most striking demonstration of this possibility comes from the ISIS-2 trial (ISIS-2 1988), in which the combination of aspirin and streptokinase was more effective than either active agent on its own though each also reduced cardiovascular mortality. The case for establishing the potential value of low intensity oral anticoagulation in primary prevention is strengthened by the relationship between factor VII activity and the incidence of CHD (Meade *et al*. 1986), bearing in mind that factor VII is one of the vitamin-K-dependent clotting factors whose activity is reduced by warfarin. Accordingly, the separate and combined effects of 75 mg of aspirin and of warfarin achieving an international normalized ratio (INR) of about 1.5 are currently being investigated in the Thrombosis Prevention Trial (Meade *et al*. 1988; Meade 1990) which, unlike the American and British doctors' trials, is based on men at considerably increased risk of CHD. The encouraging results of the RISC trial (RISC 1990) in unstable angina provide a further strong incentive to the evaluation of 75 mg of aspirin in primary prevention.

But firmly establishing the value of different antithrombotic measures is not the end of the story. The advent of the HMG co-A reductase inhibitors with their striking cholesterol-lowering properties suggests a choice between antithrombotic and lipid-lowering approaches which can only be made objectively if they are in due course directly compared, and the possibility of significant adverse effects of lipid-lowering regimes has still to be resolved (Muldoon *et al*. 1990). It is perhaps easier to see more general applicability for antithrombotic treatment, if thrombosis is the immediate arterial cause of most major episodes of CHD, whatever the more remote explanations—smoking, hypertension, obesity, or hyperlipidaemia. The indications for lipid-lowering treatment must presumably continue to be sustained hyperlipidaemia in the same way that blood-pressure-lowering agents would only be used in those with hypertension. So, while the developments of recent years have to an appreciable extent linked the lipid and thromogenic hypotheses for CHD, they probably do carry some as yet unresolved practical implications for pharmacological approaches to primary prevention.

REFERENCES

Bauer, K. A. and Rosenberg, R. D. (1987). The pathophysiology of the prethrombotic state in humans: insights gained from studies using markers of hemostatic system activation. *Blood*, **70**, 343–50.

Bauer, K. A., Kass, B. L., ten Cate, H., Bednarek, M. A., Hawiger, J. J., and Rosenberg, R. D. (1989). Detection of factor X activation in humans. *Blood,* **74,** 2007–15.

Bauer, K. A., Kass, B. L., ten Cate, H., Bednarek, M. A., Hawiger, J. J., and Rosenberg, R. D. (1990). Factor IX is activated *in vivo* by the tissue factor mechanism. *Blood,* **76,** 731–6.

Burr, M. L., Fehily, A. M., Rogers, S., Welsby, E., King, S., and Sandham, S. (1989). Diet and reinfarction trial (DART): design, recruitment, and compliance. *Eur. Heart J.,* **10,** 558–67.

Chandler, A. B., Chapman, I., Erhardt, L. R., Roberts, W. C., Schwartz, C. J., Sinapius, D., *et al.* (1974). Coronary thrombosis in myocardial infarction. Report of a workshop on the role of coronary thrombosis in the pathogenesis of acute myocardial infarction. *Am. J. Cardiol.,* **34,** 823–33.

Cook, D. G., Shaper, A. G., Pocock, S. J., and Kussick, S. J. (1986). Giving up smoking and the risk of heart attacks. *Lancet,* **ii,** 1376–80.

Davies, M. J. (1987). Thrombosis in acute myocardial infarction and sudden death. In *Thrombosis and platelets in myocardial ischemia* (eds J. L. Mehta, C. R. Conti, and A. N. Brest), Chapter 10, F A Divis, Philadelphia, PA, pp. 151–9.

Davies, M. J. and Thomas, A. (1984). Thrombosis and acute coronary-artery lesions in sudden cardiac ischemic death. *New Engl. J. Med.,* **310,** 1137–40.

DeWood, M. A., Spores, J., Notske, R., Mouser, L. T., Burroughs, R., Golden, M. S., *et al.* (1980). Prevalence of total coronary occlusion during the early hours of transmural myocardial infarction. *New Engl. J. Med.,* **303,** 897–901.

El Fawal, M. A., Berg, G. A., Wheatley, D. J., and Harland, W. A. (1987). Sudden coronary death in Glasgow: nature and frequency of acute coronary lesions. *Br. Heart J.,* **57,** 35.

Frink, R. J., Rooney, P. A., Jr, Trowbridge, J. O., and Rose, J. (1988). Coronary thrombosis and platelet/fibrin microemboli in death associated with acute myocardial infarction. *Br. Heart J.,* **59,** 196–200.

Haerem, J. W. (1974). Mural platelet microthrombi and major acute lesions of main epicardial arteries in sudden coronary death. *Atherosclerosis,* **19,** 529–41.

Hamsten, A., de Faire, U., Walldius, G., Dahlen, G., Szamosi, A., Landou, C., *et al.* (1987). Plasminogen activator inhibitor in plasma: risk factor for recurrent myocardial infarction. *Lancet,* **ii,** 3–9.

Hennekens, C. H., Buring, J. E., Sandercock, P., Collins, R., and Peto, R. (1989). Aspirin and other antiplatelet agents in the secondary and primary prevention of cardiovascular disease. *Circulation,* **80,** 748–56.

Herrick, J. B. (1912). Clinical features of sudden obstruction of the coronary arteries. *J. Am. Med. Assoc.,* **23,** 2015–20.

ISIS-2 (Second International Study of Infarct Survival) Collaborative Group (1988). Randomised trial of intravenous streptokinase, oral aspirin, both, or neither among 17187 cases of suspected acute myocardial infarction: ISIS-2. *Lancet,* **ii,** 349–60.

Kannel, W. B., Wolf, P. A., Castelli, W. P., and D'Agostino, R. B. (1987). Fibrinogen and risk of cardiovascular disease. *J. Am. Med. Assoc.,* **258,** 1183–6.

McGill, H. C. (1988). The cardiovascular pathology of smoking. *Am. Heart J.,* **115,** 250–7.

Meade, T. W. (1987*a*). Epidemiology of atheroma, thrombosis and ischaemic heart disease. In *Haemostasis and thrombosis*, 2nd edn (eds A. L. Bloom and D. P. Thomas), Churchill Livingstone, Edinburgh, pp. 697–720.

Meade, T. W. (1987*b*). The epidemiology of haemostatic and other variables in coronary artery disease. In *Thrombosis and haemostasis* (eds M. Verstraete, J. Vermylen, R. Lijnen, and J. Arnout), Leuven University Press, pp. 37–60.

Meade, T. W. (1990). Low-dose warfarin and low-dose aspirin in the primary prevention of ischemic heart disease. *Am. J. Cardiol.*, **65,** 7c–11c.

Meade, T. W. and North, W. R. S. (1977). Population-based distributions of haemostatic variables. *Br. Med. Bull.*, **33,** 283–8.

Meade, T. W., North, W. R. S., Chakrabarti, R., Stirling, Y., Haines, A. P., and Thompson, S. G. (1980). Haemostatic function and cardiovascular death: early results of a prospective study. *Lancet,* **i,** 1050–4.

Meade, T. W., Howarth, D. J., and Stirling, Y. (1984). Fibrinopeptide A and sudden coronary death. *Lancet,* **ii,** 607–9.

Meade, T. W., Mellows, S., Brozovic, M., Miller, G. J., Chakrabarti, R. R., North, W. R. S., *et al.* (1986). Haemostatic function and ischaemic heart disease: principal results of the Northwick Park Heart Study. *Lancet,* **ii,** 533–7.

Meade, T. W., Imeson, J., and Stirling, Y. (1987). Effects of changes in smoking and other characteristics on clotting factors and the risk of ischaemic heart disease. *Lancet,* **ii,** 986–8.

Meade, T. W., Wilkes, H. C., Stirling, Y,, Brennan, P. J., Kelleher, C., and Browne, W. (1988). Randomized controlled trial of low dose warfarin in the primary prevention of ischaemic heart disease in men at high risk: design and pilot study. *Eur. Heart J.,* **9,** 836–43.

Miller, G. J., Martin, J. C., Webster, J., Wilkes, H., Miller, N. E., Wilkinson, W. H., *et al.* (1986). Association between dietary fat intake and plasma factor VII coagulant activity—a predictor of cardiovascular mortality. *Atherosclerosis,* **60,** 269–77.

Miller, G. J., Cruickshank, J. K., Ellis, L. J., Thompson, R. L., Wilkes, H. C., Stirling, Y., *et al.* (1989). Fat consumption and factor VII coagulant activity in middle-aged men. An association between a dietary and thrombogenic coronary risk factor. *Atherosclerosis,* **78,** 19–24.

Morris, J. N. (1951). Recent history of coronary disease. *Lancet,* **i,** 1–7, 69–73.

Muldoon, M. F., Manuck, S. B., and Matthews, K. A. (1990). Lowering cholesterol concentrations and mortality: a quantitative review of primary prevention trials. *Br. Med. J.,* **301,** 309–14.

Peto, R., Gray, R., Collins, R., Wheatley, K., Hennekens, C., Jamrozik, K., *et al.* (1988). Randomised trial of prophylactic daily aspirin in British male doctors. *Br. Med. J.,* **296,** 313–16.

Physicians' Health Study Research Group (1989). Final report on the aspirin component of the ongoing Physicians' Health Study. *New Engl. J. Med.,* **321,** 129–35.

Poller, L. (1957). Thrombosis and factor VII activity. *J. Clin. Pathol.,* **10,** 348–50.

Rapold, H. J., Haeberli, A., Kuemmerli, H., Weiss, M., Baur, H. R., and Straub, W. P. (1989). Fibrin formation and platelet activation in patients with myocardial infarction and normal coronary arteries. *Eur. Heart J.,* **10,** 323–33.

RISC Group (1990). Risk of myocardial infarction and death during treatment with low dose aspirin and intravenous heparin in men with unstable coronary artery disease. *Lancet,* **336,** 827–30.

Rosendaal, F. R., Varekamp, I., Smit, C., Brocker-Vriends, A. H. J. T., van Dijck, H., Vandenbroucke, J. P., *et al.* (1989). Mortality and causes of death in Dutch haemophiliacs, 1973–86. *Br. J. Haematol.,* **71,** 71–6.

Stone, M. C. and Thorp, J. M. (1985). Plasma fibrinogen—a major coronary risk factor. *J. R. Coll. Gen. Pract.,* **35,** 565–9.

Trip, M. D., Cats, V. M., van Capelle, F. J. L., and Vreeken, J. (1990). Platelet hyperreactivity and prognosis in survivors of myocardial infarction. *New Engl. J. Med.,* **322,** 1549–54.

van Dantzig, J. M. and Becker, A. E. (1986). Sudden cardiac death and acute pathology of coronary arteries. *Eur. Heart J.,* **7,** 987–91.

Wilhelmsen, L., Svardsudd, K., Korsan-Bengtsen, K., Welin, L., and Tibblin, G. (1984). Fibrinogen as a risk factor for stroke and myocardial infarction. *New Engl. J. Med.,* **311,** 501–5.

Wilkes, H. C., Kelleher, C., and Meade, T. W. (1988). Smoking and plasma fibrinogen. *Lancet,* **i,** 307–8.

Yarnell, J. W. G., Baker, I. A., Sweetnam, P. M., Bainton, D., O'Brien, J. R., Whitehead, P. J., and Elwood, P. C. (1991). Fibrinogen, viscosity, and white blood cell count are major risk factors for ischaemic heart disease. *Circulation,* **83,** 836–44.

21

Coronary risk factors and non-cardiovascular disease

A. Menotti

INTRODUCTION

The advent and development of cardiovascular epidemiology after the Second World War allowed identification of the so-called coronary risk factors. Particular attention was paid to the basic, graded, independent and universal predictive, and probable causal role of smoking habits, blood pressure, and cholesterol (Gordon *et al.* 1971; Shurtleff 1974; Pooling Project Research Group 1978; Dawber 1980; Keys 1980).

Interest during the first 20 years of this new research field was focused on coronary heart disease (CHD) in recognition of its major morbid and lethal role in advanced societies. Later, the availability of long-term follow-up data, giving information mainly on causes of death, stimulated interest in the relationship of major coronary risk factors to morbid conditions and causes of death other than coronary and cardiovascular disease. All-cause mortality was also of great interest, and life expectancy emerged as an important topic of research and particularly of prediction (Keys 1980; Menotti *et al.* 1989a). Thus a by-product of studies originally designed to answer questions concerning the incidence, mortality, and prediction of CHD was that similar approaches were applied to non-cardiovascular diseases, although perhaps not in a systematic way.

Before reviewing the risk factors for non-cardiovascular diseases, it should be recalled briefly that the three main coronary risk factors have unequivocal relationships with non-CHD cardiovascular conditions. In particular, blood pressure is a universal predictor for stroke, although smoking habits and cholesterol have been variously reported both as predictors and non-predictors (Gordon *et al.* 1971; Dawber 1980; Menotti *et al.* 1989a); cholesterol may be related to atherothrombotic cerebral stroke but not to the haemorrhagic type of stroke. However, cholesterol and smoking seem to be the major risk factors for intermittent claudication (Gordon *et al.* 1971; Shurtleff 1974; Dawber 1980).

TYPOLOGY OF NON-CARDIOVASCULAR DISEASES

The relationship of the three major CHD risk factors to non-cardiovascular diseases or deaths depends upon the definition of such a subset of causes of death.

For example, the 25 year death rate from several causes has recently been reported in population samples of men originally aged 40–59 from three countries—Finland with two cohorts (East and West), the Netherlands with one cohort (Zutphen), and Italy with two cohorts (Crevalcore and Montegiorgio) (Menotti et al. 1991). There were large differences in all-cause death rates among the five groups, although the majority of them were explained by differences in CHD which ranged from 294 per 1000 in 25 years in East Finland to 113 per 1000 in Montegiorgio, Italy. Despite this, the ratio of cancer death to all-cause mortality ranged from 37 per cent in Zutphen to 20 per cent in East Finland, suggesting the existence of competing risks among different causes of death. It is likely that such differences are paralleled by differences in the relationship of risk factors to mortality, particularly when looking at all-cause mortality.

The relationship of risk factors to events is largely conditioned by the sex and age distribution of the population under consideration and by the length of follow-up. In Western societies and in middle-aged and older people, the large majority of deaths, other than those from cardiovascular disease, are from cancer. In general, non-cardiovascular deaths can be split into a few components such as cancer, chronic bronchitis, violent deaths, and others. All-cause mortality will also be considered as a relevant endpoint.

SMOKING

The statistical and possibly causal association of smoking with a number of conditions, particularly lung cancer but also chronic bronchitis, other relevant cancer sites, and possibly peptic ulcer, is so overwhelming that little can be added (Doll and Bradford-Hill 1954; Doll and Peto 1976; US Surgeon General 1989). Moreover, such relationships were largely known before the availability of long-term data from longitudinal studies originally designed for the study of coronary and other cardiovascular diseases. An example is provided by Table 21.1, which refers to 20 year old data. The role of smoking in the prediction and possible causality of several fatal conditions explains why, whatever population is considered, it is one of the most powerful direct predictors of all-cause mortality and, conversely, of life expectancy.

Table 21.1 Mortality ratio for some non-cardiovascular causes of smokers to non-smokers

Cause of death	Non-smokers	Smokers (extremes)
Cancer of lung	1.00	4.50–14.20
Cancer of larynx	1.00	6.09–11.83
Cancer of oesophagus	1.00	1.82– 8.75
Cancer of kidney	1.00	1.06–10.0
Cancer of bladder	1.00	1.36– 2.71
Chronic obstructive lung disease	1.00	2.30–24.7
Peptic ulcer	1.00	0.5 – 2.8
All-cause mortality	1.00	1.25– 1.83

Reconstructed from studies reported in *Smoking and Health* (1979).

The predominant role of smoking in lung cancer is also suggested by the fact that non-smokers usually have a negligible risk of lung cancer, which is not the case for CHD events or other conditions (Doll and Bradford-Hill 1954; Doll and Peto 1976; US Surgeon General 1989). One of the most comprehensive contributions on the relationship of smoking to mortality from chronic bronchitis is provided by a recent analysis of the Whitehall Study (Ebi-Kryston 1989).

BLOOD PRESSURE

For many years research on blood pressure and hypertension focused on the relationship with CHD, stroke, and cardiovascular diseases. Later, the availability of long-term mortality data suggested a multipotential role for this coronary risk factor. In particular, a small number of studies showed an unexpected and largely unexplained direct association between levels of blood pressure (and especially hypertension) and cancer mortality (Dyer *et al.* 1975; Raynor *et al.* 1981; Khaw and Barrett-Connor 1984).

Several variables were tested as possible confounders, but after adjusting for smoking habits, consumption of alcohol, some specific drugs (such as rauwolfia), and other possible predictors of cancer, the predictive power of blood pressure, although less prominent, remained independent and statistically significant. In one of the studies (Raynor *et al.* 1981), the association was limited to cancer of the kidney. These findings were mainly shown in American studies, but similar conclusions could be drawn by analysing data from two Italian cohorts of the Seven Countries Study, where a direct and significant association between mean blood pressure and all-site cancer mortality was found by solving multivariate models in

15–25 year follow-up data (Menotti *et al.* 1980; 1987*a*). In the latter case a 10 mmHg difference in mean blood pressure (diastolic pressure plus one third of the differential) is associated with a 5 per cent difference in cancer death risk, which increases to 22 per cent for a 20 mmHg difference.

After cancer, the most common cause of death in many societies, at least in middle-aged men, is violence. Repeated analyses at different lengths of follow-up in some Italian data showed a direct relationship of blood pressure to violent death (Menotti *et al.* 1980, 1987*a*). The explanation of this finding is not straightforward and calls for a deeper analysis. However, in some specific case reviews, it was found that some lethal road or work accidents were immediately preceded and possibly triggered by minor cardiocirculatory events.

Although the biological explanation for the above findings is incomplete, blood pressure is related in some way to about 75 per cent of adult or adult–elderly mortality through cardiovascular disease, cancer, and violent death. Analyses of blood pressure relative to other causes of death are rare. However, multivariate analysis of the Italian population samples discussed above, allowing for a number of other factors, showed a similar direct relationship of blood pressure to other causes of death including many relatively rare conditions (Menotti *et al.* 1980, 1987*a*).

The obvious conclusion is that almost any fatal event can be predicted, if not caused, by blood pressure levels and that hypertensives in particular are at a higher risk of death from any cause, not only for cardiovascular disease. As a consequence it appears that, of the known risk factors, a single measurement of blood pressure in middle-aged persons seems to be the single most efficient predictor of all-cause mortality and, conversely, of life expectancy. Thus higher blood pressure may be associated not only with a greater risk of cardiovascular events, but also with a less adaptive response of the individual to other diseases and, through still unknown mechanisms, a greater predisposition to conditions or events other than cardiovascular disease.

CHOLESTEROL

Serum cholesterol has repeatedly been demonstrated to be a major risk factor for CHD, showing a direct, graded, independent, and perhaps causal relation to the development of the disease (Gordon *et al.* 1971; Shurtleff 1974; Pooling Project Research Group 1978; Dawber 1980; Keys 1980; Martin *et al.* 1986). However, at the end of the 1970s some reports suggested that an inverse relationship existed between serum cholesterol and cancer deaths. Following the early papers, analyses from many epidemiological studies showing contrasting evidence have been published. This issue is particularly important because campaigns launched recently in several countries, aimed at reducing serum cholesterol in order to prevent CHD and other complications of atherosclerosis, could be brought into question if the reduction of cholesterol were to increase susceptibility to cancer.

In the main studies published during the last 10–12 years, the following types of results can be found (the references are only selected examples):

(1) no relationship between cholesterol and cancer (Kozarevic *et al.* 1981; Salonen 1982; Kromhout *et al.* 1988);

(2) an inverse relationship which disappears after the removal of early deaths in the first few years after the cholesterol measurement (Rose and Shipley 1980; Cambien *et al.* 1981; International Collaborative Group 1982; Sherwin *et al.* 1987) (an example is given in Table 21.2);

(3) an inverse relationship which does not disappear after the removal of early deaths (Kark *et al.* 1980; Williams *et al.* 1981; Keys *et al.* 1985; Schatzkin *et al.* 1988);

(4) relationships of different or uncertain interpretation (Tornberg 1988);

(5) a direct relationship between cholesterol and cancer (usually only for breast cancer) (Tornberg *et al.* 1988).

The current hypothesis for explaining the inverse relationship, when found, between serum cholesterol and cancer deaths suggests that pre-clinical cancers could modify lipid metabolism with the net result of reducing the level of circulating cholesterol. This hypothesis would explain how the relationship can be transformed from negative to null by excluding the early cancer deaths.

Biological explanations for the decrease in serum cholesterol, mainly in leukaemias, have recently been given in terms of an activation of the membrane low density lipoprotein receptors of the cancer cells and perhaps of other tissues as well. This mechanism would incorporate cholesterol into the cells with a consequent reduction of its serum level (Budd and

Table 21.2 Age-adjusted mortality rates per 1000 per year in a 7.5 year follow-up of the Whitehall Study.

Cause of death	Follow-up period (years)	Plasma cholesterol (mg/dl)			
		<180	180–219	220–259	260+
Non-CHD	<2	4.28	2.80	2.32	2.05
	2–7.5	3.55	3.32	3.76	3.37
All causes	<2	6.35	5.28	5.11	6.28
	2–7.5	5.35	5.41	7.51	8.04

Rates by cause, plasma cholesterol levels and duration of follow-up
Modified from Rose and Shipley 1980.

Ginsberg 1986). Another possible explanation for the inverse relationship between cholesterol and cancer is competitive mortality in the subjects with high levels of cholesterol, i.e. between CHD and cancer (and other conditions). Innovative mathematical modelling is probably needed to clarify this issue.

After the cholesterol–cancer question, what remains of the major non-cardiovascular causes of death with respect to cholesterol is a miscellany of conditions which have never been systematically investigated from this point of view. When cholesterol is studied against all-cause mortality little, if any, association is usually found (Gordon *et al.* 1971; Keys 1980), although exceptionally the relationship is positive and significant as has been found in the Multiple Risk Factor Intervention Trial (MRFIT) screenees (Kannel *et al.* 1986; Martin *et al.* 1986). This finding, of course, may depend upon the proportion of CHD within all-cause mortality. Again, the question of competing risks should be raised although it has not received a clear answer so far.

MULTIVARIATE ANALYSIS AND ALL-CAUSE MORTALITY

Some data from multivariate analysis have been discussed above, but a more systematic review is warranted together with discussion of current interest in all-cause mortality as an end-point (Keys 1980; Menotti *et al.* 1983, 1987*b*, 1989*a*, 1991; Kannel *et al.* 1986). A number of studies have shown the predictive value of smoking and blood pressure on all-cause mortality even in multivariate analyses with control for other possibly confounding factors. Examples are the Seven Countries Study (Menotti *et al.* 1989*a*, *b*), the Pooling Project (Kannel *et al.* 1986), and the follow-up of the MRFIT screenees (Kannel *et al.* 1986).

In the Seven Countries study, the results for smoking and blood pressure were obtained in the 10 year analysis by solving the multiple logistic model for the US sample, the pool of North European cohorts, and the pool of South European cohorts, allowing for four other factors as possible confounders (Keys 1980). Similar results were obtained in the 20 year follow-up analysis made in the cohorts pooled in national groups of six out of the Seven Countries (USA not available) (Menotti *et al.* 1989*a*). Blood pressure was always a significant predictor, whereas the coefficients for smoking habits were non-significant in Greece, Japan, and the Netherlands. Some of these results were confirmed in a 25 year follow-up analysis limited to the Dutch, the Finnish, and two of the Italian cohorts (Menotti *et al.* 1991). Both blood pressure and smoking were significantly related to all-cause mortality in all five components of the Pooling Project (Kannel *et al.* 1986).

Cholesterol was not a significant predictor of all-cause mortality in any of the above analyses, except in Tecumseh. This is a somewhat unexpected finding, at least for the Finnish cohorts where an overwhelming 32.2 per cent (at 10 year follow-up), 43.4 per cent (at 20 year follow-up), and 43.8 per cent (at 25 year follow-up) of deaths were from CHD which is the condition most frequently associated with serum cholesterol. In contrast, the converse was found in the analysis of 325 348 screenees of MRFIT, in which cholesterol yielded a significant predictive coefficient in a multivariate analysis with all-cause mortality as the end-point (Kannel *et al.* 1986). Some of the data discussed above are summarized in Table 21.3. Since the cholesterol–CHD relationship was clear-cut in all the above studies, the conclusion should be drawn that the relationship between cholesterol and other causes of death varies between different studies concerning different populations groups.

Only a few studies have tried to tackle the problem by simultaneously examining CHD, cardiovascular disease, cancer, non-cardiovascular disease, and all-cause mortality by means of a multivariate approach (Menotti *et al.* 1980, 1987a). For the purpose of this chapter an attempt has been made to look at these end-points in a sample of 3349 middle-aged men enrolled in Rome and followed up for 6.5 years (Table 21.4). With some differences, age and smoking were clearly shown to predict CHD, cardiovascular disease, non-cardiovascular disease, and all-cause mortality.

Table 21.3 All-cause mortality in a number of studies as a function of serum cholesterol, blood pressure, and cigarette smoking

Study	Serum cholesterol (mg/dl)	Diastolic blood pressure (mmHg)	Mean blood pressure (mmHg)	Cigarette smoking (per day)
Framingham[a]	0.32	4.76	—	4.27
Albany[a]	1.05	5.17	—	3.74
Chicago-Gas[a]	1.26	2.84	—	4.60
Chicago-West El.[a]	0.17	3.96	—	3.27
Tecumseh[a]	2.81	3.37	—	2.99
MRFIT[a]	8.25	15.64	—	28.14
SC-Finland[b]	1.00	—	9.15	6.27
SC-Netherlands[b]	0.51	—	4.17	0.71
SC-Italy[b]	1.14	—	10.40	4.70
SC-Yugoslavia[b]	0.38	—	5.13	6.29
SC-Greece[b]	−1.95	—	4.86	0.93
SC-Japan[b]	−1.35	—	4.57	1.25

t value of coefficients from multivariate models
[a] Men aged 40–59; 6 year follow-up; multiple logistic function.
[b] Men aged 40–59; 20 year follow-up; Cox model. SC, Seven Countries Study.
Data reconstructed from Kannel *et al.* (1986) and Menotti *et al.* 1989a.

Table 21.4 NFR Study in Rome: solution of Cox models with different conditions as end-points and four risk factors as covariates in a 6.5 year follow-up of 3349 men aged 46–65

Factor	CHD (n = 68)	CVD (n = 95)	Non-CVD (n = 136)	ALL (n = 231)
Age (years)	0.0482	0.0591	0.1216	0.0955
	(1.99)	(2.86)	(6.83)	(7.10)
Cholesterol (mg/dl)	0.0072	0.0053	−0.0031	0.0005
	(2.52)	(2.15)	(−1.41)	(0.29)
Systolic blood pressure (mmHg)	0.0172	0.0207	0.0055	0.0121
	(3.01)	(4.44)	(1.27)	(3.81)
Cigarettes, yes–no	0.6287	0.5201	0.5178	0.5190
	(2.48)	(2.47)	(2.94)	(3.85)

t values given in parentheses.
CVD, cardiovascular disease; Non-CVD, non-cardiovascular disease; ALL, all-cause mortality.

Blood pressure predicted CHD, cardiovascular disease, and all-cause mortality, but only marginally predicted non-cardiovascular diseases. Cholesterol had a positive and significant coefficient for coronary and cardiovascular end-points, a negligible coefficient for all-cause mortality, and a negative although non-significant coefficient for non-cardiovascular death. In this population the proportion of all-cause mortality from CHD was 29 per cent.

Taking the whole population as a reference, a decrease of 10 mmHg (from 135 to 125 mmHg) in the average systolic blood pressure would theoretically be accompanied by a decrease of 11 per cent in total mortality, and a reduction of prevalence of smoking from 50 to 25 per cent would be accompanied by a 6 per cent decrease in mortality. A combination of the above two changes would provide a 22 per cent benefit in all-cause mortality.

CONCLUSIONS

1. The three major coronary risk factors show clear although slightly different relationships with non-cardiovascular diseases and all-cause mortality in both univariate and multivariate analyses.

2. Smoking is strongly related to both non-cardiovascular conditions and all-cause mortality. Its role is partly causal, depending on the condition, and partly non-causal.

3. Blood pressure is also strongly related to non-cardiovascular disease and to all cause mortality, again in mixed fashion—causal, non-causal,

or as a precipitating factor. Some of the pathophysiological mechanisms are still unknown.

4. Serum cholesterol appears either neutral or inversely related to non-cardiovascular diseases and to all-cause mortality. A better understanding of its role should come from further investigation concerning its relationship to cancer, and the reductions in cholesterol as a consequence of co-morbidity (Nissinen *et al.* 1989; Harris *et al.* 1990).

5. The above relationship may depend upon the different nosographic mixes of all-cause mortality and upon competing risks which deserve more investigation.

REFERENCES

Budd, D. and Ginsberg, H. (1986). Hypocholesterolemia and acute myelogenous leukemia. Association between disease activity and plasma low-density lipoprotein cholesterol concentrations. *Cancer*, **58**, 1361–5.

Cambien, F., Ducimetiere, P., and Richard, J. (1981). Total serum cholesterol and cancer mortality in a middle-aged male population. *Am. J. Epidemiol.*, **112**, 388–94.

Dawber, T. R. (1980). *The Framingham study. The epidemiology of atherosclerotic disease*, Harvard University Press, pp. 1–257.

Doll, R. and Bradford-Hill, A. (1954). The mortality of doctors in relation to their smoking habits. *Br. Med. J.*, **1**, 1451–5.

Doll, R. and Peto, R. (1976). Mortality in relation to smoking: 20 years' observation on male British doctors. *Br. Med. J.*, **2**, 1525–36.

Dyer, A. R., Stamler, J., Berkson, D. M., Lindberg, H. A., and Stevens, E. (1975). High blood pressure: a risk factor for cancer mortality? *Lancet*, **i**, 1051–6.

Ebi-Kryston, K. (1989). Predicting 15 year chronic bronchitis mortality in the Whitehall study. *J. Epidemiol. Community Health*, **43**, 168–72.

Gordon, T., Sorlie, P., and Kannel, W. B. (1971). Coronary heart disease, atherothrombotic brain infarction, intermittent claudication. A multivariate analysis of some factors related to their incidence. Framingham study, 16 year follow-up. In *The Framingham study. An epidemiological investigation of cardiovascular disease. Section 27* (eds W. B. Kannel and T. Gordon), US Department of Health, Education and Welfare–National Institutes of Health, Washington, DC.

Harris, T., Makuc, D., Kleinman, J., Gillum, R., Curb, J. D., Schatzkin, A., and Feldman, J. V. (1990). Modification of the serum cholesterol–ischaemic heart disease association by physical activity in older men and women. *Circulation*, **81**, 714.

International Collaborative Group (1982). Circulating cholesterol level and risk of death from cancer in men aged 40 to 69 years. *J. Am. Med. Assoc.*, **248**, 2853–9.

Kannel, W. B., Neaton, J. D., Wentworth, D., Thomas, H. E., Stamler, J., Hulley, S. B., *et al.* (1986). Overall and coronary heart disease mortality rates in relation of major risk factors in 325 348 men screened for the MRFIT. *Am. Heart J.*, **112**, 825–36.

Kark, J. D., Smith, A. H., and Hames, E. G. (1980). The relationship of serum cholesterol to the incidence of cancer in Evans County, Georgia. *J. Chron. Dis.,* **33,** 311–32.

Khaw, K.-T. and Barrett-Connor, E. (1984). Systolic blood pressure and cancer mortality in an elderly population. *Am. J. Epidemiol.,* **120,** 550–8.

Keys, A. (ed.) (1980). *Seven Countries. A multivariate analysis of death and coronary heart disease,* Harvard University Press, pp. 1–381.

Keys, A., Aravanis, C., Blackburn, H., Buzina, R., Dontas, A. S., Fidanza, F., *et al.* (1985). Serum cholesterol and cancer mortality in the Seven Countries study. *Am. J. Epidemiol.,* **121,** 870–83.

Kozarevic, D., McGee, D., Vojvodic, N., Gordon, T., Racic, Z., Zukel, W., *et al.* (1981). Serum cholesterol and mortality. The Yugoslavia cardiovascular disease study. *Am. J. Epidemiol.,* **114,** 21–8.

Kromhout, D., Bosschieter, E. B., Brijver, M., and De Lezenne Coulander, C. (1988). Serum cholesterol and 25 year incidence and mortality from myocardial infarction and cancer. *Arch. Intern. Med.,* **148,** 1051–5.

Martin, M. J., Hulley, S. B., Browner, W. S., Kuller, L. M., and Wentworth, D. (1986). Serum cholesterol, blood pressure and mortality: implications from a cohort of 361 662 men. *Lancet,* **ii,** 933–6.

Menotti, A., Conti, S., Giampaoli, S., Mariotti, S., and Signoretti, P. (1980). Coronary risk factors predicting coronary and other causes of death in fifteen years. *Acta Cardiol.,* **35,** 107–20.

Menotti, A., Conti, S., Dima, F., Giampaoli, S., Giuli, B., Rumi, A., *et al.* (1983). Prediction of all causes of death as a function of some factors commonly measured in cardiovascular population surveys. *Prev. Med.,* **12,** 318–25.

Menotti, A., Mariotti, S., Seccareccia, F., and Giampaoli, S. (1987*a*). The 25 year estimated probability of death from some specific causes as a function of twelve risk factors in middle-aged men. *Eur. J. Epidemiol.,* **4,** 60–7.

Menotti, A., Mariotti, S., Seccareccia, F., Torsello, S., and Dima, F. (1987*b*). The determinants of all causes of death in samples of Italian middle-aged men followed-up for 25 years. *J. Epidemiol. Community Health,* **41,** 243–50.

Menotti, A., Keys, A., Aravanis, C., Blackburn, H., Dontas, A., Fidanza, F., *et al.* (1989*a*). Seven Countries Study. First 20-year mortality data in 12 cohorts of six countries. *Ann. Med.,* **21,** 175–9.

Menotti, A., Keys, A., Blackburn, H., Aravanis, C., Dontas, A., Fidanza, F., *et al.* (1989*b*). Twenty-year stroke mortality and prediction in twelve cohorts of the Seven Countries Study. *Int. J. Epidemiol.,* **19,** 309–15.

Menotti, A., Keys, A., Kromhout, D., Nissinen, A., Blackburn, H., Fidanza, F., *et al.* (1991). All causes mortality and its determinants in middle aged men of Finland, The Netherlands and Italy in a 25 years follow-up. *J. Epidemiol. Community Health*, **45,** 125–30.

Nissinen, A., Pekkanen, J., Porath, A., Punsar, S., and Karvonen, M. J. (1989). Risk factors for cardiovascular disease among 55 to 74 year-old Finnish men: a 10 year follow-up. *Ann. Med.,* **21,** 239–40.

Pooling Project Research Group (1978). Relationship of blood pressure, serum cholesterol, smoking habits, relative weight and ECG abnormalities to incidence of major coronary events: final report of the Pooling Project. *J. Chron. Dis.,* **32,** 201–306.

Raynor, W. J., Jr, Shekelle, R. B., Rossof, A. H., Maliza, C., and Paul, O. (1981). High blood pressure and 17 year cancer mortality in the Western Electric health study. *Am. J. Epidemiol.,* **113,** 371–7.

Rose, G. and Shipley, M. J. (1980). Plasma lipids and mortality: a source of error. *Lancet,* **i,** 523–6.

Salonen, J. T. (1982). Risk of cancer and death in relation to serum cholesterol. A longitudinal study in an Eastern Finnish population with high overall cholesterol levels. *Am. J. Epidemiol.,* **116,** 622–30.

Schatzkin, A., Hoover, R. W., Taylor, P. R., Ziegler, R. G., Carter, C. L., Albanes, D., *et al.* (1988). Site-specific analysis of total serum cholesterol and incident cancer in the National Health and Nutrition Examination Survey. I Epidemiologic follow-up survey. *Cancer Res.,* **48,** 452–8.

Sherwin, R. W., Wentworth, D. N., Cutler, J. A., Hulley, S. B., Kuller, L. H., and Stamler, J. (1987). Serum cholesterol levels and cancer mortality in 361 662 men screened for the Multiple Risk Factor Intervention Trial. *J. Am. Med. Assoc.,* **257,** 943–8.

Shurtleff, D. (1974). Some characteristics related to the incidence of cardiovascular disease and death. Framingham Study 18 year follow-up. In *The Framingham Study. An Epidemiological Investigation of Cardiovascular Disease.* Section 30 (eds W. B. Kannel and T. Gordon), US Department of Health Education and Welfare–National Institutes of Health, Washington, DC.

Tornberg, S. A. (1988). Serum cholesterol level and the risk of colorectal cancer. *Biomed. Pharmacotherap.,* **42,** 381–5.

Tornberg, S., Holm, L. E., and Carstensen, J. M. (1988). Breast cancer risk in relation to serum cholesterol, serum beta-lipoprotein, height, weight and blood pressure. *Acta Oncol.,* **27,** 31–7.

US Surgeon General (1979). *Smoking and health. A report of the Surgeon General,* Publ. PHS 79–50066, Department of Health Education and Welfare, Washington, DC.

Williams, R. R., Sorlie, P. D., Feinleib, M., McNamara, P. M., Kannel, W. B., and Dawber, T. R. (1981). Cancer incidence by levels of cholesterol. *J. Am. Med. Assoc.,* **245,** 247–52.

PUBLIC HEALTH

22

Strategies of prevention: the individual and the population

G. Rose

AETIOLOGY: TWO DIFFERENT QUESTIONS

The clinician asks: 'Why did this patient have a heart attack?' The public health doctor asks: 'Why do so many people have heart attacks?' These questions typify the two branches of aetiology: the causes of disease in individuals, and the determinants of its incidence rate in populations. Obviously each is relevant, but each calls for a different kind of research to provide the answers and those answers may not be the same.

Each approach to aetiology involves two further issues: susceptibility and exposure. In individuals, male sex identifies susceptibility, whereas smoking history and diet identify exposure to external causes. Both are called 'risk factors', but the distinction is important. Susceptibility cannot be changed. Its practical relevance is simply to indicate the individual's need for drug treatment or to attend to the modifiable external causes. Some risk factors, such as blood pressure and lipids, represent a complex outcome of both genetically determined susceptibility and modifiable behaviour, but in the main risk differences between individuals are due more to genetic than to modifiable factors (apart from smoking, and perhaps obesity). Thus a high level of blood cholesterol can be reduced by dietary change, but it will probably still fall in the upper part of the range for that population.

Results from migrant studies suggest that the reverse is true of risk differences between populations. Those of Asian extraction, it is true, seem to carry a high cardiovascular risk with them wherever they travel, but this is an exception, and migrants in general tend to acquire the disease rates of their adoptive countries. Incidence differences between countries, which are amazingly large, are due mainly to modifiable external factors rather than to differences in genetic susceptibility. The same must also, of course, apply to the rapid temporal changes in incidence which are occurring within so many countries: they must reflect changes in environment and behaviour.

Aetiologically there is thus a contrast: immutable genetic determinants of susceptibility play a much greater role in the risk differences between individuals within one population than in the incidence differences between populations. Conversely, the latter are much more the outcome of modifiable factors in the environment and behaviour. This creates a prior expectation of a greater potential for prevention at the population level.

PREVENTION: TWO DIFFERENT STRATEGIES

The two levels of aetiology have their counterparts in prevention. The individual or clinical approach seeks to identify and help those in whom an amalgam of genetic susceptibility and unhealthy life-style indicates unusual risk, but the public health approach seeks changes in those features of the population's behaviour or environment which are held responsible for the overall incidence rate. Thus the individual strategy is a rescue operation for individuals in need, whereas the population strategy is a radical attempt to deal with the underlying causes. The former is analogous to sending emergency aid for famine relief in the Third World: it is ethically compelling and it saves lives, but famines will continue to occur until there are changes in their underlying causes, which are economic, social, and agricultural. These radical changes are analogous to the population strategy of prevention.

Sick individuals: the 'high risk strategy'

Medicine's concern is with individuals. The main task of doctors will always be the care of sick patients, and many in fact see this as their only role, but preventive medicine is also essential because illness is unpleasant, care is expensive, and cure may be impossible. Nevertheless, even in preventive medicine doctors are naturally more attracted to a personal approach. High risk individuals are not really patients, but they are managed as though they were. Thus, for example, the care of hypertensives is really preventive medicine, but everyone speaks and thinks of it as treatment. For this to be possible, a label must first have been offered and accepted in order to justify the segregation of the high risk individuals from the 'healthy' population and their subsequent care alongside other patients.

Labelling, like diagnosis, implies a dichotomy. Medicine is heavily committed to dichotomous thinking. We speak of a risk factor as being present or absent. Screening involves recall of a high risk minority and reassurance of the rest. We say that a patient has or has not got coronary heart disease (CHD), even though pathologists tell us that it is all a matter of degree (nearly everyone has some of it). Coronary angiograms are reported as showing, for example, 'two-vessel disease'—as though coronary artery disease were either present or absent. It is nearly 40 years since Pickering produced clear evidence that hypertension is a man-made artefact, the result of an arbitrary split in a continuum. In nature, normality merges imperceptibly into abnormality, and most risk factors and diseases should be defined quantitatively and not qualitatively. He won the battle but he lost the war: medical thinking continues to espouse dichotomy.

The process of screening and high risk labelling thus necessarily involves a falsification. Nevertheless it may be quite appropriate to divide the population in this way if the purpose is to guide a decision on management which is itself necessarily dichotomous—such as giving or not giving some treatment or advice which is either not suitable or not available for everyone. But it should not be forgotten that this classification of the population is simply a matter of administrative convenience.

The large cohort studies have generally failed to identify any critical threshold level for the major risk factors (Martin *et al.* 1986; Rose and Shipley 1986): the lower the levels of blood pressure, cholesterol, and smoking, the lower is the long-term risk. If there are 'ideal' levels, then in Western populations they are rare, and a label of 'high risk' is affixed only to that proportion of the population to whom special help is to be offered. A management statement must not be confused with a prognostic statement. The public may readily misunderstand, and sometimes a screening examination with a 'normal' result can be a positive disincentive to preventive action (Kinlay and Heller 1990). This is not so much an argument against screening as a warning that the delivery of results needs to be accompanied by proper interpretation.

The point is further illustrated by our experience in the Whitehall Study of civil servants (Reid *et al.* 1976). For each participant we calculated a risk score based on smoking, blood pressure, and cholesterol, and the men were then classified into deciles of multivariate risk. Over the next 15 years the age-adjusted mortality from CHD was 10 times greater for men in the top decile relative to those in the lowest (Table 22.1 (previously unpublished)). For stroke, the difference was even larger. Men in the lowest-risk decile also had very favourable rates for cancers, especially of lung and stomach, and for respiratory disease. Their total mortality was about one-sixth of that for men in the top decile of coronary risk, which suggests that current advice on heart disease prevention should have favourable long-term effects on total mortality. It was, of course, to be expected that coronary mortality would be much reduced in the group with the lowest risk scores. The surprise was that, even in this group, CHD is still much the commonest single cause of death. Thus, although we can readily identify what we call a 'high risk' sector of the population, we cannot identify any such thing as a low risk group.

Potential benefits

It makes sense to focus preventive efforts on those who need them most, and so doctors and patients alike are better motivated. Thus, for example,

Table 22.1 15 year mortality (age-adjusted) among men in the Whitehall Study in whom values for smoking status, systolic blood pressure, and plasma cholesterol placed them in the top or bottom decile of multivariate risk

Cause of death	Percentage dead	
	Top decile	Bottom decile
All causes	36 (630)	7 (117)
CHD	17 (295)	2 (29)
Stroke	3 (53)	0.1 (2)
Cancer		
All sites	8 (141)	2 (45)
Lung	3 (57)	0.5 (9)
Stomach	1 (13)	0.2 (3)
Bronchitis/pneumonia	2 (37)	0.3 (6)

the personal and service costs of achieving a change in eating habits are unrelated to the serum cholesterol level, but the potential rewards, which are substantial for high risk individuals, are statistically small (although still real) for the many with values around the average. An even stronger argument applies to the use of drugs, whether to control blood pressure or lipid levels, or to reduce the risk of thrombosis: the adverse effects are largely independent of cardiovascular risk, but it is only in high risk individuals that we can assert with sufficient confidence that the dangers are exceeded by the benefits. Therefore there can be no place for their mass use. Finally, in these days when 'Value for money!' is the cry, it has to be recognized that the cost per unit of benefit escalates rapidly as the clientele is enlarged. All these considerations argue potently for the advantages of focused preventive efforts.

Since it appears that disease is common even among those with low risk scores (see Table 22.1), it becomes important to know how the total case burden is distributed across different levels of risk. The more that cases are concentrated among an identifiable 'high risk' group, the better for a strategy based on screening: only a minority of people then need to take action. Conversely, this approach becomes less attractive if risk is more diffused and a higher proportion of people need to take action.

Widespread awareness of this issue originated with the World Health Organization (WHO) report (WHO 1982), where results of the Framingham Study were used to show that most of the excess cholesterol-associated risk of CHD did not occur among the clinically 'hypercholesterolaemic' minority, but rather among the large numbers of men with values around or a little above the average. This illustrates an important general principle of preventive medicine: *many exposed to a small risk may generate more cases than a small number exposed to a conspicuous risk.* It also explains how a doctor can say: 'Most of my patients do not have risk factors'. It is all too easy to confuse statistical and biological normality. By definition, most people are within the statistical range of normal, but in Western populations most have (biologically speaking) high blood cholesterol levels and high blood pressure.

The efficiency of a screening strategy is further reduced by the error involved in characterizing individuals, particularly when this is based on a single examination. For example, within-subject variability for cholesterol is such that, it has been estimated, 28 per cent of middle-aged men with a single value above 6.9 mmol/l have a true (average) value below that level (Thompson and Pocock 1990). In order to avoid such frequent misclassifications, it is necessary to set the recall level for first screening examination well above the final action level and then to base the final decision on management on the mean of (say) three separate examinations. This is analogous to accepted good practice in blood pressure screening, but the costs and practical problems of implementing it are higher for a laboratory test.

The cardiovascular risks associated with raised blood pressure are rather more concentrated towards the high end of the distribution than those for raised cholesterol level, since the dose–response curve rises more sharply (particularly for stroke). Data from the Framingham Study for men and women aged 35–64 years indicate that nearly half of the excess strokes will occur among the 16 per cent of the population with the highest pressures (diastolic blood pressure, >100 mmHg) (Royal College of Physicians 1989). This implies that, for a given recall and intervention rate, the potential for benefit is greater with screening for blood pressure than for cholesterol. (The actual benefit, of course, will also reflect the relative effectiveness of intervention.)

It has often been said that smoking is the chief preventable cause of heart disease, and the evidence for this view has (rather curiously) excited much less controversy than the case against dietary factors. It has perhaps not been sufficiently realized that the public health importance of a particular cause depends as much on the prevalence of exposure as on the risk to exposed individuals. In many countries smoking is now confined to a shrinking minority, and as its prevalence falls, so does its contribution to the total burden of illness. Advice to smokers is as important as ever it was for them as individuals, but its preventive potential for the community is falling rapidly (though it is still large).

Risk can be predicted better by a multivariate than a univariate score (Table 22.2). In the Whitehall Study 42 per cent of the 15 year coronary deaths occurred among men in the top 20 per cent of multivariate risk.

Table 22.2 Distribution of 15 year coronary and all-cause deaths according to quintile of a risk score based on smoking status, systolic blood pressure, and plasma cholesterol (Whitehall Study)

Quintile of risk	Percentage of deaths	
	CHD	All causes
1	7	10
2	11	13
3	17	17
4	24	24
5	42	36

(Interestingly, almost the same was true for total mortality.) This means that a screening strategy using a single examination of these three factors would require intervention in 20 per cent of this population in order to offer help to 42 per cent of the candidates for a heart attack. Intervention in only 10 per cent would omit 75 per cent of the candidates.

Realizable benefits

Achievement of these potential benefits is limited by factors of effectiveness, feasibility, and cost.

In the WHO European trial (WHO 1986) we estimated that the observed reduction in incidence of CHD was about two-thirds of what would have been expected if the observed changes in risk factors had led to an immediate and commensurate fall in risk. From this and other evidence it seems that a combined change in the major risk factors is likely to be reasonably and fairly rapidly effective.

The more serious problem is with feasibility. At present there is a disturbing lack of evidence on the long-term risk factor changes that can be achieved and sustained under ordinary practice conditions. A smoking cessation rate of 10–20 per cent seems possible, but for cholesterol control the only evidence comes from relatively short follow-up in specialized clinics seeing selected referrals. This evidence is encouraging (Lewis and Rose 1991), but it may not be very relevant to the need to motivate and supervise ordinary people so that they will eat differently from their fellows for the rest of their lives.

Taking these problems together with the difficulties of screening those sections of the population that are most at risk, it seems unlikely that a high risk strategy could in practice achieve even half of its theoretical potential. If we accept the rather optimistic estimate from the European trial of about two-thirds effectiveness (relative to achieved risk factor reduction), taken with the earlier estimate that the 20 per cent high risk segment of the population includes about 40 per cent of future cases, we reach an overall (and probably overoptimistic) estimate of the maximum impact of a high risk preventive strategy in middle-aged men of $\frac{1}{2} \times \frac{2}{3} \times 0.4 = 13$ per cent reduction in total CHD in this group (probably less in older men and in women).

There are no realistic cost estimates for a national programme of screening and multifactorial prevention. Cost-effectiveness analyses of individual components (Lewis and Assmann 1989) suggest that general practitioners' advice against smoking is highly cost effective, and even cholesterol-lowering dietary advice calls for only half the cost of breast cancer screening per quality-adjusted life-year gained. The cost of a properly supported national programme would be high, but in relation to other accepted health service activities (not to mention governmental expenditure in other areas) it ought to be acceptable.

Outline principles for a risk factor screening programme

1. Screening without adequate advice and treatment has been shown to be a waste of time. Inded, it can do positive harm by labelling people who previously thought that they were healthy. We are in danger of forgetting this lesson. There are strong pressures, backed by lipidologists and some pharmaceutical companies, to institute mass screening for serum cholesterol, regardless of whether there are resources to deal adequately with the positive cases. But the first principle is: *no screening without adequate resources for long-term care*.

2. The second principle is that *selective screening and care are far more cost effective than mass screening*. It would cost 100 times as much to prevent one heart attack by cholesterol screening in 40 year old women as in 60 year old men (Khaw and Rose 1989).

3. The third principle is that *screening for a multifactorial disease should be multifactorial*. For cholesterol screening this means that the aim should not be to identify those with the highest cholesterol values, but those with the highest cholesterol-associated risk, for they are the ones who will receive most benefit from intervention. Thus in the population screened by the Multiple Risk Factor Intervention Trial (MRFIT) investigators (Martin *et al.* 1986), the 6 year follow-up found that the excess mortality associated with being in the top tertile of cholesterol was more than five times greater in a smoker whose blood pressure was in the top tertile than in a non-smoker with blood pressure in the lowest tertile. The importance of one risk factor or exposure depends on its context: isolated elevation of one factor may be relatively benign in individuals who are otherwise at low risk. Our aim should be to identify risk, not the individual risk factor. It

makes little sense to define fixed action cut-points for cholesterol or blood pressure.

4. The fourth principle is a consequence of the third: *prevention of multifactorial disease must be multifactorial, not unifactorial.* Doctors treating hypertension are often satisfied if they can normalize the blood pressure. Lipid clinics concentrate on controlling blood lipid levels, and diabetic clinics on blood sugar. Yet in the Medical Research Council hypertension trial (MRC 1985) we found that the difference in the incidence of stroke between smokers and non-smokers was greater than the difference between treated and control patients. Risk factors interact. To control smoking in a hypertensive, or cholesterol in a diabetic, may be as important as to control the presenting problem. Management of multifactorial diseases should be multifactorial, but this is often not the case.

Conclusion

A high risk strategy for heart disease prevention is logical and scientifically well founded, and it is attractive to doctors. Resources for adequate national implementation do not yet exist, and its long-term feasibility is unknown. It is unlikely that in any circumstances it could achieve a reduction of more than around 10–15 per cent in the total incidence of CHD in middle-aged men. However, this does not condemn it, since *an intervention should be judged by what it achieves, not by what it fails to achieve,* but it does imply that we must look elsewhere for a more substantial answer to the problems of mass cardiovascular disease.

Sick populations: the public health approach

Pickering was the first to recognize that sick individuals may represent simply the extreme of a continuum, 'disease' being a quantitative rather than a qualitative phenomenon, but he did not generalize this revolutionary concept beyond blood pressure, nor did he recognize the idea of a sick population. That idea entered cardiovascular medicine with Keys' famous diagram demonstrating a near-complete separation of the Japanese and Finnish distributions of serum cholesterol. This told us that the root of the cholesterol problem lies in a characteristic of the population as a whole. To the extent that cholesterol differences determine incidence differences, this means that both research and prevention must be concerned with populations as a whole, not merely with deviant individuals, and this is the basis of the population or public health strategy of prevention.

We now know that what Keys demonstrated for one risk factor and one pair of populations is also true of many risk factors and population differences (Rose and Day 1990). Figure 22.1 illustrates the phenomenon for body mass index, using data from the INTERSALT study (INTERSALT Cooperative Research Group 1986). This study, which was undertaken for

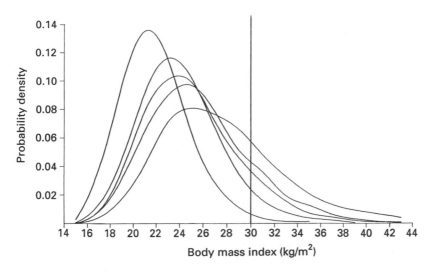

Fig. 22.1 Distributions of body mass index in five aggregated population groups of men and women aged 20–59 years, grouped according to increasing levels of the median.

a different purpose, provided high quality standardized data on some cardiovascular risk factor distributions in 52 populations from 32 countries. For convenience of presentation in the figure, the 52 data sets have been aggregated into five groups, ranked according to their median values.

Several important points emerge, of which the chief is that the distributions shift up or down as a whole. Populations behave coherently: the range of difference between individuals is constrained, so that few move very far from their society's norm. Next, these whole-population shifts are large, with dramatic consequences for the prevalence of 'overweight'. In this particular instance an important part of the differences in prevalence results from variation in skewness, which is more pronounced for body weight than for other risk variables: the latter often show a striking consistency in the coefficient of variation.

Differences between populations in the incidence of cardiovascular disease are largely secondary to these whole-distribution shifts in major risk factors, and these in turn simply reflect mass differences in behaviour (principally eating, smoking, and exercise). Similar whole-distribution shifts probably also occur within populations over time, in company with secular changes in life-style, but unfortunately there are few data sets to test this supposition.

The aim of the population strategy of prevention is to seek means for promoting favourable shifts of these population distributions of risk factors—in other words, to tackle the underlying causes of a high incidence rate. The arguments for the desirability of such an approach are over-

Table 22.3 Reductions in population mean values associated with a halving of the prevalence of high values

Variable (definition of 'high')	Required reduction in mean
Systolic BP ($\geqslant$140 mmHg)	8 mmHg
Diastolic BP ($\geqslant$90 mmHg)	4 mmHg
Overweight (BMI $\geqslant$30 kg/m^2)	2.6 kg/m^2
Sodium intake ($\geqslant$250 mmol/day)	39 mmol/d

BP, blood pressure; BMI, body mass index.

whelming. Unfortunately its realization is impeded by our scanty understanding of the determinants of population change.

Potential benefits

The high risk strategy of prevention offers attractive rewards to individuals, but its probable impact on the total burden of disease is disappointingly small. The reverse is true of the population strategy (Table 22.3). Its potential for total benefit is large because a great many people are involved, each receiving a small reduction in risk, but the expectation of reward to individuals is small. Hence the 'prevention paradox': *a preventive measure which brings much benefit to the population offers little to each individual* (Rose 1981). This paradox applies to most public health measures (e.g. immunization, car seat belts, clean air legislation). It means that, if we are realistic, personal health rewards must be a weak motivator in health education.

Applied to blood pressure, a downwards shift of 2–3 mmHg in the whole distribution, if accompanied by corresponding reductions in risk, might save as many lives as all existing antihypertensive medication (Rose 1981). Applied to serum cholesterol, each 1 per cent fall in the average level would lead (it has been estimated) to a 3 per cent fall in the incidence of CHD. Applied to alcohol intake, a fall of 30 per cent in average consumption might yield similar health benefits to the total elimination of all heavy drinking (Kreitman 1986).

Using data from the Whitehall Study we compared the relative size of predicted benefits from the population and high risk approaches to cholesterol reduction (Rose and Shipley 1990). A 10 per cent reduction in the average level for the whole population (such as has probably already been achieved in some places) would be expected to reduce coronary mortality by more than twice as much as a reduction of 10 per cent in the average for *all* members of the population with values in the top decile (which no one has yet been able to demonstrate as achievable by a screening programme).

Realizable benefits

The effectiveness of population-wide changes in coronary risk factors is amply demonstrated by the dramatic decline in coronary mortality for both men and women in a number of countries. What is not clear from such national experiences is which specific factors are responsible, nor how far they might have occurred in the absence of medical efforts.

The experience of the occupationally based WHO European trial showed that advice aimed at the three major risk factors was effective to the extent that it was accepted (Rose 1987), but that acceptance was often disappointing in a low-cost health education effort and it was not sustained when the effort ceased. Medically led mass health education certainly seemed, after many years of sustained effort, to be effective against smoking, but in general it is ineffective if the timing is not right (the population must be in a receptive frame of mind) and it is probably much less powerful than economic and social forces. In developing countries the latter are exerting a seemingly irresistible adverse effect on coronary risk factors, but in Western countries they may have provided the prime mover behind declining coronary mortality. They have been a major force behind the impressive rise in the ratio of polyunsaturated to saturated fats in some national diets, and this has probably been a major factor in the declining incidence of heart disease. Thus an important decline in national consumption of saturated fats is clearly achievable, but so far a decline in total fat intake is not!

Estimates based on results from the INTERSALT study indicate that small but highly important falls in population levels of blood pressure might be expected to follow moderate changes in salt and alcohol intake and body weight (Stamler et al. 1989; Law et al. 1991). The first of these is now being realized in some countries, but unfortunately no one has yet much success to report in the control at population level of alcoholism or overweight.

Ethics and general principles

Doctors cannot decide how people are to live. As scientific experts we can say that a cholesterol-lowering dietary change will reduce the risk of heart disease, but the decision on whether the benefit justifies the costs is a matter for those whose lives are involved. This is difficult for doctors to accept, for their role in the care of acute illness leads them to expect a decision-taking role.

The concept of a need for mass change is also difficult for the community, for we are accustomed to believing that what most people do must be all right. They can readily accept the need for moderation—avoiding extremism and conforming with the average—but the suggestion that most people are living unhealthily is too threatening to be acceptable. Therefore the first need is for a changed perception of what is normal and socially desirable. The medical rewards for healthier living are remote in time and, for most individuals, small, but given a change in social norms of sensible behaviour the social rewards for a healthier life-style can be immediate and substantial.

The first necessity is a community will to change. For this to find practical expression calls for the support of educators and the mass media (so that people are properly informed about their choices) and of the suppliers of services and facilities for healthier eating and physical exercise (so that new demands can be met). There are different views on the role of government. Most seem to believe it to be legitimate for governments to seek to enforce virtue by heavy taxes on tobacco and alcohol, or even by legislation (car safety belts). This cannot be defended, either ethically or economically. Moreover, it is hypocritical if such governments are at the same time subsidizing and protecting the tobacco industry. The proper role of government in health promotion is (1) to protect the public from unbalanced or misleading information (the food and tobacco industries apply vast sums of money to encouraging people to eat unhealthy foods, to smoke, and to drink more alcohol), (2) to pursue economic policies which at least do not make it harder for people to pursue a healthier life-style (by, for example, subsidizing the production of saturated fats), and (3) to provide services which the public needs and wants in order to implement accepted health recommendations (such as intelligible food labelling and exercise facilities).

SYNTHESIS AND CONCLUSIONS

High risk individuals need help, and this calls for screening and personal care to be provided by the medical services. But whatever it may offer to the individuals concerned, the high risk strategy is no more than an expensive rescue operation, offering disappointingly little towards solving the overall problem. This does not mean that it ought not to be pursued but only that it cannot be the main answer to the problems of a mass disease.

The two approaches (at individual and population levels) are interactive and mutually supportive, rather than rivals. Population-wide changes are essential if the attempts of individuals to change their life-styles are not to turn them into social outcasts: people do not eat or live in isolation. Conversely, health education and advice given to individuals then diffuse outwards among their families, friends, and workmates, thus making the high risk strategy far more potent than if the targeted individuals were the only beneficiaries.

There are also deeper reasons why the two approaches must be seen as two component of a single preventive strategy. High risk individuals are quantitatively but not qualitatively different people: they are simply the tail of a continuous distribution, one part of their parent population. When different populations are compared (Fig. 22.1) it is seen that they behave as coherent entities, with their risk factor distributions shifting up or down as a whole. As a result of this coherence, population mean and the prevalence of deviance are necessarily highly correlated. Thus the prevalence of obesity, hypertension, or high intakes of fat or alcohol closely reflect the *average* weight, blood pressure, and dietary habits of the population as a whole; therefore the problems of deviance cannot be understood except in their societal context, and it is most unlikely that they can ever be successfully managed as isolated phenomena.

This means for research that in order to explain the prevalence of obesity, hypertension, hypercholesterolaemia, and alcoholism we need to understand the determinants of average weight, blood pressure, cholesterol, and drinking, and the dynamics of their changes. It means for preventive policy that it may be difficult or impossible to achieve any large fall in the prevalence of risk factors except as part of population-wide changes.

This population approach to prevention takes us beyond the responsibilities of medicine. The underlying causes for the rise and fall of major diseases, and for their national and regional differences, are related to the circumstances and manner of daily life. It is the responsibility of doctors to communicate their findings and expert opinions to the public and their governments, to exhort and support, and (if possible) to set a good personal example of healthy life-style, but society, not doctors, must decide how it wishes to live and what its priorities are. The prevention of heart disease is basically a matter of social, economic, and political policy.

Recent years have seen an astonishing growth in public concern about heart disease, health, and healthy living. Our task in the medical services is to work with this change. By more effective communication of medical knowledge (and its limitations) to the public, and by accepting that prevention is an integral part of all medical practice, we can hope to see greater improvements in health than could ever be achieved by therapeutic care alone. Treatment, preventive care for individuals, public health, and social policy are interlocking parts of a single strategy for better health.

REFERENCES

INTERSALT Cooperative Research Group (1986). Intersalt study: an international co-operative study on the relation of blood pressure to electrolyte excretion in populations. 1. Design and methods. *J. Hypertension,* **4,** 781–7.

Khaw, K. T. and Rose, G. (1989). Cholesterol screening programmes: how much potential benefit? *Br. Med. J.,* **299,** 606–7.

Kinlay, S. and Heller, R. F. (1990). Effectiveness and hazards of case finding for a high cholesterol concentration. *Br. Med. J.,* **300,** 1545–7.

Kreitman, N. (1986). Alcohol consumption and the preventive paradox. *Br. J. Addiction,* **81,** 353–63.

Law, M. R., Frost, C. D., and Wald, N. J. (1991). Analysis of data from trials of salt reduction. *Br. Med. J.,* **302,** 819–24.

Lewis, B. and Assmann, G. (eds) (1989). *The social and economic contexts of coronary prevention,* Current Medical Literature, London.

Lewis, B. and Rose, G. (1991). Prevention of coronary heart disease—putting theory into practice. *J. R. Coll. Physicians*, **25**, 21–6.

Martin, M. J., Hulley, S. B., Browner, W. S., Kuller, L. H., and Wentworth, D. (1986). Serum cholesterol, blood pressure, and mortality: implications from a cohort of 361 662 men. *Lancet*, **ii**, 933–6.

MRC (Medical Research Council) Working Party on Mild to Moderate Hypertension (1985). MRC trial of treatment of mild hypertension: principal results. *Br. Med. J.*, **291**, 97–104.

Reid, D. D., Hamilton, P. J. S., McCartney, P., Rose, G., Jarrett, R. J., and Keen, H. (1976). Smoking and other risk factors for coronary heart-disease in British civil servants. *Lancet*, **ii**, 979–84.

Rose, G. (1981). The strategy of prevention: lessons from cardiovascular disease. *Br. Med. J.*, **282**, 1847–51.

Rose, G. (1987). European collaborative trial of the multifactorial prevention of coronary heart disease. *Lancet*, **i**, 685.

Rose, G. and Day, S. (1990). The population mean predicts the number of deviant individuals. *Br. Med. J.*, **301**, 1031–4.

Rose, G. and Shipley, M. (1986). Plasma cholesterol concentration and death from coronary heart disease: 10 year results of the Whitehall study. *Br. Med. J.*, **293**, 306–7.

Rose, G. and Shipley, M. (1990). Effects of coronary risk reduction on the pattern of mortality. *Lancet*, **i**, 275–7.

Royal College of Physicians (1989). *Stroke: towards better management*, Royal College of Physicians, London, p. 9.

Stamler, J., Rose, G., Stamler, R., Elliott, P., Dyer, A., and Marmot, M. (1989). INTERSALT study findings—public health and medical care implications. *Hypertension*, **14**, 570–7.

Thompson, S. G. and Pocock, S. J. (1990). The variability of serum cholesterol measurements: implications for screening and monitoring. *J. Clin. Epidemiol.*, **43**, 783–9.

WHO (World Health Organization) (1982). *Prevention of coronary heart disease: report of a WHO Expert Committee*, Tech. Rep. Ser. 678, World Health Organization, Geneva.

WHO (World Health Organization) European Collaborative Group (1986). European collaborative trial of multifactorial prevention of coronary heart disease: final report on the 6-year results. *Lancet*, **i**, 869–72.

23

Intervention in high risk groups: blood pressure

N. R. Poulter and P. S. Sever

INTRODUCTION

Prospective epidemiological data demonstrate that the increased risk of cardiovascular disease due to both systolic and diastolic blood pressure (SBP and DBP) is continuous and graded with no evidence for a J-shaped curve (MacMahon *et al.* 1990) (Fig. 23.1). Quantitatively, it is estimated that, in middle-aged men, 20 mmHg higher SBP is associated with 60 per cent higher cardiovascular mortality and, furthermore, with 40 per cent higher all-cause mortality over a 10 year period (J. Stamler, personal communication 1990). Prior to the introduction of drug therapy for severe

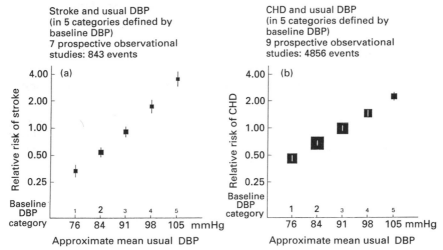

Fig. 23.1 Relative risks of (a) stroke and (b) CHD estimated from combined results. Estimates of the usual DBP values are taken from the mean DBP values 4 years post-baseline in the Framingham Study. The solid squares represent disease risks in each category relative to risk in the whole study population. The sizes of the squares are proportional to the number of events in each DBP category. The vertical lines represent 95 per cent confidence intervals for estimates of relative risk. (Reproduced with permission from MacMahon *et al.* 1990.)

hypertension, associated morbidity and mortality, mainly from stroke, coronary heart disease (CHD), congestive heart failure, and renal failure, were high. For example, data from Mayo Clinic reports of 1939 (Keith *et al.* 1939) show that those who developed papilloedema had 1, 2, and 3 year mortality rates of 80 per cent, 90 per cent, and almost 100 per cent respectively. With the introduction of drug therapy these survival rates were dramatically improved. For example, in one series 50 per cent of treated patients survived for 2 years (Swales *et al.* 1991, Fig. 10.3). The introduction of therapy changed not only the associated mortality rates but also the relative importance of the causes of death, such that congestive cardiac failure and renal disease were virtually eliminated and stroke was no longer the main cause of death (Swales *et al.* 1991, Fig. 10.4).

The results of the Veterans Administration Study (Swales *et al.* 1991, Fig. 10.4) laid to rest any doubts which may have existed about the advantages of treating moderate (DBP = 105–114 mmHg) and severe (DBP $\geqslant$115 mmHg) levels of blood pressure (BP). However, even at these levels of DBP, benefits in terms of CHD reduction were limited. This trial stimulated the Hypertension Detection and Follow-up Program (HDFP) (HDFP 1979) and many more trials which were designed to address the far more difficult and still contentious questions of if, when, and how to treat milder forms of BP elevation (Wolff and Lindeman 1966; Carter 1970; Veterans Administration Cooperative Study Group on Hypertensive Agents 1970; Barraclough *et al.* 1973; Hypertension–Stroke Cooperative Study Group 1974; US Public Health Service Hospitals Cooperative Study Group 1977; Veterans Administration–National Heart, Lung, and Blood Institute Study Group 1977; Australian National Blood Pressure Management Committee 1980; Helgeland 1980; Kuramoto *et al.* 1981; Amery *et al.* 1985; IPPPSH 1985; MRC 1985; Coope and Warrender 1986; Wilhelmsen *et al.* 1987.)

This chapter will attempt to review the results and interpretation of these trials and the implications for determining the policy of hypertension management.

THE INTERVENTION TRIALS

Results

Individually, many of the trials were insufficient in size and hence lacked the power to evaluate benefits in terms of CHD and stroke events due to lowering of BP. Consequently, the results of the trials have been subjected to several meta-analyses (Sacks *et al.* 1985; MacMahon *et al.* 1986; Herbert *et al.* 1988; Collins *et al.* 1990). The trials included in these analyses varied because of the different inclusion criteria and end-points considered. In

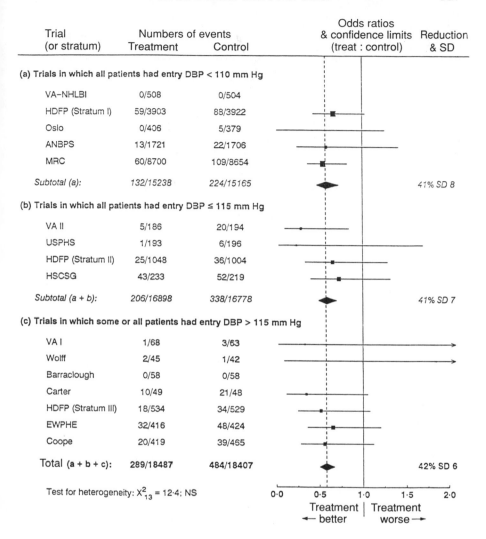

Trial (or stratum)	Numbers of events Treatment	Control	Odds ratios & confidence limits (treat : control)	Reduction & SD
(a) Trials in which all patients had entry DBP < 110 mm Hg				
VA–NHLBI	0/508	0/504		
HDFP (Stratum I)	59/3903	88/3922		
Oslo	0/406	5/379		
ANBPS	13/1721	22/1706		
MRC	60/8700	109/8654		
Subtotal (a):	*132/15238*	*224/15165*		*41% SD 8*
(b) Trials in which all patients had entry DBP ≤ 115 mm Hg				
VA II	5/186	20/194		
USPHS	1/193	6/196		
HDFP (Stratum II)	25/1048	36/1004		
HSCSG	43/233	52/219		
Subtotal (a + b):	*206/16898*	*338/16778*		*41% SD 7*
(c) Trials in which some or all patients had entry DBP > 115 mm Hg				
VA I	1/68	3/63		
Wolff	2/45	1/42		
Barraclough	0/58	0/58		
Carter	10/49	21/48		
HDFP (Stratum III)	18/534	34/529		
EWPHE	32/416	48/424		
Coope	20/419	39/465		
Total (a + b + c):	**289/18487**	**484/18407**		**42% SD 6**

Test for heterogeneity: $X^2_{13} = 12.4$; NS

0·0   0·5   1·0   1·5   2·0

Treatment | Treatment
← better | worse →

Fig. 23.2 Stroke in antihypertensive trials. (Reproduced with permission from Collins *et al.* 1990.)

the most recent of these analyses (Collins *et al.* 1990) results have been compared with data from a similar meta-analysis of prospective observational studies (MacMahon *et al.* 1990) in terms of benefits expected versus those realized for stroke and CHD events (Figs 23.2 and 23.3). This comparison is consistent with previous meta-analyses in that expected benefits of around 40 per cent in stroke reduction were realized, whilst the trial data for CHD are not consistent with previous analyses in that a significant

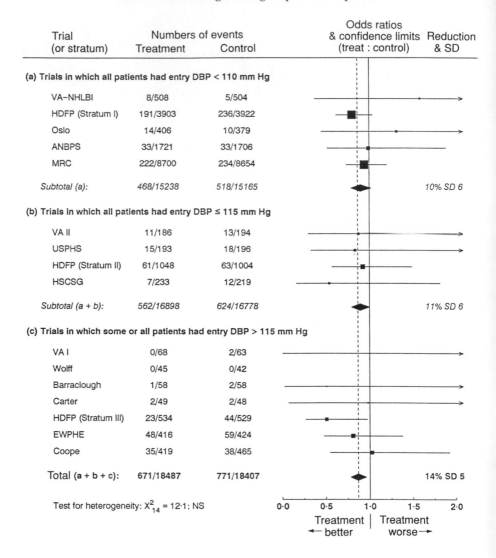

Fig. 23.3 CHD in antihypertensive trials. (Reproduced with permission from Collins *et al.* 1990.)

reduction in CHD events was now demonstrated. However, in keeping with individual trial results and previous meta-analyses, the estimated reduction in CHD events of 14 per cent is less than the 20–5 per cent predicted by the observational data. Given the ratio of CHD to stroke events attributable to elevated BP (3–4:1), this shortfall may have implications for the treatment of hypertension as practised in the trials.

Shortfall in CHD benefits?

Several arguments have been proposed to explain the shortfall in CHD benefit. The disappointing effect on CHD repeatedly shown in the individual studies suggests that the results are unlikely to be due to chance. The extensive and coherent data arising from a variety of other sources suggest that the association between elevated arterial pressure and CHD is causal. It seems unlikely that the development of CHD induced by hypertension is an irreversible effect, although it is feasible that, within the time-scale of the trials (3 years on average), this might in part explain the results. Perhaps a more likely explanation is the effect of the well-established adverse metabolic effects of the drugs used in the trials, particularly on lipids, which may counterbalance the benefits of lowering BP.

The drugs most frequently used in the trials were diuretics, with beta-blockers being the next most commonly used. Diuretics, particularly at the high dosages used in the trials, are known to have an adverse affect on low density lipoprotein cholestrol (LDL-cholesterol), triglycerides, uric acid, potassium, glucose, and insulin resistance. Since all these variables, either directly or indirectly, have an adverse effect upon CHD risk, there are strong theoretical reasons for explaining why the drugs do not produce the benefits expected from lowering BP. Beta-blockers have also been shown to impair efforts to lose weight and adversely effect high density lipoprotein cholesterol (HDL-cholesterol), triglycerides, glucose metabolism, and insulin resistance. Hence they might also be expected to be less than ideal for the primary prevention of CHD events in hypertensives. It has been argued that the small changes in serum cholesterol induced by the diuretics are biologically insignificant. However, a review of studies of diuretic-induced changes in cholesterol does not support this argument (Weidman *et al.* 1985). Because of decreasing compliance over time and the use of intention to treat analyses, the intervention trials are not the best way to evaluate the absolute size of the adverse metabolic effects induced by the agents used—such information is better acquired via carefully controlled metabolic studies. However, if we are to explain the shortfall of CHD benefits observed in the trials, the in-trial metabolic effects should be considered. Analyses of data from the Medical Research Council (MRC) trial show that, after 3 years, diuretics induced approximately a 2 per cent increase in plasma cholesterol compared with placebo (Greenberg *et al.* 1984). This must be considered in the light of the unpublished meta-analyses of the lipid-lowering trials which (in support of conclusions drawn after the Lipid Research Clinics Coronary Primary Prevention Trial (LRCCPPT) (Lipid Research Clinics Program 1984) suggest that a 1 per cent increase in serum cholesterol is associated with a 2–3 per cent increase in CHD risk. Hence total cholesterol changes alone may account for 5 per cent of the reported shortfall discussed above. If we add to this the possible impact of significant adverse effects on other risk factors, as demonstrated in the MRC trial (Greenberg *et al*. 1984) (impaired glucose tolerance, reduced serum potassium, elevated uric acid), a plausible explanation for the trial results is apparent. It is of interest that results obtained in the European Working Party on High Blood Pressure on the Elderly (EWPHE) trial (Amery *et al*. 1985) differed from the others, in that coronary mortality was significantly reduced by active treatment although total morbid and fatal CHD events were not. Explanations for this different result include chance, the older age of the patients studied, and the type of diuretics used—a potassium-sparing component (triamterene) was included. Evidence that the last explanation may apply arises from one recent study which has demonstrated the importance of low levels of serum potassium in causing ventricular fibrillation in the first 48 hours post-myocardial infarction (Nordrehaug and von der Lippe 1983).

Presumably it is data such as these which have recently persuaded the pharmaceutical industry to remove two standard thiazide diuretics from the market and to replace them with diuretics which include a potassium-sparing component.

From trials to policy?

The reports of the trials, viewed individually or collectively, have resulted in very disparate interpretations. Some have ignored the failure of traditional therapy to protect patients against CHD and continue to recommend diuretics and beta-blockers as first-line agents in the management of hypertension (Swales 1990; Ramsey and Yeo 1991). For example, in 1989 a working party of the British Hypertension Society (BHS) reviewed the trials and on the basis of that review published the following recommendations (BHS Working Party 1989).

1. Treat patients under 80 years with diastolic pressures over 100 mmHg for 3–4 months.

2. Observe patients with pressures of 95–99 mmHg every 3–6 months.

3. Use either diuretics or beta-blockers as first-line treatment.

4. Use other agents if these are contra-indicated, ineffective, or poorly tolerated.

5. Warn all patients against smoking and heavy alcohol intake.

6. Advise weight reduction in obese patients.

Interestingly, and at odds with other major consensus reports on hypertension management, advice to avoid excess salt intake was not included in this report. Whilst the role of salt as a major aetiological agent in the development of elevated arterial pressure remains controversial, studies have generally demonstrated an additive effect on BP lowering of sodium restriction and drug therapy (Beard *et al*. 1982; Dodson *et al*. 1985; Weinberger *et al*. 1988) (with the possible exception of calcium antagonists (Luft and Weinberger 1988)). This omission therefore seems inappropriate.

The remit of the BHS working party was to make recommendations based on trial data. This inevitably means that because the trials have included few patients over 80 years of age and have used DBP levels as entry criteria, no recommendations could be made for those over 80 or in relation to levels of SBP. As discussed elsewhere in this book (Chapter 7), SBP appears to be a better predictor of cardiovascular disease, which serves to highlight the possible shortcomings of being restricted to trial data when making treatment policy decisions. A further example of the limitations of trial data arise from considering the second BHS recommendation in the context of data from the Multiple Risk Factor Intervention Trial (MRFIT) (Stamler *et al*. 1989) where it was estimated that there were 678 coronary deaths attributed to DBP above 85 mmHg. From these data, observing those with DBPs in the range 95–99 mmHg, and presumably ignoring those in the range 90–94 mmHg, implies observing almost a quarter (152 of 678) and ignoring a further quarter (154 of 678) of the CHD deaths attributable to BP.

Whilst a minority would advocate drug therapy for the large numbers in this BP range (90–99), surely non-pharmacological intervention could have been recommended?

What level to treat?

It has been argued (Beaglehole *et al*. 1988; Kawachi and Purdie 1989) that the costs and side-effects of treating mild hypertension outweigh the advantages of treatment, and consequently that treatment should be deferred until DBP levels reach 105 or even 110 mmHg. Such arguments are often based on a statement in the MRC trial report (MRC 1985) that 850 patients must be treated for 1 year in order to prevent a single stroke. This estimate may grossly underestimate benefits of treatment to ordinary hypertensives, as reviewed by Simpson (1990), for the following reasons. First, the ranges of BP entry criteria in the MRC and Australian trials were 90–109 mmHg and 95–109 mmHg with mean entry levels of 98 and 100.4 mmHg respectively (Australian National Blood Pressure Management Committee 1980; 1985). However, 'actual' mean BPs (those recorded a few weeks post-randomization and on placebo) were 91 and 93 mmHg. Presumably the benefits observed in the trials relate to these lower 'actual' BP levels, and hence underestimate benefits which would accrue from lowering BPs which are genuinely as high as 98 and 100.4 mmHg. Second, the controls' mortality rates in the MRC and Australian trials were low, in part because of the study exclusion criteria and the healthy volunteer effect, and because most of the volunteers were middle-class patients who generally enjoy better cardiovascular health. Third, the intention to treat analyses makes no allowance for the effects of controls receiving active antihypertensive medication. This inevitably leads to an underestimation of benefits. Furthermore, because treatment is more likely to be initiated in those controls with highest BPs (and hence at greatest risk) and those who stop active treatment are likely to be at least risk by virtue of lower BP levels, 'on-treatment' analyses do not solve all these problems. Fourth, because inflexible drug regimens often using high dosages are inevitably followed in trials, side-effects are likely to be more prevalent and severe (with implications for compliance) than in everyday clinical practice.

In addition to these arguments, the implications of the fact that even 'mild' levels of hypertension, if left untreated, cause target organ damage must be considered. This has become clear from both prospective observational data and intervention trials. For example, over 14 per cent of mild hypertensives included at entry in Stratum I of the HDFP trial had target organ damage (HDFP 1982), and similarly the US Public Health Service Hospitals Trial (US Public Health Service Hospitals Cooperative Study Group 1977) demonstrated a 45 per cent incidence of target end-organ damage in the placebo-treated group during a 7–10 year follow-up period compared with 29 per cent in the actively treated group. Whilst intervention trial data demonstrate that the percentage benefit to those with target organ damage is greater than for those without, the HDFP follow-up data clearly underline the importance of pre-empting these problems with early intervention (HDFP 1982). Finally, trial data have shown that, if left untreated, a significant number of 'mild' hypertensives become 'moderate' hypertensives in a relatively short time (Moser 1986), demonstrating the clear benefit of treatment in preventing the progression of hypertension and by implication the increased morbidity and mortality associated with higher BP levels.

These data were not incorporated into the often quoted evaluation of benefits estimated from the MRC trial, and hence our best estimate must be that the simple ratio of 1 stroke saved for 850 treated seriously underestimates the overall benefits likely to accrue from the treatment of genuinely mild hypertension. In keeping with Simpson's (1990) suggestions, the MRC report would have been more accurate if it had stated: In this trial, which dealt with mainly middle-class people aged 35 to 64 (who are known to be in better cardiovascular health than most hypertensives) whose average DBP was 91 mmHg and in which treatment was given to those controls at most risk, 850 people had to be treated for 1 year to make a difference of one stroke between the 'treated' group and the theoretically untreated 'control' group.

How to treat?

Some major consensus reports have concluded that the benefits of treating mild hypertension in terms of reduced stroke events vindicate intervention at lower BP levels (National High Blood Pressure Education Program 1988). However, conscious of the shortfall in CHD benefits observed and that CHD prevention should be the primary aim of treatment, others have suggested that the results indicate that we should modify how we treat hypertension if we are to improve our record in this critical area (Hansson *et al.* 1989).

In essence the changes proposed tend towards a multiple risk factor approach to management—as typified by the summary of the management policy of the Hypertension Clinic, St Mary's Hospital, London (Table 23.1). It has been argued that this broader approach to hypertension management lacks the necessary supportive evidence from trials that such an approach is effective and hence worthwhile, and therefore should not yet be universally recommended. However, we believe that a review of currently available data vindicates this approach. Some of these data from BP-lowering trials merit a brief mention.

MULTIPLE RISK FACTOR MANAGEMENT: A JUSTIFICATION

Non-pharmacological intervention

From the guidelines outlined in Table 23.1, it is clear that we believe that non-pharmacological intervention should invariably be an integral part of the management of all hypertensives—either alone or in combination with drug therapy. The BP-lowering benefits for hypertensives of salt restriction, alcohol, and weight loss have been demonstrated by MacGregor *et al.* (1982), Potter and Beevers (1984), and Gillum *et al.* (1983) respectively. The effects of these three variables have been thoroughly reviewed elsewhere (Houston 1986; Saunders 1987; Staessen *et al.* 1985), and many of

Table 23.1

---

1. Confirm that the BP really is elevated—readings should be taken after a reasonable rest period (10 min) and, depending upon the level, at least two and preferably many more sets of readings should be recorded over a period of days or weeks before a decision to treat with drugs can be considered

2. Assess risk factors for hypertension:
   Increased body weight
   Excess alcohol intake
   Salt intake
      Is salt added to food?
      Are salty foods ingested?
      Is salt added to cooking?
   Family history

Table 23.1 (*contd.*)

---

3. Assess other CHD risk factors
   Lipid profile
       Is serum cholesterol >5.2 mmol/l?
       Is HDL-cholesterol <0.9 mmol/l?
       (NB high HDL raises the threshold for action on total cholesterol)
       Is serum triglyceride >1.7 mmol/l?
   Smoking
   Diabetes and glucose intolerance
   Exercise output
   Left-ventricular hypertrophy
   Oral contraceptive use

4. Explain why BP and other risk factors need 'treatment'

5. Advise the non-pharmacological approach to lowering BP by:
   Reducing body weight if overweight (decrease calories, increase exercise)
   Reducing alcohol intake if excessive (i.e. >2 units/day)
   Reducing salt intake (not adding salt to food, avoiding salty food, reducing salt added to cooking)
   Increasing intake of potassium-rich foods, e.g. figs, bananas, etc.
   Involving the spouse and/or other close family in the above measures

6. Advise on non-pharmacological approach to other CHD risk factors:
   Serum total cholesterol (reduce saturated fat intake, reduce cholesterol intake)
   HDL-cholesterol (stop smoking, increase exercise, lose weight)
   Smoking (STOP)
   Diabetes and glucose intolerance (lose weight, other standard dietary advice)
   Exercise output, e.g. walking, swimming, etc. (increase gradually)
   Canadian Airforce exercises are easy to do for patients of *all* ages
   Oral contraception (avoid if possible)
   Involve the spouse and/or close family in the above measures.

7. If BP remains elevated, initiate drug therapy and continue non-pharmacological approach to BP and other risk factors; avoid, where possible, drugs with adverse metabolic effects especially on lipid profiles (if serum total cholesterol is >5.2 mmol/l and/or HDL <0.9 mmol/l)

8. Reassess BP levels and other risk factor status frequently at first, and feed back information to the patients as to where progress has and has not been made; adjust treatment as necessary

9. In young (<45 years), severe, or refractory hypertensives, investigation for 'secondary hypertension' is recommended

10. If after several months of combined drug and non-drug 'treatment', BP levels fall to 'low' levels (e.g. DBP <75 and/or SBP <120), a gradual reduction of drug treatment could be attempted

---

these data are summarized in Chapter 29 of this volume. Furthermore, the potentially large benefits of the combined effect of these three variables in greatly reducing the need for pharmacological intervention in mild hypertensives has been demonstrated in the Hypertension Control Program (Stamler *et al.* 1987).

The benefits for cardiovascular health of stopping smoking and improving serum lipid profiles are well established and need no justification here. However, the frequency of these and other cardiovascular risk factors found in hypertensives—clustering—as shown in Table 23.2 and the interaction amongst the three major CHD risk factors as observed in prospective observational data suggest that a combined impact on these risk factors is a logical approach. Once again, it is argued that trial evidence to support such recommendations is lacking, but several large trials do lend support to the epidemiological data. The Gothenburg Study (Wilhelmsen *et al.* 1986) was considered to be 'negative' in that the incidence of CHD, stroke, and total mortality over 10 years was not significantly lower in the intervention group (who received advice on stopping smoking, dietary advice to improve blood lipid profiles, and antihypertensive medication) compared with controls. However, large reductions in levels of all three of these risk factors was achieved not only in the intervention group but also in the control group. Furthermore, it appeared from within this study that 'If serum cholesterol levels remained unchanged or even increased, the effect of BP reduction was small, whereas a substantial reduction in both risk factors produced a substantial reduction in CVD and CHD morbidity'.

The WHO European Factory Study (WHO 1986), which evaluated the effects of a prevention programme in 40 factories in four countries compared with 40 matched 'control' factories, has also been described as a negative trial (McCormick and Skrabanek 1988), but this appears to be at odds with the data. Intervention consisted of dietary advice to lower blood cholesterol levels and lose weight, advice on stopping smoking and increasing

Table 23.2 CHD risk factors

Elevated total serum cholesterol (>5.2 mmol/l)	85%[a]
Smoking	35%[b]
Low HDL-cholesterol (<0.9 mmol/l)	15%[a]
Low exercise output	>75%[a]
Glucose intolerance including diabetes	13%[c]
Synthetic oestrogens	2%[c]
Left-ventricular hypertrophy	50%[c]

Estimates of the prevalence of CHD risk factors in hypertensive subjects. Most hypertensives have at least two other risk factors.
[a] UK general practice (Poulter, personal communication).
[b] Hypertension trial (MRFIT Research Group 1982).
[c] Population survey data.

exercise, and advice or referral for treatment of hypertension. Uptake was very variable in the different countries, but nevertheless there was an overall reduction of 10.2 per cent in total CHD, 6.9 per cent in fatal CHD, and 5.3 per cent in total deaths—the trial's three predefined end-points. Importantly, this report (WHO 1986) and a subsequent reanalysis (Rose 1987) confirm that the relation between compliance and outcome for all three of these end-points was statistically significant.

More recently the 10.5 year mortality rates of the participants in the MRFIT have been published (MRFIT 1990). At 6.9 years of follow-up (the end of the trial) no significant effect on CHD mortality compared with controls had been demonstrated in the 'special intervention' group who had various combinations of elevated BP, blood cholesterol, and smoking, and who received advice to stop smoking and lower cholesterol and stepped care for BP control (MRFIT 1982). However, at 10.5 years significant reductions in CHD mortality (10.6 per cent) and all-cause mortality (7.7 per cent) were observed. Of special interest for hypertension management was the subgroup analysis of those in the 'special intervention' group with resting baseline electrocardiogram (ECG) abnormalities in whom there was higher CHD and all-cause mortality at both 6.9 and 10.5 years. This analysis may have important implications for the type of drugs used in this study (chlorthalidone and hydrochlorothiazide) as they may well be implicated in causing these adverse effects.

Pharmacological intervention

When BP cannot be adequately controlled by non-pharmacological methods, drug treatment becomes necessary. During the 1980s the stepped care policy was widely advocated with diuretics and beta-blockers as first- and/or second-line drugs, to which vasodilators such as hydralazine were added in refractory cases.

On the basis of the arguments presented earlier in this chapter, and an increasing awareness of the impact of additional CHD risk factors which tend to cluster in hypertensives (Poulter *et al.* 1989), we believe that drug selection should be incorporated as part of a multiple risk factor approach to management. For the reasons outlined above, this often means a departure from traditional therapy with diuretics and beta-blockers, and their cautious replacement by the 'newer' classes of agents such as α_1-blockers, ACE inhibitors, and calcium channel blockers. The ideal requirements of an antihypertensive are that it be effective at lowering BP, well tolerated, cheap, and compatible with a multiple risk factor approach on the basis that it is more likely to prevent all aspects of hypertension-induced cardiovascular morbidity and mortality, including CHD. The Total Treatment of Mild Hypertension Study (TOMHS) (Grimm *et al.* 1989)—the only study to compare diuretic, beta-blocker, α_1-blocker, ACE inhibitor, and calcium

Table 23.3 Impact of five classes of antihypertensive drugs on alterable cardiovascular risk factors

	Diuretic	Beta-blocker	Calcium blocker	ACE inhibitor	α-blocker
Blood pressure	+	+	+	+	+
Cholesterol	−	+/−	0	0	+
HDL-cholesterol	0	−	0	0	+
Triglycerides	−	−	0	0	+
Glucose intolerance	−	−	0	+	+
Hyperinsulinemia	−	−	0	+	+
Physical activity	0	−	0	0	0
Left-ventricular hypertrophy	0	+/0	+	+	+

+ Beneficial.
− Adverse.
0 Neutral.

antagonist with placebo—demonstrates that at equivalent dosages there is little to choose amongst the drug groups in terms of BP-lowering efficacy and tolerability. The relative 'cost' of the drugs is a very complex issue, and as shown by a recent cost–benefit analysis (Grimm 1989), rather than a simple drug cost comparison, diuretics and beta-blockers are not necessarily the cheapest drugs. Table 23.3 demonstrates the profiles of the various drug groups in relation to their effects on several cardiovascular risk factors. It is apparent that, from this viewpoint, the newer agents are more logical choices than diuretics and beta-blockers.

To counter these arguments, a commonly held view recently reported by Hampton (1987) states that 'Clinical practice must be based on the results of clinical trials not on theories derived from epidemiological observations'. Whilst this is in part reasonable, we must realize that no long-term morbidity and mortality trial of the newer agents is either in progress or planned. Furthermore, if such a study were to start tomorrow the results would not be available until well into the next century! Surely this does not commit us to persevere slavishly with diuretics and beta-blockers for at least the next 10 years.

In the absence of appropriate trial data it seems reasonable to make a best estimate of which drugs are most likely to achieve optimal CHD and stroke benefits. In the meantime, it is very important that a further trial to evaluate the long-term effects on morbidity and mortality of the newer and 'standard' agents be carried out. The great difficulties and prohibitive costs of such an exercise should not detract from the urgent need for this study, which is critical to the progress of hypertension management.

In support of expanding the choice of first-line agents, three major review bodies (National High Blood Pressure Education Program 1988; Hansson *et al.* 1989; WHO/ISH 1989) have recommended the use of the newer agents as reasonable and often preferable alternatives to diuretics and beta-blockers. We would agree with Kant, who said 'It is often necessary to make a decision on the basis of knowledge sufficient for action but insufficient to satisfy the intellect'.

CONCLUSIONS

1. Caution should be exercised in the extrapolation to the general hypertensive population of data derived from trials, in which patients are often atypical and only specific drugs at fixed dosages are used.

2. Despite a shortfall in expected CHD reduction, the intervention trials demonstrate that DBP levels of 100 mmHg and above merit treatment with antihypertensive medication. However, non-pharmacological advice to reduce body weight, alcohol intake, and salt ingestion should always be the first line in treatment and, when drugs are necessary, used as an adjunct to therapy.

3. Several trials (Australian National Blood Pressure Management Committee 1980; IPPPSH 1985; MRC 1985) demonstrate that the better the BP control achieved, the greater is the reduction in absolute risk to the patients. Furthermore, since DBP was only reduced by 5–6 mmHg compared with placebo in the trials, greater benefits than those reported may reasonably be expected in clinical practice.

4. Given knowledge of prospective observational data, it may be appropriate to set the threshold for initiating drug therapy at DBP = 95 mmHg, and to pay increased attention to levels of SBP.

5. A long-term morbidity and mortality trial, comparing the new and 'standard' agents, is urgently required. Meanwhile, the judicious introduction of the newer agents as first-line therapy seems justified on the basis of currently available evidence.

REFERENCES

Amery, A., Birkenhäger, W., Brixko, P., Bulpitt, C., Clement, D., and Deruyttere, M. (1985). Mortality and morbidity results from the European Working Party on High Blood Pressure in the Elderly trial. *Lancet,* (i), 1349–54.

Australian National Blood Pressure Management Committee (1980). The Australian therapeutic trial in mild hypertension. *Lancet,* i, 1261–7.

Barraclough, M., Bainton, D., Cochrane, A. L., Joy, M. D., MacGregor, G. A., and Foley, T. H. (1973). Control of moderately raised blood pressure: report of a co-operative randomised controlled trial. *Br. Med. J.,* 3, 434–6.

Beaglehole, R., Bonita, R., Jackson, R., and Stewart, A. (1988). Prevention and control of hypertension in New Zealand: a reappraisal. *NZ Med. J.,* **101,** 480–3.

Beard, T. C., Cooke, H. M., Gray, W. R., and Barge, R. (1982). Randomised controlled trial of a no added sodium diet for mild hypertension. *Lancet,* **ii,** 455–8.

BHS (British Hypertension Society) Working Party (1989). Treating mild hypertension: agreement from the large trials. *Br. Med. J.,* **298,** 694–8.

Carter, A. B. (1970). Hypotensive therapy in stroke survivors. *Lancet,* **i,** 485–9.

Collins, R.. Peto, R., MacMahon, S., Hebert, P., Fiebach, N. H., Eberlein, K. A., *et al.* (1990). Blood pressure, stroke, and coronary heart disease. Part 2, Short-term reductions in blood pressure: overview of randomised drug trials in their epidemiological context. *Lancet,* **335,** 827–38.

Coope, J. and Warrender, T. S. (1986). Randomised trial of treatment of hypertension in the elderly in primary care. *Br. Med. J.,* **293,** 1145–51.

Dodson, P. M., Pacy, P. J., and Cox, E. V. (1985). Long-term follow-up of the treatment of essential hypertension with a high-fibre, low-fat and low-sodium dietary regimen. *Hum. Nutr. Clin. Nutr.,* **39C,** 213–20.

Gillum, R. F., Prineas, R. J., Jeffrey, R. W., Jacobs, D. R., Elmer, P. J., and Gomez, O. (1983). Non-pharmacologic therapy of hypertension: the independent effects of weight reduction and sodium restriction in overweight borderline hypertensive patients. *Am. Heart J.,* **105**(1), 128–33.

Greenberg, G., Brennan, P. J., and Miall, W. E. (1984). Effects of diuretic and beta-blocker therapy in the Medical Research Council Trial. *Am. J. Med.,* **76**(2A), 45–51.

Grimm, R. H. (1989). Epidemiological and cost implications of antihypertensive treatment for the prevention of cardiovascular disease. *J. Hum. Hypertension,* **3** (Suppl. 2), 55–61.

Grimm, R. H., Neaton, J. D., Stamler, J., Prineas, R. H., and Cutler, J. A. (1989). The treament of 'mild' hypertension study (TOMHS): results at 1 year. Abstract 328, *2nd Int. Conf. on Preventive Cardiology and 29th Annu. Meeting of the AHA Council on Epidemiology. Washington, DC, 18–22 June 1989.*

Hampton, J. R. (1987). Mild hypertension: to treat or not to treat? *Nephron,* **47** (Suppl. 1), 57–61.

Hansson, L., Mancia, G., and Reid, J. L. (1989). *Current problems in clinical hypertension: What pressure? What patient? What treatment?* Oxford Clinical Communications, Oxford.

Helgeland, A. (1980). Treatment of mild hypertension: a five-year controlled drug trial. The Oslo Study. *Am. J. Med.,* **69,** 725–32.

HDFP (Hypertension Detection and Follow-up Program) Cooperative Group (1979). Five-year findings of the Hypertension Detection and Follow-up Program. I. Reduction in mortality in persons with high blood pressure, including mild hypertension. *J. Am. Med. Assoc.,* **242,** 2562–71.

HDFP (Hypertension Detection and Follow-up Program) Cooperative Group (1982). The effect of treatment on mortality in 'mild' hypertension. *New Engl. J. Med.,* **307,** 976–80.

Herbert, P. R., Fiebach, N. H., Eberlein, K. A., Taylor, J. O., and Hennekens, C. H. (1988). The community-based randomized trials of pharmacologic treatment of mild-to-moderate hypertension. *Am. J. Epidemiol.,* **127,** 581–90.

Houston, M.C. (1986). Sodium and hypertension: a review. *Arch. Intern. Med.*, **146,** 179–85.

Hypertension-Stroke Cooperative Study Group. Effect of antihypertensive treatment on stroke recurrence. *J. Am. Med. Assoc.*, **229,** 409–18.

IPPPSH (International Prospective Primary Prevention Study in Hypertension) Collaborative Group (1985). Cardiovascular risk and risk factors in a randomised trial of treatment based on the beta-blocker oxprenolol. *J. Hypertension*, **3,** 379–92.

Kawachi, I. and Purdie, G. (1989). The benefits and risks of treating mild to moderate hypertension. *NZ Med. J.,* **102,** 377–9.

Keith, N. M., Wagener, H. P., and Barker, N. W. (1939). Some different types of essential hypertension: their course and prognosis. *Am. J. Med. Sci.,* **197,** 332–43.

Kuramoto, K., Matsushita, S., Kuwajima, I., and Murakami, M. (1981). Prospective study on the treatment of mild hypertension in the aged. *Jpn. Heart J.,* **22,** 75–85.

Lipid Research Clinics Program (1984). The lipid research clinics coronary primary prevention trial. II. The relationship of reduction in incidence of coronary heart disease to cholesterol lowering. *J. Am. Med. Assoc.,* **251,** 365–74.

Luft, F. C. and Weinberger, M. H. (1988). Review of salt restriction and the response to antihypertensive drugs. Satellite symposium on calcium antagonists. *Hypertension,* **11,** 1229–32.

MacGregor, G. A., Best, F. E., and Cam, J. M. (1982). Double-blind randomized cross-over trial of moderate sodium restriction in essential hypertension. *Lancet,* **i,** 351–4.

MacMahon, S. W., Cutler, J. A., Furberg, C. D., and Payne, G. H. (1986). The effects of drug treatment for hypertension on morbidity and mortality from cardiovascular disease: a review of randomized controlled trials. *Prog. Cardiovasc. Dis.,* **24** (Suppl. 1), 99–118.

MacMahon, S., Peto, R., Cutler, J., Collins, R., Sorlie, P., Neaton, J., *et al.* (1990). Blood Pressure, stroke, and coronary heart disease: Part I, Prolonged differences in blood pressure: prospective observational studies corrected for the regression dilution bias. *Lancet,* **335,** 765–74.

McCormick, J. and Skrabanek, P. (1988). Coronary heart disease is not preventable by population interventions. *Lancet,* **2**(8615), 839–41.

Moser, M. (1986). Historical perspective on the management of hypertension. *Am. J. Med.,* **80** (Suppl. 5B), 1–11.

MRC (Medical Research Council) Working Party (1985). MRC trial of treatment of mild hypertension: principal results. *Br. Med. J.,* **291,** 97–104.

MRFIT (Multiple Risk Factor Intervention Trial) Research Group (1982). Multiple Risk Factor Intervention Trial: risk factor changes and mortality results. *J. Am. Med. Assoc.,* **248,** 1465–77.

MRFIT (Multiple Risk Factor Intervention Trial) Research Group (1990). Mortality rates after 10.5 years for participants in the Multiple Risk Factor Intervention Trial: findings related to a priori hypotheses of the trial. *J. Am. Med. Assoc.,* **263**(13), 1795–801.

National High Blood Pressure Education Program, National Heart, Lung and Blood Institute (1988). *Report of the Joint National Committee on detection, evaluation, and treatment of high blood pressure,* NIH Rep. 88–1088, National Institutes of Health, Bethesda, MD, pp. 1–53.

Nordrehaug, J. E. and von der Lippe, G. (1983). Hypokalaemia and ventricular fibrillation in acute myocardial infarction. *Br. Heart J.,* **50,** 525–9.

Potter, J. F. and Beevers, D. G. (1984). Pressor effect of alcohol in hypertension. *Lancet,* **i,** 119–22.

Poulter, N. R., Thom, S., and Sever, P. S. (1989). Hypertension—problem solving for the 1990's. *Mod. Med. (Postgrad. Partwork Series),* November, 1–12.

Ramsey, L. E. and Yeo, W. W. (1991). First line treatment in hypertension. *Br. Med. J.,* **302,** 352–3.

Rose, G. (1987). European collaborative trial of multifactorial prevention of coronary heart disease. *Lancet,* **i,** 685.

Sacks, H. S., Chalmers, T. C., Berk, A. A., and Reitman, D. (1985). Should mild hypertension be treated? An attempted meta-analysis of the clinical trials. *Mount Sinai J. Med.,* **52,** 265–70.

Saunders, J. B. (1987). Alcohol: an important cause of hypertension. *Br. Med. J.,* **294,** 1045–6.

Simpson, F. O. (1990). Fallacies in the interpretation of the large-scale trials of treatment of mild to moderate hypertension. *J. Cardiovasc. Pharmacol.,* **16** (Suppl. 7), S92–5.

Staessen, J., Fagard, R., and Amery, A. (1985). Blood pressure, calorie intake and obesity. In *Epidemiology of hypertension. Handbook of hypertension,* Vol. 6 (ed. C. J. Bulpitt), Elsevier, Amsterdam.

Stamler, J., Neaton, J. D., and Wentworth, D. N. (1989). Blood pressure (systolic and diastolic) and risk of fatal coronary heart disease. *Hypertension,* **13** (Suppl. I), 2–12.

Stamler, R., Stamler, J., Grimm, R., Gosch, F. C., Elmer, P., and Dyer, A. (1987). Nutritional therapy for high blood pressure. Final report of a four-year randomized controlled trial—the Hypertension Control Program. *J. Am. Med. Assoc.,* **257**(11), 1484–91.

Swales, J. D. (1990). First line treatment in hypertension. *Br. Med. J.,* **301,** 1172–3.

Swales, J. D., Sever, P. S., and Peart, S. (1991). *Clinical atlas of hypertension,* Gower Medical Publishing, London, Section 10.3.

US Public Health Service Hospitals Cooperative Study Group (1977). Treatment of mild hypertension: results of a ten-year intervention trial. *Circ. Res.,* **40** (Suppl. 1), 98–105.

Veterans Administration Cooperative Study Group on Antihypertensive Agents (1970). Effects of treatment on morbidity in hypertension: II. Results in patients with diastolic blood pressure averaging 90 through 114 mmHG. *J. Am. Med. Assoc.,* **213,** 1143–92.

Veterans Administration–National Heart, Lung, and Blood Institute Study Group for Cooperative Studies on Antihypertensive Therapy: Mild Hypertension (1977). Treatment of mild hypertension: preliminary results of a two-year feasibility trial. *Circ. Res.,* **40** (Suppl. 1), 180–7.

Weidmann, P., Uehlinger, D. E., and Gerber, A. (1985). Antihypertensive treatment and serum lipoproteins. *J. Hypertension,* **3,** 297–306.

Weinberger, M. H., Cohen, S. J., Miller, J. Z., Luft, F. C., Grim, C. E., and

Fineberg, N. S. (1988). Dietary sodium restriction as adjunctive treatment of hypertension. *J. Am. Med. Assoc.,* **259,** 2561–5.

Wilhelmsen, L., Berglund, G., Elmfeldt, D., Tibblin, G., Wedel, H., Pennert, K., *et al.* (1986). The multi-factor primary prevention trial in Goteborg, Sweden. *Eur. Heart J.,* **7**(4), 279–88.

Wilhelmsen, L., Berglund, G., Elmfeldt, D., Fitzsimons, T., Holzgreve, H., Hosie, J., *et al.* (1987). Beta-blockers versus diuretics in hypertensive men. Main results from the HAPPHY trial. *J. Hypertension,* **5**(5), 561–72.

Wolff, F. W. and Lindeman, R. D. (1966). Effects of treatment in hypertension: results of a controlled study. *J. Chron. Dis.,* **19,** 227–40.

WHO (World Health Organization) European Collaborative Group (1986). European collaborative trial of multifactorial prevention of coronary heart disease: final report on the 6-year results. *Lancet,* April 19, **ii,** 869–72.

WHO (World Health Organization)–ISH Mild Hypertension Liaison Committee (1989). Guidelines Sub-committee of the WHO/ISH Mild Hypertension Liaison Committee. 1989 guidelines for the management of mild hypertension: memorandum from a WHO/ISH Meeting. *J. Hypertension,* **7,** 689–93.

24

Reduction of cholesterol-mediated risk: the role of the doctor

B. Lewis

A comprehensive policy to control coronary heart disease (CHD) requires patient-based preventive care as well as a sound population-orientated approach. These two methods of delivery of an essentially similar package of preventive measures were first clearly defined by Rose (1985). The clinician, like the practitioner in public health, is aware of the multi-factorial nature of CHD risk; although this chapter is concerned with a single risk factor, the practising doctor seeks to identify and deal with all modifiable risk factors.

The diagnostic and therapeutic components of the clinical approach to hyperlipidaemia are precisely analogous to those by which hypertension and non-insulin-dependent diabetes are dealt with. In each instance they aim to identify and provide individual management of persons at high risk, for whom the current level of population-based measures is inadequate. The individual and population strategies for decreasing cholesterol-related risk are synergistic (Lewis *et al.* 1986)—the more effective the latter, the fewer persons will require the former—and the detection of a risk factor in a clinical setting has an educational component that is likely to enhance compliance with population-based efforts to improve health-related behaviour. In no sense are these alternative approaches.

The scientific basis for reducing elevated plasma cholesterol levels comprises concordant data from epidemiology, clinical trials (with clinical events or atheroma progression as end-points), and animal experimentation. Accumulation of cholesterol in the arterial wall is a consistent feature of atherosclerosis; this cholesterol is derived from plasma lipoproteins. Of these, low density lipoprotein (LDL) and intermediate density lipoprotein (IDL) are known to transfer from plasma into arterial initima (Nordestgaard 1991). LDL in man, and both LDL and IDL in experimental animals, are known to transfer at a fractional rate that is directly related to their plasma concentrations. In a genetically hyperlipidaemic rabbit strain, the extent of atherosclerosis is also directly and independently related to plasma concentrations of LDL and IDL (Nordestgaard 1991). Understanding the mechanisms of arterial lipid accumulation provides a theoretical rationale for the treatment of hyperlipidaemia that is consonant with the epidemiology of the cholesterol–CHD relationship.

TARGET GROUPS

The relation between plasma cholesterol and CHD incidence is continuous, graded, and curvilinear or log-linear. Rigid action limits for therapy are therefore arbitrary; however, such action limits have been proposed to simplify management of lipid problems, but always with the qualification that the patient, not merely the laboratory finding, is being treated (Study Group 1987, 1988; Lewis *et al*. 1989). In particular, all determinants of risk must be taken into account. The European recommendations for management of hyperlipidaemia include three action limits for such management: average cholesterol levels in the ranges 5.2–6.5 mmol/l, 6.5–7.8 mmol/l, and >7.8 mmol/l suggest different patterns of therapy (Study Group 1988; Lewis *et al*. 1989).

Among the 4 per cent of British men and women aged 25–59 years with cholesterol levels above 7.8 mmol/l, possibly one in four has a major monogenically inherited hyperlipidaemia such as heterozygous familial hypercholesterolaemia (prevalence about 2 per 1000), familial combined hyperlipidaemia (which is commoner on the admittedly selective basis of clinic referrals), and the comparatively uncommon remnant hyperlipidaemia and familial defective apolipoprotein B. All are associated with a high frequency of early onset CHD, and all require individualized management and follow-up for effective control.

Some 60 per cent of British adults have plasma cholesterol levels in the range 5.2–7.8 mmol/l (Mann *et al*. 1988). Among these, most are attributed to so-called common or polygenic hypercholesterolaemia, a term that until recently meant no more than the presence of cholesterol levels in the upper part of the frequency distribution, above a chosen cut-point, after excluding certain specific disorders. Some understanding of abnormal lipoprotein kinetics involved and its relation to diet has now been achieved (Lewis *et al*. 1986), and genetic polymorphism of apolipoproteins E and B has been shown to be associated with differences in mean cholesterol levels (Sing and Davignon 1985; Law *et al*. 1986). Other persons with levels of cholesterol in the range 5.2–7.8 mmol/l have familial combined hyperlipidaemia. A further cause, important to recognize because no therapy is required, is high density lipoprotein (HDL) hyperlipidaemia; an unusually high level of HDLs is relatively common among post-menopausal women, whether or not oestrogen replacement therapy is used, and among young lean athletes.

For most people with cholesterol levels of 5.2–7.8 mmol/l, the dietary recommendations offered to the population as a whole will, if fully complied with, reduce such levels substantially (Lewis *et al.* 1981). The role of the doctor is to reinforce the need for such compliance, particularly for persons with levels in the lower part of this range, and to attend to any further risk factors. Ongoing medical care is appropriate for a subset in whom overall risk is high because of the presence of multiple risk factors or the presence of overt CHD, and also for persons with cholesterol levels in the upper part of this range. Therefore, despite the high prevalence of cholesterol levels in the range 5.2–7.8 mmol/l, care for many members of this subset is not arduous and generally amounts to a single counselling session on diet and other risk factors (Study Group 1988; Lewis *et al.* 1989).

CASE FINDING

The detection of high cholesterol-related risk requires systematic cholesterol measurement; in adults this is analogous to and as necessary as routine measurement of blood pressure. It has been argued that high CHD risk can result either from the interaction between multiple risk factors or from severe hypercholesterolaemia alone (Lewis and Rose 1991); cholesterol measurement contributes to recognition of multifactorial risk and is essential to diagnosis of severe hypercholesterolaemia. Cost considerations and work-load problems have led some to argue that cholesterol measurement should be confined to persons recognized to be at high risk on other grounds. However, this would miss many people with severe hypercholesterolaemia as a sole risk factor, and the practical problems of universal testing can readily be dealt with by allocating an acceptable amount of time for preventive work in general and in occupational practice; this is coupled with the adoption of a simple system of priorities so that persons at greatest risk (based on known characteristics such as age, sex, presence of CHD, hypertension, diabetes, or obesity) are tested promptly (Lewis and Rose 1991). To do less would contravene Hippocratic principles.

Nor is it justifiable to defer cholesterol testing to middle age, though this may be more cost-effective. This practice would delay the detection of familial hypercholesterolaemia sufficiently to allow extensive coronary atherosclerosis, and often overt CHD, to develop. A large angiographic study of heterozygous familial hypercholesteroaemia in Japan suggests that coronary narrowing becomes evident in males at a mean age of 17 years and in females at a mean of 25 years (Mabuchi *et al.* 1989).

Cholesterol screening is worthless without effective ongoing management. The preferred setting is general practice. This permits comprehensive assessment and appropriate monitoring in the context of the doctor–patient relationship (Waine *et al.* 1991).

Table 24.1 Risk assessment

History
1. Personal history of cardiovascular disease, noting age of onset, functional impairment, and bypass grafting or angioplasty
2. Family history of CHD or other atherosclerosis, noting number and proximity of affected relatives and ages of onset
3. Cigarette smoking: number and duration
4. Alcohol use
5. Known diabetes, hypertension, gout

Examination
6. Weight-for-height, supplemented by manual (or caliper) assessment of abdominal skinfold thickness
7. Blood pressure
8. Presence of tendon or other xanthomas, corneal arcus

Laboratory
9. Non-fasted serum cholesterol (mmol/l)

<5.2	5.2–6.5	>6.5
Recommend COMA diet	Formal diet counselling	Measure cholesterol, triglyceride, HDL; treat and follow-up.
Counsel on any other risk factors	Counsel on other risk factors	Counsel on any other risk factors
Reassess in 10 years	Reassess in 1–5 years according to overall risk status	

CLINICAL ASSESSMENT

Table 24.1 shows a scheme for initial risk assessment in general or occupational practice (Lewis *et al.* 1989). It can be based partly on a self-completion questionnaire, together with a 20 min assessment by the doctor or a trained practice nurse. To identify patients with more severe hyperlipidaemia, for whom an aetiological diagnosis is important for prognosis and optimal therapy, the clinical characteristics shown in Table 24.2 should be borne in mind during initial and/or follow-up assessment; many such patients have serum cholesterol levels above 7.8 mmol/l, and in almost all it is above 6.5 mmol/l. Table 24.1 leads to fuller lipid assessment in a subset of those initially tested; this will reveal markedly elevated serum triglyceride in some major hyperlipidaemias.

MANAGEMENT

The first stage in management of the hyperlipidaemic person is common to all forms and all degrees of severity of lipid abnormality (Study Group 1988; Lewis *et al.* 1989). Its components can be listed as follows.

Table 24.2 Clinical features of some specific hyperlipidaemias

	Prevalence	Cholesterol (mmol/l)	Triglyceride (mmol/l)	Signs	Associations
Familial combined hyperlipidaemia	Up to 1%	7–9	2–6		CHD
Familial hypercholesterolaemia	2:1000	8–14	1–4	Tendon xanthomas	Premature CHD
Remnant hyperlipidaemia	Rare	8–14	5–15	Skin xanthomas: palmar creases, elbows	CHD Peripheral Vascular Disease
HDL	?1–2%	5–7.5	<2		CHD risk below average
Familial	Rare	5–8	4–50	Skin xanthomas: back, elbows Retinal lipaemia Hepatosplenomegaly	Pancreatitis diabetes
Chylomicronaemia syndrome[a]	Very rare	8–12	20–80	Skin xanthomas: back, elbows Retinal lipaemia Hepatosplenomegaly	Pancreatitis

[a] Treated by specific very low fat diet.

Identification and management of all modifiable CHD risk factors

This serves to reduce multifactorial risk, and in some situations correction of non-lipid risk factors may modify lipid abnormalities in the direction of reduced risk. For example, hypertriglyceridaemia often abates when excessive alcohol intake is reduced, while low HDL-cholesterol levels commonly increase following cessation of smoking or reduction of obesity.

Correction of causes of secondary hyperlipidaemia where possible

Classical secondary hyperlipidaemias which often provide a therapeutic opportunity include hypothyroidism, diabetes mellitus, and over-use of alcohol. Causes that may prove less responsive to treatment include the nephrotic syndrome, chronic renal insufficiency, bulimia, and anorexia nervosa. Other disorders that can lead to hyperlipidaemia, such as myelomatosis, obstructive jaundice, and systemic lupus erythematosus, themselves dominate the clinical picture, with the lipid disorder being an incidental finding.

Commoner than any of these is the iatrogenic group of lipid disorders due to drugs. To the extent that alternative lipid-neutral drugs can be substituted, this entity provides scope for amelioration of the hyperlipidaemia. Elevation of triglyceride and cholesterol levels, and suppression of HDL-cholesterol, may occur to varying degrees with diuretics, some beta-blockers, retinoids, corticosteroids, oestrogens (elevated triglyceride), progestogens related to testosterone (elevated cholesterol), and anabolic steroids. HDL-cholesterol may be elevated by phenobarbitone, phenytoin, rifampicin, and cimetidine, sometimes sufficiently to lead to a high serum cholesterol level.

Correction of or reduction of overweight

Weight reduction, which is necessary on several health grounds, is often effective in decreasing elevated triglyceride and cholesterol levels, and increasing their response to other lipid-lowering measures. HDL-cholesterol shows a biphasic response, decreasing initially but tending to rise above initial levels as weight stabilizes at reduced level. Weight reduction appears to influence triglyceride and cholesterol initially by virtue of the low energy intake; the long-term benefit results from a reduced adipose tissue mass. The effects of weight reduction show pronounced inter-individual variation.

The isocaloric lipid-lowering diet

The isocaloric lipid-lowering diet is common to the management of all hypercholesterolaemia and all but a small subset of hypertriglyceridaemias.

It is, together with the measures outlined above, effective and sufficient treatment for most hyperlipidaemic persons including the great majority of those with mild to moderate elevation of serum lipids (Lewis *et al.* 1981; Choudhury *et al.* 1984). Diet is also the initial therapy for severe hyper-lipidaemias; owing to the wide range of response, dietary treatment proves rewardingly effective even in some individuals with marked lipid elevation. When diet is incompletely effective and drug therapy is prescribed, diet is always continued since its effect is additive to that of medication.

In controlled institutional conditions, the multicomponent lipid-lowering diet can reduce serum cholesterol by an average of 29 per cent and LDL-cholesterol by almost 34 per cent relative to a baseline diet of nutrient composition similar to a typical Western diet (Lewis *et al.* 1981). In a long-term study of this diet, fed isocalorically to ambulant hyperlipidaemic patients attending a lipid clinic, the mean cholesterol reduction was 21 per cent and that of LDL cholesterol was 26 per cent (Choudhury *et al.* 1984). In this study intensive efforts were made to maximize dietary compliance and to enhance patients' motivation.

In addition to variation in compliance, the wide individual variation in responsiveness to this diet deserves re-emphasis. We are only beginning to understand the metabolic bases of this variation (Katan *et al.* 1988; Glatz *et al.* 1991), which may prove to stem in part from genetic polymorphism of apolipoproteins and differences in regulator gene control of apolipoprotein B production. However, the clinical implications are clear: responsiveness to diet cannot reliably be predicted from pretreatment plasma lipid levels. The corollary is that it is meaningless to attempt to define any particular lipid level as an indication for drug therapy. The therapeutic trial is the only means of assessing whether serum lipid levels can be reduced to target values by diet (Study Group 1988; Lewis *et al.* 1989). In practice, such a trial can reasonably continue for 4 months to 1 year, during which doctor and (wherever possible) dietitian make repeated efforts to enhance compliance and motivation, and to adapt the diet to individual food preferences.

The several components of the lipid-lowering diet appear to be additive wherever this has been investigated (Lewis *et al.* 1981). All are required if a maximum response is to be obtained. They comprise the following.

1. Reduction of saturated fatty acids containing 14 or 16 carbon atoms, of which palmitate (16 carbon atoms) is the most abundant. Saturated fats provide 3–20 per cent of dietary energy in different populations (15–20 per cent in most Western countries) and are the most important single dietary determinant of serum cholesterol levels. The extensive feeding experiments by Keys and coworkers yielded a regression equation in which the absolute change in serum cholesterol (in mg/dl) is 2.74 times the change in the percentage of energy derived from saturated fat (Keys *et al.* 1957). The recommended intake of saturated fat for populations and for moderately

hyperlipidaemic patients is less than 10 per cent of energy. With care, a diet providing 7–8 per cent of energy from saturated fat can be made acceptable and congenial to most patients with severe or relatively refractory hypercholesterolaemia. Stearic acid, with 18 carbon atoms, is one of the saturated fatty acids in beef fat and chocolate. It has little or no cholesterol-raising effect, but as we lack sufficient data on its effect on thrombosis and serum triglyceride it is premature to consider including it in a lipid-lowering diet. In cross-cultural food disappearance data, saturated fat availability is directly related to CHD mortality.

2. Unsaturated fats do not increase serum cholesterol when substituted for carbohydrate, and may lower it. The reduction in serum cholesterol is partly due to the reduced intake of saturated fatty acids, but in the original studies an independent cholesterol-lowering effect of polyunsaturated fatty acids of the $n-6$ class (e.g. linoleic acid) was also observed. In the Keys equation the serum cholesterol change (mg/dl) was expressed by the function -1.31 times the change in energy intake from polyunsaturated fat (Keys *et al.* 1957). Many, but not all, more recent studies indicate that mono-unsaturated fat has a cholesterol- and LDL-lowering effect similar to that of polyunsaturated fat. At usual intakes the two classes of unsaturated fat have similar effects on HDL-cholesterol. All affirmative dietary coronary prevention trials have included an increased intake of polyunsaturated fat. However, cross-cultural epidemiological evidence shows an inverse relation between CHD mortality and mono-unsaturated but not poly-unsaturated intake. In contrast, linoleic acid content in plasma or adipose tissue lipids is inversely related to CHD incidence within a population, but where the mono-unsaturated oleic acid has been investigated no association with CHD has been observed (Wood *et al.* 1987). In current dietary recommendations polyunsaturated fatty acid intake is increased from 2–4 to 6–10 per cent of energy. If there is an optimal intake of $n-3$ polyun-saturates, this is presently unknown. Since reduction of saturates implies a decreased intake of animal fats, this not insubstantial source of oleic acid will also be decreased. For this reason alone, an increased intake of plant sources of oleic acid, notably olive oil, is justified, maintaining a mono-unsaturate consumption of 12–15 per cent of energy.

3. In univariate cross-cultural data, and in a recent analysis of a longi-tudinal study (Stamler and Shekelle 1988), dietary cholesterol is at least as strongly related as saturated fat to CHD mortality. Dietary cholesterol in-creases mean serum cholesterol, LDL-cholesterol, and HDL-cholesterol. The extent of this response shows wide individual variation, consistent on repeated testing and also consistent with the serum cholesterol responsive-ness to dietary saturated fat in the same individual (Choudhury *et al.* 1984; Beynan *et al.* 1988). A reduced cholesterol intake is inevitable in a diet in which saturated fat intake is decreased, but the need to restrict cholesterol-

rich foods other than meat and milk products has been debated. While there is good reason to limit cholesterol-rich offal such as brain, tongue, and kidney, eggs and liver are valuable sources of micronutrients and should be included, in modest amounts, in therapeutic diets. The total intake of cholesterol should then be less than 250 mg/day.

4. A moderate serum-cholesterol-lowering effect of soluble fibre (pectins and gums) has been well documented. Intake of vegetables (including pulses), fruit, and oats should be substantial. However, no single food on its own (e.g. oats) has a major cholesterol-lowering effect at tolerable intake (Swain *et al.* 1990).

Lipid-lowering drugs

As with the management of hypertension and diabetes mellitus, drug therapy plays a valuable role in the management of primary hyperlipidaemia, and in some situations in treatment of secondary hyperlipidaemias which are otherwise resistant. To use such drugs where diet and other non-pharmacological measures would be effective is bad practice, as is the withholding of necessary drug treatment. At the present time lipid-lowering drugs are widely underprescribed in the treatment of cholesterol-mediated risk of CHD as a result of poor case finding in most high incidence countries. To take one example, there are of the order of 120 000 persons in the UK with familial hypercholesterolaemia. Affected men have a greater than 20-fold excess risk of definite myocardial infarction or sudden cardiac death occurring at an average age of 45 years; in women the excess risk is about six-fold and evident CHD appears at an average age of 55 years. Yet only a minority of patients with this form of hyperlipidaemia alone are receiving suitable therapy.

Indications for lipid-lowering drug therapy fall into two classes. The first comprise genetic hyperlipidaemias of severe degree that have not responded to a short trial of the measures listed above. The term 'responded' implies attainment of the target lipid levels shown in Tables 24.3 and 24.4. The initial aim of such therapy is to minimize the risk of CHD and peripheral atherosclerotic diseases by reducing levels of LDL and/or IDL to values associated with less than average risk. As stated, such values are arbitrary and need to be interpreted flexibly. The second aim is to prevent the complication of acute pancreatitis in patients with gross hypertriglyceridaemia. Pancreatitis can occur in the presence of triglyceride levels in the range 25–50 mmol/l or above. However, triglyceride levels are exceedingly labile, and in consequence levels exceeding 5 mmol/l, after effective deployment of the measures discussed above, require serious consideration for drug therapy.

The second class of indications for drug therapy is high CHD risk due to resistant hyperlipidaemia of moderate extent. Here the use of

Table 24.3 Factors influencing the choice and aims of lipid-lowering therapy

Modifiable risk factors
Cigarette smoking
Hypertension
Diabetes
Low HDL-cholesterol[a]
Obesity

Other clinical findings
Male sex
Presence of CHD
Family history of CHD

[a] 0.8–1 mmol/l (very low, <0.8 mmol/l)

Table 24.4 Therapeutic aims in hypolipidaemic treatment

	Group A	Group B
Serum cholesterol (mmol/l)	5.2–5.7	>5.2
LDL-cholesterol (mmol)	>4.0	>3.5

Group A, factors in Table 24.3 absent.
Group B, any two factors in Table 24.3 present, or any one factor present to a marked degree.

non-pharmacological measures is effective in most, but not all, patients. Trials of such measures should be far more extended: 4–12 months (Study Group 1988; Lewis *et al.* 1989). Before drug therapy is undertaken, repeated efforts are required to maximize compliance to diet and to ensure effective reduction of non-lipid risk factors. The criteria shown in Table 24.3 assist the doctor in forming a judgement concerning overall risk of cardiovascular disease.

An audit of therapy for hyperlipidaemia was carried out, reflecting the choice of treatment for patients referred to a teaching hospital lipid clinic for 1 year or more and managed according to the guidelines in this chapter. Forty-five per cent of patients with marked hypercholesterolaemia received medication, but only 9 per cent of those with milder lipid problems were so treated. Every adult with a positive diagnosis of familial hypercholesterolaemia proved to require drug therapy. This population included a number of patients referred because they were refractory to initial dietary therapy. The findings do not reflect the probable therapeutic pattern in primary care, but indicate a 'worse case' estimate based on a selected population.

1. Bile acid sequestrant resins: cholestyramine and colestipol have both been tested in controlled CHD prevention trials (the former in the definitive Lipid Research Clinics (LRC) study) and in angiographic studies of atheroma progression/regression. Their good safety record is presumably related to their non-absorbability. A recent valuable trend has been the recognition of their effectiveness in low dosage in combination with diet or with diet plus a second drug. The US National Cholesterol Education Program regards them as drugs of first choice in hypercholesterolaemia. Serum cholesterol is reduced by 20–30 per cent due to a fall in LDL. HDL may increase slightly. An untoward effect is a rise in triglyceride with larger doses, especially when baseline triglyceride is slightly elevated.

2. HMG CoA reductase inhibitors (simvastatin, lovastatin, pravastatin) are a recently introduced group of drugs acting by selective partial inhibition of cholesterol synthesis (Alberts 1988; Grundy 1988). They mark a major advance in lipid-lowering therapy. Cholesterol is lowered by 30–35 per cent and LDL-cholesterol by 35–40 per cent. Triglyceride decreases, usually more modestly, and HDL-cholesterol rises to a variable extent. Their effect on CHD incidence is currently being tested. Like the resins, reductase inhibitors are effective in lowering cholesterol in familial hypercholesterolaemia and in diet-resistant common hypercholesterolaemia. Unlike the resins, they are effective in some patients with remnant hyperlipidaemia. They have not been sufficiently tested in childhood. Because they are teratogenic in the rat, they should be avoided in women of childbearing potential unless effective contraception is assured. Side-effects include transient headache, a rare (1 in 1000) skeletal myopathy which is rapidly reversible on stopping therapy, and abnormal liver function tests in 1–2 per cent of patients.

3. Fibric acid derivatives include bezafibrate, ciprofibrate, fenofibrate, gemfibrozil, and the parent compound clofibrate. They lower triglyceride by 50–70 per cent, increase HDL by 10–20 per cent or more, and have a varying ability to lower cholesterol. Some improve glucose tolerance and are of value in resistant diabetic lipaemia. The Helsinki primary prevention trial of gemfibrozil revealed a substantial reduction in non-fatal and fatal CHD events. The two large trials of clofibrate, and two smaller ones, yielded inconsistent results. Side-effects (dyspepsia, skeletal myopathy, reduced potency, potentiation of warfarin, and abnormal liver function) are relatively infrequent. All of them appear to be class effects. Only clofibrate has been shown to increase the frequency of gallstones, though increased lithogenicity of bile has been reported for bezafibrate. In the rat, the liver shows massive peroxisomal proliferation and hepatomas develop; despite extensive study there appears to be no evidence in man

of more than minimal peroxisomal increase and no increased incidence of hepatoma.

4. Nicotinic acid in pharmacological doses (1.5–6 g/day) effectively lowers triglyceride and cholesterol, and elevates HDL-cholesterol (Illingworth 1987). It is moderately effective in secondary prevention of CHD and (on long-term follow up) in reducing total mortality (Canner *et al.* 1986). Careful guidance of the patient is the key to its successful use and a gradually progressive dose schedule is needed. Initial flushing and pruritus can largely be prevented by daily aspirin administration, and the main limiting side-effect is dyspepsia. Others are hyperuricaemia and gout, abnormal liver function and occasional hepatitis, worsening of diabetes (rare), and rashes. It is effective in familial combined hyperlipidaemia.

5. Combinations of two lipid-lowering drugs often permit lower dosage if appropriately selected to have differing modes of action and usually comprise a resin with a reductase inhibitor, a fibrate, or nicotinic acid (Study Group 1988). The risk of myopathy and rhabdomyolysis is increased considerably when a reductase inhibitor is combined with gemfibrozil or nicotinic acid (and, it should be noted, with cyclosporin and erythromycin). Two-drug therapy may be necessary in familial hypercholesterolaemia, in combined hyperlipidaemia, and (in specialist hands) to produce very low LDL levels (2.5–5 mmol/l) with a view to producing regression of atherosclerotic lesions; such use in secondary prevention should at present be regarded as experimental, but it is of great potential importance.

FUTURE DEVELOPMENTS

The single most important advance in controlling lipid-mediated risk of CHD does not depend on further research but on the systematic competent application of existing knowledge—of the aetiological role, diagnosis, and management of the commoner plasma lipid disorders. Probably no aspect of preventive medicine is better documented, yet none has so belatedly been incorporated into clinical practice. In no way does this negate the need for answers to several questions, some topical and others unresolved after decades. In this final section some of these are enumerated.

1. Is 'regression therapy', mentioned above, a tenable concept? Quantitative analysis of serial angiograms of the femoral and coronary arteries has established that lipid-lowering therapy favourably alters the natural history of atheroma and can induce partial regression. It is not necessary to learn whether a functionally significant degree of regression can be achieved. If this is the case, we shall need to define what target levels of LDL, IDL, and perhaps HDL are required to induce such changes.

2. What is the place of treatment of hypertriglyceridaemia in the control of atherosclerosis and arterial thrombosis? That low HDL cholesterol and hypertriglyceridaemia often coexist is commonplace. Is there then a 'high triglyceride, low HDL syndrome' that is a causal risk factor for CHD, analogous to the better documented 'high LDL syndrome'? To evaluate this, clinical and epidemiological data and trials on an appropriate population sample will be needed. A corollary is the laboratory, clinical, and genetic problem of distinguishing 'atherogenic hypertriglyceridaemia', reflecting elevated levels of small triglyceride-rich lipoproteins (IDL or, more specifically, Sf 12–60 particles), from large-particle hyperlipidaemia (Nordestgaard 1991). To the extent that atherogenicity is a function of the rate of entry of lipoproteins into the intima from plasma, the relevance of small particles is established, but this measurement requires methods at present beyond the capacity of routine laboratories. IDL levels are increased in at least three genetic conditions, and in diabetes and chronic renal failure, and dietary cholesterol is an important determinant. Hypertriglyceridaemia may also be atherogenic by virtue of its association with the presence of a small dense subclass of LDL.

3. Is HDL cholesterol a causal risk factor or only a powerful and consistent risk indicator? Although the former is suggested by evidence of association in some clinical trials, no trial exists that has shown that selective elevation of HDL cholesterol reduces CHD incidence. Two other negative findings may be noted. Where the HDL–CHD relation has been examined cross-culturally with analyses in a single laboratory, the findings have disagreed with those of longitudinal population studies, and among the several genetic disorders in which HDL levels are very low, some but not others show an association with CHD. The most plausible hypothesis to explain a causal HDL–CHD relationship concerns the undoubted role of HDL in the reverse transport of cholesterol to the liver from extrahepatic tissues including cells of the arterial intima. This traffic of cholesterol is essential to maintenance of cellular cholesterol balance, but it is a multi-stage process and at present we do not know which step governs its rate. Is it the activity of the peripheral HDL receptor, e.g. on arterial macrophage/foam cells? Is it the level of a minor subclass of HDL, the small apolipoprotein A-I containing particles recognized by this receptor that trigger movement of cholesterol to the cell surface, or the receptor that triggers movement of cholesterol to the cell surface, or the level of 'bulk' HDL to which this cell surface cholesterol transfers, or activity of cholesteryl ester transfer protein, or the kinetics of the VLDL–IDL–LDL system to which this protein transfers cholesteryl ester, or the activity of one of the hepatic lipoprotein receptors? HDL is a profoundly heterogeneous class of lipoproteins, and on present evidence it seems unlikely that total HDL-cholesterol is more than an index of an atherogenic process. But it is

plausible that fundamental preventive and therapeutic opportunities lie within the reverse transport process.

4. Before LDL cholesterol is taken up by macrophages in the intima, leading to foam cell formation, plasma LDL has to undergo one of a number of modifications that make it 'recognizable' by macrophage receptors. Among these is peroxidation, and it is peroxidized rather than native plasma LDL that is found in surgical specimens of human arterial intima. In hyperlipidaemic rabbits, massive doses of the antioxidant drug probucol retard atherosclerotic changes. It remains to be seen whether this drug, or free-radical scavengers including vitamins E and A, is comparably effective in man.

5. So-called 'new' risk factors for CHD (fibrinogen, factor VII, and Lp(a)) have yet to influence clinical practice. Their levels can be modified by diet and/or drugs, and the relevance of such modification to preventive practice may be considerable. At present, fibrinogen and Lp(a) measurements sharpen the assessment of risk and help decide on the level of therapy appropriate for other, demonstrably causal, risk factors.

REFERENCES

Alberts, A. W. (1988). HWG CoA reductase inhibitors—the development. *Atheroscler. Rev.,* **18,** 123–31.

Beynan, A. C., Katan, M. B., and van Zutphen, L. F. M. (1988). Hypo- and hyperresponders: individual differences in the response of serum cholesterol to changes in diet. *Adv. Lipid Res.,* 115–71.

Canner, P. L., Berge, K. G., Wenger, N. K., *et al.* (1986). Fifteen year mortality in Coronary Drug Project patients: long-term benefits with niacin. *J. Am. Coll. Cardiol.,* **8,** 1245–55.

Choudhury, S., Jackson, P., Katan, M. B., Marenah, C. B., Cortese, C., Miller, N. E., *et al.* (1984). A multifactorial diet in the management of hyperlipidaemia. *Atherosclerosis,* **50,** 93–103.

Glatz, J. F. C., Turner, P. R., Katan, M. B., *et al.* (1991). Human hypo- and hyperresponders to dietary cholesterol differ in the responsiveness of their low density lipoprotein production. Submitted for publication.

Grundy, S. M. (1988). HMG CoA reductase inhibitors for treatment of hypercholesterolemia. *New Engl. J. Med.,* **319,** 24–31.

Illingworth, D. R. (1987). Lipid lowering drugs. *Drugs,* **33,** 259–79.

Katan, M. B., *et al.* (1988). Congruence of individual responsiveness to dietary cholesterol and saturated fat in humans. *J. Lipid Res.,* **29,** 883–92.

Keys, A., Anderson, J. T., and Grande, F. (1957). Prediction of serum-cholesterol responses of man to changes in fats in the diets. *Lancet,* **ii,** 959–66.

Law, A., Powell, L. M., Brunt, H., Knott, T. J., Altman, D. G., Rajput, J., *et al.* (1986). Common DNA polymorphism within coding sequence of apo B gene associated with altered lipid levels. *Lancet,* **i,** 1301–3.

Lewis, B. and Rose, G. (1991). Prevention of coronary heart-disease—putting theory in practice. *J. R. Coll. Physicians*, **25**(1), 21–6.

Lewis, B., Assmann, G., Mancini, M., and Stein, Y. (1989). *Handbook of coronary heart disease prevention. A practical guide to the management of lipid and other risk factors in adults*, Current Medical Literature, London.

Lewis, B., Hammett, F., Katan, M. B., Kay, R. M., Merkx, I., Nobels, A., *et al.* (1981). Towards an improved lipid lowering diet. Additive effects of changes in nutrient intake. *Lancet*, **ii**, 1310–13.

Lewis, B., Mann, J. I., and Mancini, M. (1986). Deducing the risk of coronary heart disease in individuals and in the population. *Lancet*, **i**, 956–9.

Lewis, B., Turner, P. R., Rossouw, J. E., *et al.* (1986). The metabolic epidemiology of plasma cholesterol. *Lancet*, **ii**, 663–5.

Mabuchi, H., Koizumi, J., Shimuzu, M., Takeda, R., and Hokuriku FH-CHD Study Group (1989). Hokoriku FH-CHD Study Group. Development of coronary heart disease in familial hypercholesterolemia. *Circulation*, **79**, 225–32.

Mann, J. I., *et al.* (1988). Blood lipid concentrations and other cardiovascular risk factors: distribution, prevalence, and detection in Britain. *Br. Med. J.*, **296**, 1702–6.

Nordestgaard, B. G. (1991). In press.

Rose, G. (1985). Sick individuals and sick populations. *Int. J. Epidemiol.*, **14**, 32–8.

Sing, C. F. and Davignon, J. (1985). Role of apolipoprotein E polymorphism in determining normal plasma lipid variation. *Am. J. Hum. Genet.*, **37**, 268–85.

Stamler, J. and Shekelle, R. (1988). Dietary cholesterol and human coronary heart disease. *Arch. Pathol. Lab. Med.*, **112**, 1032–40.

Study Group, European Atherosclerosis Society (1987). Strategies for the prevention of coronary heart disease. *Eur. Heart J.*, **8**, 77–88.

Study Group, European Atherosclerosis Society (1988). The recognition and management of hyperlipidaemia in adults. *Eur. Heart J.*, **9**, 571–600.

Swain, J. F., Rouse, I. L., Curley, C. B., *et al.* (1990). Comparison of the effects of oat bran and lower-fiber wheat on serum lipoprotein levels and blood pressure. *New Engl. J. Med.*, **322**, 147–52.

Waine, C., *et al.* (1991). *Guidelines for the management of high blood lipids*, Royal College of General Practitioners, London, in press.

Wood, D. A., Riemersma, R., Butler, S., *et al.* (1987). Linoleic and eicosapentaenoic acids in adipose tissue and platelets and the risk of coronary heart disease. *Lancet*, **i**, 177–83.

25

Cholesterol and coronary heart disease: to screen or not to screen

N. J. Wald

INTRODUCTION

There is an intuitive appeal to screening, but not all screening is worthwhile and it is important to evaluate proposed screening procedures adequately before they are introduced into medical practice. However well intentioned the desire to adopt a new screening approach, the assessment must be rational and based on evidence. This is particularly true for coronary heart disease (CHD), a disease of such public health importance that it is essential to be sure that our strategies for prevention are well directed.

The assessment of general adult serum cholesterol measurement as a screening test for CHD is considered in this chapter. Two other possible uses of mass serum cholesterol measurement, namely as a monitoring test to assess a person's response to a dietary change aimed at lowering serum cholesterol and as a promotional exercise to individualize advice on serum cholesterol reduction, are also discussed. The case for neonatal or childhood serum cholesterol screening which might be considered for the detection of premature CHD due to familial hypercholesterolaemia is not considered.

EVALUATING SERUM CHOLESTEROL AS A SCREENING TEST FOR CHD

Any screening test must be able to distinguish persons who have a particular disorder (or will develop it in a specified period of time) from persons who do not have the disorder at the time of the test (or do not develop it over the same period of time). The greater the ability of the test to distinguish the two, the better is the test. For a quantitative screening test, such as serum cholesterol measurement, a simple way of displaying the information needed for a preliminary assessment of the test is to plot the relative frequency distributions of the screening variable (in this case serum cholesterol) in individuals who do and do not develop CHD. The

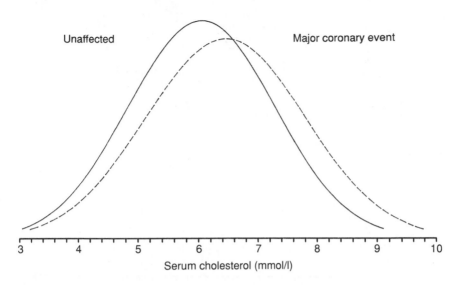

Fig. 25.1 Distribution of a single serum cholesterol measurement in 634 men who had experienced a first major coronary event and 6349 men who had not experienced such an event (unaffected) over an average of 8.6 years of observation (data from the US Pooling Project). The parameters are in mmol/l. Major coronary events: mean, 6.4692; SD, 1.3244. Unaffected: mean, 6.0657; SD, 1.2131.

less overlap between the two distributions, the better is the performance of the screening test.

Figure 25.1 shows the distributions of serum cholesterol in relation to the development of a first major coronary event (death or non-fatal infarct) in the US Pooling Project over an average of 8.6 years of observation (Pooling Project Research Group 1978). There is substantial overlap between the two distributions; the proportion of individuals with cholesterol levels above a given cut-off value who develop a major CHD event is not much greater than the proportion of those remaining unaffected with cholesterol levels above the same cut-off value. That is, in screening terminology, the detection rate (or sensitivity) is not much greater than the false-positive rate. Figure 25.2 shows the corresponding serum cholesterol distributions in the British Regional Heart Study based on an average of 7.5 years of observation (Pocock *et al.* 1989). The position is very similar: the mean cholesterol levels are a little higher, the standard deviations somewhat smaller, and the overlap slightly less. Table 25.1, based on the distributions shown in Fig. 25.2, shows the detection rate of the test and the corresponding false-positive rate at specified serum cholesterol cut-off levels. For a cholesterol cut-off of 7.5 mmol/l, for example, the detection rate would be 26 per cent and the false-positive rate 12 per cent. Taking repeat cholesterol measurements improves the performance of screening somewhat, but does

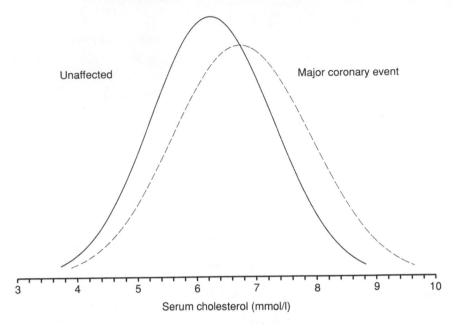

Fig. 25.2 Distribution of a single serum cholesterol measurement in 438 men who had a major coronary event and 7252 other men (unaffected) over an average of 7.5 years of observation (data from the British Regional Heart Study). The parameters are in mmol/l. CHD cases: mean, 6.766; SD, 1.151. Unaffected: mean, 6.2750; SD, 1.022.

not alter the conclusion that the measurement of serum cholesterol as a screening test for CHD in adults is poor and not to be recommended.

PERSONAL CHOLESTEROL MONITORING FOR CHD

Another reason proposed for general serum cholesterol testing is to provide people with information against which to monitor dietary changes designed to reduce their risk of CHD, in the same way that overweight people might weigh themselves at regular intervals to see if their weight-reducing diet is working. Regular measurement of this kind is intended to provide psychological reinforcement if serum cholesterol declines or a psychological reprimand if it does not.

A real reduction in cholesterol levels lowers the risk of CHD. This is shown in Table 25.2; a reduction of 0.5 mmol/l in serum cholesterol (about 10 per cent) will reduce the risk by about 30 per cent. However, repeated cholesterol measurements are only of value in monitoring an individual's risk of CHD if they provide a genuine indication of a person's change in

Table 25.1 Major CHD events (fatal and non-fatal)

Serum cholesterol (mmol/(mg/dl))	Detection rate[a] (%)	False–positive rate[b] (%)
≥ 8.5 (330)	6	1
≥ 8.0 (310)	14	5
≥ 7.5 (290)	26	12
≥ 7.0 (270)	42	24
≥ 6.5 (250)	59	41
≥ 6.0 (230)	75	61

First major coronary event: detection rate and false–positive rate according to serum cholesterol level (derived from Fig. 25.2 using data from the British Regional Heart Study).
[a] Detection rate is a synonym for sensitivity.
[b] False–positive rate is the complement of specificity (e.g. 2% false–positive rate = 98% specificity).

Table 25.2 Estimated approximate percentage reduction in risk of CHD according to changes in serum cholesterol

Serum cholesterol (mmol/l)		Reduction in risk of CHD (%)
Change	Absolute difference	
6.5–6.0	0.5 (8%)	30
6.5–5.5	1.0 (15%)	50
6.5–5.0	1.5 (23%)	65
6.5–4.5	2.0 (31%)	75

Adapted from Law and Wald 1991.

serum cholesterol. This would be so only if there were little random fluctuation around an individual's true average level, which is generally the case for weight but not for serum cholesterol. In a cohort of 14 600 people with repeat cholesterol measurements after 1 year the between-person coefficient of variation of serum cholesterol was 14.6 per cent and the within-person coefficient of variation was 7.4 per cent (Thompson and Pocock 1990). A person with a mean value of 6.5 mmol/l would thus have a within-person standard deviation of about 0.5 mmol/l (7.4% × 6.5). Figure 25.3 is a schematic illustration of the fluctuation in serum cholesterol over time in an individual with a mean value of 6.5 mmol/l. The figure illustrates that for about 68 per cent of the time the person's cholesterol will fluctuate

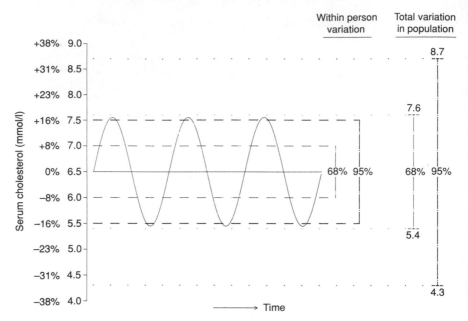

Fig. 25.3 The fluctuation in serum cholesterol for an individual with an average serum cholesterol of 6.5 mmol (approximately 250 mg/dl) showing (i) the range of values for that individual including 68 per cent of measurements (mean and 1 SD) and the range that includes 95 per cent of measurements (mean and 2 SD), and (ii) the equivalent ranges of values for the population.

within an interval of 1 mmol/l about the mean (i.e. about 1 within-person standard deviation (SD), or 0.5 mmol/l, on either side of the mean) and for 95 per cent of the time it will fluctuate within a 2 mmol/l interval around the mean value (i.e. ±2 SD or 1 mmol/l). The fluctuation in an individual's serum cholesterol over time is wide relative to the total population variation (also shown in Fig. 25.3), and the variation in CHD risk that would be inferred from a single measurement is also wide, as shown in Table 25.2. Serum cholesterol can vary by as much as 2 mmol/l from one occasion to another; if this random fluctuation were regarded as being genuine, the CHD risk might incorrectly be judged to have been reduced by 75 per cent when it had in fact not changed, or, conversely, not to have changed when it had been reduced by 75 per cent.

Table 25.3 shows the extent of serum cholesterol change that would need to be observed to exclude chance according to the number of measurements on an individual before and after a dietary change. This gives an indication of the number of measurements required and the size of the observed change needed to be reasonably certain ($p < 0.05$) that *any* true reduction in serum cholesterol had, in fact, occurred. (To estimate the size of the reduction with reasonable accuracy would require many more

Table 25.3 Percentage serum cholesterol change that would need to be observed to exclude chance ($p<0.05$) according to the number of tests before and after a dietary change

No. of tests before dietary change	No. of tests after dietary change				
	1	2	3	4	5
1	21[a]	18	17	16	16
2	18	15	13	13	12
3	17	13	12	11	11
4	16	13	11	10	10
5	16	12	11	10	9[b]

[a] For example, from 6.5 to 5.1 mmol/l.
[b] For example, from 6.5 to 5.9 mmol/l.

cholesterol measurements.) The number of initial measurements is as important as the number of subsequent ones, though in practice anyone contemplating a diet designed to lower their cholesterol is unlikely to delay doing so to obtain several baseline values. If only one initial value were obtained, even five subsequent ones would only provide assurance if the decline were 16 per cent or more. (Statistically, observing a declining trend would be a better way of detecting a change, but again this is impractical and the advantage would be small.) Even in the hypothetical case of a person having five initial and five subsequent measurements, only an observed change in serum cholesterol of 9 per cent or more would confidently exclude random fluctuation about a 'no change' state. Cholesterol monitoring is too imprecise a technique to be useful. For serum cholesterol measurements that are well above the population average the problem will be further compounded by regression to the mean, and the effect of intervention will be even more difficult to discern.

KNOWING ONE'S CHOLESTEROL

A further reason that has been put forward to justify performing a routine serum cholesterol measurement is to personalize the importance of reducing one's serum cholesterol. It is argued that, while general cholesterol testing would only confirm that most people living in Western countries would benefit by lowering their serum cholesterol, individual measurements would none the less make a person more aware of his or her own personal risk and so be more likely to adopt a diet that will lower serum cholesterol. The argument is much the same as the proposal that a smoker who has a blood test to measure carboxyhaemoglobin level (largely reflecting the carbon monoxide in cigarette smoke) may be encouraged to give up smoking. There is some evidence for this, although the effect observed was small (Jamrozik *et al*. 1984). However, it is misleading to encourage the widespread use of a test when the result of the test will not alter the advice that will be given.

A refinement of the same argument is the proposition that it is worthwhile to tailor the action to the risk—recommending more intensive dietary approaches or drug treatments for individuals with cholesterol levels in progressively higher 'bands'. The US National Cholesterol Education Program Expert Panel, for example, recommended this strategy (National Cholesterol Education Program 1988). The arguments against such recommendations are compelling, from both a theoretical and a practical perspective. The theoretical objection is that, just as cholesterol measurement in screening and as a monitoring instrument is insufficiently discriminatory to be worthwhile, categorizing individuals into cholesterol bands is similarly ineffective. Anyone classified in one band is not at sufficiently different risk of CHD to be offered different advice from someone else in an adjacent band. The argument can perhaps be illustrated by considering an analogous policy in which a population is screened to see how many cigarettes each person smoked, and then varying the intensity of advice given to each person on the importance of giving up smoking in relation to the number of cigarettes smoked—the greater the number smoked, the more intensive the counselling. This would be unlikely to attract much support even though the enquiry ('How many cigarettes do you smoke?') is simpler and cheaper than cholesterol measurement. It would probably attract no support at all if, like serum cholesterol level, the number of cigarettes smoked varied substantially within an individual from time to time (say fluctuating between 10 and 30 cigarettes per day) so that the same individual would be categorized in different bands at different times even though that person's average consumption was not materially changed.

Perhaps it is the knowledge that serum cholesterol is an important risk factor that persuades some that a form of screening, or cholesterol banding, must be worthwhile: how can a powerful risk factor fail to be a useful screening test? Again, the smoking analogy may help explain the apparent paradox. If everyone in the population smoked 20 cigarettes a day, cigarette smoking would still be an important risk factor for lung cancer, but asking people how much they smoked would be a useless screening test for the disease because it could not discriminate between those who will and those who will not develop it. If everyone smoked, but cigarette consumption varied only between 15 and 25 cigarettes per day, screening to determine cigarette consumption would have some value in distinguishing a person's risk, but it would be small and again would not be worthwhile. The position with serum cholesterol is similar, in that there is also a 'narrow window' of values over which there is only a relatively small difference in risk of CHD.

The practical reasons against cholesterol banding are academic in the face of the theoretical objections, but it is of interest to examine some of the practical implications of the US proposal. Their proposed cut-off level of 5.2 mmol/l would identify, in the UK, about three-quarters of the population aged over 34 years and these would require personal dietary counselling; their proposed cut-off level of 4.9 mmol/l for low density lipoprotein cholesterol would identify about one-fifth of the population of the same age group requiring drug treatment. The cost of the drug treatment alone would be enormous. There are about 30 million persons in the UK aged 35 years or more; if one-fifth received drug treatment, say at £350 per person per year (Table 25.4), the cost would be over £2 billion per year, increasing the present National Health Service drug expenditure by half.

Table 25.4 Costs of maintenance therapy with selected lipid lowering drugs

	Recommended adult dosage per day	Annual cost (£)
Cholestyramine (Questran)	12–24 g	456–912
Bezafibrate (Bezalip)	600 mg	116
Gemfibrozil (Lopid)	1200 mg	350
Probucol (Lurselle)	1000 mg	163
Simvastatin (Zocor)	10–40 mg	238–952

Dosages and prices taken from *MIMS*, January 1990; cited by O'Brien (1991).

CONCLUSION

Geoffrey Rose, in the 1980 Adolf Streicher Memorial Lecture cautioned the enthusiasm of screeners (Rose 1981). He drew attention to the limited public health gains that may result from the 'high-risk' prevention strategy. His assessment is confirmed by the large overlap in the cholesterol distributions among persons who do and do not develop a major CHD event and supports the conclusion that adult serum cholesterol screening is not worthwhile. In any case, there is no point in screening a population to identify a proportion who would benefit from a particular course of action if the same action would benefit everyone at no extra cost.

Data on the within-person and between-person variation in serum cholesterol values similarly reveals the inadequacy of using serial cholesterol measurements to monitor genuine changes in average cholesterol levels, Cholesterol monitoring is also not worthwhile. This is not to say that it is not worthwhile changing one's diet to reduce the risk of CHD. A substantial reduction in risk can be achieved with dietary change (Table 25.3), but measuring cholesterol does not adequately test achievement in an individual. Knowing one's serum cholesterol level may be appealing and help motivation in the short term, but with the recognition that the dietary advice is, for practical purposes, the same whatever the cholesterol level, the public is liable to feel misled about the setting up of general cholesterol testing. Cholesterol banding is also not justified; it does not sufficiently separate people into different categories, each requiring different advice, and it may encourage complacency or false reassurance to people in lower bands.

Various national and international expert committees have considered the value of cholesterol testing, for example the National Cholesterol Education Program (1988) in the USA, the European Atherosclerosis Society (1988), the British Hyperlipidaemia Association (Shepherd *et al.* 1987), the Royal College of General Practitioners (Waine 1988), the Faculty of Community Medicine of the Royal College of Physicians (Smith *et al.* 1989), and the Standing Medical Advisory Committee (1990) in the UK. Some committees recommend general screening, others recommend opportunistic testing (the testing of persons already presenting to a doctor for other reasons), and only one, Smith *et al.* 1989 recommends no screening at all. Some programmes recommend graded interventions depending upon the initial cholesterol band. Many reports state that the individual and population strategies are complementary rather than being alternatives, implying that both are worthwhile. The position is confused and without consensus apart from a well-intentioned desire to offer cholesterol testing on some basis or other. The British Standing Medical Advisory Committee on Blood Cholesterol Testing and Treatment concluded cautiously that 'some programmes of opportunistic blood cholesterol testing and treatment have the potential to make a cost-effective contribution to coronary heart disease prevention while others are likely to perform less well' (Standing Medical Advisory Committee 1990).

While the position on any matter of public policy needs to be reviewed in the light of new information, the answers to the main questions on serum cholesterol screening and on general serum cholesterol testing for other reasons are available from existing data, and conclusions can be reached from these data if they are examined in the appropriate way. It is not an issue of 'More research is needed', as some expert committees have suggested, but one of interpreting the results of research that has already been completed.

The reduction of serum cholesterol levels in the population is one of the most important public health priorities in most economically developed countries. Adult cholesterol screening, monitoring, or banding should not form part of a nation's public health programmes designed to reduce serum cholesterol and the associated morbidity and mortality. Asserting that the individual and population strategies are complementary rather than alternatives is unhelpful since there is no evidence that one adds to the effect of the other. Indeed one may subtract from the effect of the other if people with cholesterol levels below the screening cut-off level regarded themselves as 'not at risk' and therefore with no need to improve their diet. Speculation on this should not detract from the unanimous recommendation that collective public health action on dietary change is needed.

ACKNOWLEDGEMENTS

I thank Malcolm Law and Christopher Frost for their helpful comments and suggestions and Tiesheng Wu for his help preparing the three figures.

REFERENCES

European Atherosclerosis Society (1988). The recognition and management of hyperlipidemia in adults: a policy statement of the European Atherosclerosis Society. *Eur. Heart J., 9*, 571–600.

Jamrozik, K., Vessey, M., Fowler, G., Wald, N. J., Parker, G., and van Vunakis, H. (1984). Controlled trial of three different antismoking interventions in general practice. *Br. Med. J., 288*, 1499–503.

Law, M. and Wald, N. J. (1991). By how much does serum cholesterol reduction lower ischaemic heart disease mortality. In preparation.

National Cholesterol Education Program (1988). Report of the National Cholesterol Education Program Expert Panel on Detection, Evaluation and Treatment of High Blood Cholesterol in Adults. *Arch. Intern. Med., 148*, 36–69.

O'Brien, B. J. (1991). *Cholesterol and coronary heart disease: consensus or controversy?*, Office of Health Economics, London.

Pocock, S. J., Shaper, A. G., and Phillips, A. N. (1989). Concentrations of high density lipoprotein cholesterol, triglycerides, and total cholesterol in ischaemic heart disease. *Br. Med. J., 298*, 998–1002.

Pooling Project Research Group (1978). Relationship of blood pressure, serum cholesterol, smoking habit, relative weight and ECG abnormalities to incidence of major coronary events: final report. *J. Chron. Dis., 31*, 201–306.

Rose, G. (1981). Strategy of prevention: lessons from cardiovascular disease. *Br. Med. J., 282*, 1847–51.

Shepherd, J., Betteridge, D. J., Durrington, P., Laker, M., Lewis, B., Mann, J., *et al.* (1987). Strategies for reducing coronary heart disease and desirable limits for blood lipid concentrations: guidelines of the British Hyperlipidemia Association. *Br. Med. J., 295*, 1245–6.

Smith, W. C. S., Kenicer, M. B., Maryon Davis, A., Evans, A. E., and Yarnell, J. (1989). Blood cholesterol: is population screening warranted in the UK? *Lancet*, **i**, 372–3.

Standing Medical Advisory Committee (1990). *Blood cholesterol testing. Report to the Secretary of State for Health,* Department of Health, London.
Thompson, S. G. and Pocock, S. J. (1990). The variability of serum cholesterol measurements: implications for screening and monitoring. *J. Clin. Epidemiol.,* **43**(8), 783–9.
Waine, C. (1988). *The prevention of coronary heart disease,* Royal College of General Practitioners, London.

26

Assessing the evidence: risks and benefits

L. H. Kuller

The evolution of our success in reducing mortality and morbidity from cardiovascular diseases (Thom *et al.* 1985; Beaglehole 1990) has proceeded through three critical stages.

1. The first was the descriptive natural history studies (Keys 1970; Connor and Connor 1972) that documented the substantial variation in mortality, morbidity, pathology (Solberg and Strong 1983), and risk factors among populations. The importance of these risk factors was then carefully documented by further animal experimental studies (Steinberg 1989) and in unique genetically susceptible high risk populations (Brown and Goldstein 1990).

2. The analytical epidemiological studies such as the Framingham Heart Study (Gordon *et al.* 1977), the Whitehall Study (Rose *et al.* 1977), and many others (Stamler 1979) further documented the consistent relationship between the risk factors and subsequent cardiovascular and cerebral vascular diseases. A new generation of analytical epidemiological studies is now evaluating finer discriminators of the key risk factors such as lipoproteins, apoproteins, insulin, clotting factors, and certain behavioural attributes (Pyörälä 1979; Solberg and Strong 1983; Meade *et al.* 1986; Steinberg 1989).

3. Finally, randomized clinical trials have clearly documented the effectiveness of lowering total or low-density-lipoprotein cholesterol (LDL-cholesterol) on coronary heart disease (CHD) mortality, morbidity (Malenka and Baron 1989; Holme 1990; Rossouw *et al.* 1990), and the progression of atherosclerosis (Blankenhorn *et al.* 1990). We are now entering a new and exciting era that promises to have an even greater impact on cardiovascular and cerebral vascular diseases through prevention of the elevation of the risk factors or eliminating them altogether in order to minimize the extent of underlying pathology and subsequent disease in the population.

There are still a few sceptics who doubt the value of treating high blood cholesterol levels (US Congress 1989; Palca 1990). The evidence of the efficacy of treating high risk populations is overwhelming, and it is counter-productive to continue to conduct numerous clinical trials that document the benefits of lowering LDL-cholesterol in hyperlipidaemic individuals to demonstrate the incidence or reduction in mortality due to CHD.

We have previously proposed that atherosclerosis, the basic underlying pathology of CHD, be considered as an example of a common source epidemic (Kuller and Orchard 1988). The common source, i.e. the agent, is the amount and type of fat in the diet and dietary cholesterol. Environmental factors include other life-style factors such as cigarette smoking, alcohol intake, physical activity, and certain behavioural attributes.

The most important risk factors associated with the environmental determinants are obesity, body fat distribution, and insulin metabolism. Distribution of and amount of body fat, insulin resistance, and/or presence of diabetes play an important role in lipoprotein metabolism, especially triglyceride and high density lipoprotein cholesterol (HDL-cholesterol) metabolism, and probably also play a role in determining blood pressure levels.

Host susceptibility is determined by genetic influence on lipoprotein metabolism, insulin and glucose metabolism, diabetes, obesity, and vessel wall metabolism. In many cases clinical CHD depends on another critical stage, the development of a thrombus and an acute narrowing or occlusion of a coronary artery.

There are several important aspects of this model. First, without the common source, i.e. dietary intake of cholesterol and fat and relatively high blood cholesterol or LDL-cholesterol levels, the other risk factors are of much less importance in terms of the development of atherosclerosis or clinical CHD. Thus we can identify populations in the world in which cigarette smoking is prevalent and high blood pressure is very common, and yet the extent of CHD is low (Connor and Connor 1986). Second, the most successful approach to the control of the epidemic is by reducing or eliminating the causal agent, i.e. fat and cholesterol in the diet, especially in the susceptible host (Williams *et al.* 1986). Susceptibility, however, is a relative term. Individuals exposed to the same common source may respond with very different levels of total cholesterol and LDL-cholesterol (Beynen and Katan 1987) and, most important, exhibit variation in extent of atherosclerosis at any level of LDL-cholesterol or total cholesterol.

The population response to the common source can be measured by the mean and distribution of the LDL-cholesterol and total cholesterol levels in the population (Kris-Etherton *et al.* 1988), the extent of atherosclerosis (Solberg *et al.* 1980; Solberg and Strong 1983), and the subsequent incidence and mortality due to clinical cardiovascular diseases, including myocardial infarction and sudden CHD deaths. The relationship between total cholesterol or LDL-cholesterol and the risk of either atherosclerosis or CHD at the population level tends to be linear (Solberg *et al.* 1980;

Martin *et al.* 1986) and persists down to relatively low cholesterol levels (Martin *et al.* 1986).

Individuals at the high end of the distributions of blood pressure, cholesterol, etc. are at very high risk, but contribute relatively few cases to the total burden of cardiovascular disease in the population.

The association between the LDL-cholesterol or blood total cholesterol levels, extent of atherosclerosis, and especially dietary intake of cholesterol and fat is not very good at the individual level, i.e. for predicting the extent of individual's atherosclerotic disease. For example, in the Multiple Risk Factor Intervention Trial (MRFIT) (Fig. 26.1) the screenees, aged 35–57, were followed for 10 years. The CHD mortality was 1.4 per cent for men with a cholesterol level of 200–209 mg per cent and 4.3 per cent for men with a cholesterol level greater than 300 mg per cent. Therefore the relative risk was about four-fold. However, the absolute difference was only 3 per cent. Thus, over 10 years, an individual with a cholesterol level greater than 300 mg per cent would have a 4:100 chance of dying of a heart attack, while an individual with a cholesterol level of 200–209 mg per cent would have a 1:100 chance. The addition of such factors as cigarette smoking and elevated blood pressure to the risk profile (Stamler *et al.* 1989) will substantially increase the risk for a relatively small number of individuals. For the majority of individuals, however, we do not presently have the tools to determine whether any individual with a serum cholesterol level of 240 mg per cent will or will not have atherosclerotic disease until they develop some clinical manifestations. In the 10 year follow-up of the MRFIT screenees, about 25 per cent of CHD deaths occurred in individuals with screening cholesterol levels of 200 mg per cent or less and over

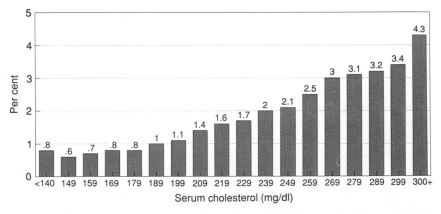

Fig. 26.1 Percentage of MRFIT screenees ($n = 361\,662$) who died from CHD by serum cholesterol level at screen after 10 years of follow-up.

half occurred in men with cholesterol levels of 240 mg per cent or less. It is an unfortunate presumption that an individual with a cholesterol level of around 200 mg per cent is immune to atherosclerosis and CHD, i.e. he is non-susceptible. Such a notion has developed from a statistical concept of relative risk rather than from an understanding of susceptibility within a common source epidemic. Unfortunately, about 60 per cent of CHD deaths occur outside hospital (Kuller *et al.* 1989), and probably about 20 per cent of new heart attacks are sudden and unexpected deaths.

Prevention of a heart attack must be the cornerstone of an effective cardiovascular programme. As has been the situation with other common source epidemics in the past, we must identify groups of individuals at risk, i.e. populations, and reduce or eliminate the common source for most in order to benefit the smaller number of individuals at risk of a heart attack, especially sudden CHD death.

There are several reasons for our inability to identify individual risk. The ability to measure differential exposure to the common source is not very good. Within-individual variability is almost as great as, if not greater than, between-individual measures of saturated fat and cholesterol in the diet (Beaton *et al.* 1979; Jacobs *et al.* 1979). We have depended on natural experiments, i.e. comparing populations differing in their possible exposure to the common source, migrant studies, or studies of unique religious or social characteristics of populations, to evaluate the exposure to the common source and disease.

The risk of developing atherosclerosis is a function of the LDL-cholesterol or total cholesterol level and the duration of exposure (Masuda and Ross 1990). Thus, with increasing age, a higher percentage of the population has extensive atherosclerotic disease and is at risk of a heart attack, accounting for the increase in CHD incidence and mortality with age.

Clearly, if the model of dose times duration in a common source epidemic is correct with regard to the development of atherosclerosis in a genetically susceptible host, then the first, most successful, approach for reducing the extent of heart attack or CHD deaths would be to prevent the rise in total or LDL-cholesterol with increasing age. Second, environmental exposures such as smoking, determinants of elevated blood pressure, etc. should be decreased, and, third, better identification of the susceptible host is important. The susceptible host can probably be better identified via specific abnormalities of lipoprotein metabolism, non-invasive methods of measuring atherosclerosis, and the study of genetic polymorphism.

The selection of specific cut-points of cholesterol as high or low is arbitrary. The basic goal of such a classification is to be able to identify subgroups of individuals who need more aggressive treatment, especially pharmacological therapy, because they are believed to be at higher risk of developing the disease and therefore warrant the cost and potential risks of pharmacological therapy (Malenka and Baron 1989).

There has been some concern about lowering blood total cholesterol or LDL-cholesterol levels and especially about the attempt to modify cholesterol levels for individuals who are not at very high risk. The primary concern has been whether lowering cholesterol will increase risk of other diseases, especially cancer, suicide, accidents, or homicide. Investigators have argued that only very high risk individuals, i.e. those with LDL-cholesterol levels greater than 160 mg per cent or with other substantial risk factors such as smoking or elevated blood pressure, should be candidates for either pharmacological or non-pharmacological treatment (Toronto Working Group on Cholesterol Policy 1990). The proponents based their arguments on three observations.

1. Most of the clinical trials that have attempted to evaluate the effects of lowering cholesterol by diet or drugs have failed to demonstrate a decrease in total mortality (US Congress 1989) and therefore, if the CHD death rates have declined in such trials, there must be an increase in other causes of death to compensate for the failure to show a decline in total mortality.

2. There is some evidence that all-cause mortality rates are higher at the lower end of the cholesterol distribution and this may relate to deaths from cancers, accidents, and respiratory and liver disease (Fig. 26.2).

3. Cholesterol is an important precursor of hormones and is involved in cell metabolism.

Many of these issues related to low cholesterol and disease were discussed at a conference in Bethesda, MD, 9–10 October 1990. The problems of using all-cause mortality as an end-point in primary prevention trials is that

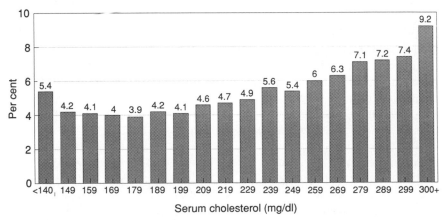

Fig. 26.2 Percentage of MRFIT screenees ($n = 361\,662$) who died from all causes by serum cholesterol level at screen after 10 years of follow-up.

probably only cigarette smoking, as a unique risk factor, and measures of socio-economic class and education are good predictors of the age-specific all-cause mortality among a random sample of healthy adults. Approximately one-third of the deaths in 'a healthy population' will be due to CHD. A 20 per cent reduction in CHD deaths in such a trial would therefore result in an approximate 6 per cent reduction in total mortality. Most primary prevention trials are therefore unlikely to show a substantial effect on all-cause mortality. In some of the trials, there may even be no difference or excess mortality from other 'causes' than cardiovascular diseases. This excess mortality would be spread over a variety of diseases, but would be especially focused on diseases associated with the major determinants of excess mortality, i.e. smoking, respiratory disease, lung cancer, accidents, suicide, etc., and with low socio-economic class.

It is probable that individuals at high risk of CHD will continue to remain at high risk of other diseases as their risk of CHD decreases (Rose and Shipley 1990). For example, individuals who have both a high LDL-cholesterol level and smoke cigarettes are at substantial increased risk of CHD mortality. If risk is reduced by lowering the LDL-cholesterol, then it is possible that they remain at excess risk of lung cancer and respiratory disease and develop these diseases during the trial. Therefore it is possible that some invididuals protected against CHD death in the intervention group may die of another at-risk disease such as cancer, diabetes, etc.

The lack of change in total mortality should therefore not be interpreted as a measure of the ineffectiveness of interventions to lower cholesterol on life expectancy, but rather that changes in many types of behaviour are required in order to reduce total mortality substantially. It is unlikely that any single intervention, except perhaps smoking cessation, will have an effect on total mortality and life expectancy in adults (Ockene *et al.* 1990).

Secondary prevention trials (Malenka and Baron 1989) include individuals who already have clinical heart disease. Most of the subsequent deaths will be due to CHD. There is a high correlation between the reduction of CHD and total mortality.

Another major problem with the evaluation of mortality in primary prevention trials is the measurement of subclinical disease at baseline. The incubation period, or perhaps the latency period to clinical diagnosis, is long for many diseases, especially cancer. Individuals with subclinical disease are likely to be recruited into clinical trials, and may develop clinical disease and die within the short time period of the trial. In MRFIT, for example, there was a substantial reduction in CHD mortality among participants who stopped smoking, but no change in lung cancer mortality over 10 years comparing ex-smokers and continued smokers, or between special intervention and the usual care groups (Ockene *et al.* 1990). It is possible that many of the smokers who developed lung cancer even 7–10 years after the trial began had subclinical disease at entry to the trial and would be unlikely to benefit from the effects of smoking cessation during the trial. Much longer follow-up of these high risk men would therefore be required to ascertain the effectiveness of smoking cessation and other interventions on cancer risk.

There is obviously a possibility that drugs used to treat hyperlipidaemia may have adverse effects that could increase mortality and morbidity (Muldoon *et al.* 1990; Dalen 1991). Furthermore, the possible adverse effects of these drugs may be noted only after many years of follow-up. Pharmacological therapy is much more effective than dietary interventions in lowering cholesterol levels, and is therefore indicated for individuals at high risk based on their cholesterol level or other risk factors. It is extremely important in all pharmacological studies of lipid lowering that audits of deaths from other causes be carefully done both during and following the trial to determine the remote possibility that excess mortality from a cancer or from some other disease is not directly related to the therapy (Wysowski and Gross 1990). The evidence to date that lipid-lowering drugs are causally related to cancer or other diseases is weak. Longer follow-up and post-trial and marketing surveillance must be continued in order to evaluate possible adverse effects.

The relationship between benefit, i.e. reduction of mortality and morbidity and potential adverse effects including cost and morbidity, is extremely important in determining the best approach to reducing cholesterol levels, especially for primary prevention of CHD. The choices include non-pharmacological therapy, drugs, or some combination of non-pharmacological and pharmacological therapy.

At any level of blood cholesterol or LDL-cholesterol there will be a distribution of individuals with varying degrees of atherosclerosis. For example, at a blood cholesterol level of 240 mg per cent, perhaps half the middle-aged men would have little atherosclerosis and would not benefit from any reduction of their blood cholesterol levels, at least within the usual time of a clinical trial, i.e. 5–10 years. They would possibly benefit in the future if the progression of atherosclerosis could be slowed. Perhaps another 25 per cent of individuals in this sample will have moderate disease and are more likely to benefit from the intervention, although again this may take a period of time, possibly after the termination of a trial. Finally, there will be 25 per cent of the population who have sufficiently extensive disease that the intervention would be effective within the 5–10 years of the study. If the intervention was 50 per cent effective in reducing CHD risk among this 25 per cent as compared with the controls, then the overall benefit in the trial would only be 50 per cent times the 25 per cent at risk, or 12.5 per cent, which is the amount of reduction observed in some clinical trials.

The percentage of individuals likely to benefit in a clinical trial will therefore depend on the distribution of the extent of atherosclerotic disease. Studies that have included individuals with very high cholesterol levels, or individuals who have subclinical or clinical CHD, will almost certainly include a high percentage of individuals with extensive coronary atherosclerosis. They are more likely to benefit in terms of a difference between the intervention and control group (Malenka and Baron 1989; Holme 1990; Rossouw *et al.* 1990), especially in short-term intervention trials. Similarly, those trials which have the greatest effect in reducing the lipid levels are most likely to see a benefit in terms of reduction of risk of disease.

In the long term, however, the prevention of the progression of atherosclerosis will have a greater impact on CHD incidence or mortality (PDAY 1990). The clinical trials usually do not follow individuals long enough to identify the clinical effects of the prevention of the progression of atherosclerosis and disease. There has been a misinterpretation of the data suggesting that intervention for individuals whose cholesterol levels are not considered to be high, i.e. greater than 240 mg per cent or LDL-cholesterol greater than 160 mg per cent, do not require change in 'the common source' or risk factors.

The second major issue is whether a low cholesterol level in the population is a marker for increased risk of other diseases, especially cancer, suicide, homicide, etc. The possible association of low cholesterol and disease has been noted primarily in analysis of large cohorts followed for many years, such as the Framingham Study (Sorlie and Feinleib 1982), NHANES (Schatzkin *et al.* 1987), the Scottish Heart Study (Isles *et al.* 1989), and MRFIT (Sherwin *et al.* 1987). For example, in the 10 year follow-up of the MRFIT screenees, the total mortality was 5.4 per cent in those with a cholesterol level less than 140 mg per cent, declining to 3.8 per cent for those with a cholesterol level between 170 and 179 mg per cent and then increasing so that men with cholesterol levels of 300 mg per cent or more had a 10 year mortality of 9.1 per cent (Fig. 26.2). In MRFIT, as well as in other studies, several diseases were noted to be related to low cholesterol levels, especially some of the cancers, such as lung cancer and colon cancer, chronic respiratory diseases, suicide, homicide, and liver disease.

There are several important steps for evaluating the relationship between low cholesterol and disease. It is necessary to determine first the reasons for the low cholesterol levels (Table 26.1), second the association of low cholesterol with other attributes that may increase or decrease the risk of disease, and third the specific diseases that might be associated with low cholesterol levels.

As noted, the distribution of cholesterol levels is a function of genetics or host susceptibility to the common source and to the other environmental factors, especially caloric balance, weight gain and loss, glucose–insulin metabolism, and alcohol consumption.

Table 26.1 Possible explanations of low blood cholesterol level

Random variation	Acute effects	Existing disease	'True' low cholesterol (persistently low)
Biological Laboratory	Weight loss Infection High alcohol intake	Liver disease Cancer	(a) Genetic factors Apoprotein polymorphisms Modification of RAS proteins
			(b) Environmental factors Diet Toxic exposures?
			Reduced β-carotene levels (increased susceptibility)
			Environmental exposures to carcinogens Cigarette smoking Occupational
			Elevated risk of cancer

The distribution of cholesterol levels in the population is, in reality, a series of cholesterol distributions for each specific genetic polymorphism such as the apo-E polymorphism (Eichner *et al.* 1989). For example, the mean cholesterol for individuals with Apo E4*3 may be 15–20 mg higher than that for individuals with Apo E3*2. An individual with a cholesterol level of 190 mg per cent might be in the 30th percentile for the Apo E3*2 polymorphism and in the 20th percentile for Apo E4*3. There are probably other polymorphisms that also affect the distribution of cholesterol levels (Goldstein and Brown 1990). The effects of any specific polymorphism on the distribution of the cholesterol in the population would be a function of the prevalence of the specific genotype or phenotype and the differences in cholesterol level between one phenotype and another. At the extreme end of the distribution there are primarily major gene effects such as familial hypercholesterolaemia (Brown and Goldstein 1990).

It is also possible that genetic polymorphisms may affect the distribution of cholesterol levels by modifying the other environmental factors, such as obesity, body fat distribution, insulin–glucose metabolism, and diabetes. It is also very possible that genetic factors that contribute to low cholesterol levels may also relate to the susceptibility to other diseases. The most likely reason for this is that lipoproteins are important in the transport of many fat-soluble substances such as retinoids and other fat-soluble vitamins and therefore may be involved in the prevention of cancer or other diseases (Peto *et al.* 1981; Russell-Briefel *et al.* 1985).

A second reason why a low cholesterol level may be related to other diseases is the direct effect of various environmental factors on cholesterol level. It is probably unlikely that a very low cholesterol level, i.e. below 150 or 140 mg per cent, in an average US or European population is primarily due to a low cholesterol or low fat diet, except perhaps among vegetarians.

The blood cholesterol level for men increases from about 180 mg per cent at age 20–24 to about 225 mg per cent at age 45–54. The LDL-cholesterol level among women increases at a later age. An important determinant of this increase in cholesterol is probably weight gain (Berns *et al*. 1989; Kuller *et al*. 1990). Men who do not gain weight or lose weight between adolescence and age 45 may not have an increase in their cholesterol level and possibly have a persistent low cholestereol level. Factors that affect weight gain, such as cigarette smoking or excess alcohol intake, as well as genetic factors that may relate to individual metabolic differences may contribute to the distribution of weight gain and the prevalence of low serum cholesterol levels.

There is also evidence that cytokines may have an acute effect on cholesterol levels and could be related to the low cholesterol levels seen among individuals with malignancy and certain infectious diseases. The immune responses early in the development of cancer may contribute to the fall in the serum cholesterol level even before the cancer is clinically apparent.

Behavioural attributes such as smoking or excess alcohol intake, low body weight, or chronic inflammatory response may relate to both low serum cholesterol levels and increased risk of disease. There are two ways of evaluating these associations. First, if low cholesterol is a risk factor for disease, then the mortality and morbidity due to that specific disease should be higher in populations that have an average low serum cholesterol level due to major differences in exposure to the common source—cholesterol and fat intake. To date there is no evidence of a clear relationship between low cholesterol in the population and the risk of such diseases as suicide, homicide, accidents, lung cancer, etc. The only direct association of possible relevance is the relationship between low cholesterol level and cerebral haemorrhage (Iso *et al*. 1989). Second, we also need a model to explain the relationship between low cholesterol and disease. The relationship should be consistent after controlling for other risk factors. Unfortunately, most of the reported studies have not evaluated other risk factors.

The study of individuals with very low cholesterol levels is very important, because some of these individuals may have unique genetic polymorphisms that result in a low cholesterol level. The identification of these polymorphisms and a further understanding of lipoprotein metabolism could provide a valuable insight into possible treatment of individuals with high cholesterol levels. For example, it may be important to carry out feeding experiments among individuals with very low cholesterol levels and to determine their response to a high fat and cholesterol diet. We may need to evaluate the effects of caloric intake or weight change on the specific genetic lipoprotein abnormalities and metabolic factors that account for the low cholesterol. It is also probable that the majority of these individuals with low cholesterol levels will have relatively little atherosclerosis. However, they might have a genetic metabolic abnormality in which their low LDL-cholesterol is a risk factor for significant atherosclerotic disease.

It is possible that individuals with low cholesterol levels who are exposed to environmental agents such as cigarette smoking or other environmental carcinogens may really have an increased risk of disease related to the association of low cholesterol and other biochemical parameters. A low cholesterol level, as noted, may result in inadequate transport of antioxidants, vitamins, etc. that may lead to an increased risk of disease given exposure to specific environmental agents. The key risk factor is environmental exposure, with the effect of low cholesterol being a measure of host susceptibility because of reduced antioxidant transport. Trying to increase the cholesterol level in these individuals without modifying environmental exposure, for example cigarette smoking, may be counterproductive. It would obviously be much more logical to attack the environmental exposures such as smoking.

In the future it may be possible to determine *in vivo* whether an individual is susceptible to the common source (dietary fat and cholesterol) in terms of the extent of atherosclerosis, and to plan specific therapies in relationship to the extent of atherosclerosis rather than on the blood cholesterol or LDL-cholesterol level or lipoprotein profile. Until we reach this goal, however, we shall continue to have to intervene on a large percentage of the population.

Atherosclerosis is a chronic pathological process that in most cases does not necessarily result in clinical disease without concomitant thrombosis. Thrombosis is probably not important in the development of clinical CHD in the absence of the underlying coronary atherosclerotic disease. Further knowledge of lipoprotein metabolism will provide a much better rationale for identifying the interrelationship among the common source, environmental factors, and the development of atherosclerotic diseases.

These new approaches will enhance our ability to categorize individuals into various risk strata and probably to provide better pharmacological and possibly non-pharmacological therapy. In the long run, however, it is probable that the relatively simplistic approach of changing dietary fat and cholesterol levels will have the largest effect on atherosclerosis and risk of CHD across the entire bood cholesterol distribution. The emphasis in the future must be more on preventing the risk factor elevations than either treating the elevated risk factors or therapies after incident clinical disease.

REFERENCES

Beaglehole, R. (1990). International trends in coronary heart disease mortality, morbidity, and risk factors. *Epidemiol. Rev.,* **12,** 1–15.

Beaton, G. H., Milner, J., Corey, P., McGuire, V., Cousins, M., Stewart, E., *et al.* (1979). Sources of variance in 24-hour dietary recall data: implications for nutrition study design and interpretation. *Am. J. Clin. Nutr.,* **32,** 2546–59.

Berns, M. A. M., DeVries, J. H. M., and Katan, M. B. (1989). Increase in body fatness as a major determinant of changes in serum total cholesterol and high density lipoprotein cholesterol in young men over a 10-year period. *Am. J. Epidemiol.,* **130,** 1109–22.

Beynen, A. C. and Katan, M. B. (1987). Individuality of the response of serum cholesterol to dietary cholesterol. In *Atherosclerosis and cardiovascular diseases* (eds S. Lenz and G. C. Descovich), MTP Press, pp. 273–8. Boston.

Blankenhorn, D. H., Johnson, R. L., Mack, W. J., El Zein, H. A., and Vailas, L. I. (1990). The influence of diet on the appearance of new lesions in human coronary arteries. *J. Am. Med. Assoc.,* **263,** 1646–52.

Brown, M. S. and Goldstein, J. L. (1990). Lipoprotein receptors: therapeutic implications. *J. Hypertension,* **8,** S33–6.

Chappell, D. A. and Spector, A. A. (1991). Lipoprotein and lipid metabolism: basic and clinical aspects. In *Lipids and Women's Health* (ed. G. P. Redmond), Springer-Verlag, New York, pp. 21–38.

Connor, W. E. and Connor, S. L. (1972). The key role of nutritional factors in the prevention of coronary heart disease. *Prev. Med.,* **1,** 49–83.

Connor, W. E. and Connor, S. L. (1986). Dietary cholesterol and fat and the prevention of coronary heart disease: risks and benefits of nutritional change. In *Diet and prevention of coronary heart disease and cancer* (eds B. Hallogren, O. Levin, S. Rossner, and B. Vessby), Raven Press, New York, pp. 113–47.

Dalen, J. E. (1991). Detection and treatment of elevated blood cholesterol. What have we learned? *Arch. Intern. Med.,* **151,** 25–8.

Eichner, J. E., Kuller, L. H., Ferrell, R. E., and Kamboh, M. I. (1989). Phenotypic effects of apolipoprotein structural variation on lipid profiles: II. Apolipoprotein A-IV and quantitative lipid measures in the Healthy Women Study. *Genet. Epidemiol.,* **6,** 493–9.

Goldstein, J. L. and Brown, M. S. (1990). Regulation of the mevalonate pathway. *Nature, Lond.,* **343,** 425–30.

Gordon, T., Castelli, W. P., Hjortland, M. C., Kannel, W. B., and Dawber, T. R. (1977). Predicting coronary heart disease in middle-aged and older persons. The Framingham Study. *J. Am. Med. Assoc.,* **238,** 497.

Holme, I. (1990). An analysis of randomized trials evaluating the effect of cholesterol reduction on total mortality and coronary heart disease incidence. *Circulation,* **82,** 1916–24.

Isles, C. G., Hole, D. G., Gillis, C. R., Hawthorne, V. M., and Lever, A. F. (1989). Plasma cholesterol, coronary heart disease, and cancer in the Renfrew and Paisley survey. *Br. Med. J.,* **298,** 920–4.

Iso, H., Jacobs, D. R., Wentworth, D., Neaton, J. D., and Cohen, J. (1989). Serum cholesterol levels and six-year mortality from stroke in 350,977 men screened for the Multiple Risk Factor Intervention Trial. *New Engl. J. Med.,* **320,** 904–10.

Jacobs, D. R., Jr, Anderson, J. T., and Blackburn, H. (1979). Diet and serum cholesterol: do zero correlations negate the relationship? *Am. J. Epidemiol.,* **110,** 77–87.

Keys, A. (ed.) (1970). Coronary heart disease in seven countries. *Circulation,* **41,** I–1.

Kris-Etherton, P. M., Krummel, D., Russell, M. E., Dreon, D., Mackey, S., Borchers, J., *et al.* (1988). The effect of diet on plasma lipids, lipoproteins, and coronary heart disease. *J. Am. Diet. Assoc.,* **88,** 1373–400.

Kuller, L. H. and Orchard, T. J. (1988). The epidemiology of atherosclerosis in 1987: unraveling a common-source epidemic. *Clin. Chem.,* **34,** B40–8.

Kuller, L. H., Traven, N. D., Rutan, G. H., Perper, J. A., and Ives, D. G. (1989). Marked decline of coronary heart disease mortality in 35–44 year-old white men in Allegheny County, Pennsylvania. *Circulation,* **80,** 261–6.

Kuller, L. H., Meilahn, E. N., Gutai, J., Cauley, J., Wing, R. R., Matthews, K. A., *et al.* (1990). Lipoprotein, estrogens, and the menopause. In *The menopause—biological and clinical consequences of ovarian failure: evolution and management* (ed. S. G. Korenman), Serono Symposia, Norwell, MS.

Malenka, D. J. and Baron, J. A. (1989). Cholesterol and coronary heart disease: the attributable risk reduction of diet and drugs. *Arch. Intern. Med.,* **149,** 1981–5.

Martin, M. J., Browner, W. S., Hulley, S. B., Kuller, L. H., and Wentworth, D. (1986). Serum cholesterol, blood pressure, and mortality: implications from a cohort of 361,662 men. *Lancet,* **ii,** 933–6.

Masuda, J. and Ross, R. (1990). Atherogenesis during low level hypercholesterolemia in the nonhuman primate. I. Fatty streak formation. *Arteriosclerosis,* **10,** 164–77.

Meade, T. W., Mellows, S., Brozovic, M., Miller, G. J., Chakrabarti, R. R., and North, W. R. S. (1986). Haemostatic function and ischaemic heart disease: principal results of the Northwick Park Heart Study. *Lancet,* **ii,** 533–7.

Muldoon, M. F., Manuck, S. B., and Matthews, K. A. (1990). Lowering cholesterol concentrations and mortality: a quantitative review of primary prevention trials. *Br. Med. J.,* **301,** 309–14.

Ockene, J. K., Kuller, L. H., Svendsen, K. H., and Meilahn, E. (1990). The relationship of smoking cessation to coronary heart disease and lung cancer in the Multiple Risk Factor Intervention Trial (MRFIT). *Am. J. Publ. Health,* **80,** 954–8.

Palca, J. (1990). Getting to the heart of the cholesterol debate. *Science,* **247,** 1170–1.

(PDAY) Pathobiological Determinants of Atherosclerosis in Youth Research Group (1990). Relationship of atherosclerosis in young men to serum lipoprotein cholesterol concentrations and smoking. *J. Am. Med. Assoc.,* **264,** 3018–24.

Peto, R., Doll, R., Buckley, J. D., and Sporn, M. B. (1981). Can dietary beta carotene materially reduce human cancer rates? *Nature, Lond.,* **290,** 201–8.

Pyörälä, K. (1979). Relationship of glucose tolerance and plasma insulin to the incidence of coronary heart disease: results from two population studies in Finland. *Diabetes Care,* **2,** 131–41.

Rose, G. and Shipley, M. (1990). Effects of coronary risk reduction on the pattern of mortality. *Lancet,* **i,** 275–7.

Rose, G., Reid, D. D., Hamilton, P. J. S., McCartney, P., Keen, H., and Jarrett, R. J. (1977). Myocardial ischaemia risk factors and death from coronary heart disease. *Lancet,* **i,** 105.

Rossouw, J. E., Lewis, B., and Rifkind, B. M. (1990). The value of lowering cholesterol after a myocardial infarction. *New Engl. J. Med.,* **323,** 1112–19.

Russell-Briefel, R., Bates, M. W., and Kuller, L. H. (1985). The relationship of plasma carotenoids to health and biochemical factors in middle-aged men. *Am. J. Epidemiol.,* **122,** 741–9.

Schatzkin, A., Hoover, R. N., Taylor, P. R., Ziegler, R. G., Carter, C. L., Larson, D. B., *et al.* (1987). Serum cholesterol and cancer in the NHANES I epidemiologic follow-up study. *Lancet,* **ii,** 298–301.

Sherwin, R. W., Wentworth, D. N., Cutler, J. A., Hulley, S. B., Kuller, L. H., and Stamler, J. (1987). Serum cholesterol levels and cancer mortality in 361,662 men screened for the Multiple Risk Factor Intervention Trial. *J. Am. Med. Assoc.,* **257,** 943–8.

Solberg, L. A. and Strong, J. P. (1983). Risk factors and atherosclerotic lesions: a review of autopsy studies. *Atherosclerosis,* **3,** 187–98.

Solberg, L. A., Enger, S. C., Hjermann, I., Helgeland, A., Holme, I., Leren, P., *et al.* (1980). Risk factors for coronary and cerebral atherosclerosis in the Oslo Study. In *Atherosclerosis V* (eds A. M. Gotto, L. C. Smith, and B. Allen), Springer-Verlag, New York, pp. 57–62.

Sorlie, P. D. and Feinleib, M. (1982). The serum cholesterol–cancer relationship: an analysis of time trends in the Framingham Study. *J. Nat. Cancer Inst.,* **69,** 989–96.

Stamler, J. (1979). Population studies. In *Nutrition, lipids, and coronary heart disease* (eds R. I. Levy, B. M. Rifkind, B. H. Dennis, and N. Ernst), Raven Press, New York, p. 72.

Stamler, J., Neaton, J. D., and Wentworth, D. N. (1989). Blood pressure (systolic and diastolic) and risk of fatal coronary heart disease. *Hypertension,* **13,** I-2–12.

Steinberg, D. (1989). The cholesterol controversy is over. Why did it take so long? *Circulation,* **80,** 1070–8.

Thom, T. J., Epstein, F. H., Feldman, J. J., and Leaverton, P. E. (1985). Trends in total mortality and mortality from heart disease in 26 countries from 1950 to 1978. *Int. J. Epidemiol.,* **14,** 510–20.

Toronto Working Group on Cholesterol Policy (1990). Asymptomatic hypercholesterolemia: a clinical policy review. *J. Clin. Epidemiol.,* **43,** 1103–12.

U.S. Congress, Office of Technology Assessment (1989). *Costs and effectiveness of cholesterol screening in the elderly, Paper 3,* Superintendent of Documents, US Government Printing Office, Washington, DC.

Williams, R. R., Hasstedt, S. J., Wilson, D. E., Ash, K. O., Yanowitz, F. F., Reiber, G. E., *et al.* (1986). Evidence that men with familial hypercholesterolemia can avoid early coronary deaths: an analysis of 77 gene carriers in four Utah pedigrees. *J. Am. Med. Assoc.,* **255,** 219–24.

Wysowski, D. K. and Gross, T. P. (1990). Deaths due to accidents and violence in two recent trials of cholesterol-lowering drugs. *Arch. Intern. Med.,* **150,** 2169–72.

27

Assessing the evidence: the role of meta-analysis

S. J. Pocock and S. G. Thompson

THE RATIONALE FOR META-ANALYSIS

There are many important issues in aetiology, prevention or treatment of cardiovascular diseases where it is unrealistic to expect any single study to provide a definitive conclusion. The key limitations of any one study are the following:

(1) its limited size, so that any statistical associations cannot be determined with sufficient precision;

(2) its specific selection of study subjects and treatment schedules, so that findings cannot be readily generalized to a broader population and class of treatments of interest.

The assessment of evidence from a collection of closely related studies of the same therapeutic, preventive, or aetiological issue has been undertaken in narrative-style reviews for many decades, but such an informal approach suffers from a reliance on subjective expert opinion, and is unable to quantify any overall statistical conclusion. Hence it has become increasingly recognized that a more objective means of combining evidence from related studies is needed to provide a clearer and less contentious overall picture. Accordingly, *meta-analysis methods* (sometimes known as *overviews*) have been developed and enthusiastically presented for a wide range of specific applications, particularly concerning cardiovascular disease. In particular, meta-analysis has enabled a clearer understanding of many therapeutic issues, such as antiplatelet therapy in the prevention of major cardiovascular morbidity and mortality, reduction in mortality due to thrombolysis after myocardial infarction, reduction in risk of stroke and coronary heart disease (CHD) by treatment of mild hypertension, and the value of rehabilitation with exercise after myocardial infarction.

The leading proponents of meta-analyses have devoted considerable energy to both the reporting and the dissemination of meta-analysis findings. However, the passionate conviction with which their case has been presented has not always been readily adopted by the broader medical fraternity, and there are many leading clinical experts (and also some medical editors) who express considerable scepticism about the meta-analysis approach, both in general and in specific examples.

Whereas meta-analysis can be defined as 'an objective quantitative method for combining evidence from separate but similar studies', there is a more critical view that meta-analysis comprises 'statistical tricks which make unjustified assumptions in producing oversimplified generalizations out of a complex of disparate studies'!

In this chapter, our aim is to provide a critical appreciation of the role of meta-analysis in clinical and epidemiological research. We hope to achieve the following:

(1) to enhance a greater sense of realism as to when and how meta-analysis can usefully be undertaken;

(2) to clarify some of the specific statistical issues that fundamentally affect all meta-analyses, paying particular attention to the potential heterogeneity between studies;

(3) to encourage a spirit of constructive criticism in the interpretation and practical application of the results of meta-analysis.

THE CRITERIA FOR A MEANINGFUL META-ANALYSIS

For a meta-analysis to make any sense, the most fundamental requirement is that all the studies included must have sufficient common ground in terms of the scientific question being studied. For instance, in clinical trial meta-analyses there are three key considerations:

similarity of treatments;
similarity of patients;
similarity of end-points.

Perhaps the greatest difficulty raised by sceptics with regard to meta-analysis concerns the clinical heterogeneity inherent in any collection of studies. No two study protocols are identical and meta-analyses often contain considerable variation in all three of the above features, so how can one justify formal statistical techniques for combining their results?

The counter-argument in support of meta-analysis requires a clear distinction between the objectives of the individual study and the meta-analysis. The individual study is concerned with a specific and precise set of circumstances, and so its conclusions, based on conventional statistical inference, are of limited generalizability. However, a meta-analysis is concerned with achieving much broader conclusions relating to a major issue of practical relevance. Consequent problems of interpretation are discussed later, but we should not dismiss lightly the worthy intent of meta-analysis to derive a coherent, objective, and global conclusion out of a mix of related studies. It is valuable to consider whether the differences between studies are so great as to overwhelm their broad commonality of intent, and this is now illustrated further with regard to the above three key features in clinical trials.

Similarity of treatments   One of the earliest meta-analyses in cardiovascular disease studied the effect on mortality of beta-blockers after myocardial infarction (Baber and Lewis 1982). It combined data from trials using different beta-blockers, on the basis that all such drugs had a common mode of action and hence it was plausible to ask questions about the generic term 'beta-blocker drugs'. However, it was thought important to separate 'early' use of beta-blocker immediately after the infarct from 'later' use commencing after the initial few days by presenting two separate meta-analyses. The underlying principle here is to define, preferably in advance, the criteria for what constitutes 'adequate' similarity of treatments.

Similarity of patients   We expect all trials in a meta-analysis are of the same disease condition, though details of patient selection may differ. For instance, in recent trials of thrombolysis after myocardial infarction there are differences in patient entry requirements (e.g. on electrocardiogram (ECG) criteria and age limits for inclusion), but these differences would not generally be considered sufficiently radical to invalidate combining the trials' results into an overall assessment of mortality reduction due to thrombolysis. A more difficult judgement arose in the meta-analysis of secondary prevention trials of antiplatelet therapy (Antiplatelet Trialists' Collaboration 1988) in that the potential benefits of aspirin and other antiplatelet drugs could relate to patients with a wide range of cardiovascular diseases, including cerebrovascular disease, myocardial infarction, and unstable angina. Here it is sensible to proceed in two stages, first presenting a combined estimate of treatment effect from trials of patients in each disease category (e.g. myocardial infarction) and then combining the results of all trials into a single overall estimate. The latter step could then be ignored (or receive less emphasis) by those readers who are unhappy with such clinical heterogeneity. Similar 'stagings' of meta-analysis arise in trials of cholesterol-lowering for prevention of cardiovascular events, where in addition to a global meta-analysis we could group trials according to (a) drug therapy or non-drug intervention and (b) primary or secondary prevention.

Similarity of end-points   It would seem essential that all trials are studying the same outcome measures of patient response. In meta-analyses of mortality or major cardiovascular events this is not usually a serious problem, even though some differences in definition or validation of events and causes of death are likely to exist. However, if outcome measures are more subjective and less well defined, there is greater scope for variation between trials. For instance, in trials of drug therapy for critical limb ischaemia it will be more difficult to obtain adequate uniformity of response criteria for outcomes such as ulcer healing and relief of rest pain. Another variation is in the length of follow-up over which events and/or deaths are observed. If the magnitude of treatment effect varies over time, then some uniformity of follow-up time is desirable. Thus, in a thrombolysis meta-analysis it is important to distinguish between short-term (e.g. up to 1 month) and longer-term mortality. However, in trials of longer-acting continuous therapy (e.g. mild hypertension trials) variation in follow-up time may be less important.

The premise that sophisticated statistical analysis can never rescue poor study design applies to meta-analysis just as it does to individual studies. Thus, the value of a meta-analysis is also totally dependent on the quality and completeness of its constituent studies. In meta-analyses of clinical trials we require each individual trial to conform to acceptable standards of clinical trial design so that serious biases are unlikely to exist and estimates of treatment differences are only subject to sampling variation. For instance, it would be unacceptable to include non-randomized trials, and we might require that the data from all trials be analysed according to the intention to treat principle. Also, in meta-analyses of drug therapy, trials which were not double-blind might be excluded if lack of blinding could influence the end-point of interest. Similarly, in meta-analyses of observational studies, we require each individual study to have taken adequate account of confounding factors and other potential biases. It has been suggested that clinical trials can be graded as to their quality (Chalmers *et al.* 1981), and in principle meta-analyses could be presented 'cumulatively' starting with the best quality trials and including others sequentially. However, in practice we would suggest predefinition of minimally acceptable standards in a single meta-analysis presentation.

A particularly important influence on the reliability of a meta-analysis is the extent to which it is able to include all studies of an acceptable standard. For instance, if one relies on published studies only, there is a serious danger of publication bias, i.e. studies with more positive findings are more likely to be published because of the selection processes used by both investigators and medical journals. Overcoming such problems is no easy matter, and some of the most notable achievements in meta-analysis, for example in antiplatelet therapy (Antiplatelet Trialists' Collaboration 1988) and breast cancer adjuvant therapy (Early Breast Cancer Trialists' Collaborative Group 1990), have been made possible by extensive collaborations of investigators in both completed and ongoing trials, who have provided up-to-date information for all trials in a unified manner appropriate for meta-analysis.

The identification of all published trials is in itself fraught with difficulty. For instance, a comprehensive literature search based on Medline requires an experienced knowledge of essential keywords (Hewitt and Chalmers 1985), but even so such Medline searches are liable to miss some published studies (Dickersin *et al*. 1985). A particularly exciting development in perinatal medicine has been the establishment of an exhaustive computerized register of all published trials, from which meta-analyses can readily be undertaken (Chalmers *et al*. 1989). Similar ongoing exercises in other clinical fields should be actively encouraged.

Overall, the unbiased selection of studies for inclusion in a meta-analysis is of great importance. One can never be fully assured that completeness is achieved, but some judgement may be exercised as to the potential bias in any given field. For instance, thrombolysis after myocardial infarction or cholesterol lowering in primary prevention are major topics of interest for which all large trials will be published regardless of their findings, whereas other less fashionable areas of research with much smaller trials (e.g. symptomatic improvement in intermittent claudication) are much more prone to publication bias.

DATA DISPLAY IN A META-ANALYSIS

The two statistical objectives of meta-analysis are as follows:

(1) to display the separate findings for each study in a uniform manner;

(2) to combine these data into an overall assessment of the strength of evidence for treatment effect, using significance tests and estimation methods.

The second and more controversial aspect is considered in the next section, but first we wish to focus on the very important contribution that consistent data display makes in understanding the overall evidence. Indeed, for many meta-analyses a well-informed insight into how to interpret such displays of the data from all the individual studies makes the reader able to reach his own sensible conclusions without having to rely on the formality of statistical techniques.

Consider the meta-analysis of antiplatelet treatment for secondary prevention of vascular disease (Antiplatelet Trialists' Collaboration 1988), and for simplicity let us confine attention to the 13 cerebrovascular trials (mostly for patients who have already had a transient ischaemic attack) and the end-point 'major cardiovascular event' which includes stroke, myocardial infarction, and other vascular death.

The most crucial achievement is to obtain reliable basic data for all trials as shown in Table 27.1.

Table 27.1 Basic data for 13 trials of antiplatelet treatment in cerebrovascular disease

	Ratio of number of patients with major cardiovascular event to total number of patients	
Trial identifier	Antiplatelet treatment group	Control group
ESPS	182/1250	264/1250
UK-TIA	348/1621	204/814
AICLA	61/400	48/204
CCSG	101/446	30/139
Swedish stroke	60/253	55/252
McMaster	49/222	57/225
Toulouse	24/284	17/156
AITIA	26/153	35/150
Toronto[a]	34/143	38/147
DCS	22/101	27/102
Stoke[b]	24/85	19/84
Tennessee[b]	21/73	25/75
German TIA	2/30	3/30

[a] Deaths only.
[b] Excluding myocardial infarction.
Adapted from Antiplatelet Trialists' Collaboration (1988).

Most meta-analyses have been based on such 'event data', for which the proportion of patients in each treatment group experiencing the 'event' is obtained. It is then necessary to choose an appropriate scale for estimating the treatment effect, for which there are three choices: odds ratios, risk ratios, or differences in proportions. The difference in proportions is often unsuitable, since larger differences can be expected in trials with higher risk subjects or longer periods of follow-up. Odds ratios and risk ratio analyses give very similar results if the proportion experiencing an event is relatively small (say, less than 20 per cent). Odds ratios are more commonly used, both because of the statistical theory for combining estimates of odds ratios and because the techniques can readily be extended to survival data in which the time of each patient's follow-up is taken into account.

The consequent visual display of odds ratios and their 99 per cent confidence intervals is shown in Fig. 27.1. Such a figure, with one row of information for each trial, is the most common display technique used in meta-analysis and has several features worth further discussion.

1. *Point estimates* of treatment effect in each trial are given by the centre of each square and the odds ratio scale is given at the foot of the figure. For instance, for the first trial (ESPS) the odds ratio derived from Table 27.1 is

$$\frac{182/(1250-182)}{264/(1250-264)} = 0.64$$

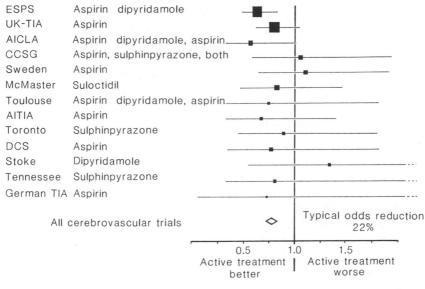

Fig. 27.1 Odds ratios (active treatment:control) for first stroke, myocardial infarction, or vascular death during the scheduled treatment period in completed antiplatelet trials: —■—, trial results and 99 per cent confidence intervals (area of ■ is proportional to the amount of information contributed); ◇ overview result and 95 per cent confidence interval (explained in the text). The solid vertical line represents an odds ratio of unity (no treatment effect).

Alternatively, this could be stated as an estimated 36 per cent reduction in odds of a major cardiovascular event attributed to antiplatelet treatment. The number of point estimates less than unity, i.e. 'active treatment better', is a crude initial guide to the overall conclusion. In this case 10 out of 13 trials had proportionately fewer events in the antiplatelet treatment groups.

2. *Confidence intervals* for each trial's estimate are a valuable means of expressing the statistical uncertainty inherent in each trial. Large trials (e.g. ESPS and the UK-TIA trial) provide more reliable estimates so that their confidence intervals are narrower, whereas other very small trials in Fig. 27.1 have very wide confidence intervals. This meta-analysis has used 99 per cent confidence limits, whereas other choices (e.g. 95 or 90 per cent) could be made. In fact, 95 per cent and 70 per cent confidence correspond to approximately two standard errors and one standard error respectively and can both be used in the same diagram (Pocock and Hughes 1990). It should be noted that confidence limits for odds ratios are not symmetric about the point estimate, but symmetry would occur with use of a logarithmic scale.

3. *The amount of information* in each trial is essentially determined by the number of events in it (both groups combined). Perversely, trials with wide confidence intervals, which contain less information, can be more noticeable to the eye when looking at Fig. 27.1. Hence, to reverse this misperception, point estimates are given at the centres of squares whose areas are proportional to the amount of information contributed. Also, it is helpful to present trials in order of amount of information, i.e. the most reliable data are given at the top of Fig. 27.1.

4. *Significance tests* for each trial can be deduced from the confidence intervals. For instance, a 99 per cent confidence interval completely on one side of unity, as in the ESPS trial, corresponds to $p < 0.01$ (two-sided test). Use of 95 per cent confidence intervals in Fig. 27.1 would have resulted in the confidence intervals of the next two trials being wholly less than unity, thus demonstrating that the three largest trials had $p < 0.05$. However, significance testing in individual trials should receive little emphasis in meta-analyses since it tends to make an artificial distinction between 'significant' and 'non-significant' trials. Also, any 'meta-analysis of p values' is an inefficient method of combining evidence which fails to allow for the fact that statistical significance depends on both the observed magnitude of the effect and the size of the trial.

5. *Evidence for statistical heterogeneity* between trials can be informally assessed by studying the degree of overlap among the confidence intervals. For instance, in Fig. 27.1 no two confidence intervals are distinct, and indeed all intervals cover odds ratios from around 0.6 to 0.8. This would suggest that there is no substantial evidence for statistical heterogeneity.

Thus a thorough inspection of individual trial findings, as in Fig. 27.1, can reveal a great deal about the nature of a particular meta-analysis before one proceeds to more formal statistical analysis.

STATISTICAL METHODS FOR COMBINING EVIDENCE

In reaching an overall statistical conclusion from a meta-analysis, one concentrates on the point estimates of treatment effect in the trials, taking account of the amount of information in each trial. One hopes that there is no evidence of any real differences between the point estimates beyond what could be attributed to random (sampling) variation, and in the absence of such statistical heterogeneity there exist standard 'fixed-effect' methods for obtaining a weighted average of the point estimates of the trials.

In fact, there are a number of closely related statistical methods for this fixed-effect approach. Without going into technical details, it is worth giving a brief outline of the alternatives.

1. *Woolf's method* produces a weighted average of the logarithmic odds ratios, with the weights being inversely proportional to the variances of the logarithmic odds ratios (Woolf 1955). This method is simple to calculate, producing an overall point estimate and confidence interval on the logarithmic scale from which estimates for the odds ratio can be obtained by taking antilogarithms. The method is reliable, except when the meta-analysis is largely based on trials with very small numbers of events.

2. The *Mantel–Haenszel method* produces a weighted average of the odds ratios, with the weights being approximately proportional to the variances of the odds ratio (Mantel and Haenszel 1959). While it is simple to obtain a pooled point estimate of the odds ratio, the most reliable formula for obtaining an overall confidence interval is more complicated (Robins *et al.* 1986). However, with modern computing packages such as StatXact, such calculational difficulties can be overcome.

3. The *Peto method* obtains for each trial the expected number of events in the active treatment group, under the null hypothesis that active treatment has no effect. For instance, if a trial has equal numbers of patients in active treatment and control this expected number is half the total number of events observed in both groups. The total cumulative number of observed events across all trials in the active treatment group can then be compared with the total number of expected events in the active treatment group, and formulae are available which enable the difference between observed and expected totals to be converted into an approximate overall odds ratio estimate together with a confidence interval. Collins *et al.* (1985) give an explanatory example.

In practice, all three fixed-effect methods usually produce remarkably similar pooled estimates and confidence intervals, particularly if a meta-analysis is based on a reasonably substantial totality of data. Comparable fixed-effect methods exist for other measurement scales such as risk ratios, differences in proportions, or differences in means of a quantitative outcome measure.

It should be noted that none of these methods is simply pooling the data of all the trials together as if they were from one huge trial. The separate identity of each trial is preserved, and it is the estimates of effect from each trial that are combined in an appropriately weighted manner.

In the antiplatelet therapy example in Fig. 27.1 the pooled odds ratio estimate is 0.78 with 95 per cent confidence interval from 0.68 to 0.88. This can be re-expressed as an estimated 22 per cent reduction in the odds of a cardiovascular event, due to antiplatelet therapy, with a 95 per cent confidence interval from 12 to 32 per cent, as shown by the diamond-shape at the foot of Fig. 27.1.

The interpretation of this combined estimate would be straightforward if we were prepared to assume that all the trials were homogeneous, in the sense that all were really estimating the same true magnitude of treatment effect. However, any meta-analysis will contain some clinical heterogeneity between trials. For instance, the antiplatelet trials are of different drugs and have some differences in patient entry criteria, length of follow-up, and recording of cardiovascular events. Hence it is more plausible that the trials differ sufficiently to be estimating different true magnitudes of effect. The extent to which this matters in terms of statistical heterogeneity can be assessed by performing a statistical test of heterogeneity (DerSimonian and Laird 1986). Such a heterogeneity test examines whether the individual trial point estimates vary about the overall pooled estimate to a greater extent than could be expected by the chance (sampling) error attributable to each trial's limited size. In the antiplatelet example the heterogeneity test has $p = 0.3$, indicating no evidence of statistical heterogeneity between the trials.

However, the interpretation of any non-significant heterogeneity test requires caution. Heterogeneity tests lack statistical power, so that usually they can only detect marked statistical differences between trials. For instance, if the true odds ratios in the antiplatelet trials varied between 0.7 and 0.9, say, it would be rather unlikely that a formal heterogeneity test would reveal such subtle differences. Thus lack of statistical evidence for heterogeneity does not establish that the trials are homogeneous.

A particularly interesting example is a meta-analysis (overview) of the two aspirin primary prevention trials in US physicians (Steering Committee of the Physicians' Health Study Research Group 1989) and British physicians (Peto *et al.* 1988). The larger US trial showed a 41 per cent reduction in the odds of non-fatal myocardial infarction (95 per cent confidence interval, 26–53 per cent reduction), whereas the British trial had only an observed 2 per cent reduction in odds (95 per cent confidence interval, 13 per cent reduction to 12 per cent increase). The heterogeneity test is significant ($p = 0.03$), and this discrepancy between trial findings may have been accentuated by the early closure of the more significant trial. Clearly, some apprehension remains as to how to interpret the combined estimate of 33 per cent odds reduction and a high level of statistical significance ($p = 0.0002$), particularly in view of the major differences in trial designs and the fact that non-fatal myocardial infarction was not a prespecified primary end-point.

Therefore in most meta-analyses it is realistic to assume that the inherent clinical heterogeneity amongst the trials is liable to result in some modest degree of statistical heterogeneity, which may well be undetectable by formal testing. Given the clinical common ground that justifies a meta-analysis, we could argue that different trial circumstances may often lead to modest differences in true magnitudes of effect, but that the direction of effect is likely to be the same in all trials.

Such a realistic scenario regarding heterogeneity affects how we interpret the fixed-effect methods.

1. The *overall significance test* for treatment effects (e.g. the Mantel–Haenszel test) is valid in examining departure from the global null hypothesis that every trial has no true difference between treatment and control groups. However, if we have a mix of trials, of which some contain 'effective' treatments and others do not, we might still reach a highly significant overall test. Thus overall significance does not automatically enable a blanket conclusion that the treatment effect existed in all the different trial circumstances. A certain leap of faith is required in order to infer any general conclusion of widespread efficacy, and the plausibility of such broad extrapolation of a 'significant' meta-analysis will depend particularly on the degree of clinical homogeneity across the trials.

2. The *overall point estimate* of treatment effects is an estimate of a weighted average of the (possibly different) true treatment effects in the individual trials. In that sense, it is wise to consider it as estimating a 'typical' odds ratio that can be achieved by such a mode of therapy in the broad class of patients encompassed in the meta-analysis. As such, it can be a useful simple guide to the overall degree of treatment benefit. However, it is not an accurate estimate of the treatment benefit to be achieved in any particular trial circumstance. That would be a naive oversimplification ignoring the variety of treatments and patients included in the meta-analysis.

3. The *overall confidence interval* for the treatment effect expresses the degree of statistical precision achieved in the weighted average point estimate of a 'typical' effect. It takes into account the random (sampling) variation within each trial, but does not allow for any potential variation in magnitude of true effect between trials (or between treatments or types of patient). Thus we might argue that this confidence interval is artificially narrow in terms of extrapolating to future patients since it fails to consider the inherent clinical heterogeneity which might plausibly result in some statistical heterogeneity. Nevertheless, such confidence intervals are a useful expression of the overall weight of evidence upon which the point estimate is based.

In an informal literature search of recent published meta-analyses of treatment in cardiovascular disease, we have found little evidence of statistical heterogeneity despite the substantial clinical heterogeneity present in some of them. This is partly due to the lack of statistical power inherent in such tests, but on a more positive note it may reflect the fact that many therapeutic policies in cardiovascular disease have a consistent benefit that applies to a broad class of patients. This general lack of serious statistical heterogeneity adds some plausibility to the fixed-effect methods for combining trial evidence in the cardiovascular field, provided that the caveats mentioned above are not forgotten.

However, statistical heterogeneity has been found in some other applications of meta-analysis, such as prophylactic sclerotherapy for portal hypertension (Pagliaro *et al.* 1989), use of diuretics in preventing toxaemia in pregnancy (Collins *et al.* 1985), and the relation between low serum cholesterol and cancer (Law and Thompson 1991). Random effects models (DerSimonian and Laird 1986) have been proposed to incorporate such heterogeneity into the overall estimates of association. By assuming that the available studies in the meta-analysis are a random sample from a hypothetical population of studies, it is possible to express heterogeneity in terms of a between-study variance in treatment effects. This is then considered in addition to the usual sampling variation within trials in deriving an estimate of the average effect across all trials. Such random effect methods can be used in any meta-analysis, but in the absence of statistical heterogeneity they will agree closely with the fixed-effect methods.

If heterogeneity is present, random effects methods will produce wider confidence intervals and usually a less pronounced level of statistical significance, thus incorporating an appropriate degree of statistical caution. However, random effects methods give more even weight to the different studies (i.e. they take less account of study size), and this can unduly emphasize data from small studies which are often more prone to both design flaws and publication bias. Also, the rather peculiar premise that the studies themselves are a random sample, and the inability to estimate the between-study variance with precision are further weaknesses that inhibit the placing of too much reliance on random effects models. Perhaps we should recommend that they be used as an adjunct to fixed-effects methods when a meta-analysis is based on a substantial number of studies which exhibit some degree of statistical heterogeneity.

More importantly, if statistical heterogeneity exists, we could question the meaningfulness of any overall estimate. Our efforts might be better directed towards obtaining an understanding of *why* heterogeneity is present, since we appear to have violated the underlying premise that the studies have sufficient common ground to merit combining their evidence.

The statistical methods described in this section have been illustrated only by clinical trial meta-analyses. However, the same set of techniques can be applied equally well to meta-analyses of aetiological associations in observational epidemiology. A greater variation in study designs, including grossly different study samples and different ways of expressing associations and adjusting for confounders, may be encountered in observational study applications. This may increase the prospect of the presence of statistical heterogeneity, which inhibits the usefulness of a straightforward fixed-effect method of analysis in observational meta-analyses.

DISCUSSION AND CONCLUSIONS

It has long been recognized that (a) the narrow perspective and limited size of any single study of a therapeutic or aetiological issue and (b) the potentially distorted perspectives of informal literature reviews have both been deterrents to the ability to extend medical research findings into widely used health practices. The proponents of meta-analysis have pressed their objective methodology for overviewing evidence as a major new achievement (Mann 1990). For instance, Tom Chalmers has stated that 'meta-analysis is going to revolutionize how sciences, especially medicine, handle data. And it's going to be the way many arguments will be ended'.

Both the scale and the objectivity of meta-analysis have the scope to remove the idiosyncratic ways in which many medical issues are evaluated. Some supposed advances receive undue emphasis because excessive attention is focused on the most significant in a collection of studies, while other important advances have gone unrecognized because of the paucity of evidence available in any one study. The strengths of meta-analysis have been highlighted in a substantial number of cardiovascular disease applications, especially in the identification of modest but important therapeutic advances applicable to large numbers of patients (Yusuf et al. 1988).

However, we fear that the forceful, at times dogmatic, and potentially oversimplistic style adopted in some meta-analysis presentations has had rather a negative reception by some clinical opinion-leaders, who perhaps feel that insufficient attention is being given to interpretation, particularly as regards clinical heterogeneity. On the other hand, too much attention on study differences can be a destructive pastime which seriously interferes with the task of using the common ground across related studies to derive the overall evidence that practitioners believe is of relevance to their patients and their health policies.

One important consideration is to ensure that meta-analysis findings are not extrapolated beyond the patient and treatment circumstances within which they were derived. For instance, in an unpublished meta-analysis of cholesterol-lowering trials it has been inferred that each 1 per cent reduction in serum cholesterol results in an estimated 2 per cent reduction in coronary events. This finding was given considerable emphasis in a recent report concerning UK national policy on cholesterol screening and intervention (Standing Medical Advisory Committee 1990). However, this meta-analysis estimate cannot be automatically extrapolated to the new class of cholesterol-lowering drugs (co-reductase inhibitors) which can reduce mean serum cholesterol by about 30 per cent, nor can it be extrapolated to policies of cholesterol reduction in the elderly, since neither issue is adequately represented in the evidence in the trials.

In summary, meta-analysis is a valuable technique which has rightly helped in the assimilation of evidence and the determination of policy in a wide range of cardiovascular disease issues. In this chapter, our aim has been to provide a constructive critique of both practical and statistical issues in meta-analysis. Our overall conclusion is that meta-analysis should not be viewed as an exact statistical science guaranteed to provide simple statistical answers to complex clinical issues. Meta-analysis should instead be viewed as a *descriptive semi-quantitative* technique which should be applied judiciously and self-critically, paying due regard to the strengths, weaknesses, and variations in the individual studies comprising the meta-analysis.

REFERENCES

Antiplatelet Trialists' Collaboration (1988). *Br. Med. J.,* **296,** 320–31.

Baber, N. S. and Lewis, J. A. (1982). *Br. Med. J.,* **284,** 1749–50.

Chalmers, I., Inken, M., and Keirse, M. J. N. C. (1989). *Effective care in pregnancy and childbirth,* Oxford University Press.

Chalmers, T. C., Smith, H., Blackburn, B., Silverman, B., Schroeder, B., Reitman, D., *et al.* (1981). *Controlled Clin. Trials,* **2,** 31–49.

Collins, R., Yusuf, S., and Peto, R. (1985). *Br. Med. J.,* **290,** 17–23.

DerSimonian, R. and Laird, N. (1986). *Controlled Clin. Trials,* **7,** 177–88.

Dickersin, K., Chan, S. S., Chalmers, T. C., Sacks, H. S., and Smith H. (1985). *Controlled Clin. Trials,* **6,** 306–17.

Early Breast Cancer Trialists' Collaborative Group (1990). *Treatment of early breast cancer,* Oxford University Press.

Hewitt, P. and Chalmers, T. C. (1985). *Controlled Clin. Trials,* **6,** 168–77.

Law, M. and Thompson, S. G. (1991). *Cancer Causes and Control,* **2,** 253–61.

Mann, C. (1990). *Science,* **249,** 476–80.

Mantel, N. and Haenszel, W. (1959). *J. Natl Cancer Inst.,* **22,** 719–48.

Pagliaro, L., Burroughs, A. K., Sorensen, T. I. A., Labrec, D., Morabito, A., and Amico, G. D. (1989). *Gastroenterol. Int.,* **2,** 71–84.

Peto, R., Gray, R., Collins, R., Wheatley, K., Hennekens, C., Jamrozik, K., *et al.* (1988). Randomised trial of prophylactic daily aspirin in British male doctors. *Br. Med. J.,* **296,** 313–19.

Pocock, S. J. and Hughes, M. D. (1990). *Statist. Med.,* **9,** 657–71.

Robins, J., *et al.* (1986). *Biometrics,* **42,** 311–23.

Standing Medical Advisory Committee (1990). *Blood cholesterol testing,* Department of Health, London.

Steering Committee of the Physicians' Health Study Research Group (1989). *New Engl. J. Med.,* **321,** 129–35.

Woolf, B. (1955). *Ann. Hum. Genet.,* **19,** 251–3.

Yusuf, S., Wittes, J., and Friedman, L. (1988). *J. Am. Med. Assoc.,* **260,** 2088–93, 2259–63.

28

Secondary prevention of coronary heart disease: drug intervention and life-style modification

L. Wilhelmsen and S. Johansson

Patients who have already suffered a coronary heart disease (CHD) event such as myocardial infarction or angina pectoris are at considerably increased risk of recurrent fatal or non-fatal events compared with healthy individuals of the same age (Weinblatt *et al*. 1968; Hagman *et al*. 1988). Protection by female sex does not continue after an infarction; prognosis is similar for men and women (Johansson *et al*. 1984). The likelihood of a recurrent event is greatest during the period immediately following infarction, after which risk levels off. A post-infarction clinic in Göteborg, Sweden, has followed a large unselected series of infarct patients below age 65 after discharge from hospital. Mortality after 5 years was 19 per cent and after 10 years was 33 per cent (Ulvenstam *et al*. 1985). Fifty per cent of patients neither suffered another infarction nor died during a 10 year follow-up. Thus, although early prognosis seems poor, long-term prognosis may be reasonable.

Infarction usually occurs as a consequence of coronary atheromatosis (or spasm in a few instances) with thrombosis superimposed on that lesion, often as a result of a rupture of the plaque. Long-term prognosis is apparently dependent upon progress of atherosclerosis, and the sudden, so far unpredictable, occurrence of a new thrombus with new infarction or sudden death.

Prognosis during the first 2–3 years after infarction is mainly influenced by myocardial factors: number of previous infarcts, size of infarction, and presence of congestive heart failure, as well as ventricular arrhythmias. During long-term follow-up 'primary' risk factors such as elevated low density lipoprotein cholesterol (LDL-cholesterol) levels, elevated blood pressure, diabetes mellitus, and tobacco smoking become increasingly important.

In few diseases have clinical trials had such an impact on treatment as in the acute and long-term follow-up of infarct patients. Several overviews have been published. In the present chapter we aim to review these trials based on the overviews. The importance of applying beneficial treatments to an appropriate number of patients, as well as avoiding treatments with negative effects, is stressed. The analysis indicates a large potential benefit to a large number of patients of even moderate percentage treatment effects.

In contrast with primary prevention, drug interventions are more acceptable in secondary prevention because the benefit–side-effect potential is usually much greater. Although secondary prevention deals with patients who already have CHD, trials show that substantial benefit can be achieved. This indicates the importance of rapid processes like thrombosis for coronary events or a relatively rapid healing (regression?) of atherosclerotic plaques.

Patients with clinical CHD tend to be more strongly motivated to make life-style changes, and moderate reductions in risk factor levels can have substantial effects on their markedly increased absolute risk compared with age-matched healthy counterparts.

In the following, treatments in hospital, which often have long-term effects on prognosis, will be considered first followed by interventions during longer-term follow-up. The contribution is restricted to myocardial infarction mainly because most clinical trials have been conducted in this patient group. However, similar effects of long-term interventions are to be expected also among patients with stable (and unstable) angina pectoris.

INTERVENTIONS IN HOSPITAL

Results of trials are summarized in Table 28.1.

Thrombolytic drugs

The use of streptokinase in acute myocardial infarction was reported by Fletcher *et al.* (1958), but a number of early clinical trials in several countries failed to show a beneficial effect of that therapy. Inadequate patient numbers in the studies may be an explanation. A new era started when DeWood *et al.* (1980) confirmed the importance of coronary thrombosis in the development of myocardial infarction. Over the past 25 years intra-coronary and intravenous thrombolytic agents such as streptokinase, tissue-plasminogen activator (tPA), or anisolyated plasminogen-streptokinase activator complex (APSAC) have been compared with standard treatment in more than 30 randomized clinical trials involving a total of about 41 000 patients with suspected acute myocardial infarction. In the streptokinase studies the overall early mortality (about 2–5 weeks) was 12.8 per cent (2614/20 371) in the control group and only 10.0 per cent

Table 28.1 Effects on mortality of acute interventions in randomized clinical trials of myocardial infarction

Interventions	No. of trials	No. of patients in trials	Mortality effect (%) (95% confidence interval)
I.v. streptokinase	31	41 000	−24 (−20 to −29)
I.v. t-PA given <6 h	5	6500	−26 (−11 to −39)
I.v. APSAC given <6 h	9	2000	−52 (−33 to −65)
Aspirin	2	17 600	−21 (−13 to −28)
I.v. nitrates	10	2000	−35 (−18 to −49)
I.v. beta-blockers	27	27 000	−13 (− 2 to −25)
Lidocaine	10	8500	+11 (−16 to +46)
Calcium-channel blockers	28	19 000	+ 6 (− 4 to +18)

I.v., intravenous.

(2062/20 634) in the treatment group. The estimated reduction in risk of death was 24 per cent (95 per cent confidence interval, −20 per cent to −29 per cent; $p < 0.0001$) (Yusuf et al. 1988a). Improvements in ejection fraction and wall movement, and a decrease in enzyme indices of infarct size have also been reported.

Treatments with tPA given within 6 hours of onset of pain have resulted in a reduction in mortality of about 26 per cent (95 per cent confidence interval, −11 per cent to −39 per cent; $p < 0.001$) according to Yusuf et al. (1988a). The same authors combined data from all available trials of APSAC on a total of about 2000 patients and reported a 52 per cent reduction in mortality (95 per cent confidence interval, −33 per cent to −65 per cent; $p < 0.001$). The recent ISIS-3 trial did not demonstrate any difference in mortality of the 3 thrombolytic drugs (unpublished). Hence there is no evidence that any one of the drugs is superior to the others. All the thrombolytic drugs have a substantial effect on short-term mortality after acute myocardial infarction.

A problem with both intravenous and intracoronary streptokinase treatment has been reports of increased risk of reinfarction compared with those treated with placebo (3.3 per cent compared with 2.4 per cent; $p < 0.001$). In this context it is interesting to note that in the Second International Study of Infarct Survival (ISIS-2) these extra reinfarcts were completely prevented by additional treatment with aspirin (ISIS-2 1988).

A follow-up 12–15 months after thrombolytic therapy indicates that the early mortality reduction also persists long term, and that the early increased reinfarction rate among streptokinase-treated patients does not influence long-term mortality to any appreciable extent (Simoons et al. 1985; ISIS-2 1988). Because of the antigenic properties of streptokinase and APSAC these drugs should not be used if the patient has been treated with these drugs in the previous 1–2 years.

Antiplatelet agents

The acute effect of aspirin was studied in the ISIS trials (ISIS Pilot Study Investigators 1987; ISIS-2 1988). Mortality was reduced by 21 per cent (809/8679 in the aspirin group compared with 1013/8679 in the control group; 95 per cent confidence interval, −13 per cent to −28 per cent; $p < 0.0001$). In addition, there was a 44 per cent reduction in non-fatal myocardial infarction ($p < 0.001$) and a 36 per cent reduction in non-fatal stroke ($p < 0.01$). The effects of aspirin were shown to be additional to those of streptokinase in the ISIS-2 trial, and the combined use resulted in a 42 per cent reduction in mortality (ISIS-2 1988).

Nitrates

Nitrates, especially used in the acute setting and as intravenous infusions, reduce oxygen demand and myocardial wall stress by reducing afterload and preload, and may also have an effect by relieving coronary spasm. In about 2000 patients randomized to either nitroglycerine or nitroprusside, mortality was reduced by 35 per cent (95 per cent confidence interval, −18 per cent to −49 per cent; $p < 0.001$) (Yusuf *et al.* 1988a).

Intravenous beta-blockers

Many studies have indicated reductions in infarct size when beta-blockade is given prior to or immediately after an experimental myocardial infarction. As many as 27 randomized acute trials, including about 27 000 patients, have presented data on mortality and non-fatal myocardial infarction. Mortality reduction amounts to 13 per cent (95 per cent confidence interval, −2 per cent to −25 per cent; $p < 0.02$) according to Yusuf *et al.* (1988a). Non-fatal reinfarction and non-fatal cardiac arrests in hospital were reduced by about 19 per cent (95 per cent confidence interval, −5 per cent to −33 per cent; $p < 0.01$) and 16 per cent (95 per cent confidence interval, −2 per cent to −30 per cent; $p < 0.02$) respectively. All these end-points taken together amount to a 16 per cent reduction in the risk of serious complications, which is strongly significant. Analyses of the causes of deaths in the First International Study of Infarct Survival (ISIS-1) suggest that the reduction in mortality is due chiefly to prevention of cardiac rupture and ventricular fibrillation (ISIS-1 1988). Whereas intravenous nitrates may be given even to patients with very large and complicated myocardial infarctions, the tendency has been more conservative regarding intravenous beta-blockade although studies indicate that adverse effects are relatively uncommon (Held 1986).

Lidocaine

Lidocaine has long been used in coronary care units to prevent ventricular fibrillation. More than 8000 patients have been included in randomized trials (McMahon and Yusuf 1987). The incidence of ventricular fibrillation and fatal asystole among untreated patients was 1.4 per cent and 0.2 per cent respectively. The risk of developing ventricular fibrillation was reduced by 36 per cent (95 per cent confidence interval, -57 per cent to -6 per cent) with a doubling in the risk of fatal asystole ($p = 0.06$). Overall mortality showed an 11 per cent increase (non-significant (n.s.)). It may be that ventricular fibrillation could be prevented in some cases with high risk of such events, whereas this effect may be offset by an increased mortality from asystole in other groups of patients. The previous widespread use of lidocaine in acute myocardial infarction has now been reduced.

Calcium-channel blockers

Like beta-blocker agents the calcium blockers have beneficial effects in experimental myocardial infarction, if given prior to coronary occlusion, by reducing oxygen demand, lowering blood pressure, and reducing contractility. However, clinical experience has not been rewarding. An overview of 19 000 patients randomized in 28 trials showed mortality in the actively treated group to be 873/8870 compared with 825/8889 in the placebo group with a 6 per cent *higher* mortality in the actively treated group (95 per cent confidence interval, -4 per cent to $+18$ per cent, n.s.) according to Held *et al.* (1989). There was no evidence of a beneficial effect on infarct size or development, or on rate of reinfarction. Thus calcium-channel blockers do not seem to have preventive effects in myocardial infarction.

LONG-TERM INTERVENTIONS

Results of trials of pharmacological interventions are summarized in Table 28.2. Effects of interventions on risk factors such as plasma lipids are not listed in the table because of different effects due to variations in the magnitude of the intervention.

Lipids

Increased low density lipoprotein in plasma, whose effect is modified by levels of high density lipoprotein, is the most important risk factor for myocardial infarction and is also a risk factor for recurrence after an infarction—a secondary risk factor (Coronary Drug Project Research

Table 28.2 Effects on the mortality of long-term pharmacological interventions in randomized clinical trials of myocardial infarction

Interventions	No. of trials	No. of patients in trials	Mortality effect (%) (95% confidence interval)
Anti-arrhythmics	8	3700	+15 (+ 4 to +28)
Beta-blockers	25	23 000	−22 (−16 to −30)
Calcium-channel blockers	3	6534	+ 1 (− 6 to + 9)
Anticoagulants	6	4500	−15 (− 6 to −23)
Antiplatelets	10	18 500	−11 (− 2 to −20)

Group 1978; Ulvenstam *et al.* 1984). The relative risk of high cholesterol is smaller among infarct patients than in the general healthy population, but the excess risk attributable to increases in cholesterol levels is greater among survivors of myocardial infarction because the absolute risk of cardiac events is so much higher in these patients. Thus a cholesterol-lowering intervention among infarct patients could potentially prevent many cardiac events. Several randomized controlled clinical trials have been undertaken to determine whether diet or lipid-lowering drugs can reduce mortality in both the general population and post-infarct patients. However, many trials have been too small. An overview indicates a significant positive benefit of such interventions on CHD incidence (Holme 1990).

The pooling of lipid-lowering trials showed that 1667 out of 19 813 subjects suffered a CHD event in the treated group compared with 2191 out of 20 506 in the control group, which is a 23 per cent risk reduction (95 per cent confidence interval, −18 per cent to −28 per cent; $p < 0.0001$) according to the summary by Yusuf *et al.* (1988*b*).

The results of Brensike *et al.* (1984), Blankenhorn *et al.* (1987), and Brown *et al.* (1990), as well as those of Buchwald *et al.* (1990), support the effect in demonstrating reductions in the progression of coronary athero-sclerosis and, in the two last-mentioned studies, in the incidence of cardio-vascular events also.

It is important to advise patients on a prudent diet as soon as possible after an infarction and to remember the importance of repeated education and counselling. Depending upon the specific lipid disturbance, various hypolipaemic drugs may be given. However, for patients with more serious prognosis because of complications such as severe congestive heart failure and/or arrhythmias, other forms of interventions may receive higher *immediate* priority.

Hypertension

Several studies have shown that hypertension, treated or untreated, continues to be a risk factor after an infarction. It should be emphasized that blood pressure falls with infarction: the larger the infarction the greater the fall in blood pressure (McCall *et al.* 1979). It is logical to assume that reduction of elevated blood pressure would reduce cardiac events, but although several large trials in the general population have been performed the effect so far has been more modest than that regarding stroke (Collins *et al.* 1990). Overall, there were 885 deaths among 18 487 treated patients compared with 1014 among 18 407 controls, which is a 13 per cent reduction (95 per cent confidence interval, -3 per cent to -19 per cent; $p < 0.003$). The risk reduction for stroke was 40 per cent. No formal clinical trial comparing antihypertensive treatment with placebo has been performed in post-infarct patients. However, patients with a history of myocardial infarction who were randomly assigned to the antihypertensive treatment group in the American Hypertension Detection and Follow-up Program (Browner and Hulley 1989) had significantly reduced total mortality compared with controls.

The present approach is to treat infarct patients with the same criteria as is used in the general population with the aim of normalizing blood pressure. It is probable that patients with more or less extensive coronary stenoses are more sensitive than other people to critical blood pressure reductions, and it might therefore be advisable to reduce blood pressure more gradually when starting treatment in order to preserve coronary blood flow.

The type of antihypertensive treatment may also be important. Diuretics may affect myocardial potassium and magnesium levels and cause arrhythmias, and dosages of these agents should therefore be as low as possible. Beta-blockers, which have been found to be cardioprotective, have a natural place in the treatment of hypertensive infarct patients. Calcium-channel blockers, which are often effective in lowering blood pressure, have not had the encouraging effects on mortality expected, and are not recommended. Angiotensin-converting-enzyme-inhibitors have theoretical advantages because of their efficacy in advanced heart failure and recently reported effects in human myocardial infarction (CONSENSUS Trial Study Group 1987; Pfeffer *et al.* 1988; Sharpe *et al.* 1988).

Tobacco smoking

Tobacco smoking is a strong risk factor both for a first myocardial infarction and for fatal and non-fatal recurrences. It is advisable to stop smoking from many points of view but, so far, no controlled trial with post-infarction patients has been performed; such trials are, in fact, not feasible. Observational studies comparing smokers who continued to smoke after an infarction with smokers who quit suggest that cessation is associated with about 40 per cent lower mortality and morbidity (Åberg *et al*. 1983). Available data also indicate that this was not due to differences in other prognostic factors. Patients should be encouraged to stop smoking as soon as possible after their infarction, and should be strongly advised not to start after the natural cessation period in the coronary care unit. Those who continue to smoke after an infarction have greater difficulties in stopping later on. Even if results on morbidity and mortality after infarction are not based upon controlled trials, they indicate that this intervention is among the most powerful measures in this disease.

Diabetes mellitus

Diabetes mellitus is a risk factor for myocardial infarction as well as a strong predictor of mortality after an event (Ulvenstam *et al*. 1985). There is some evidence that improved control of the condition lowers the incidence of complications and probably also improves the prognosis, but a controlled trial has not been conducted. Non-pharmacological measures such as weight reduction, a prudent diet, and treatment of other risk factors are of particular importance in diabetic post-infarction patients.

Physical training

Low levels of physical activity, especially during leisure time, have been reported to be a risk factor for myocardial infarction in some, but not all, prospective studies in the general population (Johansson *et al*. 1988). The effects of physical training after infarction have been tested in several trials, but none has been statistically significant for mortality on its own. The nine randomized trials have been pooled, and overall there were 126 deaths among 1388 patients allocated to exercise and 152 deaths among 1321 patients allocated to the control group ($p = 0.05$) (Collins *et al*. 1984). No effect on non-fatal reinfarction was seen in these trials. Since compliance has been low to modest, the results tend to underestimate the possible effects of exercise.

There are several contra-indications to physical training, including congestive heart failure, exercise-induced arrhythmias, angina pectoris at low levels of exercise, and orthopaedic problems which make training impossible. However, physical training for half an hour three times a week at a level of 40–60 per cent of maximum exercise capacity appears to be of value. In addition to its beneficial effects on mortality, exercise also increases patients' working capacity, lowers blood pressure, and improves overall feelings of well-being (Bonanno and Lies 1974; Wilhelmsen *et al*. 1975; Goldberg *et al*. 1984).

Anti-arrhythmic drugs

Recurrent tachycardia and ventricular fibrillation are adverse prognostic signs after an infarction. Prompt recognition and treatment of these arrhythmias may prevent the development of severe ventricular dysfunction due to inadequate cardiac output. Thus it seems appropriate to try to abolish arrhythmias, including ventricular ectopic beats, by anti-arrhythmic treatment. However, several trials with anti-arrhythmic drugs have so far not yielded encouraging effects (rather the opposite) on mortality in post-infarct patients. A report of the effects in six long-term trials of anti-arrhythmic drugs indicated an increased mortality with such treatment (Furberg 1983). The IMPACT trial also showed a non-significantly higher mortality on active drug (IMPACT 1984). The recent Cardiac Arrhythmia Supression Trial (CAST) had a sensitive design to detect effects because only patients who responded to anti-arrhythmic therapy with reduced ventricular premature beats were included. However, the study showed a significantly *increased* mortality on the two anti-arrhythmic drugs encainide and flecainide compared with placebo (CAST 1989). The pooled effect on mortality in all eight trials is an increase of 15 per cent (95 per cent confidence interval, +4 per cent to +28 per cent; $p < 0.02$). Thus current experiences do not support the use of anti-arrhythmic agents for prophylaxis of sudden death in asymptomatic infarct patients.

Beta-blockers

Few interventions have attracted as much interest during the past 15 years as treatment of CHD patients with beta-blockers. The pooled evidence, including over 23 000 patients in longer-term treatment, indicates substantial benefit from such treatment. Mortality among 12 140 patients allocated to beta-blocker therapy was 7.6 per cent compared with 9.4 per cent among the 11 551 controls; the risk reduction was 22 per cent (95 per cent confidence interval, −16 per cent to −30 per cent; $p < 0.001$) according to Yusuf *et al.* (1988a). The effect is mainly seen in sudden deaths, a notion that was put forward in the early days of beta-blockade after myocardial infarction (Wilhelmsson *et al.* 1974).

Non-fatal reinfarctions were also reduced by about 27 per cent with 5.6 per cent in the beta-blocker group compared with 7.5 per cent among controls ($p < 0.001$) according to Yusuf *et al.* (1985).

Initially feared adverse effects such as heart block and induction of congestive heart failure have not been major problems when patients are appropriately monitored. When these complications occur, they are easily reversible by appropriate treatment or discontinuation of the beta-blocker. Patients with obstructive lung disease have to be excluded from the treatment. About 70 per cent of post-infarction patients aged up to 70 years of age do not have contra-indications to beta-blocker therapy (Åberg *et al*. 1984). A preventive effect with regard to mortality and morbidity can be expected for at least 2–3 years. The effect is more pronounced in patients at higher risk of death, whereas it has been difficult to show any reduction in mortality in those at low risk.

Calcium-channel blockers

Animal experiments have indicated beneficial effects on the ischaemic myocardium from various calcium-channel blocking agents. However, in human myocardial infarction, several trials have not shown any reduction in mortality or morbidity. In fact, in an overview of long-term trials, Held *et al*. (1989) found a mortality of 409 out of 3266 patients (12.5 per cent) versus 399 deaths out of 3268 (12.2 per cent) of placebo-treated patients (95 per cent confidence interval, −6 per cent to +9 per cent). In the combined acute and long-term trials the mortality was 254 out of 2409 calcium-blocked patients (10.5 per cent) versus 235 out of 2396 (9.8 per cent) placebo-treated patients. These differences are not statistically significant. While there are differences in function of the various calcium blockers, their effects on mortality and morbidity in the post-infarct patients seem rather similar (Held *et al*. 1989). The results indicate caution with regard to the prophylactic use of calcium channel-blocking drugs after myocardial infarction.

Anticoagulants

Peroral anticoagulants were commonly used in infarct patients 20–30 years ago at the time when patients were kept bedridden for 2–3 weeks or even longer. Most of the trials that were peformed in the beginning were non-randomized and small, and their validity was questioned. None of the trials individually provided clear evidence of benefit. Previous data have been pooled by Chalmers *et al*. (1977), Peto (1978), and Mitchell (1981). The conclusion is that anticoagulants reduce mortality. A recently published well-conducted Norwegian randomized trial of 1214 patients showed a clear benefit of warfarin versus placebo on both mortality and reinfarction (Smith *et al*. 1990). The pooled mortality reduction is 15 per cent (95 per cent confidence interval, −6 per cent to −23 per cent; $p < 0.001$). It is not known to what extent warfarin and similar anticoagulants convey any benefit in addition to that gained by aspirin, and the combination may lead to increased bleeding complications.

Platelet active drugs

All the long-term trials of antiplatelet agents in secondary prevention have been reviewed by the Antiplatelet Trialists Collaborative Group (1988) and Yusuf *et al.* (1988*a*). In the 10 post-infarction trials on a total of 18 441 patients, antiplatelet treatment reduced the risk of vascular death by 11 per cent (7.9 per cent in the active group compared with 8.8 per cent in the control group; $p <0.01$) and non-fatal myocardial infarction by 31 per cent (5.5 per cent and 7.4 per cent respectively; $p <0.0001$), and there was also a significant reduction of non-fatal strokes by 42 per cent ($p <0.0001$). The overview data indicated that aspirin is as effective as its combination with dipyridamol or sulphinpyrazone. Aspirin treatment is also very cheap. A problem is that the data do not answer the question of dose; from 160 to 1300 mg/day has been used in the trials. The lower dosage level, which is associated with less adverse effects such as gastro-intestinal symptoms and bleeding, seems to be as effective as the higher doses. However, from a theoretical point of view even lower doses, around 50 mg per day or less, are sufficient to induce a proper beneficial balance between thromboxane A_2 and prostacyclin I_2, and such low doses may later become recommended.

Coronary surgery

No clinical trial has specifically looked at the effect of bypass surgery in patients after a myocardial infarction, but subgroup analyses of trials in angina patients who have also suffered a myocardial infarction indicate positive effects (Califf *et al.* 1989). Thus, indications for surgery are generally the same as in uncomplicated angina pectoris. Post-infarct patients do not seem to run higher operative risks than angina patients when ordinary precautions are taken.

Psychological factors

Psychological factors including behavioural pattern and social factors, such as lack of social contacts, are associated with increased risk of myocardial infarction and an increased risk of recurrence (Ruberman *et al.* 1984; Wiklund *et al.* 1988). Irrespective of the pre-infarction social status, an infarction is a serious threat to the individual and can often be described as an 'ego infarction'. Appropriate treatment to improve the quality of life is important, and such treatment has been shown in some trials to lower the rate of recurrence (Friedman *et al.* 1984; van Dixhoorn *et al.* 1987).

Quantitative aspects of treatment and secondary prevention

The trial results cited above generally refer to single interventions. Apart from the combined effects of streptokinase and aspirin in acute infarction, little is known as to whether the effects are additive. The trial results point towards major effects on mortality in acute myocardial infarction and during 2–4 years of follow-up. It is generally believed that modern hospital treatment of myocardial infarction has had important effects on mortality in the acute phase. However, relatively few studies have looked at this with standardized methodology, taking other prognostic variables into account. It also has to be remembered that hospital mortality cannot be analysed without knowledge of out-of-hospital mortality, as well as taking the duration of hospitalization into account. A considerable proportion of total mortality from myocardial infarction and sudden coronary death in a population takes place out of hospital—before any medical care can be given. As previously shown by us (Wilhelmsen *et al.* 1989) the majority of these cases would not be detected by any screening procedure aimed at finding cases with clinically overt CHD. Estimations from both the Myocardial Infarction Register and a prospective population study among middle-aged men arrive at about 20 per cent of sudden death cases previously having had myocardial infarction or angina pectoris (Wilhelmsen *et al.* 1989). The Myocardial Infarction Register indicates a very small reduction of inhospital mortality during the period 1970–85. In parallel, a clear reduction of the 2 year mortality after discharge from hospital has been recorded, and this decline in mortality may well have been achieved by the consistent use of beta-blockade in about 70 per cent of infarct cases (Åberg *et al.* 1984).

It is important not only to demonstrate mortality reductions in clinical trials but also to apply beneficial interventions and avoid adverse effects in as many patients as possible.

Table 28.3 exemplifies effects on mortality in clinical trials, an estimation of the proportion of infarct patients which may be candidates for the treatment in question, and estimated effects on total in-hospital mortality

Table 28.3 Estimated effects on in-hospital mortality of acute interventions in patients with myocardial infarction

Interventions	Relative effect on mortality (%)	Treated patients (%)	Absolute effect[a] on mortality (%)
Thrombolysis (streptokinase, t-PA, APSAC)	−30	70	−2.5
I.v. beta-blockers	−13	20	−0.3
I.v. nitrates	−35	30	−1.3
Calcium-channel blockers	+ 6	10	+0.13[b]

[a] In-hospital mortality without intervention estimated as 12 per cent.
[b] Non-significant; see Table 28.1.

among patients with myocardial infarction up to 75 years of age. Hospital mortality has been estimated as 12 per cent without intervention. The percentage of infarct patients that can be given a drug is related to age, and contra-indications to the treatment. These practices may markedly influence the outcome of the entire group of patients.

It can be seen that thrombolytic therapy, used in 70 per cent of patients, would reduce mortality by 2.5 per cent from 12.0 to 9.5 per cent. The use of intravenous nitrates in 30 per cent of patients would reduce mortality by 1.3 per cent. Other examples are given in the table.

As previously mentioned, in several instances we do not know whether the interventions are additive; if they were, the true mortality would theoretically fall from 12 per cent to about 7 per cent.

The estimated effects on mortality of various interventions during a 2 year follow-up after myocardial infarction, not including the acute phase, are given in Table 28.4. It is evident that beta-blockers, anticoagulant drugs, and antiplatelet drugs carry important preventive potentials, whereas use of anti-arrhythmic drugs and calcium blockers may cause increased mortality.

Table 28.5 summarizes the number of lives saved (or lost) by various treatments. It takes into account different percentages of infarct patients that can be given the treatment in question. A 12 per cent in-hospital mortality and a 10 per cent 2 year mortality after an infarction is assumed.

We believe that about 50 per cent of patients are candidates for thrombolytic therapy, intravenous beta-blockade, and intravenous nitrates in the acute phase. We know from own experiences that 70 per cent of a non-selected infarct population can be given beta-blockade after an infarction (Åberg *et al.* 1984), and we estimate that 90 per cent can be given aspirin.

Table 28.4 Estimated effects of long-term interventions on 2 year mortality after myocardial infarction

Interventions	Relative effect on mortality (%)	Treated patients (%)	Absolute effect[a] on mortality (%)
Anti-arrhythmics	+15	5	+0.08
Beta-blockers	−22	70	−1.5
Calcium-channel blockers	+ 1	10	+0.01[b]
Anticoagulants	−15	20	−0.3
Antiplatelets (aspirin)	−11	95	−1.0

[a] 2 year mortality estimated as 10 per cent.
[b] Non-significant; see Table 28.2.

Table 28.5 Examples of treatment effects: number of saved/lost lives from various percentages of infarct patients treated[a]

Percentage treated	5	20	50	70	90
Acute treatment					
Thrombolysis	—	−220	−540	−760	—
I.v. beta-blockers	—	− 90	−230	−330	—
I.v. nitrates	—	−250	−630	—	—
During 2 years after MI					
Anti-arrhythmics	+20	+ 90	—	—	—
Beta-blockers	—	−130	−330	−460	—
Anticoagulants	—	− 90	−230	−320	—
Aspirin	—	− 70	−170	−230	−300

[a] In a population of 10 million persons 30 000 infarct patients per year are estimated to be candidates for treatment.
MI, myocardial infarction.

The calculations indicate substantial differences in the number of lives saved according to the proportion of infarct patients given the treatment in question. Most of the interventions are also highly cost-effective.

SUMMARY

Knowledge of the causes and natural history of CHD has contributed to our management of patients with established disease. There is increasing recognition that acute treatment as well as long-term secondary prevention play a vital role in the management and rehabilitation of survivors of myocardial infarction. In this chapter we have summarized the results of risk factor modification and clinical trials in common use on morbidity and mortality after infarction and estimated quantitative effects on mortality of various interventions. The trial results point towards substantial effects in the early phase of infarction, and during 2–4 years of follow-up. Risk factor modification has a considerable influence mainly on long-term outcome. The preventive measures reviewed were basically originated in single interventions, and potential additive effects have so far not been evaluated by formal trials except for streptokinase and aspirin. In terms of improving short- and long-term event-free survival in infarct patients, current knowledge points to a combination of pharmacological interventions and early risk factor modification.

ACKNOWLEDGEMENTS

This work was supported by grants from the Swedish Heart and Lung Foundation and the Knut & Alice Wallenberg Foundation. The excellent secretarial help by Ms Ingela Thorlin is acknowledged.

REFERENCES

Åberg, A., Bergstrand, R., Johansson, S., Ulvenstam, G., Vedin, A., Wedel, H., *et al.* (1983). Cessation of smoking after myocardial infarction. Effects on mortality after 10 years. *Br. Heart J., **49**, 416–22.
Åberg, A., Bergstrand, R., Johansson, S., Ulvenstam, G., Vedin, A., Wedel, H., *et al.* (1984). Declining trend in mortality after myocardial infarction. *Br. Heart J., **51**, 346–51.
Antiplatelet Trialists' Collaboration (1988). Secondary prevention of vascular disease by prolonged antiplatelet treatment. *Br. Med. J., **296**, 320–31.
Blankenhorn, D. H., Nessim, S. A., Johnson, R. L., Sanmarco, M. E., Azen, S. P., and Cashin-Hemphill, L. (1987). Beneficial effects of combined colestipol–niacin therapy on coronary atherosclerosis and coronary venous bypass grafts. *J. Am. Med. Assoc., **257**, 3233–40.
Bonanno, J. A. and Lies, J. E. (1974). Effects of physical training on coronary risk factors. *Am. J. Cardiol., **33**, 760–4.
Brensike, J. F., Levy, R. I., Kelsey, S. F., Passamani, E. R., Richardson, J. M., Loh, I. K., *et al.* (1984). Effects of therapy with cholestyramine on progression of coronary arteriosclerosis: results of the NHLBI Type II Coronary Intervention Study. *Circulation, **69**, 313–24.
Brown, G., Albers, J. J., Fisher, L. D., Schaefer, S. M., Lin, J.-T., Kaplan, C., *et al.* (1990). Regression of coronary artery disease as a result of intensive lipid-lowering therapy in men with high levels of apolipoprotein B. *New Engl. J. Med., **323**, 1289–98.
Browner, W. S. and Hulley, S. B. (1989). Clinical trials of hypertension treatment: implications for subgroups. *Hypertension, **13** (Suppl. I), I-51–6.
Buchwald, H., Varco, R. L., Matts, J. P., Long, J. M., Fitch, L. L., Campbell, G. S., *et al.*, for the POSCH Group (1990). Effect of partial ileal bypass surgery on mortality and morbidity from coronary heart disease in patients with hypercholesterolemia. *New Engl. J. Med., **323**, 946–55.
Califf, R. M., Harrell, F. E., Jr, Lee, K. L., Rankin, J. S., Hlatky, M. A., Mark, D. B., *et al.* (1989). The evolution of medical and surgical therapy for coronary artery disease. A 15-year perspective. *J. Am. Med. Assoc., **261**, 2077–86.
CAST (Cardiac Arrhythmia Suppression Trial) Investigators (1989). Preliminary report: effect of encainide and flecainide on mortality in a randomized trial of arrhythmia suppression after myocardial infarction. *New Engl. J. Med., **321**, 406–12.
Chalmers, T. C., Matta, R. J., Smith, H., Jr, and Kunzler, A. M. (1977). Evidence favouring the use of anticoagulants in the hospital phase of acute myocardial infarction. *New Engl. J. Med., **297**, 1091–6.

Collins, R., Yusuf, S., and Peto, R. (1984). Exercise after myocardial infarction reduces mortality: evidence from randomized controlled trials (abstract). *J. Am. Coll. Cardiol.*, **3**, 622A.

Collins, R., Peto, R., McMahon, S., Hebert, P., Fiebach, N. H., Eberlein, K. A., *et al.* (1990). Blood pressure, stroke, and coronary heart disease. Part 2, Short-term reductions in blood pressure: overview of randomized drug trials in their epidemiological context. *Lancet,* **i,** 827–38.

CONSENSUS Trial Study Group (1987). Effects of Enalapril on mortality in severe congestive heart failure. Results of the Cooperative North Scandinavian Enalapril Survival Study (CONSENSUS). *New Engl. J. Med.,* **316**, 1429–35.

Coronary Drug Project Research Group (1978). Natural history of myocardial infarction in the Coronary Drug Project: long-term prognostic importance of serum lipid levels. *Am. J. Cardiol.,* **42**, 489–98.

DeWood, M. A., Spores, J., Notske, R., Mouser, L. T., Burroughs, R., Golden, M. S., *et al.* (1980). Prevalence of total coronary occlusion during the early hours of myocardial infarction. *New Engl. J. Med.,* **303**, 897–902.

Fletcher, A. P., Alkjaersig, N., Smyrniotis, F. E., and Sherry, S. (1958). The treatment of patients suffering from early myocardial infarction with massive and prolonged streptokinase therapy. *Trans. Assoc. Am. Coll. Physicians,* **71,** 287–96.

Friedman, M., Thoresen, C. E., Gill, J. J., Powell, L. H., Ulmer, D., Thompson, L., *et al.* (1984). Alteration of type A behavior and reduction in cardiac recurrences in postmyocardial infarction patients. *Am. Heart J.,* **108,** 237–48.

Furberg, C. D. (1983). Effect of antiarrhythmic drugs on mortality after myocardial infarction. *Am. J. Cardiol.,* **52,** 32–6C.

Goldberg, L., Elliott, D. L., Schutz, R. W., and Kloster, F. E. (1984). Changes in lipid and lipoprotein levels after weight training. *J. Am. Med. Assoc.,* **252,** 504–6.

Hagman, M., Wilhelmsen, L., Pennert, K., and Wedel, H. (1988). Factors of importance for prognosis in men with angina pectoris derived from a random population sample. Multifactor Primary Prevention Trial, Gothenburg, Sweden. *Am. J. Cardiol.,* **61,** 530–5.

Held, P. (1986). Central haemodynamics in acute myocardial infarction. Natural history, relation to enzyme release and effects of metoprolol (thesis). *Acta Med. Scand.,* Suppl. 709.

Held, P., Yusuf, S., and Furberg, C. D. (1989). Calcium channel blockers in acute myocardial infarction and unstable angina: an overview. *Br. Med. J.,* **299,** 1187–92.

Holme, I. (1990). An analysis of randomized trials evaluating the effect of cholesterol reduction on total mortality and coronary heart disease incidence. *Circulation,* **82,** 1916–24.

IMPACT Research Group (1984). International mexiletine and placebo anti-arrhythmic coronary trial. I. Report on arrhythmia and other findings. *J. Am. Coll. Cardiol.,* **4,** 1148–63.

ISIS Pilot Study Investigators (1987). Randomized factorial trial of high dose streptokinase, of oral aspirin and of iv aspirin in acute myocardial infarction. *Eur. Heart J.,* **8,** 634–42.

ISIS-1 Collaborative Group (1988). Mechanisms for the early mortality reduction produced by beta-blockade started early in acute myocardial infarction. *Lancet,* **i,** 921–3.

ISIS-2 Collaborative Group (1988). Randomized trial of intravenous streptokinase, oral aspirin, both, or neither among 17 187 cases of suspected myocardial infarction: ISIS-2. *Lancet*, **i**, 397–401.

Johansson, S., Bergstrand, R., Ulvenstam, G., Vedin, A., Wilhelmsson, C., Wedel, H., *et al.* (1984). Sex differences in preinfarction characteristics and long-term survival among patients with myocardial infarction. *Am. J. Epidemiol.*, **119**, 610–23.

Johansson, S., Rosengren, A., Tsipogianni, A., Ulvenstam, G., Wiklund, I., and Wilhelmsen, L. (1988). Physical inactivity as a risk factor for primary and secondary coronary events in Göteborg, Sweden. *Eur. Heart J.*, Suppl. I, 8–19.

McCall, M., Elmfeldt, D., Vedin, A., Wilhelmsson, C., Wedel, H., and Wilhelmsen, L. (1979). Influence of a myocardial infarction on blood pressure and serum cholesterol. *Acta Med. Scand.*, **206**, 477–81.

McMahon, S. and Yusuf, S. (1987). Effects of lidocaine on ventricular fibrillation, asystole, and early death in patients with suspected acute myocardial infarction. In *Acute coronary care* (eds R. M. Califf and G. S. Wagner), Martinus Nijhoff, Boston, MA, pp. 51–60.

Mitchell, J. R. A. (1981). Anticoagulants in coronary heart disease: Retrospect and prospect. *Lancet*, **i**, 257–62.

Peto, R. (1978). Clinical trial methodology. *Biomed. Pharmacother.*, **28** (special issue), 24–36.

Pfeffer, M. A., Lamas, G. A., Vaughan, D. E., Parisi, A. F., and Braunwald, E. (1988). Effect of captopril on progressive ventricular dilatation after anterior myocardial infarction. *New Engl. J. Med.*, **319**, 80–6.

Ruberman, W., Weinblatt, E., Goldberg, J. D., and Chandhary, B. S. (1984). Psychosocial influences on mortality after myocardial infarction. *New Engl. J. Med.*, **311**, 552–9.

Sharpe, N., Murphy, J., Smith, H., and Hannan, S. (1988). Treatment of patients with symptomless left ventricular dysfunction after myocardial infarction. *Lancet*, **i**, 255–9.

Simoons, M. L., Serruys, P. W., Brand, M., Bär, F., deZwaan, C., Res, J., *et al.* (1985). Improved survival after early thrombolysis in acute myocardial infarction. *Lancet*, **ii**, 578–81.

Smith, P., Arnesen, H., and Holme, I. (1990). The effect of warfarin on mortality and reinfarction after myocardial infarction. *New Engl. J. Med.*, **323**, 147–52.

Ulvenstam, G., Bergstrand, R., Johansson, S., Vedin, A., Wilhelmsson, C., Wedel, H., *et al.* (1984). Prognostic importance of cholesterol levels after myocardial infarction. *Prev. Med.*, **13**, 355–66.

Ulvenstam, G., Åberg, A., Bergstrand, R., Johansson, S., Pennert, K., Vedin, A., *et al.* (1985). Long-term prognosis after myocardial infarction in men with diabetes. *Diabetes*, **34**, 787–92.

van Dixhoorn, J., Duivenvoorden, H. J., Staal, J. A., Pool, J., and Verhage, F. (1987). Cardiac events after myocardial infarction: possible effect of relaxation therapy. *Eur. Heart J.*, **8**, 1210–14.

Weinblatt, E., Shapiro, S., Frank, C. W., and Sager, R. V. (1968). Prognosis of men after myocardial infarction: mortality and first recurrence in relation to selected parameters. *Am. J. Publ. Health*, **58**, 1329–47.

Wiklund, I., Odén, A., Sanne, H., Ulvenstam, G., Wilhelmsson, C., and

414   *Secondary prevention of coronary heart disease*

Wilhelmsen, L. (1988). Prognostic importance of somatic and psychosocial variables after a first myocardial infarction. *Am. J. Epidemiol.*, **128**, 786–95.

Wilhelmsen, L., Sanne, H., Elmfeldt, D., Grimby, G., Tibblin, G., and Wedel, H. (1975). A controlled trial of physical training after myocardial infarction. *Prev. Med.*, **4**, 491–508.

Wilhelmsen, L., Johansson, S., Ulvenstam, G., Welin, L., Rosengren, A., Eriksson, H., *et al.* (1989). CHD in Sweden: mortality, incidence and risk factors over 20 years in Gothenburg. *Int. J. Epidemiol.*, **18** (Suppl. 1), S101–8.

Wilhelmsson, C., Vedin, J. A., Wilhelmsen, L., and Tibblin, G. (1974). Reduction of sudden deaths after myocardial infarction by treatment with alprenolol. *Lancet*, **ii**, 1157–9.

Yusuf, S., Peto, R., Lewis, J., Collins, R., and Sleight, P. (1985). Betablockade during and after myocardial infarction: an overview of the randomized trials. *Prog. Cardiovasc. Dis.*, **27**, 335–71.

Yusuf, S., Wittes, J., and Friedman, L. (1988a). Overview of results of randomized clinical trials in heart disease. 1. Treatments following myocardial infarction. *J. Am. Med. Assoc.*, **260**, 2088–93.

Yusuf, S., Wittes, J., and Friedman, L. (1988b). Overview of results of randomized clinical trials in heart disease. II. Unstable angina, heart failure, primary prevention with aspirin and risk factor modification. *J. Am. Med. Assoc.*, **260**, 2259–63.

The prim
hypertension a
pres

The primary
and prevention of tha
which is a major dise
many developing c

Most would agre
tion of disease
cannot provid
in the foll

Twas
Th

RATIONALE FC
OF H

There are at least six reasons why *prevention* of hypertension shou..
major public health objective.

1. Although treatment of hypertension, once it is present and detected, can lower risk of uncontrolled high blood pressure, mortality and morbidity are unlikely to be lowered to that of persons maintaining normal pressure in adult life.

2. The predominant form of antihypertensive treatment—pharmacological therapy—while a definite step forward compared with past neglect of all but the most severe hypertension, is itself not free of risk, especially when used on a mass scale and for decades.

3. Waiting until hypertension appears before there is concern with blood pressure level means that many persons could develop frank disease (and its complications) long before detection and treatment.

4. Failure to prevent the disease means an unending perspective of continued high incidence, requiring massive efforts to detect, treat, and control it.

5. Populations experiencing significant rise of blood pressure with age and the consequent significant occurrence of hypertension also tend to have pressures above optimal for most of the adult population. Thus prevention of hypertension is tied to the broader population-wide problem of average blood pressure at a level that carries excess risk of morbidity and premature mortality.

6. Rise of blood pressure with age, which can move people from 'normal' to 'high' levels of blood pressure, is not an inevitable human condition,

rise could eliminate epidemic hypertension
_se burden in industrialized countries as well as in
_untries.

that in general and in almost all circumstances, preven-
_r disability is better than treatment, especially if treatment
_e a 'cure'. This thought is by now folk wisdom, as embodied
_wing verse by Sir Derrick Dunlop:

a dangerous cliff as they freely confessed,
_ugh the walk near its crest was so pleasant,
_ut over its terrible edge there had slipped
A Duke and full many a peasant;
So the people said something would have to be done,
But their projects did not at all tally:
Some said, 'Put a fence round the edge of the cliff',
Some, 'An ambulance down in the valley'.

No matter how good the ambulance, or the hospital to which the fallen duke or peasant is rushed, restoring the victim to sound health may be costly, painful, and only partially successful. These probabilities are valid not only for accidents but also for a chronic disease such as hypertension. The several definitive trials on drug treatment for hypertension have indeed demonstrated both ability to normalize pressure and benefit from such treatment (Collins *et al*. 1990). The largest saving has been in stroke, with treatment resulting in an average reduction in incidence of about 40 per cent. The stroke rate in hypertensives with blood pressure lowered successfully through pharmacological therapy was close to that experienced by the normotensive population with a similar level of blood pressure. But coronary incidence, although reduced in the treated group in most trials, was still greater than expected from epidemiological observations of those with equivalent pressure among normotensives (Collins *et al*. 1990). The reasons for this difference are not fully understood. They may relate to the short length of the trials and the longer time required to reverse the effects of hypertension on atherosclerosis. They may also relate to negative effects of drug or drug dose, particularly on lipids, as well as on glucose, uric acid, and potassium. This question is discussed elsewhere in this book (Chapter 23). But since the major cause of death among hypertensives in these trials was coronary disease, this failure to realize fully the benefit expected in reducing coronary death by successfully lowering blood pressure highlights the question of action *before* hypertensive disease is established, i.e. primary prevention.

For those who are most likely candidates for development of the disease, for example those with high normal pressure (i.e. systolic pressure (SBP) of 130–139 mmHg or diastolic pressure (DBP) of 80–89 mmHg), a reactive policy of 'wait and see' carries definite risks. First, there is a high probability of the development of frank hypertension which, in the general population, may go undetected, untreated, or uncontrolled for an indefinite period. In a randomized trial on primary prevention of hypertension conducted by our group, in the short space of 5 years one in every five in the control group went from 'high normal' to sustained hypertension (R. Stamler *et al.* 1989). Second, the extra risk associated with blood pressure in the high normal range is not due only to the greater probability of developing frank hypertension with its higher morbidity (Smith 1977; J. Stamler *et al.* 1959) and mortality. Even if these individuals remain at 'high normal' pressure, that level in itself is not optimal and increases cardiovascular risk. The largest body of evidence on this issue is to be found in the 10 year mortality data for nearly 350 000 men age 35–57 screened in the USA in the 1970s for possible eligibility in the Multiple Risk Factor Intervention Trial (MRFIT) (Table 29.1) (R. Stamler 1990). Cardiovascular mortality for men with screening SBP of 130–139 mmHg was almost twice the rate in those with pressures under 110 mmHg (relative risk 1.89). Although the death rate in these men with high normal pressures was lower than for those with definite hypertension, there were so many of them among the screenees that they contributed a large number of the observed deaths and accounted for about a quarter of the excess cardiovascular deaths related to above-optimal SBP. It should be noted that mortality risk increased in this cohort at *every* level of SBP above the optimal low of <110 mmHg. It should also be noted that only about 6 per cent of the men had

Table 29.1 Baseline SBP and age-adjusted 10 year cardiovascular mortality for MRFIT primary screenees

SBP (mmHg)	No. of men	Deaths	Rate per 1000	Relative risk	Excess deaths	Percentage of all excess deaths[a]
<110	21 379	202	10.5	1.00	0.0	0.0
110–119	66 080	658	11.0	1.05	33.0	1.0 ⎫
120–129	98 834	1324	14.3	1.36	375.6	11.5 ⎬ 35.1
130–139	79 308	1576	19.8	1.89	737.6	22.6 ⎭
140–149	44 388	1310	27.3	2.60	745.7	22.8 ⎫ 41.0
150–159	21 477	946	38.1	3.63	592.8	18.2 ⎭
160–169	9308	488	44.8	4.27	319.3	9.8 ⎫
170–179	4013	302	65.5	6.24	220.7	6.8 ⎬ 23.9
≥180	3191	335	85.5	8.14	239.3	7.3 ⎭

Men free of myocardial infarction history at baseline ($N = 347978$)
[a] Excess deaths is defined as the difference between the number of observed deaths and the number that would have occurred if the lowest rate (i.e. for those with SBP <110 mmHg) had prevailed.

such low pressures. Blood-pressure-related excess risk was present for more than 90 per cent of the cohort. Such risk was, and is, a population-wide problem, and not just a problem for the 20–25 per cent with frank hypertension.

Furthermore, there is a close association between prevalence of hypertension and level of blood pressure in the general population, as exemplified by data from the 52 centres of the INTERSALT collaborative study on electrolytes and blood pressure (INTERSALT 1988; Rose and Day 1990). In the seven centres with low median SBP (under 110 mmHg), prevalence of hypertension was only 5.2 per cent. Prevalence increased stepwise with every 5 mmHg higher median SBP in the population samples until, for the five centres with the highest average SBP (≥125 mmHg), hypertension was present in more than a quarter of those surveyed.

That the pattern of a rise in blood pressure with age, high average pressure, and high prevalence of hypertension is not the normal inevitable fate of man is again illustrated in INTERSALT data. In four remote populations, the Yanomamo and Xingu Indians of Brazil, Papua New Guinean highlanders, and rural villagers in Kenya, whose shared exposures differed greatly from the rest of INTERSALT (see below), median SBP and DBP were low, the slope of SBP with age ranged from −1.5 to +2.4 mmHg per 10 years (compared with +5.0 mmHg for the rest of INTERSALT), and hypertension prevalence was less than 1 per cent in three of the centres and 5 per cent in the Kenyan centre, a sample of a population beginning to experience exposure to changing life-style. While there are no doubt multiple factors accounting for the blood pressure differences between these four populations and the more typical pattern, surely there are important lessons to be drawn from the differing blood pressure patterns in such populations—lessons with potential benefit for the human population generally (Page *et al.* 1974; Shaper 1974).

MASS EXPOSURES INFLUENCING BLOOD PRESSURE PATTERNS

History has shown that epidemic diseases—as well as population patterns of risk factors—have their roots in mass exposures experienced by populations.

Decades of research, through animal experimentation, clinical observation, epidemiological studies, and intervention, have identified the following major exposures—unprecedented in terms of human evolution—that have shaped the present pattern of blood pressure dominant in today's world:

• high salt intake;
• low potassium intake;
• high ratio of dietary sodium to potassium;

- overweight;
- high alcohol intake.

The large body of scientific evidence relating these factors to blood pressure has been extensively reviewed elsewhere (NRC 1989, Chapters 15, 16, and 21), and detailed discussion is beyond the scope of this book. For sodium, there is strong and largely consistent evidence for a positive association with blood pressure from animal experimental studies (NRC 1989, Chapter 15), clinical observations (Ambard and Beaujard 1904; Kempner 1944), including use of diuretic therapy, randomized controlled trials (Hofman *et al.* 1983; Cutler *et al.* 1991), and epidemiological studies between and within populations (Dahl 1960; Gleibermann 1973; Froment *et al.* 1979; Elliott 1991). Evidence for a relation (inverse) between potassium and blood pressure is more recent than that for sodium, but encompasses animal evidence, particularly for a protective effect in sodium-induced hypertension (Meneely and Ball 1958), epidemiological evidence between and within populations (INTERSALT 1988; NRC 1989, Chapter 15), including a possible protective effect against stroke in man (Khaw and Barrett-Connor 1987), and some but not all, human experimental studies (NRC 1989, Chapter 15; Whelton *et al.* 1991). For overweight, the relation of body mass and obesity to blood pressure has been extensively examined in human populations in a wide range of cultural settings, and in virtually every epidemiological study, both cross-sectional and prospective, there is a positive and significant association with blood pressure (R. Stamler *et al.* 1978; NRC 1989, Chapter 21; INTERSALT 1988; J. Stamler 1991). This finding is confirmed in clinical trials, either attempted unifactor trials or in combination with other interventions including reduced sodium intake (Andrews *et al.* 1982; R. Stamler *et al.* 1987, 1989; NRC 1989, Chapter 21). Finally, for alcohol, large population studies have generally found positive relations with blood pressure, although there is debate whether this occurs across the range of intakes or only at higher levels of intake (3–4 + drinks per day) (Dyer *et al.* 1981; INTERSALT 1988; NRC 1989, Chapter 16). These findings on the pressor effect of alcohol are also supported by clinical observation (NRC 1989, Chapter 16).

In the present author's estimation, the concordance of experimental evidence, both animal and human, and of observational data, leads to a judgement of causality for these life-style factors. These may not be the only features of modern life that impact on blood pressure, and others may be important (e.g. the dietary intakes of calcium and magnesium, and the amount and type of dietary protein and fat, carbohydrate, fibre, physical activity, stress, etc.), although the evidence is not ample or consistent enough, and does not have sufficiently convincing validity of measurement, to attribute to them an independent causal role in regard to blood pressure and the incidence of hypertension. However, there is sufficient evidence to justify their continued investigation.

The research data on modern mass exposures outlined above have provided the scientific foundations for a realistic strategy of prevention of hypertension. In the millennia of man's past, prior to the agricultural revolution, salt was uncommon and the usual diet was low in salt and high in potassium (Denton 1982). Man's evolution was in adaptation to these dietary features and included, for example, multiple complex mechanisms for retaining sodium against possible deficiencies. Man generally needed to be physically active in order to ensure a food supply, and overweight could not have been common. While alcohol use has a history of at least 5000 years, it was often associated mainly with periodic celebration and regular high intake was not common, at least in man's earlier history (NRC 1989, Chapter 16). All this has changed radically in a relatively very short time— too short for man to have re-adapted to the present high salt, low potassium, excess calorie, and excess alcohol intake.

The new mass exposures have had an influence at two levels: in raising blood pressure over the course of adulthood for *most* people exposed, and in raising pressure to frank hypertensive levels for a sizeable proportion (10–30 per cent of adults in most societies and often a majority in older persons). The impact of these new multiple mass exposures is illustrated in the recent INTERSALT study described below (INTERSALT 1988).

THE INTERSALT STUDY

INTERSALT is an international co-operative cross-sectional study of the relation of electrolytes and other factors to blood pressure and high blood pressure. The study is unique in several aspects. It was the largest undertaking of its type: 10 079 men and women aged 20–59 years were studied in 52 centres in 32 countries, covering a wide range of cultures and eating habits. The size of the study and the standardization of procedures resulted, in effect, in 52 simultaneous studies, each of approximately 200 persons randomly selected from defined populations. These features permitted investigation both within populations and across populations, including combination of local findings for study-wide results.

Blood-pressure-related factors in individuals in INTERSALT: findings and implications

SBP in individuals was significantly related to the major variables noted earlier: intake of sodium, intake of potassium (inversely), the sodium-to-potassium ratio, body mass, and high alcohol intake. Multiple regression analyses within each centre yielded coefficients that expressed the relation of each of these variables to the blood pressure of individuals in the centre. When combined, these within-centre coefficients resulted in study-wide

Table 29.2 How much lower would the average population SBP be with improved life-styles?

Life-style variable	INTERSALT median (approximate)	Improved level	Predicted SBP difference
Sodium (mmol/day urinary excretion)	170	70	−2.2
Potassium (mmol/day urinary excretion)	55	70	−0.7
Na/K	3.1	1.0	−3.4 ⎫
Body mass index (kg/m²)	25.0	23.0	−1.6 ⎬ −5.0

estimates of the independent effect of each variable on blood pressure. Table 29.2 shows the levels of sodium, potassium, and body mass found in the study, and also indicates, on the basis of combined centre regression coefficients, the effect on SBP that could be predicted with improved levels of these variables. (The effect on DBP was in the same direction, although of smaller magnitude.)

For example, if the average daily intake of sodium in the population (found to be close to 170 mmol/day in INTERSALT) were lower by 100 mmol (about 1 teaspoon of salt) and if potassium were moderately higher at 70 mmol/day instead of the 55 mmol/day observed, giving a sodium-to-potassium ratio of 1.0 instead of the 3.0 seen in INTERSALT, the estimate is an average population SBP lower by 3.4 mmHg. With the addition of lower average body mass the total expected difference in average systolic pressure would be 5 mmHg (Table 29.2). If, also, prevalence of heavy drinking (≥300 ml of absolute alcohol per week, or 3–4 average drinks per day) were zero instead of the approximately 13 per cent reported, the potential—with improved levels of all these factors—is estimated to be average SBP lower by at least 5.4 mmHg. (Because of the methodological limitations of a single cross-sectional assessment, this is likely to be a low estimate (Liu *et al.* 1979; Elliott *et al.* 1988; Collins *et al.* 1990).)

A clinician, observing a patient in his/her office, will note that SBP may change by 2, 3, 5, or even 10 mmHg from one measurement to the next. Understandably, that clinician will call such differences small in magnitude and consider them unimportant for health. However, a difference in average population pressure of these dimensions is not the same as an individual difference in a clinical setting—the same numerical difference in a population has an important effect on long-term risk.

The large amount of data available from prospective population studies gives an estimate of the percentage reduction in mortality that corresponds to a 2, 3, or 5 mmHg lower average SBP (J. Stamler *et al.* 1989; R. Stamler

Table 29.3 Potential for lower mortality with lower average population SBP

Average SBP (mmHg) lower by:	Difference in mortality (%)		
	Coronary deaths	Stroke deaths	All deaths
2	−4	−6	−3
3	−5	−8	−4
5	−9	−14	−7

Based on combined multiple regression coefficients from five population studies: 360 000 male screenees for MRFIT, men in the Whitehall Civil Servants Study, men in the Western Electric Company Study, 40 000 men and women in the Chicago Heart Association Detection Project in Industry, and men and women in the Framingham Study.

1991). This estimate is summarized in Table 29.3. For each 2 mmHg difference in average population SBP, the estimated difference is 4 per cent in coronary mortality, 6 per cent in stroke mortality, and 3 per cent in all deaths. For a 5 mmHg lower SBP, coronary death is lower by 9 per cent, stroke death by 14 per cent, and all deaths by 7 per cent. These differences are likely to be underestimates of the impact of blood pressure on mortality since they are based on measurements made on a single occasion only (Collins *et al.* 1990; MacMahon *et al.* 1990), but none the less they provide a qualitative idea of the potential for prevention associated with improved levels of the life-style factors shown in Table 29.2.

It should be noted here that these mortality findings are for *whole-*population samples, including people at all levels of blood pressure. In this regard it is of interest that when the INTERSALT regression analyses were repeated, this time excluding all those defined as hypertensive (SBP ⩾ 140 mmHg or DBP ⩾ 90 mmHg or on antihypertensive medication), the sodium–SBP coefficient was virtually unchanged, i.e. the higher the sodium level, the higher is the SBP across the blood pressure range. This finding reinforced the concept that the blood pressure problem is a *population-wide* problem, resulting from long-term exposure to which the vast majority are susceptible.

A major cross-centre finding of the INTERSALT study was that for most, but not all, population samples, both SBP and DBP rose with age. This rise (upward slope), averaging 5+ mmHg SBP per 10 years, was linked significantly, independent of other major factors, with average sodium intake in the population. From multiple regression analyses it was estimated that if the average daily population sodium intake was lower by 100 mmol, increase in pressure between age 25 and age 55 would, on average, be less by at least 9 mmHg for SBP and by about 5 mmHg for

DBP (INTERSALT 1988). From the long-term population studies, such a difference in average SBP at age 55 predicts a 16 per cent lower coronary mortality, 23 per cent lower stroke mortality and 13 per cent lower all-cause mortality.

The exceptions to the typical rise with age were the four remote centres noted earlier, who had a low 24 hour sodium excretion of <1–51 mmol, sodium-to-potassium ratios of <0.01–1.8 and body mass indices of 21.2–23.4. Two of these remote centres reported no alcohol intake, and in the other two 9 per cent and 31 per cent reported alcohol use (compared with 53 per cent in the rest of INTERSALT). Among these four, Kenya (a population in transition) showed the largest rise in pressure (+2.4 mmHg SBP and +1.3 mmHg DBP in 10 years) and had highest values of sodium, sodium-to-potassium ratio, and alcohol intake.

From a logical viewpoint, there is an obvious link between an increase in blood pressure in adult years and the prevalence of hypertension in middle and older age. If, on average, pressure generally remained at young adult levels, hypertension would indeed be rare and would no longer be a public health problem. Clearly, prevention of a rise in the average pressure in the population would be synonymous with prevention of the current phenom-enon of epidemic hypertension. In INTERSALT, there was a positive relationship between slope of blood pressure with age and prevalence of hypertension in those who had reached age 50–59. If the 52 centres are divided into approximate quintiles of slope of SBP with age, prevalence of hypertension in those 50–59 years is 14.9 per cent in the lowest quintile and 41.3 per cent in the highest quintile (Table 29.4). The correlation co-efficient between slope of SBP with age and prevalence of hypertension at age 50–59 was 0.68 when all 52 centres were included and 0.51 when the four remote centres were excluded ($p < 0.01$).

It was noted earlier that the prevalence of hypertension was also closely linked with the average pressure of the whole population. It is reasonable to conclude that the same exposures leading to rise of pressure with age and higher average pressures in the population are also key factors leading to the occurrence of frank hypertension, and efforts to prevent the disease

Table 29.4 Quintiles of slope of SBP in 10 years and prevalence of hypertension at ages 50–59, (INTERSALT)

10 year SBP slope (mmHg)	No. of centres	Prevalence of hypertension (%)
−1.5 to +3.0	11	14.9
+3.1 to +4.2	10	35.1
+4.3 to +5.2	10	40.8
+5.3 to +6.0	10	43.3
+6.1 to +13.3	11	41.3

must deal with these mass exposures. Rose and Day (1990) have recently demonstrated more generally that this connection between the high risk (or 'deviant') section of the population and the risk status of the 'normal' population applies to many problems facing public health. Using INTER-SALT data, they note that the higher the average sodium intake in a population, or the higher the average body mass, or the higher the average alcohol intake, the greater the proportion of very high levels of these factors. These relationships between the average and the proportion at high levels held even if those at the highest levels were removed when calculating average population values. These findings have a similar message: the way a society lives will affect the status and risk in both the 'normal' population and the proportion at particularly high risk.

Sodium as a key risk factor

In presenting the INTERSALT study results above, emphasis has been on the *combined* effect of the major risk factors demonstrated to relate to blood pressure—high sodium, low potassium, high sodium-to-potassium ratio, overweight, high alcohol intake. In this total configuration, all of which needs to receive attention in prevention efforts, a key role for sodium intake was indicated. Even in those centres where low body mass may have blunted the effect of the observed high salt intake, prevalence of hypertension in older ages was high. In addition to the four remote populations, eight other centres (Colombia, Ladakh, Osaka, Tochiga, Beijing, Nanning, Tianjin, and South Korea) had body mass indices below 23.0 kg/m^2, but the sodium intake in the eight was high (average of 190 mmol/day). Prevalence of hypertension for those aged 50–59 years in these high sodium centres was 24.8 per cent, a significant public health burden. Similar results were reported for alcohol intake. Even in those centres where the percentage reporting drinking was low, but there was a high sodium intake (average of 171 mmol/day) (Beijing, New Delhi, South Korea, and Taiwan), hypertension prevalence at ages 50–59 was again sizeable, namely 30 per cent. With the data available in INTERSALT, there is only a limited possibility of turning the question around to ask whether low salt intake protected against the other risk factors, since apart from the four centres in remote populations, there *was* no group of centres with low sodium intake.

The findings for the Kenya centre mentioned earlier are of particular interest. Although blood pressure was low, this sample had slightly higher pressures than the other three remote centres and 14 per cent of the population were hypertensive at age 50–59. While there may be other factors contributing to the incidence of hypertension in such non-industrialized populations (e.g. hypertension secondary to kidney disease, multiple nutritional deficiencies, etc.), the changes in life-style in Kenya towards a nutrition pattern similar to that of most of the industrialized world and the simultaneous changes towards a less favourable blood pressure pattern have implications for prevention in wide areas of the world.

Some methodological notes on INTERSALT

Estimates of the effect of sodium intake on blood pressure, although qualitatively appropriate, were probably quantitative underestimates because of the methodological limitations inherent in this type of cross-sectional study. These limitations can be briefly summarized as follows. Urinary sodium excretion over a 24 hour period reflects only current and not lifelong salt intake; it is only a single day's record of a pattern with a large daily variation in most populations, so that the usual intake may be misrepresented. Statistical steps taken to account for this variability are unlikely to overcome this source of underestimation of associations. There also may well have been variable incompleteness of the urine collection, and salt intake may have recently changed for health reasons, particularly in people with high blood pressure. In addition, many hypertensives were on medication so that recorded pressures were below 'true' pressures. All these limitations serve to reduce estimates of the real association between salt and blood pressure.

A recent study illustrates how just one such limitation—incompleteness of 24 hour urine collection—results in an underestimation of the sodium–blood pressure relationship. In the North London Study (Elliott *et al*. 1988), use of an ingested PABA marker made it possible, through urinalysis of excreted PABA, to identify those who provided complete versus less than complete 24 hour collections. Although the relatively small study size makes for wide confidence limits, the regression coefficient for the sodium–SBP relationship was three to four times greater in those assessed to have complete or near-complete collections than in those with incomplete 24 hour samples.

With all the limitations noted, even if the coefficients derived from the INTERSALT study are taken at face value, without taking account of the probable underestimation of their size, their implications for public health and public policy as well as for medical care are of major importance. Based on INTERSALT data, Rose and Day (1990) have estimated that a 5 mmHg lower average population SBP would mean a prevalence of hypertension lower by 5 percentage points, so that if current prevalence is 15 per cent (as is estimated in the UK), the new prevalence would be 10 per cent, a reduction of one-third. The INTERSALT data cited (Table 29.2) projected such a 5 mmHg lower population SBP by improvement in the major life-style factors shown to be related to blood pressure, indicating the potential for the prevention of hypertension in a significant proportion of the population. The implications for the general population of a 5 mmHg lower average SBP have already been cited. Changing the deleterious mass exposures leading to excess blood-pressure-related risk can be expectd not only to reduce incidence of hypertension, but also to reduce morbidity and mortality for the large majority of adults.

IS CHANGE FEASIBLE IN THE MAJOR
BLOOD-PRESSURE-RELATED MASS EXPOSURES?

Is it reasonable and practical to propose the kind of changes needed to reduce average blood pressure in the population and to prevent hypertension in a sizeable proportion of those now headed in that direction? For example, is reduction of daily sodium intake by 80–100 mmol, say, a feasible goal in the USA or the UK? The US National Research Council of the National Academy of Science recently proposed an immediate goal of not more than 6 g of salt per day (about 105 mmol of sodium), and a possible future of not more than 4.5 g of salt per day (about 80 mmol) (NRC 1989, Chapter 15). This would mean reducing the current salt intake in the USA by about half. That this is feasible, over time, is suggested both by data from INTERSALT and current American experience. In half the INTERSALT centres (apart from the four low salt population samples), at least 15 per cent of the sample had a sodium excretion level of less than 100 mmol in the single 24 hour collection on the day they were studied. Even though repeat collections would probably reduce this proportion, the finding does indicate that moderate and not high salt intake is a goal that *could* be reached in modern society, given appropriate steps to achieve it. Since an estimated 75 per cent of sodium intake in countries like the USA and the UK comes from processed foods (including bread, pre-cooked, canned, or frozen vegetables and meat dishes, etc.) (NRC 1989, Chapter 15), substantial reduction of *average* salt consumption would require a major change by the food industry. Some changes are occurring currently in the USA in response to growing willingness of consumers to reduce salt intake, although there is resistance from some commercial interests (J. Stamler 1990). However, the trend is to increase the number of low salt or 'no salt added' products. To continue and enlarge this change, wider participation by food producers is needed, together with government action supporting accurate package labelling that includes sodium content, and continued public and professional education. Starting with healthier nutrition patterns early in life to avoid high salt foods from childhood on is an important part of achieving the desired adult pattern.

On a population-wide basis, some important changes have already taken place, particularly in countries with very high salt intake. Earlier studies in Japan (Dahl 1960) reported intake as high as 400 mmol of sodium per day (23 g of salt) in some communities. In contrast, in the three Japanese INTERSALT centres, median sodium intake, although still high, was under 200 mmol/day in two centres and 201 mmol in the third, reflecting a mass public health effort to reduce past very high salt intake and the related high prevalence of hypertension and high stroke incidence and mortality.

Of course, the experience of the four low salt centres in INTERSALT underlines the physiological feasibility of a diet markedly lower in salt intake, even well below the goal of 4.5 g considered as a future objective by the National Academy of Science. Populations in these four centres had average sodium excretion ranging from less than 1 mmol to 51 mmol per day, and were essentially healthy, with a level of physical activity higher than most of the other study populations (Mancilha-Carvalho *et al.* 1989).

Regarding the safety of an average population salt intake of 4.5 g, there is no evidence to suggest that this recommendation—still well above the usual physiological need—carries hazard. As with other public health measures, there will be a few individuals for whom low salt intake would not be appropriate (e.g. patients with salt-losing nephritis), but such persons are likely to be under medical supervision and individually prescribed diets.

As to increase in potassium intake, achievement of a population average of 70–80 mmol per day (approximately a 50 per cent increase above the average observed in INTERSALT) is certainly feasible. Of the 48 INTERSALT centres (not counting the four remote populations), eight already had mean intake in that range and another nine centres had a mean daily intake of 60–69 mmol. However, a sizeable improvement in the sodium-to-potassium ratio is unlikely to be achieved unless a major reduction also takes place in salt intake, since there is a practical limit to which potassium level is likely to be increased using natural foods. Nor is there evidence that potassium supplementation, through pills, is a safe long-term solution. A combined nutritional pattern of lower salt intake and increase of potassium-rich fruits and vegetables is a reasonable and practical direction for an improved sodium-to-potassium ratio.

An increased intake of fruit and vegetables—as a substitute for foods of high caloric density—also has the advantage of being useful in prevention or reduction of overweight. Again, such a pattern begun in early childhood is critical, since avoidance of overweight is easier to achieve than its reversal, once established. Increased caloric expenditure is an important part of the equation for avoiding or controlling overweight, and in several countries there has been a remarkable growth in health clubs and other forms of physical activity. These changes, like many other improvements in life-style (e.g. cessation of smoking) are not being made equally in all social strata, so that to influence population average, special consideration of practical ways to help implement such changes in those less affluent and with less education is needed.

In the USA, the present trend is for a modest reduction in alcohol intake. Data on whether there has been any sizeable reduction in *heavy* drinking, which has been more consistently linked with blood pressure elevation than has light drinking, are not available. But the more the public, as well as health professionals, are made aware of the pressor effect of alcohol, especially high intakes, the more likely the present trend can be intensified.

IS PRIMARY PREVENTION OF HYPERTENSION FEASIBLE?

Until the changes in the key mass exposures described above are implemented over time in the general population, definitive evidence of ability to reduce the epidemic of hypertension (as well as improve overall population blood pressure level) will not be available. However, based on the accumulation of data on the effects of today's mass exposures on blood pressure, there is every reason to believe that prevention of hypertension is a challenge 'whose time has come'. Acting on that premise, our group organized the first randomized controlled trial on the primary prevention of hypertension (R. Stamler *et al.* 1989). The 5 year trial utilized multifactorial nutritional–hygienic intervention to test the ability to reduce the incidence of hypertension in the group randomly assigned to such a programme compared with a control group monitored semi-annually. Participants were working men and women aged 30–44, designated as hypertension prone because of high normal DBP (80–89 mmHg as an average of multiple measurements at a second screen). If pressures were in the range 80–84 mmHg, the additional criteria for eligibility were pulse above 80 beats/min and/or overweight (10–49 per cent over desirable weight). The goals for the intervention group were (1) reduction in overweight of at least 4.5 kg, with a fat-modified diet of the American Heart Association type, (2) reduction in daily sodium intake to 1800 mg (78 mmol of sodium or 4.5 g of salt), (3) reduction of alcohol intake to no more than two drinks per day (26 g alcohol), and (4) increases in moderate isotonic physical exercise for periods of 30 minutes at least 3 days per week. Blood pressure was recorded semi-annually in both the intervention and monitored (control) groups, at the work site and in the clinical office setting, by technicians unaware of the group assignment. In end-point assessment, definition of hypertension was initiation of antihypertensive drug therapy by the participant's personal physician or sustained elevation of DBP (a rise in the work site value to over 90 mmHg, followed by a mean level in excess of 90 mmHg for the remainder of the trial).

About a quarter of the intervention group met and maintained the weight loss goal of reduction by at least 4.5 kg. The net change in weight in the whole intervention group was −2.7 kg. Sodium intake in the intervention group was reduced by a quarter, with close to 20 per cent achieving the goal of 4.5 g or less of salt daily. The sodium-to-potassium molar ratio decreased from 2.5 to 1.9. No change in that ratio was seen in the control group. A small reduction in alcohol was reported (−2.2 g daily), as was an

Table 29.5 5 year incidence of hypertension: Primary Prevention of Hypertension Trial

Group	No. in group	No. (percentage) of hypertensives
Life-style Intervention Group	102	9 (8.8)
Control (Monitored) Group	99	19 (19.2)
	$\chi^2 = 3.68$, $p = 0.027$	

increase in regular physical activity (confirmed in the intervention group by performance results in treadmill testing) (Liao *et al.* 1987).

Overall, life-style changes in the intervention group were modest. None the less, these changes had a significant effect on incidence of hypertension (Table 29.5). During the 5 years of the trial, incidence of hypertension was more than twice as high in the monitored group as in the intervention group (19.2 per cent versus 8.8 per cent). Hypertension developed earlier in the monitored group. An additional finding was that incidence of hypertension was particularly high among smokers in the monitored group: 28.9 per cent compared with 8.0 per cent in the intervention group, with a significant odds ratio of 3.9. Net reduction in trial average blood pressure was modest, but was larger in the intervention group than in the control group, significantly so in three of the four comparisons (DBP at work site and office, and SBP at the annual office visits). There was a relationship between the amount of life-style change, particularly weight loss, and the amount of blood pressure reduction in the intervention group. Later primary prevention trials reported generally concordant findings (HPT 1990; TOHP 1990).

While these results are encouraging, it seems reasonable to suggest that life-style changes would have been easier and larger (and incidence of hypertension in the intervention group lower) if the whole community had been moving in the same direction. In the early 1980s, when this trial began, making the right food choices in the supermarket was more difficult than it is today. The trial experience illustrates the need for combining a strategy aimed at those at highest risk of becoming hypertensive (like those with high normal pressure in this study) with the population-wide strategy discussed above. The effort to move the *whole* population towards lower healthier blood pressure levels through improved life-style is bound to make it easier to reduce risk in the high risk groups as well.

A brief word is added here on the relevance of these improved life-styles not only for the *primary* prevention of hypertension but for its *secondary* prevention as well. What is meant by secondary prevention in this case is the return of blood pressure to normal level in those who are already hypertensive. Simultaneously with the Primary Prevention of Hypertension Trial, our group together with colleagues in Minnesota, organized a 4 year randomized controlled trial among hypertensives being treated pharmacologically and whose pressures had been normal for at least 1 year prior to start of the trial (R. Stamler *et al.* 1987). The main aim of this trial (the Hypertension Control Program) was to see whether nutritional changes, essentially the same as those prescribed in the Primary Prevention of Hypertension Trial, would maintain normal pressure without medication in a sizeable portion of the hypertensives randomized to such nutritional intervention. A control group, also made up of hypertensive who were well controlled pharmacologically, was not offered nutritional therapy and was similarly removed from medication early in the trial to see if any carry-over effect of previous successful drug treatment, by itself, was sufficient to maintain normal pressure. Careful frequent monitoring of blood pressure and strict rules on return to medication with pressure rise protected patients in both groups from uncontrolled blood pressure elevation. The main end-point comparison was the proportion in each of the two groups that remained normotensive without pharmacological treatment. The final results were a clear finding that nutritional therapy, focused on decreasing salt, increasing potassium, reducing overweight, and reducing excess alcohol intake, could maintain normal pressure in a significant proportion of hypertensives. Among the 97 patients in the intervention group, 39 per cent remained normotensive without drugs throughout the 4 years. In contrast, only 4 per cent of the 44 patients in the control group were able to maintain normal pressure without pharmacological treatment, a highly significant difference compared with the intervention group. The experience of life-style modification in this group, which was already hypertensive, was in keeping with that of the primary prevention programme. The results of both trials indicate the potential benefits if such improvements become the norm in the general population.

CONCLUSION

There are now findings from decades of research on the mass exposures producing high average population blood pressure, rise of pressure in adult years, and high prevalence of hypertension. Applying these findings is an undertaking that has both obstacles and exciting potential, and above all need, but as yet there is no clear-cut public policy either for the primary prevention of hypertension or for a shift towards a lower healthier average population blood pressure. Public policy and resources have been focused (with good and important results) on detection and treatment (mainly pharmacological) of those at highest risk, i.e. those with hypertension. Although government agencies and expert committees have made nutritional recommendations in regard to salt intake, overweight, and consumption of alcohol, these have mainly been for those who are already hypertensive.

We need to make the next step forward, namely for a public policy committed to the goal of primary prevention of hypertension and achievement of optimal levels of pressure in the general population.

ACKNOWLEDGEMENTS

It is a pleasure to acknowledge the many colleagues around the world who brought into being and carried out the INTERSALT study described here. Principal investigators of INTERSALT are Professor Geoffrey Rose, London School of Hygiene and Tropical Medicine, and Professor Jeremiah Stamler, Northwestern University Medical School, Chicago. Co-investigators are Dr Paul Elliott and Professor Michael Marmot, London School of Hygiene and Tropical Medicine, Professor Alan Dyer and the present author, Northwestern University Medical School, and Professor Hugo Kesteloot, Catholic University, Leuven. Other colleagues in the study are cited in the publications listed in the references. INTERSALT has been supported by grants from the US National Heart, Lung, and Blood Institute (NHLBI), the Heart Foundations of Canada, Great Britain, The Netherlands, and Japan, the Wellcome Trust, the World Health Organization, the Belgian National Research Foundation, the Parastatal Insurance Co., Belgium, the Council on Epidemiology and Prevention and the International Society of Hypertension (of the International Society and Federation of Cardiology), and the Chicago Health Research Foundation. Field work in 52 centres was supported by organizations in the respective countries. The NHLBI supported the two trials cited here, the Primary Prevention of Hypertension Trial and the Hypertension Control Program, the latter conducted jointly with Dr Richard Grimm and Dr Reuben Berman of the University of Minnesota. The Multiple Risk Factor Intervention Trial (MRFIT) was also funded by NHLBI. The author is pleased to acknowledge the co-operation of Dr James Neaton and Deborah Wentworth of the MRFIT Coordinating Center, University of Minnesota, headed by Dr Marcus Kjelsberg.

As always, it is a pleasure to thank Dr Jeremiah Stamler, with whom the author has had the good fortune to cooperate over many years in scientific research focused on prevention, including in several of the studies cited here.

REFERENCES

Ambard, L. and Beaujard, E. (1904). Causes de l'hypertension arterielle. *Arch. Gen. Med.*, **1**, 520–33.

Andrews, G., MacMahon, S. W., Austin, A., and Byrne, D. G. (1982). Comparison of drug and non-drug treatments. *Br. Med. J.*, **284**, 1523–6.

Collins, R., Peto, R., MacMahon, S., Hebert, P., Fiebach, N. H., Eberlein, K., *et al.* (1990). Blood pressure, stroke and coronary heart disease. Part 2. Short-term reductions in blood pressure: overview of randomised drug trials in the epidemiological context. *Lancet*, **335**, 827–38.

Cutler, J. A., Follmann, D., Elliott, P., and Suh, I. (1991). An overview of randomized trials of sodium reduction and blood pressure. *Hypertension*, **17** (Suppl. I), I-27–33.

Dahl, L. (1960). Possible role of sodium intake in the development of hypertension. In *Essential hypertension—an international symposium* (eds P. Cottier and K. D. Bock), Springer-Verlag, Berlin, pp. 53–65.

Denton, D. (1982). *The hunger for salt. An anthropological, physiological and medical analysis*, Springer-Verlag, Berlin.

Dyer, A. R., Stamler, J., Paul, O., Berkson, D. M., Shekelle, R. B., Lepper, M. H., *et al.* (1981). Alcohol, cardiovascular risk factors and mortality. The Chicago experience. *Circulation*, **64**, (Suppl. III), 20–7.

Elliott, P. (1991). Observational studies of salt and blood pressure. *Hypertension*, **17** (Suppl. I), I-3–8.

Elliott, P., Forrest, R. D., Jackson, C. A., and Yudkin, J. S. (1988). Sodium and blood pressure: positive associations in a North London population with consideration of the methodological problems of within-population surveys. *J. Hum. Hypertension*, **2**, 89–95.

Froment, A., Milon, H., and Gravier, C. (1979). Relationship of sodium intake and essential hypertension. Contribution of geographical epidemiology. *Rev. Epidemiol. Sante Publ.*, **27**, 437–54.

Gleibermann, L. (1973). Blood pressure and dietary salt in human populations. *Ecol. Food Nutr.*, **2**, 143–56.

Hofman, A., Hazebroek, A., and Valkenberg, H. A. (1983). A randomized trial of sodium intake and blood pressure in newborn infants. *J. Am. Med. Assoc.*, **250**, 370–3.

HPT (Hypertension Prevention Trial) Research Group (1990). The Hypertension Prevention Trial: three-year effects of dietary changes on blood pressure. *Arch. Intern. Med.*, **150**, 153–62.

INTERSALT Cooperative Research Group (1988). INTERSALT: an international study of electrolyte excretion and blood pressure. Results for 24 hour urinary sodium and potassium excretion. *Br. Med. J.*, **297**, 319–28.

Kempner, W. (1944). Treatment of kidney disease and hypertensive vascular disease with the rice diet: 1. *NC Med. J.*, **5**, 125–33.

Khaw, K.-T. and Barrett-Connor, E. (1987). Dietary potassium and stroke-associated mortality. A 12-year prospective population study. *New Engl. J. Med.*, **316**, 235–40.

Liao, Y., Emidy, L. A., Gosch, F. C., Stamler, R., and Stamler, J. (1987).

Cardiovascular responses to exercise of participants in a trial on the primary prevention of hypertension. *J. Hypertension,* **5,** 317–21.

Liu, K., Cooper, R., McKeever, J., McKeever, P., Byington, R., Soltero, I., *et al.* (1979). Assessment of the association between habitual salt intake and high blood pressure: methodological problems. *Am. J. Epidemiol.,* **110,** 219–26.

MacMahon, S., Peto, R., Cutler, J., Collins, R., Sorlie, P., Neaton, J., *et al.* (1990). Blood pressure, stroke, and coronary heart disease. Part 1, Prolonged differences in blood pressure: prospective observational studies corrected for the regression dilution bias. *Lancet,* **335,** 765–74.

Mancilha-Carvalho, J. J., Baruzzi, R. G., Howard, P. F., Poulter, N., Alpers, M. P., Franco, L. J., *et al.* (1989). Blood pressure in four remote populations in the INTERSALT study. *Hypertension,* **14,** 238–46.

Meneely, G. R. and Ball, C. O. T. (1958). Experimental epidemiology of chronic sodium chloride toxicity and the protective effect of potassium chloride. *Am. J. Med.,* **25,** 713–25.

NRC (National Research Council) Committee on Diet and Health, Food and Nutrition Board, Commission on Life Sciences (1989). *Diet and health—implications for reducing chronic disease risk,* National Academy Press, Washington, DC, pp. 413–30, 563–92.

Page, L. B., Damon, A., and Moellering, R. C. (1974). Antecedents of cardiovascular disease in six Solomon Island Societies. *Circulation,* **49,** 1132–46.

Rose, G. and Day, S. (1990). The population mean predicts the number of deviant individuals. *Br. Med. J.,* **301,** 1031–4.

Shaper, A. G. (1974). Communities without hypertension. In *Cardiovascular disease in the tropics* (eds A. G. Shaper, M. S. P. Hutt, and Z. Fejfar), British Medical Association, London, pp. 77–83.

Smith, W. M. (1977). Treatment of mild hypertension. Results of a ten-year intervention trial. US Public Health Service Hospitals Cooperative Study Group. *Circul. Res.,* **40,** 98–105.

Stamler, J. (1990). The politics of salt. Presented at the Conference on Hypertension in Blacks, Los Angeles, CA.

Stamler, J. (1991). Epidemiologic findings on body mass and blood pressure in adults. *Annals of Epidemiology,* **1,** 347–62.

Stamler, J., Lindberg, H. A., Berkson, D. M., Shaffer, A., Miller, W., Poindexter, A., *et al.* (1959). Epidemiolgical analysis of hypertension and hypertensive disease in the labor force of a Chicago utility company. In *Hypertension,* Vol. VII, *Drug action, epidemiology and hemodynamics—Proc. Council for High Blood Pressure Research, American Heart Association* (ed. F. R. Skelton), American Heart Association, New York, pp. 23–50.

Stamler, J., Rose, G., Stamler, R., Elliott, P., Dyer, A., and Marmot, M. (1989). INTERSALT study findings: public health and medical care implications. *Hypertension,* **14,** 570–7.

Stamler, R. (1990). The blood pressure problem: risks and their reduction. *Cardiovasc. Risk Factors,* **1,** 71–9.

Stamler, R. (1991). Implications of the INTERSALT Study. *Hypertension,* **17,** I-16–20.

Stamler, R., Stamler, J., Riedlinger, W. F., Algera, G., and Roberts, R. H.

(1978). Weight and blood pressure. Findings in hypertension screening of 1 million Americans. *J. Am. Med. Assoc.*, **240**, 1607–10.

Stamler, R., Stamler, J., Grimm, R., Gosch, F. C., Elmer, P., Dyer, A., *et al.* (1987). Nutritional therapy for high blood pressure. Final report of a four-year randomized controlled trial—the Hypertension Control Program. *J. Am. Med. Assoc.*, **257**, 1484–91.

Stamler, R., Stamler, J., Gosch, F. C., Civinelli, J., Fishman, J., McKeever, P., *et al.* (1989). Primary prevention of hypertension by nutritional-hygienic means. Final report of a randomized, controlled trial. *J. Am. Med. Assoc.*, **262**, 1801–7.

TOHP (Trial of Hypertension Prevention) Collaborative Research Group (1990). Phase I. Results of the Trial of Hypertension Prevention (Abstract). *Circulation*, **82**, III-553.

Whelton, P. K., Thaker, G. K., Klag, M. J., Seidler, A. P., and Appel, L. J. (1991). Role of potassium supplementation in the treatment and prevention of hypertension (Abstract). *Hypertension,* **17**, 434–5.

30

From observation to policy: cholesterol

B. M. Rifkind

The main reason for forging a national policy for the prevention of coronary heart disease (CHD) in the USA is the toll that it exacts. Several yardsticks give some idea of the extent of this. An estimated 1 250 000 heart attacks occur each year in the USA, of which about 0.5 million result in death. About 800 000 are first heart attacks while 450 000 are recurrent attacks. About half (250 000) the deaths occur suddenly (within 1 hour of onset of symptoms). Heart disease deaths, of which CHD accounts for two-thirds, become the leading cause of death in males by approximately age 40, and in females by approximately age 65 or 70. The estimated cost to the economy attributed to CHD in 1985 was $48.9 billion, of which direct health costs constituted $12.9 billion and indirect costs constituted $36 billion.

National policy for the prevention of CHD has been long in the making. Scientific data relating the amount and type of fat eaten to heart disease appeared in the 1950s, and by 1961 the American Heart Association was advocating dietary changes to reduce heart attack risk (Stephen and Wald 1990). Numerous reports from the USA and from many other countries subsequently appeared; Truswell (1983) identified over 40 such reports, most of which advocated some form of restriction or modification in the intake of dietary fat. Despite this impressive consistency a clear national policy did not emerge in the USA until recently. What led to this was the emergence of a sufficiently coherent and persuasive science base, especially the provision of clinical trial evidence for the benefits of cholesterol-lowering.

THE SCIENCE BASE

Many different lines of evidence incriminate cholesterol in atherogenesis and CHD. Studies of the pathology of the early or more advanced atherosclerotic lesion showed cholesterol to be a prominent component. Lesions which resemble human atherosclerosis were produced in many different experimental animal species, including the non-human primate, by inducing hypercholesterolaemia, usually through manipulation of dietary fat intake. Spontaneously occurring forms of hypercholesterolaemia, as in the WHHL rabbit, also lead to severe atherosclerosis and myocardial ischaemia. Human genetic disorders implicated certain cholesterol-rich lipoproteins as atherogenic; disorders such as familial hypercholesterol- aemia, familial combined hyperlipidaemia, and familial dysbetalipopro- teinaemia, each due to a different genetic abnormality, lead to raised plasma concentrations of atherogenic lipoproteins, and are characterized by the frequent development of premature CHD and other atherosclerotic disease.

Studies of the structure and metabolism of the plasma lipoproteins continued apace over the past three decades and, together with the more recent addition of cell biology research of the arterial wall, are gradually providing an understanding of the genesis of the atherosclerotic lesion and its subsequent development.

These diverse approaches complemented a large number of epidemio- logical studies which showed the level of plasma cholesterol, specifically low density lipoprotein cholesterol (LDL-cholesterol), to be a major and independent risk factor for CHD and, together with the animal, patho- logical, clinical genetic, and metabolic studies, identified the intake of saturated fat and cholesterol as important dietary determinants of plasma cholesterol levels.

Many regarded this impressive array of information as a sufficient basis to proceed to the development and implementation of policies to reduce cholesterol levels in order to decrease the risk of CHD. However, others held that it was necessary to confirm by means of clinical trial(s) that cholesterol-lowering is beneficial and that any accompanying risk is suf- ficiently outweighed by its benefits.

CLINICAL TRIALS

To conduct a satisfactory trial of cholesterol-lowering is demanding. The chronic nature of the disease and the low annual event rate, especially in a primary prevention context, mean that large numbers of individuals have to be recruited and followed for long periods of time. The trials are correspondingly expensive and operationally difficult. Although many cholesterol-lowering trials preceded it, often with encouraging findings, it was only after the results of the Coronary Primary Prevention Trial (CPPT) appeared that a major shift in professional and public attitudes and behaviour occurred (Lipid Research Clinics Program 1984*a, b*). This study showed a reduction in its primary end-point of coronary death and/or non- fatal myocardial infarction, together with corresponding reductions in other manifestations of cardiac ischaemia such as angina or progression to coronary bypass surgery. For each 1 per cent of reduction in cholesterol there was an approximate 2 per cent reduction in the incidence of CHD. These results were consistent with the trends seen in prior (and subsequent) cholesterol-lowering studies. For example, from a meta-analysis by Yusuf *et al.* (1988) of 22 randomized trials, of which nine were of primary prevention and 13 of secondary prevention, it was reported that an overall 23 per cent reduction, which was highly significant, occurred in the risk of non-fatal myocardial infarction plus CHD deaths, and that this reduction was directly related to both the degree and duration of lowering of cholesterol levels. For a standard reduction in cholesterol level for a fixed duration, there was no apparent heterogeneity in the reduction of CHD observed in the drug or diet intervention trials, in the primary or secondary prevention trials, or in fatal or non-fatal CHD events. Cardiac mortality *per se* was also reduced.

The reduction in the clinical end-points seen in these studies is complemented by the results of six controlled angiographic trials in which marked cholesterol-lowering, with or without an increase in high density lipoprotein (HDL), showed significant reductions in coronary atherosclerosis progression and greater stabilization and regression of lesions (Rifkind and Grouse 1990). These angiographic studies may be particularly influential in persuading cardiologists as to the efficacy of cholesterol-lowering.

An important and as yet unresolved issue remains from analysis of the clinical trials. According to Yusuf *et al.* (1988) several of the trials show, usually statistically non-significant, excesses in non-cardiovascular mortality. In particular, trials using clofibrate show a significant excess in perioperative deaths due to gallstones or acute pancreatitis. With these exceptions, Yusuf *et al.* (1988) report that the trials show no systematic excess in mortality due to other non-coronary deaths either for all drugs or for any particular class of agent. While not completely dismissing an adverse effect of lowering cholesterol, they wrote that the absolute increase in non-CHD deaths is consistent with chance. However, Muldoon *et al.* (1990), in a meta-analysis restricted to primary prevention trials, found total mortality not to be affected by treatment and reported a significant increase in deaths for accidents, suicides, and violence. Unfortunately the statistical power of each of the individual studies to assess total and especially non-cardiovascular mortality is low, the number of cases involved is small, and the causes of death are diverse and seemingly unrelated. It is difficult to draw conclusions, and the issue must be regarded as unresolved. It is less of an issue in the secondary prevention context in which most deaths are due to CHD.

ESTABLISHING A CONSENSUS

The strength of the case for the role of cholesterol in CHD thus rests on evidence derived from many approaches, from each of which a large amount of information has been assembled. A downside of this, however, is the sheer volume and diversity of the research findings, and the difficulty in translating them across the disciplines and rendering them into a coherent whole.

The National Institutes of Health (NIH) Consensus Development Conference process is designed to grapple with such problems. Its purpose has been described as to evaluate the evidence on some aspect of biomedical technology or on a controversy in treatment and diagnosis and to produce a clear concise message for clinicians and the public. The consensus process borrows from three models (Mullen and Jacoby 1985):

(1) the judicial process, where evidence is heard by knowledgeable but impartial judges or by juries of peers;

(2) the scientific meeting, where experts discuss their work with peers in a collegial manner;

(3) the town meeting, where a forum is provided for all interested persons to express their views.

The Consensus Conference on Lowering Blood Cholesterol to Prevent CHD was conducted along these lines (Consensus Conference 1985). The consensus panel was representative of the many disciplines that feed into the cholesterol science base and included a lay representative. Its conclusions were unanimous. The panel wrote that elevated blood cholesterol is a major cause of CHD and that it had been established beyond reasonable doubt that reducing definitely elevated blood cholesterol levels (specifically blood levels of LDL-cholesterol) will reduce the risk of heart attacks due to CHD. They stated that this had been most conclusively demonstrated in men with elevated blood cholesterol levels but that much evidence justified the conclusions that similar protection will be afforded in women with elevated levels.

The panel recommended treatment of individuals with high blood cholesterol (above the 75th percentile), the so-called high risk strategy. Further, they were persuaded that the blood cholesterol levels of most Americans are undesirably high, in large part because of high dietary intake of calories, saturated fat, and cholesterol, and that all Americans (except children under the age of 2 years) be advised to take a moderate fat diet. In order to implement these recommendations it was also recommended that new and expanded programmes be planned to educate physicians, other health professionals, and the public in the significance of elevated blood cholesterol and the importance of treating it. To provide a focus for the development of such programmes the NHLBI was recommended to initiate a national cholesterol education programme that would enlist participation by and contributions from all interested parties at the national, state, and local levels.

A transatlantic consensus

The European Atherosclerosis Society (EAS) with membership from 19 European countries, including the UK, published its conclusions and recommendations in its Strategies for the Prevention of Coronary Heart Disease (EAS 1987). The British Cardiac Society (BCS) Working Group on Coronary Heart Disease Prevention also published its report (BCS 1987). These two policy statements joined that of the US Consensus Conference, the striking feature being the extent to which they agreed on many major issues that hitherto had been controversial (Brook and Rifkind 1989). For example, the panels each recommended complementary and simultaneous high risk and total population approaches to the reduction of cholesterol and management of other risk factors.

THE NATIONAL CHOLESTEROL EDUCATION PROGRAM

The National Cholesterol Educational Program (NCEP) describes its mission as the reduction of CHD morbidity and mortality related to elevated blood cholesterol (Lenfant 1986). This has been accomplished through the development of a national education effort and through extensive coordination with other government agencies and intermediate groups in the private sector.

NCEP Panel reports

Early on, the NCEP recognized several key health policy areas that required attention and addressed them through the establishment of four panels:

1. The Laboratory Standardization Panel;
2. The Expert Panel on Detection, Evaluation, and Treatment of High Blood Cholesterol in Adults;
3. The Expert Panel on Population Strategies for Blood Cholesterol Reduction;
4. The Expert Panel on Blood Cholesterol Levels in Children and Adolescents.

Laboratory Standardization Panel

The Laboratory Standardization Panel (LSP) noted considerable inaccuracies in cholesterol testing in the United States and made the following recommendations (NCEP 1988*a*).

- Accurate and precise cholesterol measurements are needed for the uniform interpretation of cholesterol values to assess a person's risk for CHD and to monitor treatment.
- All clinical laboratories in the USA should adopt uniform cholesterol cut-points for identifying adults at high risk for CHD. This requires national standardization of cholesterol measurements. In order to use the new recommended cut-points properly, the laboratory must minimize method-specific biases and also achieve adequate precision of cholesterol measurement by specific attention to method-instrument and calibration procedures.
- Bias (deviation from the true value) of cholesterol measurement methods currently in use should not exceed ±5 per cent from the true value and should be no greater than ±3 per cent from the true value within 5 years. Precision appears to be less of a problem.
- The newly available portable chemistry analysers for cholesterol measurement should have further evaluation before they are adopted for routine use for patients.
- Cholesterol measurements made by all clinical laboratories in the USA can and should be standardized so that the cholesterol values are traceable to the Centers for Disease Control (CDC) reference method or to the National Institue of Standards and Technology (NIST) definitive method. Laboratories can accomplish this goal and improve the accuracy and precision of their cholesterol measurements by using certified reference materials currently available from NIST, CDC, or the College of American Pathologists (CAP) to evaluate their cholesterol measurement methods and/or instruments.

In a subsequent report the LSP recommended the detailed technical and organizational elements needed to assure the overall reliability of cholesterol measurement (NCEP 1990*a*).

Various steps have been taken to implement these and related recommendations. In particular, a National Reference Method Laboratory Network has been established throughout the USA under the aegis of the CDC–NHLBI Cholesterol Standardization Program. These reference laboratories can be accessed by clinical laboratories and by manufacturers of cholesterol equipment and reagents in order to standardize their materials through cholesterol methodologies traceable to the reference or definitive methods.

Expert Panel on Detection, Evaluation, and Treatment of High Blood Cholesterol in Adults

This panel, often known as the Adult Treatment Panel (ATP), dealt with the high risk approach to lowering blood cholesterol levels (NCEP 1988*b*),

Table 30.1 Initial classification based on total cholesterol

<5.2 mM/l (<200 mg/dl)	Desirable blood cholesterol
5.2–6.2 mM/l (200–239 mg/dl)	Borderline high blood cholesterol
≥6.2 mM/l (≥240 mg/dl)	High blood cholesterol

Table 30.2 Classification based on LDL-cholesterol

<3.4 mM/l (<130 mg/dl)	Desirable LDL-cholesterol
3.4–4.1 mM/l (130–159 mg/dl)	Borderline high risk LDL-cholesterol
≥4.1 mM/l (≥160 mg/dl)	High risk LDL cholesterol

Their goal was to establish criteria that define the candidates for medical intervention and to provide guidelines on how to detect, set goals for, treat, and monitor these patients over time.

Major features of their recommendations were as follows.

- The initial classification of individuals is based on total cholesterol (Table 30.1). LDL-cholesterol is the basis for subsequent classification and decision-making about initiating dietary or drug therapy (Table 30.2).
- Patients with LDL-cholesterol equal to or greater than 4.1 mM/l (160 mg/dl) are considered at high risk for CHD and should be treated.
- Patients with a borderline LDL-cholesterol of 3.4–4.1 mM/l (130–159 mg/dl) should also be treated to lower their cholesterol if they have definite CHD or at least two other CHD risk factors (Table 30.3).
- Dietary treatment is the cornerstone of therapy, and maximum efforts at dietary therapy should be continued even if drug treatment is needed.

Table 30.3 Other CHD risk factors

Male sex

Family history of premature CHD (definite myocardial infarction or sudden death before age 55 in a parent or sibling)

Cigarette smoking (currently smokes more than 10 cigarettes per day)

Hypertension

Low HDL-cholesterol concentration (below 35 mg/dl confirmed by repeat measurement)

Diabetes mellitus

History of definite cerebrovascular or occlusive peripheral vascular disease

Severe obesity (≥30% overweight)

The recommendations and cut-points of the report were meant to apply to all adults aged 20 years and above. The aim was to have a single set of cut-points for men and women and, because cholesterol levels are lower in younger people, to minimize drug use in this group. However, there is room for modifications based on the judgement of the physician and the preference of the patients, particularly in the case of young adults, the elderly, and women.

The impact of these guidelines on medical practice will be considerable. Applying them to the nationally representative serum total cholesterol and lipoprotein data for adults aged 20–74 from the second National Health and Nutrition Examination Survey (1976–80), it was estimated that 41 per cent of adults should have lipoprotein analysis after an initial measurement of serum total cholesterol (Sempos *et al.* 1989). Furthermore, it was estimated that 80 per cent of those who need lipoprotein analysis, or 36 per cent of all adults aged 20–74 years, are candidates for medical advice and intervention for high blood cholesterol levels. This translates to approximately 40 million Americans aged 20–59 years and an additional 24 million aged 60 years and older. These numbers will impose a heavy load on the medical system.

The cholesterol distribution varies from country to country, to some extent, because of different dietary fat intakes. In the UK the mean cholesterol is considerably higher than in the USA (Mann *et al.* 1988). Strict application of the US guidelines in the UK would thus result in a higher proportion of the population being designated at high risk and requiring appropriate attention. It would seem reasonable to select different cut-points for different populations with the intent of keeping the proportion of the population designated as high risk down to a manageable number. This is biologically defensible on the basis that there is a continuous relationship between the serum cholesterol levels and CHD risk and that there is no categorical level that defines high risk. Furthermore, if the population has higher cholesterol values, presumably this is due to a higher saturated fat and cholesterol intake and this can be dealt with by the population approach which is designed to shift the cholesterol distribution to lower levels. However, it is quite unjustified to select the very high cut-points for drug treatment that were recently advocated by a Scottish group, so denying many very high risk individuals the benefit of treatment (Scottish Home and Health Department 1990).

The need for simplicity A principle which has strongly influenced the ATP was the need to keep its guidelines as simple as possible compatible with the scientific evidence and the safety of the patient. Cholesterol diagnosis and management will be primarily in the hands of internists and primary care practitioners. Relatively rare disorders should generally be referred to a specialist.

Naturally there have been various criticisms of the ATP Guidelines. Some of them have considerable import for health policy.

High density lipoprotein It has been suggested that the initial screen should include an HDL-cholesterol measurement rather than be confined to total cholesterol. It is argued that individuals with so-called desirable (<5.2 mM/l or <200 mg/dl) total cholesterol may have a low HDL-cholesterol and so may still be at elevated risk for CHD. The ATP decided against this approach mainly on the bases that there is considerable uncertainty regarding how to treat low HDL-cholesterol levels effectively and that clinical trial evidence is encouraging but not conclusive as to whether raising low HDL-cholesterol levels helps prevent CHD. Another concern is that, in contrast to screening for total cholesterol, screening for lipoprotein levels including HDL-C, is usually performed in fasting subjects.

Hypertriglyceridaemia In contrast with the US guidelines, those of the EAS included a significant component based on classification and treatment of patients according to triglyceride levels. The ATP held that, though there is much evidence incriminating hypertriglyceridemia (often together with low HDL levels), in CHD there is still insufficient understanding to justify the inclusion of triglycerides as a primary target in a national education programme. The concerns include the very large number of additional candidates for treatment that would be generated, many of whom would end up requiring drug therapy, given the difficulty in maintaining weight loss as a primary means of controlling elevated triglycerides.

Secondary prevention While the ATP did recommend that attention should be paid to patients with manifestations of CHD and more aggressive therapy should be used, it is arguable that this large and important group of patients was insufficiently highlighted. Opinion is growing, especially in the light of the impressive results of the angiographic studies, that this group should be highlighted for attention (Rossouw *et al.* 1990). Other considerations in favour of this are the large number of heart attacks that could be potentially prevented in individuals with prior CHD given their high risk of subsequent infarction, the fact that they are already in the medical care system, and the likelihood that they would be compliant with therapy. Cost estimates suggest that concentration on this group would be economical. Also, about half of all coronary events occur in individuals with prior manifestations of CHD so that a significant proportion of the overall community burden of CHD could be prevented by such an approach.

The Expert Panel on Population Strategies for Blood Cholesterol Reduction

As indicated earlier, there have been many US and other national reports recommending alteration of the national diet with a view to reducing serum cholesterol levels and, thereby, the rate of CHD. What distinguishes the

Report of the Expert Panel on Population Strategies for Blood Cholesterol Reduction (NCEP 1990*b*) was its appearance at a time of intense public interest in cholesterol and its specific recommendations directed towards the many players in this field, such as the US public, health professionals, the food industry, government agencies, and educational programmes. The report stressed its consistency with the high risk guidelines and in fact recommended a similar diet. The central recommendation of the panel was the following nutrient intakes for healthy Americans above the age of 2 years:

- less than 10 per cent of total calories from saturated fatty acids;
- an average of 30 per cet of total calories or less from all fat;
- dietary energy levels needed to reach or maintain a desirable body weight;
- less than 300 mg cholesterol per day.

The panel believed that implementation of their recommendations, if adopted, would help most Americans lower their levels of cholesterol and would result in an approximate reduction of 10 per cent or more in the average blood cholesterol level and, in turn, to a reduction of 20 per cent or more in CHD rates. These recommendations concerning nutrient intake were regarded as appropriate for the general population including healthy women and individuals 65 years of age and older. The panel also wrote that as healthy children joined in the eating patterns of other family members they should also follow the nutrient recommendations. The panel directed the following recommendations to specific groups.

- *Health professionals* should both practice and advocate the recommended eating patterns, ensure that education of future health professionals includes appropriate nutrition education, and work with industry, government voluntary groups, and health care agencies to facilitate adoption of the recommending eating patterns.
- *The food industry*, food and animal scientists, and food technologists should increase efforts to design, modify, prepare, promote, label, and distribute good tasting safe foods that are lower in fatty acids, total fat, and cholesterol.
- *Government agencies* should provide consistent co-ordinated nutrition statements and policies emphasizing low saturated fatty acid, low fat, and low cholesterol eating patterns, should expand and standardize food-labelling requirements to identify clearly the content of saturated fatty acids, total fat, cholesterol, and total calories, and should take other steps to improve the consumer comprehension necessary to achieve the recommended patterns.
- *Educational programmes* at all levels should incorporate curricula that

emphasize background, benefits, and methods of achieving eating patterns that are low in saturated fatty acids, total fat, and cholesterol. This recommendation includes all levels of schools, vocational programmes (especially in culinary art), colleges, universities, and health professionals.

Some may doubt whether it is reasonable to expect changes in the national diet as a result of such recommendations. In fact, there are many pointers that change is indeed feasible and is occurring. For example, a comprehensive review of 171 US studies published between 1920 and 1984 that assessed individual dietary intake (Stephen and Wald 1990) found total fat intake rising from approximately 34 per cent of energy intake in the 1940s to 40–42 per cent in the late 1950s to the 1960s, and then steadily falling to approximately 36 per cent of total energy intake in 1984. The decrease in total fat intake was accompanied by a decline in saturated fat intake and an increase in polyunsaturated fat intake. It was concluded that the US population is capable of dietary change and was beginning to make such changes even before the move to a healthier life-style gained nationwide popularity.

A similar review of 95 studies of individual fat consumption in the UK (Stephen 1990) showed fat to account for 30 per cent of energy intake until the 1930s when values began to rise to 34–35 per cent by 1939. After a drop due to rationing in the Second World War, the rise continued to a plateau of 39–40 per cent through the 1960s and 1970s. A fall of 1–2 per cent has occurred since 1980. Little information was available on the type of fat consumed. The author contrasted this with the US experience and suggested that it may explain the different pattern of heart disease mortality between the two countries.

Another indicator of change involves the fast food industry. This industry accounts for a significant amount of the food eaten in the USA and is commencing to make important changes. For example, the McDonald's chain now offers a low fat milkshake and yogurt, 1 per cent instead of 2 per cent fat milk, margarine instead of butter, and no-fat and no-cholesterol apple and blueberry muffins. The fat content of a popular chicken dish has been decreased by 5 per cent, and french fries are now cooked in a low saturated fat vegetable oil. A lean hamburger, with only 9 per cent fat compared with the usual 20 per cent fat, is also being consumer-tested.

Food labelling   Adequate food labels are needed by a public that is shifting to the recommended diets and particularly by individuals being treated for high cholesterol levels. The US Congress has recently legislated to improve the food label. It deems a food as misbranded or mislabelled unless it bears nutrition information that provides (1) the serving size or other common household unit of measure customarily used, (2) the number of servings or other units per container, (3) the number of calories per serving and derived from total fat and saturated fat, and (4) the amount of total fat, saturated fat, cholesterol, and other nutrients. The legislation directs the issuance of regulations which set forth the circumstances under which nutrition and health claims may and may not be made for foods. It regulates the presentation of claims, requiring that, if the level of either cholesterol or saturated fat is disclosed, both must be disclosed and in immediate proximity to each other, and prohibiting a label from stating that the food is high in dietary fibre unless it is low in total fat, or the label discloses the level of total fat in immediate proximity.

Cholesterol screening

If large numbers of individuals are to be identified on the basis of their cholesterol levels as high risk subjects for treatment, then a large proportion of the adult population has to be screened. The slogan of the NCEP directed to American adults is to 'Know your cholesterol level'. Cholesterol screening *per se* does not require the individual to be fasting, which provides an opportunity for it to be done without prior interaction with the persons involved. New methods using portable chemical analysers can provide results quickly, near painlessly, and at quite low cost. The NCEP panels that have addressed the question prefer that screening be performed in the doctor's office or some equivalent setting (opportunistic screening). However, public (mass) screening provides an alternative to opportunistic screening and has its place if it is properly done (NHLBI 1989). The Population Panel report (NCEP 1990) describes the rationale for public screening as its educational value as well as its case-finding role. With respect to the latter, public screening programmes can be particularly helpful in detecting high risk individuals who might otherwise not be found. Their educational function is served if they provide screened individuals with health information about cholesterol beyond simply providing their 'cholesterol number'. This should be in the form of printed information, and a knowledgeable staff should include guidance regarding appropriate follow-up contingent on blood cholesterol and other CHD risk factor levels.

The Expert Panel on Blood Cholesterol Levels in Children and Adolescents

That atherosclerosis has its origins in childhood or early adult life can hardly be doubted, a view recently reinforced by the preliminary findings of the Pathological Determinants of Atherosclerosis in Youth (PDAY) study in which the percentage of the intimal surface involved with atherosclerotic lesions in both the aorta and the right coronary artery was found to be positively associated with the serum very low density lipoprotein, and low density lipoprotein cholesterol concentrations (PDAY 1990). Rather the questions are to what extent and by what means cholesterol-lowering should be a goal in childhood. Some advocate universal cholesterol screening in childhood, while others hold that the population approach should be the main strategy with screening confined to children from high risk families. Newman *et al.* (1990) have recently presented their case against cholesterol screening in childhood and point to the poor predictive value of childhood cholesterol levels for levels in early adulthood or later in life. They are also concerned with the expense of screening and intervention, and that labelling of children and family conflicts could occur. The Expert Panel on Blood Cholesterol Levels in Children and Adolescents has compared the advantages and disadvantages of the different approaches; its recent report recommended selective screening of potentially high risk children (NCEP 1991).

MONITORING THE IMPACT OF THE NCEP

National prevention programmes require assessment. A growing number of physicians are convinced of the benefit of reducing elevated blood cholesterol levels and are treating patients accordingly (Schucker *et al.* 1987*a*). Changes have occurred in drug prescribing: between 1983 and 1988 there was a five-fold increase in dispensing of prescriptions for lipid-lowering drugs by retail pharmacies (Wysowski *et al.* 1990).

From 1983 to 1989 visits to physicians for high blood cholesterol levels increased nine-fold (NDTI 1990). The National Heart, Lung, and Blood Institute (NHLBI) and the Food and Drug Administration (FDA) jointly conduct a telephone survey at intervals on samples of the US public which has also shown gains of public awareness and action (Schucker *et al.* 1987*b*).

Data on serum cholesterol levels are derived from the periodic National Health and Nutrition Examination Survey (NHANES) of representative samples of US populations. Between 1960–2 and 1976–80 age-adjusted mean serum cholesterol levels decreased by 3–4 per cent (NCHS–NHLBI 1987).

Data to monitor national food consumption trends are available from various sources. For example, the National Food Consumption Surveys periodically conducted by the US Department of Agriculture (USDA) collect their information mainly through household interviews (Sims 1988). Food disappearance data are assembled from production and domestic food use statistics. The USDA Continuing Survey of Food Intakes by Individuals (CSFII) and the Health and Nutrition Examination Surveys (HANES) of the National Center for Health Statistics (NCHS) rely to a considerable extent on 24 hour dietary recalls. Assessment of many studies of individual dietary fat intake has been carried out by Stephen and Wald (1990). Each of these surveys has strengths and weaknesses (NRC 1989). For example, some are not designed to represent the entire US population, the 24 hour dietary recall method is vulnerable to the significant variation which occurs in daily nutrient intake, and food disappearance data may not accurately reflect the food actually consumed. Furthermore, all surveys are dependent on the quality of nutrient composition data.

Overall reductions in the consumption of total and saturated fat compatible with decreased consumption of foods such as meat, eggs, whole milk, and butter have been noted in some, though not all, of the surveys.

The ultimate criteria for measuring the preventative impact of a cholesterol reduction programme are its effects on coronary mortality and morbidity. However, many factors other than cholesterol-lowering can affect mortality and morbidity, so that it is difficult to attribute any improvements to cholesterol change *per se*. Coronary mortality has declined in the USA for all four of the major race–sex groups from 1968 to 1985 (Sempos *et al.* 1988), although since 1976 the rate of decline has slowed in black men and women and in white women. The decline, which has been observed in populations in other countries, is leading to a widening in the social inequalities of health status within populations (Beaglehole 1990). Measuring trends in morbidity is more difficult because of changes in admission policies, enzyme tests, and hospital reimbursement systems (Beaglehole 1990), and results are not consistent. Nevertheless there is evidence that incidence rates have fallen in a number of centres.

REFERENCES

BCS (British Cardiac Society) (1987). *Report of British Cardiac Society Working Group on coronary disease prevention*, British Cardiac Society, London.
Beaglehole, R. (1990). International trends in coronary heart disease mortality, morbidity, and risk factors. *Epidemiol Rev., 12*, 1–15.
Brook, J. G. and Rifkind, B. M. (1989). Cholesterol and coronary heart disease prevention—a transatlantic consensus. *Eur. Heart J., 10*, 702–11.
Consensus Conference (1985). Statement on lowering blood cholesterol to prevent heart disease. *J. Am. Med. Assoc., 253*, 2080–6.
EAS (European Atherosclerosis Society) (1987). Strategy for the prevention of coronary heart disease: a policy statement for the European Atherosclerosis Society. *Eur. Heart J., 8*, 77–88.
Lenfant, C. (1986). A new challenge for America: the National Cholesterol Education Program. *Circulation, 73*, 855–6.
Lipid Research Clinics Program (1984a). The Lipid Research Clinics Coronary Primary Prevention Trial Results. I. Reduction in incidence of coronary heart disease. *J. Am. Med. Assoc., 251*, 351–64.
Lipid Research Clinics Program (1984b). The Lipid Research Clinics Coronary

Primary Prevention Trial Results. II. The relationship of reduction in incidence of coronary heart disease to cholesterol lowering. *J. Am. Med. Assoc.*, **251**, 365–74.

Mann, J. I., Lewis, B., Shepherd, J., Winder, A. F., Fenster, S., Rose, L., *et al.* (1988). Blood lipid and other cardiovascular risk factors: distribution, prevalence, and detection in Britain. *Br. Med. J.*, **1**, 1702–6.

Muldoon, M. F., Manuck, S. B., and Matthews, K. A. (1990). Lowering cholesterol concentrations and mortality: a quantitative review of primary prevention trials. *Br. Med. J.*, **301**, 309–14.

Mullen, F. and Jacoby, I. (1985). The town meeting for technology. The maturation of consensus conferences. *J. Am. Med. Assoc.*, **254**, 1068–72.

NCEP (National Cholesterol Education Program) Laboratory Standardization Panel (1988*a*). Current status of blood cholesterol measurement in clinical laboratories in the United States. *Clin. Chem.*, **34**, 193–201.

NCEP (National Cholesterol Education Program) (1988*b*). Report of the Expert Panel on Detection, Evaluation, and Treatment of High Blood Cholesterol in Adults. *Arch. Intern. Med.*, **148**, 36–69.

NCEP (National Cholesterol Education Program) Laboratory Standardization Panel (1990*a*), *Recommendations for improving cholesterol measurement*, Publ. 90–2964, National Institutes of Health, Bethesda, MD.

NCEP (National Cholesterol Education Program) (1990*b*). *Report of the Expert Panel on Population Strategies for Blood Cholesterol Reduction*, Publ. 90–3046, National Institutes of Health, Bethesda, MD.

NCEP (National Cholesterol Education Program) (1991). *Report of the expert panel on blood cholesterol levels in children or adolescents*, Publ. 91–2732, National Institutes of Health, Bethesda, MD.

NCHS–NHLBI (National Center for Health Statistics–National Heart, Lung, and Blood Institute) Collaborative Lipid Group (1987). Trends in serum cholesterol levels among US adults aged 20 to 74 years. *J. Am. Med. Assoc.*, **257**, 937–42.

Newman, T. B., Browner, W. S., and Hulley, S. B. (1990). The case against childhood cholesterol screening. *J. Am. Med. Assoc.*, **264**, 3039–43.

NHLBI (National Heart, Lung, and Blood Institute) (1988). Recommendations regarding public screening for measuring blood cholesterol. Summary of an NHLBI Workshop, October 1988. *Arch. Intern. Med.*, **149**, 2650–4.

NDTI (National Disease and Therapeutic Index) (1990). *Diagnosis: January 1989–December 1989, Plymouth Meeting, PA*, IMS America.

NRC (National Research Council) (1989). *Diet and health: implications for reducing chronic disease risk*, National Academy Press, Washington, DC.

PDAY (Pathobiological Determinants of Atherosclerosis in Youth) Research Group (1990). Relationship of atherosclerosis in young men to serum lipoprotein concentrations and smoking. Preliminary report. *J. Am. Med. Assoc.*, **264**, 3018–24.

Rifkind, B. M. and Grouse, L. D. (1990). Cholesterol redux. *J. Am. Med. Assoc.*, **284**, 3060–1.

Rossouw, J. E., Lewis, B., and Rifkind, B. M. (1990). The value of lowering cholesterol after myocardial infarction. *New Engl. J. Med.*, **323**, 1112–19.

Schucker, B. H., Bailey, K., Heimbach, J. T., Mattson, M. E., Wittes, J. T., Haines, C. M., *et al.* (1987*a*). Change in public perspective on cholesterol and heart disease: Results from two national surveys. *J. Am. Med. Assoc.,* **258,** 3527–31.

Schucker, B. H., Wittes, J. T., Cutler, J. A., Bailey, K., Mackintosh, D., Gordon, D. J., *et al.* (1987*b*). Change in physician perspective on cholesterol and coronary heart disease. Results from two national surveys. *J. Am. Med. Assoc.,* **258,** 3521–6.

Scottish Home and Health Department and Scottish Health Services Advisory Council (1990). *Prevention of coronary heart disease in Scotland*, HM Stationery Office, Edinburgh.

Sempos, C., Cooper, R., Kovar, M., and McMillen, M. (1988). Divergence of the recent trends in coronary mortality for the four major race/sex groups in the United States. *Am. J. Public Health,* **78,** 1422–7.

Sempos, C., Fulwood, R., Haines, C., Carroll, M., Anda, R., Williamson, D. F., *et al.* (1989). The prevalence of high blood cholesterol levels among adults in the United States. *J. Am. Med. Assoc.,* **262,** 45–52.

Sims, L. S. (1988). Contributions of the US Department of Agriculture. *Am. J. Clin. Nutr.,* **47,** 329–32.

Stephen, A. M. (1990). Trends in individual fat consumption in the United Kingdom, 1900–1985. *Circulation,* **8,** 347.

Stephen, A. M. and Wald, N. J. (1990). Trends in individual consumption of dietary fat in the United States, 1920–1984. *Am. J. Clin. Nutr.,* **52,** 457–69.

Truswell, A. S. (1983). The development of dietary guidelines. *Food Technol. Aust.,* **35,** 498–502.

Wysowski, D. K., Kennedy, D. L., and Gross, T. P. (1990). Prescribed use of cholesterol-lowering drugs in the United States; 1978–1988. *J. Am. Med. Assoc.,* **263,** 2185–8.

Yusuf, S., Wittes, J., and Friedman, L. (1988). Overview of results of randomized clinical trials in heart disease II. Unstable angina, heart failure, primary prevention with aspirin and risk factor modification. *J. Am. Med. Assoc.,* **260,** 2259–63.

31

From observation to policy: smoking

D. Simpson and K. Ball

THE EARLY DAYS

Starting first as a habit practised by males, cigarette smoking spread rapidly in the UK, as it did in North America and Western Europe, during the first decade of this century. Women followed men in smoking habits later on, until by the 1950s the average daily smoking prevalence among men in these areas was frequently over 50 per cent, with women not far behind.

The first major campaign against cigarette smoking in the UK followed the second report of the Royal College of Physicians, *Smoking and health now* (RCP 1971) when the College launched Action on Smoking and Health (ASH). Earlier reports had been less certain about the effect of smoking on coronary heart disease (CHD) than on lung cancer and chronic bronchitis. The first report (RCP 1962) only stated that smoking probably plays a significant part in rendering men in early middle age more liable to CHD. But by 1971 the evidence was much clearer, although little action was being taken to control the UK's largest single cause of death when compared with the USA, Australia, and Canada, where coronary rates were steadily falling. It was said that a New York taxi driver knew more about diet and heart disease than many British physicians, probably because of the pioneering work of cardiologists like Paul White, Ancel Keys, and Jerry Stamler who had persuaded the American Heart Association to make forthright statements on heart disease prevention.

The British Heart Foundation was founded in 1961 to promote research and at that time did not consider that prevention was one of its responsibilities. An article in the *Lancet* in 1973 (Turner and Ball 1973) reflected the frustration of a number of British doctors. In 1976 a Joint Working Party of the Royal College of Physicians and the British Cardiac Society chaired by Professor Gerry Shaper produced a report on the prevention of CHD (RCP–BCS 1976). It accepted that 'more than half of the excess mortality in smokers is due to cardiovascular disease'. In 1979 the Coronary Prevention Group was formed and together with ASH and other bodies including the British Medical Association, and more recently the British Heart Foundation and the British Thoracic Society, have been increasing pressure to control cigarette smoking. As a result tobacco consumption has fallen by a quarter in the last 10 years, and at last we are beginning to see a fall in the death rates from CHD, as well as from lung cancer, especially in younger men.

CIGARETTE SMOKING: A MAJOR PREVENTABLE CAUSE OF CHD

It is now widely accepted that cigarette smoking (along with inappropriate diet) is one of the two major preventable causes of CHD, and in the UK it is responsible for about 40 000 premature deaths each year. The report *The health consequences of smoking* (US Surgeon General 1983) summarized the main conclusions which are probably relevant for all industrial countries. These included the following.

1. Cigarette smoking is a major cause of CHD in the USA for both men and women: it should be considered the most important of the known modifiable risk factors for CHD.
2. Overall, cigarette smokers experience a 70 per cent greater CHD death rate than non-smokers.
3. The risk of developing CHD increases with increasing exposure to cigarette smoke, as measured by the number of cigarettes smoked daily, the total number of years one has smoked, the degree of inhalation, and an early age of initiation.
4. Women who use oral contraceptives and who smoke increase their risk of a myocardial infarction by about ten-fold compared with women who neither use oral contraceptives nor smoke.
5. The CHD mortality ratio for smokers compared with non-smokers is greater for younger than for older age groups.
6. Unless the smoking habits of Americans change, perhaps 10 per cent of all persons now alive may die prematurely of heart disease due to smoking.

Since these conclusions are now widely accepted, in this chapter we shall look at some of the more controversial or undecided aspects of the relation of smoking to cardiovascular disease.

DOES PASSIVE SMOKING CAUSE CHD?

Studies have shown that the risk of lung cancer is raised by between 30 and 53 per cent in non-smokers exposed to environmental tobacco smoke (ETS) (Wald *et al*. 1986). Glantz and Parmley (1991) reviewed 10 epidemiological studies and found that all but one also showed an increased risk of CHD in exposed non-smokers, although statistical significance usually was not reached. A survey of 513 non-smoking black and white women from Evans County, Georgia, who were married to smokers showed a relative risk for cardiovascular mortality of 1.59 with 95 per cent confidence intervals of 0.99–2.57 (Humble *et al.* 1990). In the Multiple Risk Factor Intervention Trial (MRFIT) non-smoking husbands with smoking wives had an increased but non-significant risk of fatal or non-fatal CHD events, with a relative risk of 1.61 (confidence interval 0.96–2.71, $p = 0.07$) (Svendsen *et al.* 1987). A New Zealand study, which showed increased risk for exposure to spouses who smoked, estimated that passive smoking could cause as many as 243 deaths each year from CHD compared with 30 deaths from lung cancer (Kawachi *et al.* 1989). A large study in the west of Scotland showed a relative mortality for CHD of 2.27 (confidence interval 1.21–3.35, $p = 0.008$) for non-smokers exposed to ETS (Hole *et al.* 1989). Clearly, much more work needs to be done to clarify this issue. The consistency of the increase in all but one of the studies makes it unlikely to be a chance finding, although it is recognized that positive results are more likely to be reported than negative ones. The relationship could be due to confounding factors, although these were adequately controlled for in the Scottish cohort study. However, if these findings are confirmed, CHD caused by ETS will be seen to be one of our major environmental health hazards.

IS SMOKING AN IMPORTANT CAUSE OF STROKES?

Strokes cause about 70 000 deaths a year in the UK and are the third major cause of mortality, but it is only recently that cigarette smoking has been confirmed to be an important cause. A New Zealand study of men and women aged 35–64 showed that smoking up to 20 cigarettes a day increased the risk 3.3 times, and 5.6 times for heavier smokers (Bonita *et al.* 1986). If hypertension was also present, the risk for smokers increased nearly 20-fold compared with those who neither smoked nor had hypertension. In the Medical Research Council study of the treatment of mild hypertension (MRC 1988), smoking was consistently an outstanding risk factor for strokes, especially in women where the rate was increased nearly four times. A meta-analysis of 32 studies by Shinton and Beevers (1989) showed that the overall risk of stroke associated with cigarette smoking was 1.5 (confidence interval 1.4–1.6). Considerable differences were seen in relative risks of the different types of stroke: cerebral infarction, 1.9; cerebral haemorrhage, 0.7; subarachnoid haemorrhage, 2.9. The relative risk decreased from 2.9 for those aged less than 55 years to 1.1 for those aged more than 75 years, an age effect noted in many of the studies. One survey which confirmed the presence of cerebral ischaemia with computerized tomography demonstrated a relative risk for smokers of 5.7 (confidence interval 2.8–12.0) compared with non-smokers (Donnan *et al.* 1989).

Several studies have noted the marked effect of smoking on the risk of subarachnoid haemorrhage. One large survey of women showed that the risk of cigarette smokers was 5.7 times that of non-smokers, but for those who both smoked and used oral contraceptives the risk increased 22 times (Petitti and Wingerd 1978).

There are various mechanisms by which smoking could increase the risk of cerebral ischaemia. Smoking is known to increase platelet stickiness and fibrinogen levels and therefore blood viscosity. Cerebral blood flow has been shown to be reduced in chronic smokers.

DOES SMOKING CAUSE CARDIOVASCULAR DISEASE IN THE THIRD WORLD?

As the tobacco companies see their trade declining in their traditional markets, they are turning increasingly to the developing world. In most developing countries, smoking and other forms of tobacco use are increasing, encouraged by the massive promotional activities of the multinational tobacco companies.

This rapid increase in smoking in some developing countries is already leading to growing epidemics of lung cancer, particularly in China, India, and Malaysia. Since adequate nutrition is also necessary for the development of CHD, many developing countries have not yet shown a comparable rise in heart attacks which were virtually absent until recently. Vint (1937) found no cases of CHD in a thousand autopsies in Kenya in 1936–7, and Davies (1948) found only one case of myocardial infarction in 2994 autopsies in Kampala between 1931 and 1946. Even in South Africa, where lung cancer is quite common among blacks, very few deaths are due to CHD. Today changes in the living habits of middle class Africans are leading to an increase in CHD. In Khartoum CHD was rarely diagnosed 30 years ago, but now it is said to be one of the commonest causes of death in the professional and business community (Sirag 1990). A survey showed that 64 per cent of doctors and teachers are cigarette smokers (Alarabi 1990). Likewise, in Nairobi, where there has always been a high prevalence of CHD in the Asian community, more cases are now being found in native Africans (Wangai 1991). In natives of Southeast Asia, and especially those migrating to the industrialized West, CHD associated with smoking is an important public health problem.

As living standards improve in developing countries and the transnational tobacco companies press their promotional activities, it is all too likely that deaths from cardiovascular disease will join those from lung cancer to produce a horrendous epidemic which will cause immense strains on their limited health resources.

The World Health Organization (WHO) has estimated that, at present, tobacco causes about 2.5 million premature deaths per annum world-wide, having risen more than ten-fold since 1950, when the annual burden was around 0.2 million deaths. The WHO consultancy on statistical aspects of tobacco-related mortality, chaired by Richard Peto FRS and with Dr Alan Lopez as scientific secretary, estimates that even at present rates of consumption, global annual mortality from tobacco will rise to 3.0 million during the 1990s and to 10 million sometime in about the 2020s. With consumption projected to rise still further, the actual figures may well be much greater.

HOW SOON DOES STOPPING SMOKING REDUCE THE RISK?

Although there is no doubt that cigarette smokers who stop smoking reduce their risk of a coronary attack, the findings of different surveys vary in the rapidity with which it occurs. The US Surgeon General reported in 1983 that 'Cessation of smoking results in a substantial reduction in CHD death rates compared with those persons who continue to smoke' (US Surgeon General 1983). Mortality from CHD declines rapidly after cessation. Approximately 10 years following cessation the CHD death rate for those ex-smokers who consumed less than a pack of cigarettes daily is virtually identical with that of lifelong non-smokers. Some reports such as the Framingham Study showed a swift effect, suggesting that 'smoking has a non-cumulative transient, reversible triggering effect rather than a direct influence on atherogenesis' (Gordon et al. 1974). In their study of British doctors Doll and Peto (1976) found that the risk among current smokers was 3.5 times that of lifelong non-smokers. After 5 years the risk was virtually halved to 1.9 and after 5–9 years the risk approached that of non-smokers (1.3), although it remained at this level for up to 15 years. However, the British Regional Heart study reported a much slower improvement after cessation of smoking (Cook et al. 1986).

Smokers who quit after a myocardial infarction showed a marked and rapid reduction of relapse compared with continuing smokers in most studies, although it must be accepted that in some cases they may have been lighter smokers who were also more concerned with other aspects of health such as diet and exercise. A study of Swedish women who had survived a myocardial infarction revealed that those who stopped smoking had a cumulative 5 year survival rate of 85 per cent compared with 73 per cent for those who continued to smoke ($p \leqslant 0.5$), although there was no difference in their pre-infarction characteristics (Johansson et al. 1985).

This certainly indicates that stopping smoking is one of the most effective therapies to be prescribed after a heart attack. The first dose should be administered in the coronary care unit with strong follow-up in a non-smoking medical ward.

Thus there is very strong evidence that cigarette smoking is an important factor in the cause of a whole spectrum of cardiovascular diseases. Although further studies may refine the picture, it is clearly essential to control the largest single cause of CHD in this country which is in itself the cause of more than a quarter of all deaths. Some of the key areas in the prevention and control of cigarette smoking are outlined in the remainder of this chapter.

MODEL TOBACCO POLICY

The Royal College of Physicians, the International Union Against Cancer (UICC), the WHO, and the many other expert organizations which have examined the problems of tobacco and ill health have recommended how tobacco should be controlled in order to reduce the disease, disability, and premature death which it causes. Among the measures which are consistently recommended in their reports, which form the essentials of a model tobacco control policy, are the following:

(1) stopping all forms of promotion of tobacco products;
(2) regular price rises through taxation;
(3) public education and public information programmes;
(4) strong prominent health warnings on packs;
(5) controlling smoking in public places;
(6) banning sales to children;
(7) reducing emission levels of toxic components;
(8) encouraging tobacco farmers to change to other crops.

The most essential requirement for a successful policy is that it is backed up by the force of law. Obtaining the best tobacco policy requires good baseline data, top-level interdisciplinary advisory groups to guide the formation and implementation of a model Tobacco Act, and a strong 'watchdog' body to monitor implementation and to counteract industry attempts to sabotage it. The policy should be agreed by the government as a whole, at cabinet level, to ensure that the health ministry is supported by other departments of government.

Adequate resources should be made available for tactical advertising to counter the tobacco industry's own activities in this area, for regular public attitude surveys, and for extensive public information and education programmes.

There have been successful and total bans on all tobacco promotion in a number of countries, notably in Scandinavia. The most recently enacted bans, in both cases as part of a comprehensive act to implement all the essential components of a model tobacco policy, have been in Canada (1989) and New Zealand (1990). In addition, an ingenious policy adopted by a number of Australian states has been a partial advertising ban coupled with a levy on each pack of cigarettes sold which is diverted into a special health promotion fund. This is used to pay for health education, public information programmes, and medical research, and, most uniquely, to replace the sponsorship of sporting and cultural events so dominated by the cigarette companies as a means of circumventing restrictions on advertising.

More detailed comments are offered on three areas of policy: dealing with tobacco advertising, taxation, and reducing the toxicity of cigarettes.

Tobacco advertising

All cigarettes are intrinsically the same: tubes of paper with chopped dried tobacco leaves inside which, when ignited, produce smoke containing several thousand chemicals. Many of these are known carcinogens and other highly toxic compounds. It is virtually entirely due to advertising that one brand of cigarettes is perceived as having different characteristics from another.

Cigarette advertisers never voluntarily draw attention to the toxic chemicals or the unique and substantial risks involved in inhaling the smoke from a cigarette. Instead, advertisements are exclusively concerned with creating an image intended to appeal to a particular group of people. Information provided from within the advertising industry, some of it exposed inadvertently or reluctantly, shows that strenuous efforts are made to aim certain advertisements at young people, to reassure smokers about their fears of the health risks of smoking, and to associate smoking in general, and individual brands in particular, with positive concepts and images.

Tobacco promotion maintains the social acceptability of tobacco use. Health education cannot deliver its message to the public—especially to young people—at face value as long as huge sums are spent each year associating cigarettes with success, glamour, independence, sports, and all sorts of other desirable, positive images. The tobacco industry always tries to persuade governments that self-regulation is better than legislation. Experience shows that it is indeed better—for the industry—but it is far from effective. The experience of the UK, where successive 'voluntary agreements' on advertising have merely led to more examples of tobacco industry ingenuity in circumventing the intentions of the government, is a sad testimony to this fact.

The main shortcomings of voluntary agreements on tobacco advertising are as follows.

1. They tend to be highly selective in nature: many significant types of promotion are excluded from being regulated.
2. Different government departments are involved, often pulling in opposite directions. For example, the ministry responsible for sport would like as much sponsorship of sport from private industry as possible, but tobacco sports sponsorship will have precisely the opposite effect to the policy of the health ministry, which tries to ensure that tobacco is not linked with the healthy and exciting qualities associated with sport.
3. The voluntary nature of the system means that the companies have little to lose by breaching the agreement and nothing at all to lose by refusing to agree to more stringent measures, as long as no real threat of legislation exists.
4. The many rounds of meetings involved with ministers, officials, and other organizations (advertising industry, retailers, etc.) mean that negotiations for new voluntary agreements can take a matter of years, thus giving plenty of time to plan how to circumvent the restrictions being negotiated. In addition, the government negotiators are worn down to such a degree that the industry's ultimate concessions in the talks tend to be perceived as being of far greater significance than they really are.
5. Being one of the parties to the voluntary agreement on cigarette advertising, the health ministry is effectively neutralized. From being the obvious point from which improvements, from the health point of view, could be initiated, encouraged, and executed, the health ministry is forced into the position of arbiter between health on one side and the tobacco industry on the other.

Raising price through taxation

It is widely accepted in the UK that regular increases in cigarette taxation were the most effective single measure causing the steady decline in consumption during the 1980s.

In virtually every country, no matter what type of economy it has, the government can go on increasing taxation in real terms with the combined result that consumption will fall but the government will still make more money, in real terms, from taxation. Consumer expenditure on cigarettes, adjusted for inflation, varies according to the price of an average packet of 20 cigarettes. Most of the price increases of cigarettes are caused by tax increases, because the process of cigarette manufacture becomes ever more mechanized and efficient, thus keeping below the general level of price inflation.

The government receives more cigarette tax revenue if it increases the duty on cigarettes, despite the fact that such tax/price rises cause less cigarettes to be sold. When the price is allowed to fall (by the government failing to increase the duty), even with consumers spending more money on cigarettes, the government's income falls also. Eventually a point of diminishing returns would be reached, but even in the UK, where prices are comparatively high and consumption has been falling for some years, economists calculate that this point lies many years in the future.

Increases in tobacco tax are borne more by the wealthier smokers than the poorer ones, since smokers who can more easily afford the new increased prices are more likely to maintain the same smoking habits after a rise in price, whereas smokers with less money will tend to give up or cut down their consumption.

Reducing the emission levels of toxic components

Lowering the tar emission levels of cigarettes has been shown to produce a significant reduction in the incidence of lung cancer caused by smoking, and a number of Western governments are also attempting to reduce carbon monoxide yields in view of evidence which suggests that carbon monoxide plays a role in causing heart disease in smokers. Nicotine emission levels have also been reduced in the West, though below a certain nicotine level habitual cigarette smokers may smoke more cigarettes to compensate. A cigarette with low tar and low carbon monoxide levels, but a medium nicotine level, has been suggested as the least dangerous product for those who continue to smoke.

This area of tobacco policy should never be seen as anything but an interim measure to be taken while every effort is made to eliminate all use of tobacco. While lower-tar cigarettes may reduce the risk of lung cancer, this 'lower' risk still remains far larger than any risk which could be considered acceptable, and there is no conclusive evidence that tar reduction lowers the substantial risks of cardiovascular disease and chronic obstructive airways disease caused by smoking.

Most important of all, on no account should the tobacco industry be permitted to determine the way that emission policy is implemented. If the public is educated about the relative dangers of low tar and high tar cigarettes, there is a risk that many continuing smokers will persuade themselves that as long as they smoke a low tar brand, they will be 'safe'. Instead, the toxicity of individual brands should be progressively reduced without notice to smokers.

In many countries, such as the USSR and many developing nations, significant reductions of future lung cancer mortality could be effected by setting upper limits for tar levels and regularly reviewing and lowering them. Sales-weighted tar levels can be reduced relatively quickly and cheaply, especially if the government takes legal powers to enforce compliance to the limits, as they commonly do for pharmaceuticals. Differential tax rates favouring the lower-tar brands may be considered, a system used success-fully in the UK in the 1970s.

The WHO (1979) and the UICC (1980) have suggested the goal of a market range of cigarettes between 5 and 15 mg of tar. The UICC recom-mends 'to progressively eradicate high-tar brands from the market, starting with all brands over 25 mgs; then 20 mgs; then 15 mg'. The European Community has called for all 12 member states to set an upper limit of 15 mg of tar per cigarette, falling to 12 mg in 1995.

THE INTERNATIONAL TOBACCO INDUSTRY

Apart from the reduction of toxicity, all other tobacco control measures are designed to reduce tobacco consumption. For obvious reasons, these measures are fiercely resisted by one of the world's largest and most powerful industries. Apart from the USSR, some of the Central and East European nations, and the People's Republic of China, the tobacco market in the rest of the world is dominated by just six multinational tobacco companies. In developing countries there is often little or no local know-ledge of tobacco control policy and little informed or co-ordinated action by government.

The sheer might of the tobacco companies may be gauged from a few figures for BAT Industries PLC, the conglomerate built on the world-wide tobacco operations of British American Tobacco. Its 1989 total group sales were over £21 billion, dwarfing the entire economic activities of many a developing country (BAT 1989). For example, this level of turnover ex-ceeded the combined gross domestic products of Bangladesh, Kenya, Costa Rica, and Papua New Guinea. Even BAT's tobacco division alone recorded sales of over £8 billion in 1989, with record profits of £945 million. The salary and other emoluments of the company chairman were over £601 000 for the year, more than twice the amount of the grant (£241 500) given by the Department of Health to the head office of ASH to fund its activities for 1989–90. It is hardly surprising that the major tobacco com-panies are so successful in preventing the poorer countries from taking effective action to curb tobacco use.

In 1979, the WHO Expert Committee Report *Controlling the Smoking Epidemic* stated that:

It must be recognised that the tobacco industry has presented, and will continue to present, a formidable barrier to smoking control . . . and no worthwhile progress can be achieved unless governments are prepared to put the interests of public health before those of private tobacco enterprise, and to secure appropriate action by state-owned industry.

The international tobacco industry's irresponsible behaviour and its massive advertising and promotional campaigns are, in the opinion of the Committee, direct causes of a substantial number of unnecessary deaths. (WHO 1979)

The tobacco industry has to be recognized as a major enemy to public health.

In 1971, the Royal College of Physicians declared that smoking was 'as important a cause of death as were the great epidemic diseases that affected previous generations' and concluded that 'action to protect the public against the damage done to so many of them by cigarette smoking would have more effect upon the public health in this country than anything else that could now be done in the whole field of preventive medicine' (RCP 1971). Today, that statement remains lamentably true not just for the UK, but for the vast majority of the world.

REFERENCES

Alarabi, M. (1990). The Third World struggle against tobacco—the Sudan experience. *The Global War. Proc. 7th World Conf. Tobacco and Health, Perth, Western Australia, 1–5 April 1990* (eds B. Durston and K. Jamrozik), pp. 372–3. Health Department of Western Australia, Perth.

BAT (1989). *BAT Industries annual report and accounts*, BAT Industries, London.

Bonita, R., Scragg, R., Stewart, A., Jackson, R., and Beaglehole, R. (1986). Cigarette smoking and risk of premature stroke in men and women. *Br. Med. J.,* **296,** 6–8.

Cook, D. G., Shaper, A. G., Pocock, S. J., and Kussick, S. J. (1986). Giving up smoking and the risk of heart attacks. *Lancet,* **ii,** 1376–80.

Davies, J. N. P. (1948). Pathology of Central African natives. *East Afr. Med. J.,* **25,** 454–67.

Doll, R. and Peto, R. (1976). Mortality in relation to smoking: 20 years' observations on male British doctors. *Br. Med. J.,* **2,** 1525–36.

Donnan, G. A., McNeil, J. J., Adena, M. A., Doyle, A. E., O'Malley, H. M., and Neill, G. C. (1989). Smoking as a risk factor for cerebral ischaemia. *Lancet,* **ii,** 643–7.

Glantz, S. A. and Parmley, W. W. (1991). Passive smoking and heart disease. *Circulation,* **83,** 1–12.

Gordon, T., Kannel, W. B., McGee, D., and Dawber, T. R. (1974). Death and coronary attacks in men after giving up smoking. *Lancet,* **ii,** 1345–8.

Hole, D. J., Gillis, C. R., Chopra, C., and Hawthorne, V. M. (1989). Passive smoking and cardiorespiratory health in a general population in the West of Scotland. *Br. Med. J.,* **293,** 423–7.

Humble, C., Croft, J., Gerber, A., Casper, M., Hames, C. G., and Tyroler, H. A. (1990). Passive smoking and 20-year cardiovascular disease mortality among nonsmoking wives, Evans County, Georgia. *Am. J. Public Health,* **80,** 599–601.

Johansson, S., Bergstrand, R., Pennert, K., Ulvenstam, G., Vedin, A., Wedel, H., *et al.* (1985). Cessation of smoking after myocardial infarction in women. *Am. J. Epidemiol.,* **121,** 823–31.

Kawachi, I., Pearce, N. E., and Jackson, R. T. (1989). Deaths from lung cancer and ischaemic heart disease due to passive smoking in New Zealand. *NZ Med. J.,* **871,** 337–40.

MRC (Medical Reseach Council) Working Party (1988). Stroke and coronary heart disease in mild hypertension: risk factors and the value of treatment. *Br. Med. J.,* **1,** 1565–70.

Petitti, D. B. and Wingerd, J. (1978). Use of oral contraceptives, cigarette smoking and risk of subarachnoid haemorrhage. *Lancet,* **ii,** 234–6.

RCP (Royal College of Physicians) (1962). *Smoking and health,* London, Pitman.

RCP (Royal College of Physicians) (1971). *Smoking and health now,* London, Pitman.

RCP–BCS (Royal College of Physicians–British Cardiac Society) (1976). Prevention of coronary heart disease. *J. R. Coll. Physicians,* **10** (3).

Shinton, R. and Beevers, G. (1989). Meta-analysis of relation between cigarette smoking and stroke. *Br. Med. J.,* **298,** 789–94.

Sirag (1990). Personal communication.

Svendsen, K. H., Kuller, L. H., Martin, M. J., and Ockene, J. K. (1987). Effects of passive smoking in the Multiple Risk Factor Prevention Trial. *Am. J. Epidemiol.,* **126,** 783–95.

Turner, R. and Ball, K. (1973). Prevention of coronary heart disease. A counter-blast to present inactivity. *Lancet,* **ii,** 1137–40.

UICC (Union Internationale Contre le Cancer) (1980). *Guidelines for smoking control,* UICC Tech. Rep. Ser. 52, UICC, Geneva.

US Surgeon General (1983). *The health consequences of smoking,* US Department of Health and Human Services, Rockville, MD.

Vint, F. W. (1937). Post-mortem findings in the natives of Kenya. *East Af. Med. J.,* **13,** 332–40.

Wald, N. J., Nanchahal, K., Thompson, S. G., and Cuckle, H. S. (1986). Does breathing other people's smoke cause lung cancer? *Br. Med. J.,* **293,** 1217–21.

Wangai (1991). Personal communication.

WHO (World Health Organization) Expert Committee on Smoking Control (1979). *Controlling the smoking epidemic,* WHO, Geneva.

32

Monitoring coronary heart disease in the community: why and how?

H. Tunstall-Pedoe

INTRODUCTION

The beginning of the rise in coronary heart disease (CHD) mortality in most Western industrialized countries preceded the development of the techniques which might now be used to monitor and explain it. Similarly, the large unplanned dietary changes that occurred in Europe during the Second World War, and which are now thought to have lowered mortality rates from cardiovascular disease, also prompted more comment and investigation 20 or 30 years later than they did at the time. During the 1950s and 1960s, some now classical epidemiological studies demonstrated that individual coronary risk could be estimated to a large extent through measurement of risk factors such as cigarette smoking, blood pressure, and serum cholesterol (Pooling Project Research Group 1978; Dawber 1980). These factors were shown to vary between countries with differing CHD mortality (Keys 1980), and the risk factor theory of CHD became established.

At the beginning of the 1970s this risk factor theory was used to mount prevention projects, some of which were based in whole communities (Puska *et al.* 1981). At the end of the 1970s came the realization that some national mortality rates, most notably those of the USA, were undergoing a significant decline (Stern 1979; Ragland *et al.* 1988). The need to monitor planned community experiments (Salonen *et al.* 1986, 1989) and to explain spontaneous change made imperative the accurate measurement of trends in population cardiovascular event rates, along with the monitoring of the presumed risk factors concerned. A major watershed was reached at the 'Conference on the Decline of Coronary Heart Disease Mortality', held by the American National Institutes of Health in Bethesda in 1978 (Havlik and Feinleib 1979). It appeared that the decline was largely unexplained. The acknowledged experts of the country that had undertaken more research in this area than the rest of the world put together were unable to explain the size and timing of the decline in terms of known coronary risk factors and what was happening to incidence. It was thought that part of the problem was that the funding of scientific study, of causes and mechanisms, had not necessarily resulted in the standardized collection over several years of mortality, morbidity, and risk factor data that would readily yield the answers to the obvious questions that were being asked.

The Bethesda conference gave rise directly to a World Health Organization (WHO) initiative in 1989. This study of the 'Trends and determinants of cardiovascular disease' (Tunstall-Pedoe 1985; WHO MONICA Project 1988a), later given the acronym of MONICA for 'MONItoring CArdiovascular disease', cross-fertilized the experience of the WHO registers for stroke (Aho *et al*. 1980) and heart attack (WHO 1976; Tunstall-Pedoe *et al*. 1975; Tunstall-Pedoe 1978), mounted by the European Office of the WHO in the 1970s, with the experience of the Americans in large controlled trials and field studies. Although actively encouraging the WHO, the Americans, after carrying out a feasibility study, decided to go their own way in the Atherosclerosis Risk in Communities (ARIC) Study which contains a surveillance element but involves cohort studies (ARIC 1988, 1989), and is not strictly compatible with MONICA. The monitoring of cardiovascular disease therefore follows several different strands. This chapter attempts an overview of this problem subject.

MONITORING AND VALIDATING MORTALITY RATES

The interest in monitoring and validation arose from differences and trends in routine mortality data which have now been extensively researched in many countries (e.g. Morris 1951; Smith and Tunstall-Pedoe 1984; Hughes 1986; WHO MONICA Project 1987; Nicolosi *et al*. 1988; Najem *et al*. 1990). Thom at the United States National Institutes of Health studied trends over aggregated time periods in many different countries (Thom 1989). Pisa and Uemura, from the WHO in Geneva, used data from a number of countries which satisfied certain criteria of reliability, such as absence of large numbers of vague death certificate diagnoses (Pisa and Uemura 1982; Uemura and Pisa 1985). They reported recently that the proportion of heart disease deaths (International Classification of Diseases (ICD) codes 410–429) attributed to ischaemic heart disease (410–414) varies markedly between countries, and that the broad category (ICD 410–429) would be a more consistent disease category for international comparison (Uemura and Pisa 1988).

The necropsy rate, the medico-legal system, and the coding of disease all vary between countries, so that, for example, the change in disease coding from ICD Revision 8 to ICD Revision 9 in 1978–9 produced a larger 'blip' in the trends in the USA than elsewhere (Duggar and Lewis 1987; Heathcote *et al*. 1989) (Fig. 32.1). Whilst fixed national differences may bias the

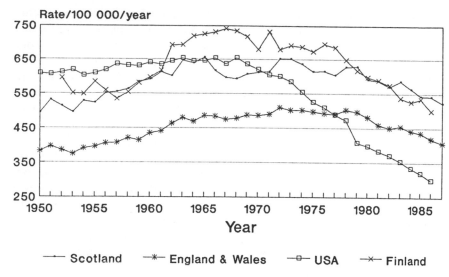

Fig. 32.1 Trends in CHD mortality in four countries during the period 1950–87: annual rate per 100 000 men aged 40–69. Age-standardized rates from WHO.

comparison of rates, it is changes in local practice, such as diagnostic and investigative practices, that are more likely to prejudice trends; for example, it is a common observation that necropsy rates are falling.

The MONICA Project (and a number of other community studies) attempts to validate cause of death in those deaths which are attributed to CHD (all MONICA centres) and those attributed to stroke (not all centres). Interesting differences have become apparent between countries in the ease with which this validation can be made (Tunstall-Pedoe 1988, 1989). The availability of data varies according to local conventions on privacy. For example, one enthusiast recently suggested that his city would be ideal for MONICA because it had such a high necropsy rate, but he admitted under questioning that death certificates had to be issued before the necropsy was done, and that local laws would preclude anyone from going from the death certificate to obtain a copy of the necropsy report! This kind of problem seems to be common in Central Europe, and makes validation of death certificate diagnoses almost impossible. The result can be that a local investigator collects data on all the deaths which he or she considers may have been diagnosed as CHD and then finds that the official statistics indicate a larger number of deaths, a difference that cannot then be explained. This is a major problem for some MONICA centres.

Lack of access to personal information prevents the investigator from finding out if there was a previous history of angina or myocardial infarction. This not only affects the allocation of a diagnostic category, but also determines whether the death can be classified as a 'first event'.

Other problems for investigators are how to deal with doubtful events, or events with insufficient data. While a mortality study linked with a medical and legal system that provides good information will collect complete data on a large proportion of deaths, there is nevertheless the problem that in every study there are a significant number of fatalities where the evidence for CHD is marginal but where there is no strong evidence for a competing pathology either. Then there are those deaths where the victim had multiple pathology including some coronary artery disease, and the decision as to which single cause of death should dominate may be arbitrary. A decision has to be made on whether or not to include in the final tally these doubtful cases or cases with 'insufficient data'. The final results of validation are therefore dependent on the medical and forensic system in operation, and must, unfortunately, be influenced to some extent by the original death certificate diagnosis, which means that the validation exercise is not completely independent. In MONICA Project test exercises, which have been administered now for many years (Tunstall-Pedoe 1988, 1989), it has been found that in ambiguous cases MONICA coders tend to agree with the clinician's death certificate diagnosis. Basically the same case histories of symptoms, signs, and test results, presented years later in disguise, with different clinical diagnoses, are coded differently with a bias towards the clinical diagnosis, whose validity is allegedly being established!

What the so-called validation of death certificates does do is to show the proportion of deaths in which necropsy, symptoms, or previous history figure, and how this proportion varies over time and between centres.

One interesting challenge for monitoring is whether the proportion of 'sudden deaths' has changed over a period of decades. A change would imply that the natural history and presentation of CHD had changed as it became less common, and there is evidence to suggest this (Kuller *et al.* 1986; Folsom *et al.* 1987). An alternative hypothesis might be that the disease is unchanged, but that out-of-hospital resuscitation attempts, medico-legal constraints, and even the financial advantages of listing someone as 'transferred to hospital' (or coronary care unit) may be distorting the figures. Routine administrative data may be inadequate to answer these questions, which can be better addressed by careful monitoring studies.

REGISTRATION OF MYOCARDIAL INFARCTION

Whilst death is a unique event, unlikely to be overlooked and warranting a specific diagnosis in all but the very old, non-fatal infarction offers the twin problems that it may be so mild that no-one, including the patient, notices (Grimm *et al.* 1987) or it may be recurrent, creating problems in defining when one event ends and the next begins (Tunstall-Pedoe 1989).

Although clinical criteria agree on the most severe cases, there is sufficient disagreement on milder cases for diagnostic criteria to have a considerable impact on event rates and case fatality (Tunstall-Pedoe 1978). The mounting of heart attack registers in the 1960s (Frank *et al*. 1963; McNeilly and Pemberton 1968; Armstrong *et al*. 1972; Kinlen 1973), an idea proposed early by Morris (1957) led to a WHO European Office initiative at the end of that decade (WHO 1971, 1976). The emphasis at that time was on exploring the potential and the limitations of acute coronary care. Most of the registers ceased operation after one or more years, but some continued (Elmfeldt *et al*. 1975), and the methodology was applied and survived in intervention studies (Puska *et al*. 1981; Salonen *et al*. 1986, 1989).

The diagnostic criteria of the first generation of registers were rather more descriptive than definitive, being based on older criteria (WHO 1959), and the collaborative report gives much food for thought as to whether all registers were registering the same thing (WHO 1976), particularly as the grounds for registration were 'suspicion of the diagnosis'. A decade later, a need was felt to tighten up the criteria by employing quantitative electrocardiographic coding using the Minnesota Code (Blackburn *et al*. 1960; Prineas *et al*. 1982). The new WHO criteria have been shown in New Zealand to produce different numbers of 'definite' cases of myocardial infarction from those produced using the old criteria (Beaglehole *et al*. 1987). Because the old criteria left a lot to local judgement, the conversion factor derived from New Zealand may not be applicable everywhere. Some MONICA investigators whose centres changed from the old to the new WHO criteria claimed verbally that the new criteria made no difference.

The Minnesota Coding of the electrocardiogram (ECG) means allocating each abnormality a class of severity. In the evolutionary changes of the peri-infarction ECG consecutive graphs may be allocated different codes although the differences are not great: the Minnesota Coding Manual (Prineas *et al*. 1982) recommends application of visual serial change rules after routine coding. These rules appeared after the drafting of the MONICA Protocol and were rejected by the MONICA Project Principal Investigators with some potential loss of specificity (Wolf *et al*. 1988), but with the advantage that the separate codes for consecutive graphs can be entered into a computer algorithm which determines the MONICA ECG code without any further procedures (WHO MONICA Project 1990*a*). The conventional 12 leads adopted by American and British cardiologists are now in general use internationally, but there are still national differences in paper speed which mean that MONICA ECG test records have to be produced at both 25 and 50 mm/s.

It is unfortunate that cardiac enzyme tests were not standardized either nationally or internationally when the MONICA Project began. Population monitoring shows that the introduction of more sensitive enzyme tests such as creatinine phosphokinase into a population can have an impact on the measured myocardial infarction rates (Burke *et al*. 1989*a*).

Agreement on a 'definite' category of myocardial infarction gives greater potential for comparison than existed previously, and this has been accepted as the end-point for comparison in MONICA. However, this excludes large numbers of 'possible' cases, most of whom have had a coronary event. The frequency of these possible cases is closely linked to the sources of event-finding that are being used (Martin *et al*. 1988). However, the proportion of definites is influenced as much by the frequency and immediacy of diagnostic testing as by the severity of the infarct (McGuinness *et al*. 1976).

Although coronary event registration using the MONICA methodology is now being pursued in 26 countries, the methodology, critical comment, and exploration of alternative methods have come from a smaller number (e.g. Tunstall-Pedoe 1977; Gillum 1978, 1987*a*; Gillum *et al*. 1982; Martin *et al*. 1987*a, b*; Beaglehole *et al*. 1988; Dobson *et al*. 1990).

REGISTRATION OF STROKE

Strokes are less common than coronary events in most industrialized countries, and occur at an older age. The diagnosis is largely clinical, and the equipment needed for diagnostic imaging is far less available than the portable ECG. Strokes are of several aetiologies, and they also may be missed or may emerge into the milder manifestations of transient ischaemic attack. The first generation of WHO registers showed that the coding of type of stroke was less reliable than the coding of stroke (Aho *et al*. 1980), and similar problems are being encountered in MONICA (Asplund *et al*. 1988). However, some centres now have the imaging equipment required to validate stroke diagnoses. Interest in stroke is considerable, as many countries are facing the problems of an aging population.

MEDICAL CARE

There is controversy as to how far mortality rates reflect risk factor changes on the one hand versus medical care on the other (Neutze and White 1987; Higgins and Luepker 1988). Monitoring of coronary events cannot now be done without taking into account the dramatic changes that have occurred in the medical care of coronary disease. Intermittent recording of coronary care was part of the 'core' MONICA Project, and some centres have been recording continuously. Because of the timing of the project, started before their introduction, MONICA has the potential for showing the impact of thrombolytic therapy and of semi-automatic defibrillators in ambulances, quite apart from being able to compare acute coronary care in different cities (Arveiler *et al.* 1990). Continuous recording of coronary care data is now recommended for all MONICA centres.

Whilst it is easy to obtain, from hospital records, details of the hospital medical care of coronary cases reaching hospital alive, it is more difficult to study pre-hospital acute care or the medical care, if any, of fatal cases outside hospital. It is also difficult to monitor the chronic management of coronary risk factors and of the milder manifestations of coronary disease in the general population.

ANGINA PECTORIS

Most community studies have concentrated on myocardial infarction and coronary deaths. But angina pectoris is also of great interest, because of its considerable economic cost and also because it is the precursor of perhaps 40 per cent of acute coronary events. However, it is difficult to study on a community-wide basis because many cases are undetected, and it may be that only a minority reach specialist clinics. The absence of data on angina pectoris from monitoring studies is striking. Should such studies be mounted, there would be a dichotomy between the angina coming to clinical attention and that potentially discoverable through the Rose Questionnaire (Rose *et al.* 1977; Cook *et al.* 1989). The variability of angina (Rose 1968) and the problems identified in community studies in the early 1970s (Fulton *et al.* 1972; Duncan *et al.* 1976) may explain why the study of angina is not more widely attempted.

BLOOD PRESSURE

Hypertension is considered to be a risk factor, but is also classified as a disease. Changes in population distributions are of major importance, but comparisons of population blood pressure levels across time and space are fraught with difficulty. Doctors or nurses need to be retrained to measure blood pressure for epidemiological purposes. Conditions of measurement need to be standardized, as the result can be influenced by the posture of the patient, the room temperature, the preceding procedures, the novelty of measurement for the patient, the sex and status of the observer, and whether the observer is wearing a white coat. There is no universal agreement on what blood pressure cuff sizes to use (Croft and Cruickshank 1990) or even what machine.

The observer using the standard mercury sphygmomanometer has problems of digit preference and of knowledge of the result influencing the reading (WHO MONICA Project 1990*b*), whilst the random-zero machine, designed to cope with these problems, has been accused of biased readings (O'Brien *et al.* 1990). Numerous automatic machines are now available, but they are unlikely to show the consistency over time and space shown by the century-old mercury column. It is of great interest to epidemiologists to be able to plot secular changes in blood pressure in the population over time (Drizd *et al.* 1986), but they must be confident that apparent changes are likely to be genuine.

CHOLESTEROL

It is important to know what is happening to blood cholesterol values in the population (Beaglehole *et al.* 1979), but standardization of measurement is difficult and techniques have changed over time, creating further problems of comparability (Kalsbeek *et al.* 1988). Plasma measurements produce different results from serum depending on the amount and nature of the anticoagulant (Laboratory Methods Committee of the Lipid Research Clinic Program 1977; Cloey *et al.* 1990). Enzymatic methods of cholesterol measurement are now widely used, so that the standard method established by the Lipid Research Clinics protocol in the USA is now being superseded (NHLI 1974). Integration of laboratories into quality control schemes is essential; two schemes used by epidemiologists are the Center for Disease Control in Atlanta, and the WHO Lipid Laboratory in Prague. Standardization of total cholesterol measurement is easier than that for high density lipoprotein cholesterol (HDL-cholesterol), as the lyophilized specimens that are distributed do not behave like the fresh specimens on which HDL-cholesterol is usually measured. Although time of day and fasting status do not appear to affect the results of cholesterol measurement, posture and prolonged use of the tourniquet (Crombie *et al.* 1987) will do so.

The first MONICA population surveys showed that cholesterol values in different populations are now much closer together than they were in the Seven Countries Study (Keys 1980), emphasizing the importance of accurate measurement (WHO MONICA Project 1988*b*, 1989). Despite attempted standardization, the results from some MONICA centres were omitted from the collaborative report (WHO MONICA Project 1988*b*); the quality control report exposes some of the problems (WHO MONICA Project 1990*c*).

SMOKING

Smoking habits are elicited by questionnaire. Unfortunately, there is no standard questionnaire, nor is there an international standard on how to report results, although MONICA is attempting this using a questionnaire from the WHO classic *Cardiovascular survey methods* (Rose *et al.* 1982; WHO MONICA Project 1990*a*).

Biochemical validation of data on smoking suggests that the proportion of smoking 'deceivers' in the population is low (Woodward and Tunstall-Pedoe 1992), but this proportion increases in circumstances where people are being pressurized to quit and are too addicted to do so. Thiocyanate has been widely used for this purpose, but it has been abandoned as a 'core' data item in MONICA because the mean values were found to vary too much between populations—in non-smokers. Of the alternative validation techniques, cotinine has the advantage of high sensitivity and specificity but is expensive to assay, whilst measurement of expired air carbon monoxide is now cheap, quick, and simple (Irving *et al.* 1987; Jarvis *et al.* 1987). Because it is not known which inhaled component of tobacco smoke is atherothrombotic, there is no indication of which test for smoking would best measure coronary risk. Although the size and constituents of cigarettes smoked, and the style of smoking, vary in time and place, the crude indicator of consumption is likely to remain the self-reported number of cigarettes a day. Therefore this sets a problem of how to classify subjects who do not smoke every day.

OBESITY

Measurement of height and weight is relatively simple, but in many countries good data on the height and weight of population samples are not routinely available. Standardization over time and place means following the same conventions on which outer garments and footwear are to be removed before measurement. Height and weight, and their combinations such as body mass index, reflect obesity indirectly; frame size and muscularity are confounding factors. Many studies have used skinfold thicknesses at various points on the body surface (Lohman 1981; Haines *et al.* 1987). More recently, waist and hip circumferences have been used to reflect central obesity (Gillum 1987*b*; WHO MONICA Project 1990*a*), because intra-abdominal fat is now thought to be metabolically different from subcutaneous fat and its amount to be more closely related to problems such as diabetes, blood pressure, and atheroma (see Chapter 15).

EXERCISE

Exercise is acknowledged to be important, but is difficult to measure. Self-reported exercise is a crude measure, and specific activities vary so much by culture that detailed questionnaires cannot be transferred readily.

Whilst exercise to the point of breathlessness may be a useful indication of severity in young people, in the middle-aged it may be more of an indication of heart or lung disease rather than life-style! Similarly, self-reporting of physical activity at work is not an accurate measure because it is subjective. Exercise testing has been employed in some cardiovascular surveys, but adds considerably to their cost, duration, and complexity. Several attempts have been made to develop and promote an international validated questionnaire or test (Andersen *et al.* 1978; Wilson *et al.* 1986), but none appears to be in widespread use. In the MONICA study, exercise is considered an optional study because of these difficulties in measurement.

NUTRITION

Nutrition is another area where the reach is far greater than the grasp. Many countries do not have good food tables, and all food tables change over time. Weighed food intakes are considered to be the gold standard for the assessment of diet, but because of daily intake variation the weighing needs to be continued for 7 days or more in order to characterize an individual's average diet. Both the recording of weighed food intakes and their coding and analysis are very time-consuming. Few countries run such studies on national population samples either on a regular basis or at all (McDowell *et al.* 1981; Cohen *et al.* 1987).

Alternatives to weighed 3 or 7 day intakes are food diaries, 24 hour recall and food frequency questionnaires, or questions about specific dietary habits. Each method has its own characteristics, and problems arise when comparing results from different measures (Cameron and Van Staveren, 1988; Pietinen *et al.* 1988; Life Sciences Research Office 1989). Food frequency questionnaires have been widely employed in cardiovascular surveys where they can be included within a standard questionnaire (Yarnell *et al.* 1983).

In the MONICA Project, diet was yet another important risk factor whose standardization proved too difficult to be made a core item, although an optional study on diet, sponsored by the European Community, has been adopted by a number of MONICA centres (De Backer *et al.* 1983; Knuiman *et al.* 1985).

Increasing use is now being made of chemical and biochemical markers for specific dietary factors. Fatty acid analysis of tissue is one example (Smith *et al.* 1986), and analysis of the urine for electrolytes is another (Smith *et al.* 1988). Gamma glutamyl transpeptidase is used as a crude indicator of alcohol intake, and of course blood cholesterol, a risk factor in its own right, reflects dietary behaviour to a certain extent.

PSYCHO-SOCIAL FACTORS

Although widely considered to be important, psycho-social factors are another area where cross-cultural standardization is difficult. For that reason, the core MONICA protocol could include only questions on years of education and on marital status. Although each country has a socio-economic classification of its work-force and a social security system, these vary so much that cross-sectional comparisons are hazardous, nor is it easy to design questions on culture and ethnicity. In cardiovascular epidemiology, the type A personality dominated the field for many years, and eventually resulted in simplified questionnaires such as the Bortner questionnaire. There is now increasing interest in other risk factors such as social support, and a number of questionnaires covering different fields of interest are being promoted by different interest groups (Marmot 1988).

OTHER FACTORS

The long-term monitoring of CHD and risk factors is limited to those factors which are identified and measurable. Some factors are not recognized, or are inaccessible, or involve techniques of assay which are, initially, too cumbersome and unreliable for mass epidemiological use. Examples of factors which only now are becoming more accessible to epidemiological survey work are those concerned with haemorheology and haemostasis (Baker *et al.* 1988; Lee *et al.* 1990). An example of a previously unrecognized and still largely inaccessible factor is the foetal and neonatal environment, reflected in birthweight, placental weight, and weight in infancy (Barker *et al.* 1989, and see Chapter 5).

THE WHO MONICA PROJECT

The WHO MONICA Project recently celebrated its half-way point, in that event registration is to continue for 10 years and the 5 year point was reached for the latest starters in 1990. There are 26 countries involved in the project, fielding some 50 populations (depending on the definition) from 38 centres. Each centre is free to publish its own data, but also submits core data items to the MONICA Data Centre in Helsinki, where quality and consistency checks are carried out and collaborative reports are eventually produced. Necessarily, there is a protracted delay in the production of these reports, which follow much later than local results. Each MONICA study finds its own local funding, so that co-ordination and discipline are different from that in a multicentre study with central funding. The central protocol has to be adapted to the local medical and political system. This is particularly apparent not only in the methods used for event-finding for registration, but also in the methods of sampling the population for the population surveys, with the sampling frames varying by country.

Longitudinal data are available only from those MONICA centres which began registration early, so that collaborative reports initially concern only cross-sectional data. These reports are proving of considerable interest, although it should be remembered that the project was designed primarily for longitudinal measurement within each centre, with less emphasis on comparability between centres.

The recent publications of two MONICA conferences (WHO MONICA Project 1988c, d) and the contributions to the American conference (Higgins and Luepker 1989) show the amount of work being done in this area, even apart from the main collaborative publications (WHO MONICA Project 1987, 1988a, b, 1989).

OTHER LONGITUDINAL STUDIES

In the USA, a number of longitudinal studies have been running either independently or in association with preventive programmes. A good example is the Minnesota Heart Survey, which preceded and influenced the MONICA Project. Whereas MONICA registers all events over 10 years, the Minnesota study covers a large conurbation and looks at what is happening to coronary events in specific years (Burke *et al.* 1989b).

CONCLUSION

The long-term objective of many monitoring projects is to explain the trends in cardiovascular mortality. Since their inception, however, it has been realized that, by measuring event rates, medical care, and the levels and trends of coronary risk factors and their treatment, these projects are providing additional essential information for health service planning and audit. A survey of different countries (Tunstall-Pedoe, unpublished) has shown that those carrying out monitoring projects like MONICA (such as Scotland, Northern Ireland, and Belgium) can characterize risk factor levels and trends in some key communities, while those not sponsoring such monitoring studies (such as England and the Netherlands) may have no recent risk factor data at all or none on a recurrent basis with which they can plan their preventive programmes.

REFERENCES

Aho, K., Harmsen, P., Hatano, S., Marquardsen, J., Smirnov, V. E., and Strasser, T. (1980). Cerebrovascular disease in the community: results of the WHO Collaborative Study. *Bull. WHO*, **58**, 113–20.

Andersen, K. L., Masironi, R., Rutenfranz, J., and Seliger, V. (1978). *Habitual physical activity and health*, WHO Regional Publ., Eur. Ser. 6, WHO, Copenhagen.

ARIC (Atherosclerosis Risk in Communities) Study Protocol (1988). *Manual 3. Surveillance component procedures*, Collaborative Studies Co-ordinating Centre, University of North Carolina, Chapel Hill, NC.

ARIC (Atherosclerosis Risk in Communities) Study Investigators (1989). The decline of ischaemic heart disease mortality in the ARIC Study Communities (prepared by G. Heiss). *Int. J. Epidemiol.*, **18**, S88–98.

Armstrong, A., Duncan, B., Oliver, M. F., Julian, D. G., Donald, K. W., Fulton, M., *et al.* (1972). Natural history of acute coronary heart attacks. A community study. *Br. Heart J.*, **34**, 67–80.

Arveiler, D., Cambou, J. P., Nuttens, M. C., Bingham, A., Hedelin, G., Ruidavets, J. B., *et al.* (1990). Acute coronary care and treatment of myocardial infarction in the three French MONICA registers. *Rev. Epidémiol. Santé Publique*, **38**, 429–34.

Asplund, K., Tuomilehto, J., Stegmayr, B., Wester, P. S., and Tunstall-Pedoe, H. (1988). Diagnostic criteria and quality control of the registration of stroke events in the MONICA Project. *Acta Med. Scand.*, Suppl. 728, 26–39.

Baker, I. A., Sweetnam, P. M., Yarnell, J. W. G., Bainton, D., and Elwood, P. C. (1988). Haemostatic and other risk factors for ischaemic heart disease and social class: evidence from the Caerphilly and Speedwell Studies. *Int. J. Epidemiol.*, **17**, 759–65.

Barker, D. J. P., Winter, P. D., Osmond, C., and Margetts, B. (1989). Weight in infancy and death from ischaemic heart disease. *Lancet*, **ii**, 577–80.

Beaglehole, R., LaRosa, J. C., Heiss, G. E., Davis, C. E., Rifkind, B. M., Muesing, R. M., *et al.* (1979). Secular changes in blood cholesterol and their contribution to the decline in coronary mortality. In *Proc. Conf. on the Decline in Coronary Heart Disease Mortality, National Heart Lung and Blood Institute, 24–25 October 1978* (eds R. J. Havlik and M. Feinleib), NIH Publ. 79–1610, US Department of Health, Education, and Welfare, Washington, DC, pp. 282–97.

Beaglehole, R., Stewart, A., and Butler, M. (1987). Comparability of old and new World Health Organization criteria for definite myocardial infarction. *Int. J. Epidemiol.*, **16**, 373–6.

Beaglehole, R., Dobson, A., Hobbs, M., Jackson, R., Jamrozik, K., Alexander, A., *et al.* (1988). Comparison of event rates among three MONICA centres. *Acta Med. Scand.*, Suppl. 728, 53–9.

Blackburn, H., Keys, A., Simonson, E., Rautaharju, P., and Punsar, S. (1960). The electrocardiogram in population studies. A classification system. *Circulation*, **21**, 1160–75.

Burke, G. L., Edlavitch, S. A., and Crow, R. S. (1989a). The effects of diagnostic criteria on trends in coronary heart disease morbidity: the Minnesota Heart Survey. *J. Clin. Epidemiol.*, **42**, 17–24.

Burke, G. L., Sprafka, H. M., Folsom, A. R., Luepker, R. V., Nosted, S. W., and Blackburn, H. (1989*b*). Trends in CHD mortality, morbidity and risk factor levels from 1960 to 1986: Minnesota Heart Survey. *Int. J. Epidemiol.,* **18** (Suppl.), S73–81.

Cameron, M. E. and Van Staveren, W. A. (eds) (1988). *Manual on methodology for food consumption studies,* Oxford Medical Publications, New York.

Cloey, T. C., Bachorik, P. S., Becker, D., Finney, C., Lowry, D., and Sigmund, W. (1990). Reevaluation of serum-plasma differences in total cholesterol concentration. *J. Am. Med. Assoc.,* **263**, 2788–9.

Cohen, B. B., Barbano, H. E., Cox, C. S., Feldman, J. J., Finucane, F. F., Kleinman, J. C., *et al.* (1987). Plan and operation of the NHANES I Epidemiological Followup Study, 1982–84. *Vital and Health Statistics,* Ser. 1, No. 22, Department of Health and Human Services PHS 87–1324, US Government Printing Office, Washington, DC.

Cook, D. G., Shaper, A. G., and Macfarlane, P. (1989). Using the WHO (Rose) angina questionnaire in cardiovascular epidemiology. *Int. J. Epidemiol.,* **18,** 607–13.

Croft, P. R. and Cruickshank, J. K. (1990). Blood pressure measurement in adults: large cuffs for all? *J. Epidemiol. Community Health,* **44,** 170–3.

Crombie, I. K., Smith, W. C. S., Tavendale, R., Clark, E. C., and Tunstall-Pedoe, H. (1987). Venous occlusion and estimation of serum constituents. *Lancet,* **ii,** 975.

Dawber, T. R. (1980). *The Framingham Study. The epidemiology of atherosclerotic disease,* Harvard University Press.

De Backer, G., Tunstall-Pedoe, H., and Ducimetiere, P. (eds) (1983). *Surveillance of the dietary habits of the population with regards to cardiovascular diseases,* Euronut Report 2, Wageningen.

Dobson, A., Alexander, H. M., al-Roomi, K., Gibberd, R. W., Heller, R. F., Malcolm, J. A., *et al.* (1990). Methodological issues in interpreting trends in MONICA event rates. *Rev. Epidémiol. Santé Publique,* **38,** 397–402.

Drizd, T., Dannenberg, A. L., and Engel, A. (1986). Blood pressure levels in persons 18–74 years of age in 1976–80, and trends in blood pressure from 1960 to 1980 in the United States. *Vital and Health Statistics,* Ser. 11, No. 234, Department of Health and Human Services Publ. PHS 86–1684, US Government Printing Office, Washington, DC.

Duggar, B. C. and Lewis, W. F. (1987). Comparability of diagnostic data coded by the 8th and 9th revisions of the International Classification of Diseases. *Vital and Health Statistics,* Ser. 2, No. 104, Department of Health and Human Services Publ. PHS 87–1378, US Government Printing Office, Washington, DC.

Duncan, B., Fulton, M., Morrison, S. L., Lutz, W., Donald, K. W., Kerr, F., *et al.* (1976). Diagnosis of new and worsening angina pectoris. *Br. Med. J.,* **1,** 981–5.

Elmfeldt, D., Wilhelmsen, L., Tibblin, G., Vedin, J. A., Wilhelmsson, C. E., and Bengtsson, C. (1975). Registration of myocardial infarction in the City of Goteborg, Sweden. *J. Chron. Dis.,* **28,** 173–86.

Folsom, A. R., Gomez-Marin, O., Gillum, R. F., Kottke, T. E., Lohman, W., and Jacobs, D. R. (1987). Out-of-hospital coronary deaths in an urban population— validation of death certificate diagnosis. *Am. J. Epidemiol.,* **125,** 1012–18.

Frank, C. W., Sager, R. V., Seiden, G. E., Shapiro, S., and Weinblatt, E. (1963). The HIP study of incidence and prognosis of coronary heart disease. Criteria for diagnosis. *J. Chron. Dis.,* **16,** 1293–1300.

Fulton, M., Duncan, B., Lutz, W., Morrison, S. L., Donald, K. W., Kerr, F., *et al.* (1972). The natural history of unstable angina. *Lancet,* **i**, 860–5.

Gillum, R. F. (1978). Community surveillance for cardiovascular disease. Methods, problems, applications—a review. *J. Chron. Dis.,* **31**, 87–94.

Gillum, R. F. (1987*a*). Acute myocardial infarction in the United States 1970–1983. *Am. Heart J.,* **113**, 804–11.

Gillum, R. F. (1987*b*). The association of the ratio of waist to hip girth with blood pressure, serum cholesterol and serum uric acid in children and youths aged 6–17 years. *J. Chron. Dis.,* **40**, 413–20.

Gillum, R. F., Prineas, R. J., Luepker, R. V., Taylor, H. L., Jacobs, D. R., Kottke, T. E., *et al.* (1982). Decline in coronary deaths: a search for explanations. The Minnesota Mortality and Morbidity Surveillance Program. *Minnesota Med.,* **65**, 235–8.

Grimm, R. H., Tillinghast, S., Daniels, K., Neaton, J. D., Mascioli, S., Crow, R., *et al.* (1987). Unrecognised myocardial infarction: experience in the Multiple Risk Factor Intervention Trial (MRFIT). *Circulation,* **75** (Suppl. II), 6–8.

Haines, A. P., Imeson, J. D., and Meade, T. W. (1987). Skinfold thickness and cardiovascular risk factors. *Am. J. Epidemiol.,* **126**, 86–94.

Havlik, R. J. and Feinleib, M. (eds) (1979). *Proc. Conf. on the Decline in Coronary Heart Disease Mortality, National Heart Lung and Blood Institute, 24–25 October 1978,* NIH Publ. 79–1610, US Department of Health, Education, and Welfare, Washington, DC.

Heathcote, C. R., Keogh, C., and O'Neill, T. J. (1989). The changing pattern of coronary heart disease in Australia. *Int. J. Epidemiol.,* **18**, 802–7.

Higgins, M. W. and Luepker, R. V. (eds) (1988). *Trends in coronary heart disease mortality. The influence of medical care,* Oxford University Press.

Higgins, M. and Luepker, R. V. (eds) (1989). Trends and determinants of coronary heart disease mortality. *Int. J. Epidemiol.,* **18** (Suppl. 1).

Hughes, K. (1986). Trends in mortality from ischaemic heart disease in Singapore, 1959–1983. *Int. J. Epidemiol.,* **15**, 44–9.

Irving, J. M., Clark, E. C., Crombie, I. K., and Smith, W. C. S. (1987). Evaluation of a portable measure of expired air carbon monoxide. *Prev. Med.,* **17**, 109–15.

Jarvis, M. J., Tunstall-Pedoe, H., Feyerabend, C., Vesey, C., and Saloojee, Y. (1987). Comparison of tests used to distinguish smokers from non-smokers. *Am. J. Public Health,* **77**, 1435–8.

Kalsbeek, W. B., Kral, K. M., Wallace, R. B., and Rifkind, B. M. (1988). Comparing mean levels of total cholesterol from visit 2 of the Lipid Research Clinics Prevalence Study with the Second National Health and Nutrition Examination Survey. *Am. J. Epidemiol.,* **128**, 1038–53.

Keys, A. (ed.) (1980). *Seven countries. A multivariate analysis of death and coronary heart disease.* Harvard University Press.

Kinlen, L. J. (1973). Incidence and presentation of myocardial infarction in an English community. *Br. Heart J.,* **35**, 616–22.

Knuiman, J. T., Pietinen, P., De Backer, G., and Ducimitiere, P. (1985). *The MONICA Project: optional study on the surveillance of the dietary intake of the population with regard to cardiovascular diseases,* EURONUT Rep. 6.

Kuller, L. H., Perper, J. A., Dai, W. S., Rutan, G., and Traven, N. (1986). Sudden death and the decline in coronary heart disease mortality. *J. Chron. Dis.,* **39**, 1001–19.

Laboratory Methods Committee of the Lipid Research Clinics Program (1977). Cholesterol and triglyceride concentration in serum/plasma pairs. *Clin. Chem.*, **23**, 60–3.

Lee, A. J., Smith, W. C. S., Lowe, G. D. O., and Tunstall-Pedoe, H. (1990). Plasma fibrinogen and coronary risk factors: the Scottish Heart Health Study. *J. Clin. Epidemiol.*, **43**, 913–19.

Life Sciences Research Office, Federation of American Societies for Experimental Biology (1989). Nutrition monitoring in the United States, Department of Health and Human Services Publ. PHS 89–1255, US Government Printing Office, Washington, DC.

Lohman, T. G. (1981). Skinfolds and body density and their relation to body fatness. A review. *Hum. Biol.*, **53**, 181–225.

Marmot, M. (1988). Psychosocial factors and cardiovascular disease: epidemiological approaches. *Eur. Heart J.*, **9**, 690–7.

Martin, C. A., Hobbs, M. S. T., and Armstrong, B. K. (1987*a*). Identification of non-fatal myocardial infarction through hospital discharge data in Western Australia. *J. Chron. Dis.*, **40**, 1111–20.

Martin, C. A., Hobbs, M. S. T., and Armstrong, B. K. (1987*b*). Estimation of myocardial infarction mortality from routinely collected data in Western Australia. *J. Chron. Dis.*, **40**, 661–9.

Martin, C. A., Hobbs, M. S. T., and Armstrong, B. K. (1988). Measuring the incidence of acute myocardial infarction: the problem of possible acute myocardial infarction. *Acta Med. Scand.*, Suppl. 728, 40–7.

McDowell, A., Engel, A., Massey, J. T., and Maurer, K. (1981). Plan and operation of the Second National Health and Nutrition Examination Survey 1976–80. *Vital and Health Statistics*, Ser. 1, No. 15, Department of Health and Human Services Publ. PHS 81–1317, US Government Printing Office, Washington, DC.

McGuiness, J. B., Begg, T. B., and Semple, T. (1976). First electrocardiogram in recent myocardial infarction. *Br. Med. J.*, **2**, 449–51.

McNeilly, R. H. and Pemberton, J. (1968). Duration of last attack in 998 cases of coronary artery disease and its relation to possible cardiac resuscitation. *Br. Med. J.*, **3**, 139–42.

Morris, J. N. (1951). Recent history of coronary disease. *Lancet*, **i**, 69–73.

Morris, J. N. (1957). *Uses of epidemiology* (1st edn), Livingstone, London.

Najem, G. R., Hutcheon, D. E., and Feuerman, M. (1990). Changing patterns of ischaemic heart disease mortality in New Jersey 1968–82 and the relationship with urbanization. *Int. J. Epidemiol.*, **19**, 26–31.

Neutze, J. M. and White, H. D. (1987). What contribution has cardiac surgery made to the decline in mortality from coronary heart disease? *Br. Med. J.*, **294**, 405–9.

NHLI (National Heart and Lung Institute) (1974). *Lipid Research Clinics Program manual of operations*, Vol. 1: *Lipid and lipoprotein analysis*. Publ. NIH 75–628, Department of Health, Education, and Welfare.

Nicolosi, A., Casati, S., Tailoi, E., and Polli, E. (1988). Death from Cardiovascular Disease in Italy, 1972–1981: decline in mortality rates and possible causes. *Int. J. Epidemiol.*, **17**, 766–72.

O'Brien, E., Mee, F., Atkins, N., and O'Malley, K. (1990). Inaccuracy of the Hawksley random zero sphygmomanometer. *Lancet*, **336**, 1465–8.

Pietinen, R., Uusitalo, U., Vartiainen, E., and Tuomilehto, J. (1988). Dietary survey of the FINMONICA project in 1982. *Acta Med. Scand., Suppl.* 728, 169–77.

Pisa, Z. and Uemura, K. (1982). Trends of mortality from ischaemic heart disease and other cardiovascular diseases in 27 countries, 1968–87. *World Health Statist. Q.,* **35,** 11–47.

Pooling Project Research Group (1978). Relationship of blood pressure, serum cholesterol, smoking habits, relative weight and ECG abnormalities to incidence of major coronary events: final report of the Pooling Project. *J. Chron. Dis.,* **31,** 201–306.

Prineas, R. J., Crow, R. S., and Blackburn, H. (1982). *The Minnesota Code Manual of electrocardiographic findings: standards and procedures for measurement and classification,* John Wright, Boston, MA.

Puska, P., Tuomilehto, J., Salonen, J., Nissinen, A., Virtamo, J., Björkqvist, S., *et al.* (1981). *Community control of cardiovascular diseases. The North Karelia Project,* WHO, Copenhagen.

Ragland, K. E., Selvin, S., and Merrill, D. W. (1988). The onset of the decline in ischemic heart disease mortality in the United States. *Am. J. Epidemiol.,* **127,** 516–31.

Rose, G. (1968). Variability of angina—some implications for epidemiology. *Br. J. Prev. Social Med.,* **22,** 12–15.

Rose, G., McCartney, P., and Reid, D. D. (1977). Self-administration of a questionnaire on chest pain and intermittent claudication. *Br. J. Prev. Social Med.,* **31,** 42–8.

Rose, G. A., Blackburn, H., Gillum, R. F., and Prineas, R. J. (1982). *Cardiovascular survey methods,* Monogr. Ser. 56, WHO, Geneva.

Salonen, J. T., Kottke, T. E., Jacobs, D. R., and Hannan, P. J. (1986). Analysis of community-based cardiovascular disease prevention studies—evaluation issues in the North Karelia Project and the Minnesota Heart Health Program. *Int. J. Epidemiol.,* **15,** 176–82.

Salonen, J. T., Tuomilehto, J., Nissinen, A., Kaplan, G. A., and Puska, P. (1989). Contribution of risk factor changes to the decline in coronary incidence during the North Karelia Project: a within-community analysis. *Int. J. Epidemiol.,* **18,** 595–601.

Smith, W. C. S. and Tunstall-Pedoe, H. (1984). European regional variation in cardiovascular mortality. *Br. Med. Bull.,* **40,** 374–9.

Smith, W. C. S., Tavendale, R., and Tunstall-Pedoe, H. (1986). Simplified subcutaneous fat biopsy for nutritional surveys. *Hum. Nutr. Clin. Nutr.,* **40C,** 323–5.

Smith, W. C. S., Crombie, I. K., Tavendale, R. T., Gulland, S. K., and Tunstall-Pedoe, H. (1988). Urinary electrolyte excretion, alcohol consumption, and blood pressure in the Scottish heart health study. *Br. Med. J.,* **297,** 329–30.

Stern, M. (1979). The recent decline in ischaemic heart disease mortality. *Ann. Intern. Med.,* **91,** 630–40.

Thom, T. J. (1989). International mortality from heart disease: rates and trends. *Int. J. Epidemiol.,* **18,** S20–8.

Tunstall-Pedoe, H. (1977). *A coronary heart attack register in East London.* MD Thesis, University of Cambridge.

Tunstall-Pedoe, H. (1978). Uses of coronary heart attack registers. *Br. Heart J.,* **40,** 510–15.

Tunstall-Pedoe, H. (1985). Monitoring trends in cardiovascular disease and risk factors: the WHO MONICA Project. *WHO Chron.*, **39**, 3–5.

Tunstall-Pedoe, H. (1988). Problems with criteria and quality control in the registration of coronary events in the MONICA Study. *Acta Med. Scand.*, Suppl. 728, 17–25.

Tunstall-Pedoe, H. (1989). Diagnosis, measurement and surveillance of coronary events. *Int. J. Epidemiol.*, **18**, S169–73.

Tunstall-Pedoe, H., Clayton, D., Morris, J. N., Brigden, W., and McDonald, L. (1975). Coronary heart attacks in East London. *Lancet*, **ii**, 833–8.

Uemura, K. and Pisa, Z. (1985). Recent trends in cardiovascular disease mortality in 27 industrialized countries. *World Health Statist. Q.*, **38**, 142–62.

Uemura, K. and Pisa, Z. (1988). Trends in cardiovascular disease mortality in industrialized countries since 1950. *World Health Statist. Q.*, **41**, 155–78.

WHO (World Health Organization) (1959). *Hypertension and coronary heart disease: classification and criteria for epidemiological studies. First report of the Expert Committee on Cardiovascular Diseases and Hypertension*, WHO Tech. Rep. Ser. 168, WHO, Geneva.

WHO (World Health Organization) (1971). *Ischaemic heart disease registers. Report of the Fifth Working Group (including a second revision of the operating protocol)*, WHO, Copenhagen.

WHO (World Health Organization) (1976). Myocardial infarction community registers. *Public Health in Europe No. 5*, WHO, Copenhagen.

WHO MONICA Project Principal Investigators (1987) (prepared by J. Tuomilehto, K. Kuulasmaa, and J. Torppa). WHO MONICA Project: geographic variation in mortality from cardiovascular diseases *World Health Statist. Q.*, **40**, 171–84.

WHO MONICA Project Principal Investigators (1988*a*) (prepared by H. Tunstall-Pedoe). The World Health Organization MONICA Project (monitoring trends and determinants in cardiovascular disease): a major international collaboration *J. Clin. Epidemiol.*, **41**, 105–13.

WHO MONICA Project (1988*b*) (prepared by A. Pajak, K. Kuulasmaa, J. Tuomilehto, and E. Ruokokoski). Geographical variation in the major risk factors of coronary heart disease in men and women aged 35–64 *World Health Statist. Q.*, **41**, 115–40.

WHO MONICA Project (1988*c*). *Proc. 2nd Int. MONICA Congr. Acta Med. Scand.*, Suppl. 728.

WHO MONICA Project (1989). A worldwide monitoring system for cardiovascular disease. *World Health Statist. Ann. 1989*, 27–149.

WHO MONICA Project (1990*a*). *MONICA manual*, Cardiovascular Diseases Unit, Geneva.

WHO MONICA Project (1990*b*) (prepared by H. W. Hense, K. Kuulasmaa, A. Zaborskis, *et al.*). Quality assessment of blood pressure measurements in epidemiological surveys. The impact of last digit preference and proportions of identical duplicate measurements *Rev. Epidémiol. Santé Publique*, **38**, 463–8.

WHO MONICA Project (1990*c*). Methods of total cholesterol measurement in the baseline survey of the WHO MONICA Project (prepared by A. Doring, A. Pajak, M. Ferrario, D. Grafnetter, and K. Kuulasmaa). *Rev. Epidémiol. Santé Publique*, **38**, 455–61.

WHO MONICA Project (1990*d*). *Proc. 3rd Int. MONICA Cong. Rev. Epidémiol. Santé Publique,* **38**(5, 6).

Wilson, P. W., Paffenberger, R. S., Jr, Morris, J. N., and Havlik, R. J. (1986). Assessment methods for physical activity and physical fitness in population studies: report of an NHLBI workshop. *Am. Heart J.,* **111,** 1177–92.

Wolf, H. K., Rautaharju, P. M., MacKenzie, B. R., Gregor, R. D., and Milsom, D. S. (1988). The consequences of reviewing serial changes in the Minnesota code for diagnosis of acute myocardial infarction. *Acta Med. Scand.* Suppl. 728, 48–52.

Woodward, M. and Tunstall-Pedoe, H. (1992). Biochemical evidence of persistent heavy smoking after a coronary diagnosis despite reported reduction: results from the Scottish Heart Health Study. *Eur. Heart J.,* in press.

Yarnell, J. W. G., Fehily, A. M., Milbank, J. E., Sweetnam, P. M., and Walker, C. L. (1983). A short dietary questionnaire for use in an epidemiological survey: comparison with weighed dietary records. *Hum. Nutr. Appl. Nutr.,* **37A,** 103–12.

33

Changing individual behaviour

M. Kornitzer

For many years the main activity of physicians was care of the sick. Treatments were aimed at relieving symptoms and, if possible, curing the sickness. Compliance with drug treatment in these chronically ill subjects did not seem a major problem, although a chronic sickness state which was almost symptomless like hypertensive disease posed a real challenge to physicians in terms of long-term, even lifelong, compliance with advice. Studies on random samples of clinic patients showed that only 55 per cent of patients complied with physicians' advice (Davis 1968). When moving from curative to preventive medicine, problems related to compliance with advice can be seen from a different perspective.

1. Compliance with advice in screening for the preclinical stage of a disease such as X-ray examination for lung tuberculosis, or compliance with preventive action which does not modify life-style, such as immunization. In the 1960s, psychologists (e.g. Leventhal 1965) studied the acceptance of new preventive health practices relating in a very simple model the level of fear or anxiety to the acceptance of preventive action: high levels of fear were paralysing, whereas some degree of realistic fear could lead to changes.

2. Modification of life-style such as eating or smoking habits or compliance with drug treatment for hypertension during a given time period, usually 5–6 years, within the framework of the unifactorial controlled trials in the prevention of coronary heart disease (CHD) which took place during the 1960s and 1970s.

3. The simultaneous modification of different life-styles leading to coronary risk factors like high serum cholesterol or obesity (nutritional patterns), high blood pressure (salt and alcohol consumption, excess calories), cigarette smoking, and sedentary behaviour. Within the perspective of the major multifactorial controlled trials of the 1970s, the goal was short term: modification of life-styles during the trial period by means of an intervention programme.

4. The ultimate goal, which emerged during the 1970s and 1980s, was a permanent modification of risky behaviour at the population level

which would lead to a slow but continuous decrease in the incidence of CHD. This approach needed in depth studies of the major unhealthy life-styles acquired during adolescence and the mechanism by which such life-styles could be permanently modified at the individual and population level. Population-wide benefits were likely to be more beneficial in terms of cost efficiency.

We shall focus this brief review on the modification of risky behaviour at the individual level within multifactorial randomized controlled trials in the primary prevention of CHD.

These trials were launched in order to confirm the coronary risk factor concept which emerged from the observational long-term cohort studies in the USA and Europe. In summary, high serum cholesterol, high blood pressure, and cigarette smoking appeared in all these studies as the major coronary risk factors. A second concept emerged: multifactorial coronary risk assessed by means of a multilogistic estimate. By this estimate 'high risk' subjects carried a risk of major coronary events 10–20 times higher than that for the lowest risk subjects. In the controlled trials a very simple concept had to be proved: given an intervention or 'experimental' group, the reduction of one or several risk factors, compared with the control group, would lead to a significant reduction in CHD incidence at the end of the trial. In most of these trials the focus was on decrease of coronary risk rather than on the techniques by which life-styles were modified. These were simple, if not simplistic.

In 1970, the World Health Organization (WHO) convened a meeting in Rome to determine whether the multifactorial coronary risk concept could be proved by means of multifactorial trials. Two apparently opposing concepts were submitted. The first was the population approach, in which attempts were made to modify the coronary risk factors at the population level. At that time the Stanford group was already engaged in a controlled trial in California (Stern *et al.* 1976), and a group in Finland decided to launch a quasi-experimental trial comparing the province of North Karelia (with the highest coronary mortality) with another control province (Puska *et al.* 1981). The individual approach was focused on life-style modifications in high risk subjects.

Table 33.1 lists the seven multifactorial trials started in the 1970s. Four of these trials, taken together, formed the WHO European Collaborative Trial in the Multifactorial Prevention of Coronary Heart Disease (WHO 1974). A further two, the Oslo Study (Hjermann 1983) and the Multiple Risk Factor Intervention Trial (MRFIT) (Benfari 1981), were directed at high risk middle-aged males free from CHD.

The Oslo Study was a bifactorial 5 year controlled trial involving 1232 male subjects at high risk of CHD because of their high serum cholesterol and smoking behaviour. The intervention techniques were straightforward:

Table 33.1 Multifactorial preventive trials: the individual approach

High risk subjects	High risk subjects + population	
Oslo trial	Göteborg Trial	
MRFIT	UK Trial	
	Belgian Heart Disease	WHO
	Prevention Project	Collaborative
	Rome Trial	Trial
	Polish Trial	

subjects were informed individually by one physician, the same for the whole trial, during a 10–15 min talk about the risk factor concept. All smokers were urged to stop smoking and were advised to change their eating habits. Dietary advice based on each man's dietary records, body weight, and blood lipids was given individually for about 30 min by a specially trained dietitian. Advice included a reduction in saturated fats and a modest increase in polyunsaturated fats. In those with elevated body weight, a reduction in total energy intake was also recommended. Dietary and antismoking counselling was repeated every 6 months. The net average reduction in serum cholesterol over the 5 year period was 10 per cent (mean pre-trial values had to be between 7.5–9.8 mmol/l). Tobacco consumption was 45 per cent lower in the intervention group than in the control group; however, only 24 per cent of the smokers in the intervention group stopped smoking completely compared with 17 per cent in the control group. The 5 year CHD incidence was significantly reduced (by 47 per cent) in the intervention group compared with the control group. This trial showed that in subjects selected on the basis of their coronary high risk status individual counselling twice a year could modify nutritional patterns and reduce serum cholesterol, modify smoking habits, and significantly reduce CHD incidence. Moreover, the intervention programme had a carry-over effect: 3–4 years after the end of the trial the effect of the intervention on cholesterol level was maintained (Hjermann *et al.* 1986). We should consider the possibility that this kind of intervention programme could have a sustained effect on nutritional behaviour in high risk subjects. This was not the case for the modification of smoking behaviour.

Compared with this European trial, the American MRFIT had a more ambitious goal: trying to modify during a 6 year period the coronary risk profile in over 12 000 subjects at very high risk, which was assessed by means of a multilogistic estimate. Life-style modification was based on an individual approach extended to group sessions. Ten group sessions were to be the cornerstone of the integrated prevention programme. All risk

factors were tackled simultaneously and an extended intervention programme was devised for the duration of the trial. Briefly, the objectives of
the intervention were based on the following:

- awareness and information acquisition on the part of the participants;
- behavioural changes in any one or all of the intervention modalities;
- change in the risk factor level.

Behavioural techniques were based on self-monitoring, goal-setting, and
contracting in consultation with the interventionist, support and positive
reinforcement from the health worker, and training of spouses to provide
positive encouragement. The total time per session was between 90 and
120 min. This intervention programme was based on new concepts of life-
style modification from the field of experts in health behaviour (Benfari
1981). This trial was 10 times larger than the Oslo Study with a large
manpower input based on the latest concepts in individual life-style modification. For each of the three major risk factors, goals were set concerning their modification over the trial period: these goals were not reached
for two of the three major risk factors, serum cholesterol and blood
pressure. After 4 years follow-up, serum cholesterol differences averaged
50 per cent of that predicted, and diastolic blood pressure difference
averaged 67 per cent of that predicted. Only difference in smoking reduction between the special intervention group (SI) and the usual care
group (UC) exceeded prediction. In fact the 4 year difference of serum
cholesterol between SI and UC was only 4 per cent, and the 4 year
difference in diastolic blood pressure was also 4 per cent. The difference in
smoking cessation was 20 per cent after adjustment for thiocyanate levels
(Neaton *et al.* 1981).

MRFIT started in the mid-1970s in the USA at a time when usual care in
the prevention of CHD in high risk subjects was already well advanced, at
least for nutritional advice concerning serum cholesterol reduction and
high blood pressure drug treatment. In fact, the small differences for these
two risk factors were mainly due to the good care received by subjects in
the reference group from their general practitioners. This suggests that,
with a conventional approach, general practitioners were capable of reducing high serum cholesterol and high blood pressure in a preventive
effort. No significant differences between SI and UC were observed for all-
cause mortality ($+1.9$ per cent) or coronary mortality (-7.1 per cent) at
the end of this 6 year trial (MRFIT 1982). Mortality rates after 10.5 years
follow-up showed no statistical differences for CHD mortality, cardiovascular mortality, and all-cause mortality, although in males without electrocardiogram (ECG) abnormalities, coronary and all-cause mortality were
significantly lower in the special intervention group (MRFIT 1990).

Both the Oslo Study and MRFIT, the two trials directed solely at high risk subjects, contributed to the confirmation of the risk factor concept: life-style modification is feasible in high risk subjects and it induces a decrease in CHD incidence when differences between risk factor modifications in intervention and control groups are substantial. These trials also point to the fact that the key risk factor that should be changed in order to see a decrease in CHD incidence is serum cholesterol level.

The Göteborg Primary Prevention Trial (Wilhelmsen *et al.* 1986) was a population-based 10 year study where high risk subjects were screened out of a random population sample and offered individual counselling in special out-patient clinics. In fact, counselling was given on a group basis of 7–10 males (with their spouses). Sessions were first on a weekly basis, and later were held fortnightly. No figures were given concerning the number of males receiving individual advice out of the 10 004 who were screened. After 4 years of follow-up there was almost no change in serum cholesterol compared with baseline in the intervention group (from 6.46 to 6.42 mmol/l). After 10 years there was a reduction in serum cholesterol of 6.8 per cent in both the intervention and control groups. No differences were observed in the reduction of blood pressure, and a difference of 3.3 per cent, in favour of the intervention group, was observed in abstention from smoking. In terms of end-points there were no significant differences between intervention and control groups for all-cause mortality, fatal CHD, non-fatal CHD, and total CHD. It is not clear why, in this trial, individual counselling in high risk subjects by specialists in health counselling in out-patient clinics with, apparently, long experience failed to induce substantial changes in the major coronary risk factors, although it is probable that the results presented are diluted by the number of subjects in the intervention group who did not receive any personal advice (Wilhelmsen 1990). It seems clear from this trial that intervention in high risk subjects alone as a small subgroup of the total population will not influence CHD incidence at the population level.

The WHO European Collaborative Trial in the Multifactorial Prevention of Coronary Heart Disease (WHO 1989) was the only one combining face-to-face counselling in high risk subjects with a 'population strategy' in lower-risk subjects. This so-called 'factory trial' was set up in four countries: the UK, Belgium, Italy, and Poland. The concept of the trial is known: it is based on the random allocation of pairs of factories (60 881 males aged 40–59 years) to an intervention or control group. Strictly speaking, this was not a primary prevention trial as subjects with angina or ischaemic ECG modifications were also included.

The trial's statistical analysis was based on 'an intention to treat' concept. It took a pragmatic or public health approach in that, if successful, the programme would be immediately applicable to the middle-aged working population of the four countries. Life-style modification was aimed at eating habits, smoking, and sedentary behaviour, whereas drug treatment was essential for high blood pressure control. Subjects were defined as high risk according to a risk score. The percentage of subjects given individual advice varied as follows: UK, 12 per cent; Belgium, 21 per cent; Italy, 32 per cent; Poland, 34 per cent. Lower-risk men received advice through the mass media: conferences, posters, and booklets on coronary risk factors. In Belgium and the UK modifications were obtained in the preparation of food in some canteens of the intervention factories. High risk subjects received personal advice at the work site, except in Poland where they were referred to special out-patient clinics. Advice at the work site was given by the factory physicians in the UK, by specially trained physicians in Belgium, and by factory physicians and project team doctors in Italy. The frequency of individual sessions varied from country to country, with the highest frequency during the first 2 years (four sessions in Italy, and three sessions in Belgium). In Italy lower-risk subjects also received face-to-face advice, but on a less intense basis. Success of behavioural modification was monitored periodically by means of the net evolution (intervention factory minus paired-off control factory) of the multilogistic risk estimate in random samples and high risk groups. In Italy, nutritional modification was confirmed by fatty acids assays on red blood cells (Angelico *et al.* 1982). In Belgium, modification of smoking behaviour was confirmed by serum thiocyanate (Kornitzer *et al.* 1983*a*).

Figure 33.1 shows that face-to-face counselling of high risk men had a greater impact on risk factor modification compared with the 'mass media' approach adopted for the lower-risk group during the whole of the trial.

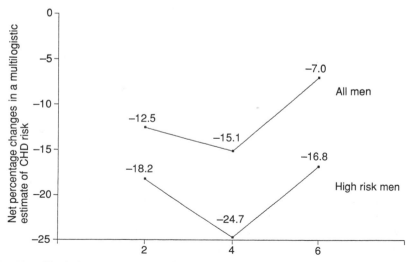

Fig. 33.1 Evolution over time of the net modifications of the coronary risk factor profile in all men (or random samples) and high risk men. (After Kornitzer and Rose 1985.)

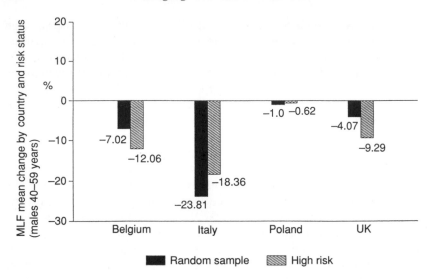

Fig. 33.2 Mean net change by country in the coronary risk factor profile in all men (or random samples) and high risk men in each of the four countries.

This is confirmed, at least for the UK and Belgium, although in Italy the mean change in the multiple logistic function (MLF) of the random samples was more pronounced than that of the high risk subjects (Italy was the only country where all subjects had face-to-face counselling) (Fig. 33.2). At the end of the trial the effect of the intervention programme was less pronounced. The Belgian trial showed a continuous decrease in the impact of the prevention programme over time, although even at the end of the trial face-to-face counselling still had a favourable effect on the multiple logistic risk estimate in the intervention factories (Figs 33.3 and 33.4).

One of the major problems in the control of cardiovascular diseases is long-term adherence to drug treatment advice in hypertensives. In the Belgian trial, hypertension had to be treated by general practitioners following recommendation from the physicians attached to the trial, as prescription of medication was not allowed at the work site. After 2 years 86 per cent of subjects with baseline untreated hypertension had consulted their general practitioner and drug therapy was started in 52 per cent of them. After 2 years follow-up, there was a decrease of 4.4 per cent in the systolic blood pressure in the control group compared with a decrease of 13.2 per cent in the intervention group (De Backer *et al.* 1979). However, at the end of the 6 year multifactorial trial, the blood pressure distribution of the intervention and control groups was again comparable, and there was no difference in the percentage of treated patients, posing the problem of both the responsibility of the medical profession and compliance with the drug regimen by the subjects (De Backer *et al.* 1983). The Belgian

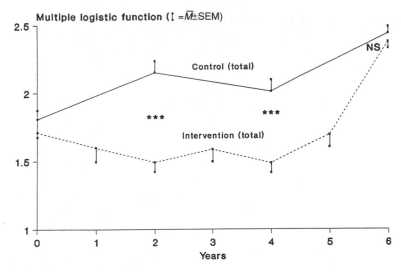

Fig. 33.3 Change in coronary risk predictors during the trial (*** p<0.001). (Reproduced with permission from Kornitzer *et al.* 1983c.)

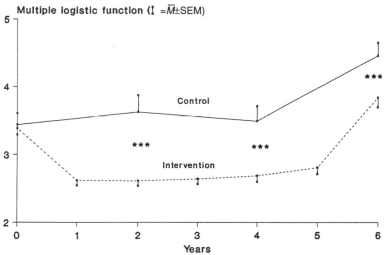

Fig. 33.4 Change in coronary risk predictors in the high risk subgroup (***p<0.001). (Reproduced with permission from Kornitzer *et al.* 1983c.)

Heart Disease Prevention Programme also looked at the possible influence of psycho-social and cultural factors on the modification of coronary risk factors by individual counselling in high risk subjects. In this trial abstention of smoking was not related to social class or study level; neither was there any relation between type A behaviour, scales of neuroticism or extraversion, and the 6 year smoking cessation rate. With regard to modification of serum cholesterol, the highest reduction was observed in blue-collar workers (−15.7 per cent) and the smallest in white-collar workers (−10.8 per cent), whereas no relation was observed with type A behaviour or with scores of neuroticism and extraversion (Kornitzer *et al.* 1983*b*). Observation of the modification of the coronary risk factor profile over the 6 year period of the trial (by means of the MLF) revealed an important relation with culture: in the Flemish-speaking high risk subjects from the north of Belgium net reduction of MLF averaged 19.2 per cent, whereas in the French-speaking subjects this reduction was only 4 per cent. The largest net MLF reduction was observed in white-collar workers (−24.1 per cent) and the smallest in executives (−8.2 per cent). Type B subjects had a net MLF reduction of 27.1 per cent, whereas type A subjects showed a reduction of only 7.6 per cent (Kornitzer *et al.* 1984). It seems that coronary risk factor modification is easier to achieve in Flemish speakers, white-collar workers, and type B subjects.

As a whole, the WHO Collaborative Trial showed non-significant differences for all-cause mortality (−5.3 per cent), total CHD (−10.2 per cent, $p = 0.07$), fatal CHD (−6.9 per cent), and non-fatal myocardial infarction, (−14.8 per cent, $p = 0.06$). For total CHD and non-fatal myocardial infarction, differences came close to significance (WHO 1986). Only in the Belgian trial was there a significant difference between intervention and control factories for all-cause mortality (−17 per cent, $p < 0.05$) and total CHD (−24 per cent, $p < 0.05$) (Kornitzer *et al.* 1983*c*).

When looking at regressions of change in CHD incidence on differences in compliance (MLF risk factor change) over the 40 pairs of factories the results are significant for three pre-trial end-points: fatal CHD, total CHD, and total deaths (Table 33.2). In other words, the differences in these end-points can be explained by mean differences in the MLF over

Table 33.2 Regressions of change in incidence p_1-p_C on differences in compliance (MLF risk factor change) and initial differences in risk (initial MLF_1 − initial MLF_C)

Outcome	Difference in MLF at entry: slope (SE)	Difference in compliance: slope (SE)
Fatal CHD	0.65[a] (0.25)	0.60[a] (0.25)
Non-fatal MI	0.72 (0.40)	0.64 (0.45)
Total CHD	1.23[a] (0.46)	1.18[a] (0.53)
Total deaths	1.98[a] (0.56)	1.41[a] (0.60)
Non-CHD deaths	1.18[a] (0.49)	0.63 (0.52)

The incidence rate and MLF score are both person per 6 years
MI, myocardial infarction.
[a] $p < 0.05$ (two-tailed test).
Reproduced with permission from Rose (1987).

time: advice on CHD was effective to the extent that it was accepted (Rose 1987). However, the intervention programme did not seem to have an impact on major risk factor changes in many of the intervention factories. In Italy, where face-to-face counselling was given to all subjects, the risk factor changes were the most important of the four countries. However, the Italian trial included only two pairs of factories and lacked the statistical power to show an impact on reduction of the new CHD events. Although evolution of the coronary risk profile in the UK and Belgium was not very different, the impact on the CHD event was quite different. One possible explanation is that in the UK influence on the MLF was mainly due to cessation or reduction of smoking in the intervention factories, whereas in Belgium the main effect on the MLF was through a reduction of serum cholesterol. As the Oslo Study had shown, it could well be that a major impact on CHD would only be obtained in those multifactorial trials where serum cholesterol was *substantially* reduced.

Finally, the kind of work site intervention programme proposed by the WHO European Collaborative Trial does not seem to have a lasting effect on risk factor modification. In the Belgian Heart Disease Prevention Project, differences between intervention and control factories in total and cardiovascular mortality were markedly reduced at 10 year follow-up (De Backer *et al*. 1988). In that trial, where the 'population approach' extended to 79 per cent of the intervention group with preventive activities during the first 3 years only, no carry-over effect was observed. At 6 years, risk factor modifications were not sustained except in the high risk men. The Italian arm of the trial, where face-to-face counselling was given to all participants, showed better results at 6 years in terms of risk factor modification, with a favourable impact after the end of the trial at 8.5 years follow-up (Research Group of the Rome Project of Coronary Heart Disease Prevention 1986). The only other trial comparing the effect of the population approach with that of face-to-face advice on a short-term basis (2 year follow-up) was the Stanford Three Community Study (Stern *et al*. 1976). This study was the first to show that counselling individuals or small groups concerning eating patterns had a more pronounced effect on behaviour modification than the community approach in terms of reduction of saturated fats and cholesterol intake.

The multifactorial trials of the 1970s were not initiated in the first place to test concepts or models concerning the modification of individual lifestyles but to provide additional proof of the validity of the multifactorial origin of CHD observed in the cohort studies. It was assumed that, provided that a substantial decrease in individuals' coronary risk factors was obtained in a high proportion of the intervention group compared with the reference group over the length of the trial, a significant difference in CHD incidence between the two groups would be observed.

All seven multifactorial trials aimed at individual life-style modification

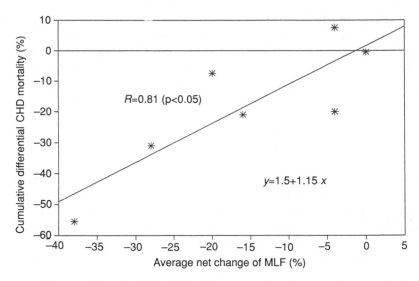

Fig. 33.5 Regression of CHD differential mortality (between intervention and control groups) on the average net change of the MLF in the seven multifactorial trials listed in Table 33.1.

(supplemented by a mass media approach in the WHO Collaborative Trial) lend strong support to the validity of the risk factor concept. We related average net difference in the multilogistic risk estimate over time in the seven trials from Table 33.1 with cumulative coronary mortality after 5–10 years follow-up: the correlation is 81 per cent significant at the $p < 0.05$ level (Fig. 33.5). For an average difference of 10 per cent in the multiple logistic function, there is a difference of 10 per cent in coronary mortality.

Various models of life-style modifications emerged during the 1960s and 1970s: the Health Belief Model (Rosenstock 1974; Becker and Maiman 1975; Berkanovic 1976), a model based on social learning (Bandura 1977), and the social support model, reviewed by Ritter (1990). Given that modification of eating and smoking habits would favourably modify the incidence of coronary mortality at the population level, it remains to apply these new health behaviour concepts in order to bring a lifelong modification of life-style leading to a reduction of coronary risk factors at the individual and population level. Provided that the medical schools impart information and skills in primary prevention of coronary heart disease to future primary care physicians so that they are able to cope with the largely inadequate life-style at the individual and population level, they could play a crucial role (Mittelmark *et al.* 1988). This is the challenge to the medical profession in the industrialized countries at the end of the twentieth century.

REFERENCES

Angelico, F., Amadeo, P., Guccione, P., Montali, S., Menotti, A., Ricci, G., *et al.* (1982). Dietary and red blood cell fatty acid changes after a four-year dietary intervention in the Rome Project of Coronary Heart Disease Prevention. *Clin. Ter. Cardiovas.,* **1**, 1–10.

Bandura, A. (1977). *Social learning theory*, Prentice-Hall, Englewood Cliffs, NJ.

Becker, M. H. and Maiman, L. A. (1975). Sociobehavioural determinants of compliance with health and medical care recommendations. *Med. Care,* **13**, 10–24.

Benfari, R. C. (1981). The Multiple Risk Factor Intervention Trial (MRFIT). III The model for intervention. *Prev. Med.,* **10**, 426–42.

Berkanovic, E. (1976). Behavioral science and prevention. *Prev. Med.,* **5**, 92–1055.

Davis, M. S. (1968). Physiologic, psychological and demographic factors in patient compliance with doctor's orders. *Med. Care,* **6**, 115–22.

De Backer, G., Dramaix, M., Kornitzer, M., Kittel, F., and Vuylsteek, K. (1979). Psychosoziale Aspekte des Hochdrucks. *Schwerpunkt Med.,* **4**, 49–56.

De Backer, G., Van Hemeldonck, A. M., Kornitzer, M., Kittel, F., and Dramaix, M. (1983). Erkennung und Kontrolle der arteriellen Hypertonie: Die Erfahrungen des belgischen Präventionsprojektes gegen Herzkrankheiten. *Schwerpunkt Med.,* **1**, 30–3.

De Backer, G., Kornitzer, M., Dramaix, M., Kittel, F., Thilly, C., Graffar, M., *et al.* (1988). The Belgian Heart Disease Prevention Project: 10-year mortality follow-up. *Eur. Heart J.,* **9**, 238–42.

Hjermann, I. (1983). A randomized primary preventive trial in coronary heart disease: the Oslo Study. *Prev. Med.,* **12**, 181–4.

Hjermann, I., Holme, I., and Leren, P. (1986). Oslo Study diet and antismoking trial, results after 102 months. *Am. J. Med.,* **80** (Suppl. 2A), 7–11.

Kornitzer, M. and Rose, G. (on behalf of the WHO Collaborative Group) (1985). WHO European Collaborative Trial of Multifactorial Prevention of Coronary Heart Disease. *Prev. Med.,* **14**, 272–8.

Kornitzer, M., Vanhemeldonck, A., Bourdoux, P., and De Backer, G. (1983*a*). Belgian Heart Disease Prevention Project: comparison of self-reported smoking behaviour with serum thiocyanate concentrations. *J. Epidemiol. Community Health,* **37**, 132–6.

Kornitzer, M., Kittel, F., Dramaix, M., and De Backer, G. (1983*b*). Psychosocial variables in relation with coronary risk status modification. In *Biobehavioral bases of coronary heart disease* (eds T. M. Dembroski, T. H. Schmidt, and G. Blümchen), Karger, Basel, pp. 459–72.

Kornitzer, M., De Backer, G., Dramaix, M., Kittel, F., Thilly, C., Graffar, M., *et al.* (1983*c*). Belgian Heart Disease Prevention Project: incidence and mortality results. *Lancet,* **i**, 1066–70.

Kornitzer, M., De Backer, G., Kittel, F., and Dramaix, M. (1984). The Belgian Heart Disease Prevention Project: influence of psychosocial variables and mode of delivery of advice on coronary risk factor modification. In *Rep. 3rd Int. Conf. on System Science in Health Care* (eds W. van Eimeren, R. Engelbrecht, and C. D. Flagle), Springer-Verlag, Berlin.

Leventhal, H. (1965). Fear communications in the acceptance of preventive health practices. *Bull. NY Acad. Med.*, **41**, 1144–68.

Mittelmark, M. B., Luepker, R. V., Grimm, R., Kottke, T. E., and Blackburn, H. (1988). The role of physicians in a community-wide program for prevention of cardiovascular disease: the Minnesota Heart Health Program. *Public Health Rep.*, **103**, 360–5.

MRFIT (Multiple Risk Factor Intervention Trial) Research Group (1982). Multiple risk factor intervention trial. Risk factor changes and mortality results. *J. Am. Med. Assoc.*, **248**, 1465–77.

MRFIT (Multiple Risk Factor Intervention Trial) Research Group (1990). Mortality rates after 10.5 years for participants in the multiple risk factor intervention trial. Findings related to a priori hypotheses of the trial. *J. Am. Med. Assoc.*, **263**, 1795–801.

Neaton, J. D., Broste, S., Cohen, L., Fishman, E. L., Kjelsberg, M. O., and Schoenberger, J. (1981). The Multiple Risk Factor Intervention Trial (MRFIT). VII A comparison of risk factor changes between the two study groups. *Prev. Med.*, **10**, 519–43.

Puska, P., Tuomilehto, J., Salonen, J., Nissinen, A., Virtamo, J., Björkqvist, S., *et al.* (1981). *Community control of cardiovascular diseases. Evaluation of a comprehensive community programme for control of cardiovascular diseases in North Karelia, Finland 1972–1977.* WHO, Copenhagen.

Research Group of the Rome Project of Coronary Heart Disease Prevention. (1986). Eight-year results from the Rome Project of Coronary Heart Disease Prevention. *Prev. Med.*, **15**, 176–91.

Ritter, C. (1990). Social supports, social networks, and health behaviours. In *Health behaviour, emerging research perspectives* (ed. D. S. Gochman), Plenum, New York, pp. 149–59.

Rose, G. (on behalf of the WHO Collaborative Group) (1987). European Collaborative Trial of Multifactorial Prevention of Coronary Heart Disease. *Lancet*, **i**, 685.

Rosenstock, I. M. (1974). The health belief model and preventive health behaviour. *Health Educ. Monogr.*, **2**, 354–86.

Stern, M. P., Farquhar, J. W., Maccoby, N., and Russell, S. H. (1976). Results of a two-year health education campaign on dietary behaviour. The Stanford Three Community Study. *Circulation*, **54**, 826–33.

Wilhelmsen, L. (1990). Personal communication.

Wilhelmsen, L., Berglund, G., Elmfeldt, D., Tibblin, G., Wedel, H., Pennert, K., *et al.* (1986). The multifactor primary prevention trial in Göteborg, Sweden. *Eur. Heart J.*, **7**, 279–88.

WHO (World Health Organization) European Collaborative Group (1986). European Collaborative Trial of Multifactorial Prevention of Coronary Heart Disease: final report on the 6-year results. *Lancet*, **i**, 869–72.

WHO (World Health Organization) Collaborative Group (1974). An international controlled trial in the multifactorial prevention of coronary heart disease. *Int. J. Epidemiol.*, **3**, 219–24.

WHO (World Health Organization) Regional Office for Europe (1989). *WHO Collaborative Trial in the Multifactorial Prevention of Coronary Heart Disease*, WHO, Copenhagen.

34

Community programmes in coronary heart disease prevention and health promotion: changing community behaviour

H. Blackburn

BACKGROUND

The population strategy of cardiovascular disease (CVD) prevention aims at reducing the average levels and distributions of risk factors for whole communities (Rose 1981). This requires changes in the risk behaviour of substantial numbers of people, brought about by change in community norms and environments to encourage healthy living patterns and to discourage unhealthy ones. It is assumed that the favourable environment achieved will ensure the least exhibition of population susceptibility, and that educational strategies, promoted through community-wide campaigns, will lead to favourable changes in health behaviour throughout the community. The community is a critical unit for health interventions, lying as it does between individual and small group medical strategies and regional or national policy and programmes for prevention. Population-wide strategies for CVD prevention were first laid out formally by a WHO Expert Committee headed by Geoffrey Rose (WHO 1982).

First-generation community programmes in coronary heart disease (CHD) prevention have been carried out over the last two decades in Finland, the USA, and elsewhere. Their designs, organizational methods, and education programmes are published, along with results of programme effects. Evidence about long-term changes in community risk factor levels and disease rates is not yet available from all programmes. Nevertheless, many of the concepts, methods, and educational components of these pioneering programmes are already in use by second-generation community research projects and are widely disseminated among current public health programmes.

What then is the status of health promotion programmes in facilitating community changes in health? What are the roles in community health promotion programmes of public and private agencies, of individuals and groups, of direct education and mass communication, of government and of the health care system? What are the major future applications and needs for new knowledge? The recent experience of community-based programmes in CVD prevention provides many relevant answers.

Contributions of first-generation community studies

In brief, first-generation community CVD prevention programmes found that middle-class communities were highly receptive to well-conceived programmes, that broad educational strategies for community change could be implemented, and that they were replicable. Population awareness of the need and potential for prevention was greatly increased, health-related activities in the community were significantly enhanced, and behavioural change was documented among a large proportion of citizens. It has not been possible to determine precisely how much and what kind of intervention is required to change risk in whole communities, but the intervention has been described and its goals achieved. The communities were entered successfully, leaders and volunteers were organized, and health messages were delivered; physicians and health professionals were included effectively; a majority of adults were recruited to heart health centres and many participated in direct education programmes for eating patterns, physical activity, and smoking; large segments of the youth in communities were involved in health-related activities.

Early reports of programme effect are encouraging, but it remains uncertain whether the educational–motivational strategies used were themselves sufficiently powerful to induce, or the evaluation strategies were sufficiently sensitive to detect, a major acceleration of the already remarkable upturn in healthy behaviour and downturn in CVD risk widely observed in American communities and elsewhere. Nevertheless, major implications for public health have emerged from the completed community demonstration programmes. Tested effective programme components are available. Much can now be said about the contributions to changes in community health behaviour of individuals and groups, of government and legislation, of industry and commerce, of direct education and mass communication strategies, and of medical care and public health systems. Much has been learned, as well, about practical schemes for evaluating community-based health promotion programmes.

The original assumptions and hypotheses made about community change, some lessons learned about design and intervention, and the state of the art of community-based health promotion will be briefly considered in this chapter. Comments will also be made on future research needs and new directions for programme design, evaluation, and intervention. Strategies for personal risk reduction and policy and practice for health promotion at national and international levels are considered elsewhere in this volume.

THE HYPOTHESES, ASSUMPTIONS, AND
THEORY BASE OF COMMUNITY PROGRAMMES

The criteria originally applied for undertaking such major, community-based CHD prevention programmes at all still hold (Blackburn 1983):

• the disease is common and often fatal;

• strong causal relationships exist between risk factor levels and disease risk;

• socio-cultural determinants of disease risk are predominant;

• the potential benefit of intervention is demonstrated;

• the safety of intervention is well established;

• important community control of the socio-cultural environment exists;

• tested and acceptable population strategies of health promotion are needed (thus research programmes) or available (thus public health applications).

At the outset, in the 1970s, we hypothesized (1) that community-based educational programmes would be feasible and, once implemented, (2) would enhance awareness and community thinking about the potential of CHD prevention, (3) that campaigns would lead to active citizen participation which, in turn, (4) would modify health behaviour, (5) that these changes would lead in time to a reduction of community risk and rates of CVD, (6) that the changes would be maintained, and (7) that the programmes would be incorporated into the community (Jacobs *et al.* 1986).

A conceptual framework, based on educational and behavioural theory current at the time, was used to plan the community strategies and to analyse their effects (Farquhar 1978). Since no single theory accounted for the variety of disease end-points, risk behaviour, and risk characteristics involved, or for the many educational strategies required among subgroups in the community, several models were employed for planning and evaluation. A central role was played by *social learning theory*: the idea that personal behaviour is learned through social influences in the community, at the work site, and in the family, and that behaviour is changed as a result of awareness of the need to change, as well as individuals' incentives and perceived ability to change (Bandura 1977). Mass communication of health messages was guided by the *diffusion of innovation model* which describes how health information is diffused, with lag times between awareness and adoption of new behaviour among different segments of the community (Green 1975). The *persuasion model* considered ways in which people perceive the relevance of health information and the motivations to which individuals and groups respond (Hovland *et al*. 1953; McGuire 1973). Concepts of *peer influence* and *health beliefs* also helped guide many personal self-help strategies devised for health promotion. Finally, *systems theory* dealt with the effectiveness and interaction of the several educational strategies throughout community networks (Farquhar *et al*. 1985).

The results to date suggest that the educational, behavioural, and communication theories, and the general hypotheses proposed, at least up to the outcomes of risk and disease, were largely confirmed.

DESIGN AND EVALUATION OF COMMUNITY PROGRAMMES

Overall outcome evaluation: status and implications

Evaluation is essential to the sound operation and understanding of community health programme effects. The major limitation has been the relatively small number of non-randomized community units involved. This was considered practically necessary at the outset, but in the end it makes the interpretation of community programme effects complex (Jacobs *et al*. 1986; Farquhar *et al*. 1990). The variability found in average risk factor levels among cluster samples of communities, and between years, was greater than anticipated from the well-known individual variability of these values. Low level correlations of risk factors within clusters led, when extended over many people, to very large 'design effects' which reduced power to detect programme effects. Systematic and random errors in measurement reduced power further. The changing composition of American communities created by migration contributed to reduced response rates and exposure to programmes. Mainly, however, American society overall has changed rapidly in awareness of and attention to high blood pressure and cholesterol values. Habitual diet, physical activity habits, and smoking patterns in the community have evolved with vertiginous speed. This dynamic has reduced the power to detect with confidence the hypothesized differences or any acceleration of changes due to focused community programmes.

One result of these limitations may be the tendency to interpret as significant the education effects suggested by individual-level (cohort) analyses in the face of equivocal community-level (cross-sectional) results. There is also a risk of claiming as treatment effects what in reality represents random variations among community clusters. Therefore community programmes need to examine both cohort and cross-sectional effects, but always to consider the community as the primary unit of intervention and analysis. Individual effects are mainly of interest for their consistency with, and explanation of, any population effects found.

Implications for future community programmes

The chief lesson for future community programmes from these design limitations is that allocation of more communities to each condition is the major need—that 'magic number' determines power. The power of the first-generation CVD community programme designs was barely adequate to detect changes of public health significance (e.g. average risk factor differences of the order of 2–5 per cent). For their designs to detect such differences with confidence, a larger treatment effect would be required. The ability to detect a difference in programme effect increases dramatically with the number of units compared, while power increases relatively less by increasing the number of persons sampled within units (Jacobs *et al.* 1986). The contributions of more frequent surveys, or comparisons of more homogeneous communities, are also relatively minor. Statisticians now hold out, enticingly, the potential of other ways to reduce dependence on the number of community units and to improve future efficiency of community programme evaluations through 'numerical solutions' (based on iterations of distributions within communities rather than comparisons of differences in respect to theoretical distributions). Such analytical methods may help to account for the fact that community samples are not truly independent and identically distributed.

These painfully acquired lessons on design have important implications for future public health programmes, particularly for the energy required in their implementation and evaluation. Even programmes having 'new and improved design', yet using traditional end-points of risk factor and disease change, may become prohibitively expensive for constrained research budgets. When larger numbers of communities are compared the cost is raised immensely, and a practical problem arises of finding numbers of comparable units amenable to randomization. The US Commit Project of the National Cancer Institute, for example, has 11 communities randomized to smoking interventions and 11 to control, while CATCH, a multifactor intervention in youth populations, has 96 school units in four towns, randomized to three conditions. These current demonstrations should offer much needed evidence about the feasibility and effects of newer designs for community programmes.

Alternative strategies for greater efficiency also may require focus on communities where disease rates and risk are unusually high, where 'background' intervention and change are less advanced, and where resources are already in place for systematic surveillance. Thus new, compelling, and focused questions about health change, along with innovative design and improved techniques of measurement, are all essential for future community health programmes. If these new designs and interventions prove more feasible and effective, and less costly, the investigative and public health scenes in health promotion should be vastly stimulated anew to address many urgent and practical health needs of communities.

Education programme design and evaluation: status and implications

The status of programme, or 'process', evaluation of community health programmes was advanced greatly by the experience of American community-based demonstration projects. Traditionally, evaluation has focused on programme effects on the health behaviour of individuals. It must now consider the extent to which a programme reaches a significant proportion of the community, including those most in need of it. The American experience has led to helping community programmes identify their goals at the outset, even determining that some goals, such as risk factor and disease change, were neither reasonable nor feasible to test. The need to demonstrate links between health programme components, the 'reach' of specific exposures into the community, and their behavioural effects is now widely appreciated.

Future needs

Future evaluations for community programmes need improved indicators of community-wide change, such as unobtrusive measures of exposure and of changes in food, alcohol, and tobacco consumption. Refinements in survey methods are also needed for evaluation under unfavourable social circumstances, along with ways of improving the validity of self-report measures in telephone and face-to-face interviews. Critically important is the need for widespread and appropriate training in programme evaluation of public health and community personnel at all levels.

THE STATUS AND ROLE OF EDUCATIONAL PROGRAMMES

Comprehensive community health promotion programmes bring to bear several major educational strategies: direct education, community organization, and mass communication. Each of these may contain, in turn, policy interventions of a specific local nature. These strategies are usually staged in sequence (Mittlemark *et al*. 1986): (1) alerting the community to the problem; (2) educating the community about solutions; (3) motivating the community to change; (4) organizing the community to implement programmes; (5) measuring community effects; (6) maintaining effects in the community.

Direct education

Educational strategies involving formal classes, risk factor screening, or self-help programmes are cost-accountable, if not always cost-effective, components of community programmes. Adult classes generally achieve significant change in individual knowledge and behaviour, particularly when built into existing institutional and educational programmes. But recruitment to adult classes is not highly successful, often involving only about 5 per cent of target populations. Furthermore, classes are labour-intensive.

Risk factor screening with education

Many authoritative bodies, including WHO Expert Committees on Prevention of Coronary Artery Disease (WHO 1982) and Community Programs (WHO 1985), as well as the US National Cholesterol Education Program (NCEP 1990), continue to recommend screening for high risk as a cost-effective method of prevention. However, they counsel that it be carried out only in the context of a wide community campaign to include physicians and public awareness of the importance of elevated risk factors, along with broad access to treatment programmes for risk reduction. The Minnesota Heart Health Program (MHHP) has demonstrated that systematic community screening approaches can achieve a wide population-based response, and that a single exposure with an intensive educational component results in measurable health action and risk change (Murray *et al.* 1986). The majority of adults in middle-class American communities (more than 60 per cent) can be recruited to such undertakings. The cost of screening is accountable and within the range of many individual or government payment plans.

Professional education: role of physicians and the medical system

Community-based strategies have involved physicians early and in positions of authority. Their leadership results in more systematic screening and preventive care, with improved identification and treatment of the high risk individual (Luepker and Rastam 1990). However, the priorities of the clinic and other barriers to preventive practice largely determine whether physicians actually implement screening and follow-up procedures or use effective hygienic interventions (Kottke *et al.* 1987). Nevertheless, in the detection, treatment, and control of hypertension in the USA, most classical barriers to preventive practice have fallen away and effective blood pressure control is now widely diffused. Similar changes are under way for medical roles in community strategies for lowering blood cholesterol levels among the general population and in those found at high risk (NCEP 1990). Dietary and smoking cessation advice are practices that have largely failed to spread in routine medical use compared with the rapid and complete adoption of pharmacological and other 'high tech' innovations. Thus the physician and medical care are impaired by a broader conceptual or 'systems' problem that reduces the effective practice of prevention and health promotion. It seems that professional training and incentives must improve before preventive practice will change widely. Therefore, a population strategy of graduated education, motivation, and policy change should include physicians and other health professionals. Meanwhile, society moves ahead 'on its own' with a widening practice of healthy behaviour and increasing demand for healthy environments. Perhaps it is indeed true that 'Where the people lead, their leaders soon will follow'.

School-based youth–parent health programmes in the community
The basic assumption of youth health promotion programmes remains unchallenged: youth behaviour is less entrenched than adult behaviour and therefore is more amenable to primary prevention strategies. Evidence indicates that most health behaviour is established by the time students complete high school. Moreover, programmes based on parent–child interventions appear to be widely feasible among American schools and families. Thus primary prevention efforts centred on childhood and adolescence are recommended.

School-based programmes for health promotion have a rich literature and experience. Their theory base has been extensively tested in programmes designed to redirect rebellious health-compromising behaviour towards healthy independent decision-making. Stone *et al*. (1989) have summarized the major contributions to youth health promotion from current programmes widely accepted among school administrators and educators. School health education curricula have been upgraded to include more student participation and skills development: enhancement of self-knowledge, self-control, personal and social responsibility, and 'self-efficacy'. Skills-based curricula are emphasized over knowledge-based ones. Peer-led student approaches have made significant inroads into youthful thinking and behaviour. The effects of exposure to these newer programmes, with and without 'booster sessions', are variable but promising. Long-lasting effects are demonstrated on cognition and health behaviour patterns, and on the rate of adoption of cigarette smoking (Perry *et al*. 1989a). Programmes designed to involve student–parent interaction were demonstrated by the MHHP to be acceptable and effective up to the sixth grade (Perry *et al*. 1989b). Parents can be recruited by students to adult programme activities, influencing family-wide decisions on eating, exercise, and smoking behaviour.

The North Karelia Study demonstrated an added contribution to changes in youthful behaviour by combining school health programmes with community-wide strategies (Puska *et al*. 1982). This experience points ———— environmental effect on youth which is now being translated ———— at individuals and communities can effectively change ———— the environment, as well as individual health behaviour ———— a). Therefore involvement of the educational community ———— munity programmes and leaders is an important new el- ———— programmes (Perry *et al*. 1990).

Implications for future youth programmes

Designs for the new generation of youth programmes recently initiated continue to target the social environment but also include a larger number of randomized units (Perry *et al.* 1990). Community-wide health strategies directed towards youth now need to include not only physical health but mental, psychological, social and spiritual domains. The assumptions of youth programmes remain that young people *can* and *do* respond to healthy goals and can acquire self-regulating skills. Because the community is the smallest unit in which all the layers of influence to promote health among youth can be found, combined school and community programmes continue to be a recommended approach to preventing the major health problems of society at an early stage.

Dynamic changes are under way in youth health practices, as evidenced, for example, by the rapid increase of the use of smokeless tobacco by young people. Therefore resources for surveillance to detect changes such as these are needed, leading, in turn, to programmes appropriate to the audience and to the changed issues. There is clearly a great need and opportunity for health promotion resource centres.

Future research needs for youth health promotion have been clearly set out (Harlan, in Stone *et al.* 1989):

Strategies for communities with different ethnic, education and income levels; models that are affordable and are acceptable to educators; studies on the transferability of school programmes; 'booster' designs and the effects of small, frequent interventions over longer periods; and studies of the degree to which healthy behaviours and risk factor changes achieved in youth extend into later life.

Mass communication in community health programmes

Health communication to mass audiences has developed in parallel with the population strategy of prevention in public health. Until recently, theory about communication for health promotion in the community stressed the limitations of mass media as a primary effector of change and emphasized their complementary function to community organization and direct educational strategies. Clearly, general awareness about and credibility of a health programme depend prominently on mass communication. The MHHP, for example, secured almost complete saturation of the community with awareness of its programmes within 2 years, and this could be explained mainly by the effects of the mass media (Finnegan *et al.* 1989). But the mass media were also particularly effective in the Stanford Heart Disease Prevention Program in directing people to community facilities and in actually encouraging and teaching changed behaviour, in addition to providing the general awareness function (Maccoby *et al.* 1977; Flora *et al.* 1989).

Community-wide media campaigns are particularly amenable to periods of intensive activity that coincide appropriately with other community activities (e.g. 'hypertension month', 'quit smoking day', and seasonal emphases on physical activity and healthy eating patterns). These can be evaluated readily by rapid surveys before, during, and after the intervention. Part of the community health communication effort is to create 'health news' of interest to local channels and to prepare materials for dissemination through those channels. Promotional campaigns are highly visible locally and their activities have many side-effects. However, the differing complexity of communities and their media channels requires different strategies for using newspapers, radio, and television.

Because communities are heterogeneous, media messages must be oriented to specific groups defined by age, sex, or other demographic factors. Groups may also require special attention based on their knowledge levels about a health topic. This is supported by MHHP findings of a 'knowledge gap', suggesting that, in the absence of certain conditions, campaigns may cause the 'information rich' to grow richer, and the 'information poor' to remain static or grow poorer, requiring intensive campaigns to overcome their ignorance (Viswanath 1990). Recently, formative evaluation has helped to prevent major programme failures. Bandura's social learning theory (Bandura 1977) has helped, particularly by suggestions that the more complex the behaviour, the more individuals seek information from multiple channels, and the less complex the behaviour, the greater the influence of a single channel.

The first-generation community CVD prevention programmes demonstrated the advantages of local media strategies. They tend to reduce the 'noise' and fragmentation of communications as found in larger regions. Local public service announcements (PSAs) also provide advantages that are missing at the regional level. Health issues 'make news' locally, and programme directors are able to deal personally with the media as a local industry. All this results in programmes tailored to specific community needs and mores. Finally, use of local media offers the advantage of wide visibility and community involvement that cannot be matched by health promotion through the national media (which must work, for example, against the huge advertising budgets of industry!).

Future applications of the media
The MHHP experience has led to emphasis on the planning *process* for health communications rather than on specific complex media strategies or 'high tech' materials preparation. The recommended process begins by establishing measurable media objectives for the community. It continues by analysing audiences to determine specific campaign targets, and then identifies key messages and media channels likely to have an effect on the segments identified. The media strategies are then integrated with other

campaign approaches under way in the community, particularly with direct education and community organization. Finally, a specific community blueprint is produced for scheduling all media tasks, deadlines, and responsibilities, for developing the materials, and then for implementing and evaluating the programme.

Community organization: status and role in community programmes

Bracht (1990) has summarized the role and advantages of organizing the community for health promotion:

- The burden of chronic or environmentally induced disease cuts across most sectors of the community. The causes of these diseases are complex and rooted for the most part in cultural phenomena.
- Community approaches affect the social milieu of individuals and are oriented towards changing the norms, values and policies surrounding behaviour.
- Community approaches are better integrated into the total community, since interventions are built into existing community structures.
- Community approaches better ensure longevity of change because the social context of behavior proscribes certain activities and local ownership generates continuing responsibility.
- Community approaches are generally more comprehensive and ensure better allocation and coordination of scarce health resources.
- Community approaches reflect shared responsibility for health and move away from individual strategies only or victim blaming. Community approaches actually augment individuals' capacity for change.

The usual six stages of community organization described by Rothman (1970) and Bracht (1990) include community analysis, design, initiation, implementation, maintenance and consolidation, and dissemination and reassessment.

Status

Success in organizing communities was a hallmark of the community-based CVD health promotion programmes of the 1970s and 1980s. This was realized through receptive communities, stable institutions, and strong leaders who understood their communities. But formal community analysis at the outset, plus innovative programme planning, are thought to have contributed to the success of programmes in varied situations such as rural Eastern Finland (Puska *et al.* 1981), urban industrial Rhode Island (Carleton *et al.* 1987), upper middle-class suburbia in Northern California (Farquhar 1990), and solid middle-class communities of the upper Midwest (Blackburn *et al.* 1984). It was possible to involve community leaders in active planning, operation, and maintenance. A central assumption was that programmes should belong to the community, first in a partnership and finally in 'ownership', direction, maintenance, and funding by the community.

Community environmental programmes and the role of industry

A cardinal principle of public health, which probably also applies to the promotion of community health behaviour change, is the need to maximize environmental influences and minimize individual decision-making and the need for personal commitment. To the extent that an individual's health action is rendered easier, or even automatic, its likelihood of being effective is greater. For example, it seems probable that reduction in saturated fatty acid intake in the population is more likely to be affected by a gradual change in the fat composition of foods commonly purchased than by customers making conscious decisions to select low fat products. Wherever possible, policy, economic incentives, and, on occasion, regulations can be used to create environments that encourage the availability and use of more healthy products.

The MHHP was particularly active in devising such environmental strategies, while local commercial firms were central to providing healthier choices. More than half the adult community participated. Restaurant programmes were particularly effective in reaching working men and grocery programmes in reaching home-makers (Mullis *et al.* 1987). The voluntary institution of smoke-free work sites organized by industry had a major influence on smoking during working hours. Industry-sponsored physical activity competitions and smoking cessation contests were also an integral part of long-term community incorporation of public health strategies. These environmental change aspects of a community-based campaign are among the more attractive and promising for the future, and are susceptible to appropriate voluntary and regulatory approaches (Bracht 1990). In the MHHP community-based organizations, councils and task forces were ultimately the essential mechanisms by which programme ownership was transferred early on, and by which the health messages and programmes were maintained and incorporated in educated communities.

Government and policy interventions in community-based programmes: background, status, and role

Clearly, individual responsibility for personal health and the health of one's family is an essential element of disease prevention in the community. However, a strategy based solely on individual responsibility fails to recognize the powerful social impediments or encouragements to individual success. The first impediment is inadequate knowledge. Knowledge about CVD risk and risky behaviour, and about the potential for prevention and the importance of individual and preventive strategies, is largely the province of the highly educated reading public. Large segments of the community remain unaware; access to information and to preventive care is unevenly distributed. Incentives are also lacking for preventive medical practice. In the USA medical care is geared towards 'high tech' procedures of diagnosis and treatment rather than careful listening and counselling. Only a relatively small proportion of the population receives any form of primary preventive care, even if it purportedly has access to it. Moreover, the concept of individual responsibility for health does not adequately take into account that, motivation aside, highly informed interest, skills, and leisure are required to select, for example, food products that, when consumed regularly, are more and less healthy. Individual responsibility, even when citizens are informed, operates with difficulty in the presence of an environment that encourages unhealthy eating, smoking, drinking, and physical activity habits. Though the tide is now turning, affluent industrial cultures have long promoted excesses of consumption.

In a free society a natural 'tension' exists between an individual's rights and individual and group responsibility. People's tendencies to 'kill themselves', in whatever fashion, must be taken account of within democratically developed social policy and health legislation, while better ways are sought to counter traditions of 'rugged individualism' on health matters. Rose's prevention paradox implies that health promotion penalizes the many for the benefit of the few and emphasizes the individual cost of the population prevention strategy (Rose 1981, 1985). But social responsibility for public health entails greater information, education, and motivation of citizens, as well as more available choices; it embraces influences that lie largely outside the control of individuals (e.g. the composition of food products and the safety of the environment). Access to information and to alternatives, as well as to preventive services, needs to be assured by society. Nevertheless, in most democratic free-enterprise systems, the strategy of primary prevention and health promotion remains mainly educational and motivational or medically based rather than policy based. It includes relatively few efforts by the community to create environments more conducive to healthy behaviour.

Classically, public health policies have tended to passive restraints as the model for health change. For example, governments require automobile manufacturers to include air bags and automatic seat belts in new cars rather than requiring that drivers and passengers wear seat belts. In this approach, human fallibility is taken into account while policy-makers seek to make the world 'impervious to folly'. The educational approach, in contrast, seeks a public motivated to make health-promoting changes. While the education strategy is morally consistent and necessary for community programmes, it may be rendered more effective by a policy and public health approach that uses unobtrusive safety and health measures (Jeffery *et al.* 1990).

Policy interventions have been much less emphasized at the community level than at the national level of health promotion strategy. In the first-generation community intervention programmes, for example, it was assumed at the outset that the education–motivational approach was the more appropriate and ethical strategy. We believed that if better-informed communities eventually wanted to develop regulatory approaches this would be a desirable side-effect of our programmes. However, we avoided initiating regulatory strategies through policy interventions because of their apparent conflict with the assumptions of the educational model. Current experience, and a new 'public will', now suggest that policy interventions are, in fact, highly appropriate to community-based prevention strategies and might well be mounted in parallel with educational–motivational campaigns. Their goals and effects are complementary.

For the moment, however, even the newer community-based life-style strategies continue to assign much of the burden of change to the individual. A shift of focus to reducing, by policy change, many widespread practices that are life-threatening, while enhancing life-supportive practices, should redirect the currently misplaced emphasis on achieving 'responsible' individual behaviour and its purported difficulty. For example, local communities may more appropriately be considered to have a 'youth tobacco access problem', approachable in part by regulation, than a 'youth smoking problem', approachable mainly by education. Policy interventions may also be designed to improve access to benefits, or to make preventive practice more economical, as well as to encourage the development of more healthy products by industry. They may be a partial answer to another major paradox: while unhealthy personal behaviour is medically discouraged for individuals, the whole of society legalizes, tolerates, and even encourages the same practices in the population.

The future of policy interventions

Policy options that are currently unrealized are available for influencing health behaviour at a community level. For tobacco and alcohol use alone they are numerous (Forster *et al.* 1990). By exercising these options, communities can achieve rational decisions made locally under conditions where the local leaders and legislators are relatively strong, while industrial, advertising, and lobbying groups are relatively weak. For example, when a community deliberately decides that its children simply should not have free access to tobacco and alcohol, no amount of (irrelevant) calls to 'free-enterprise' or smoke-screens about the fine points of 'legalities' and 'individual rights' can successfully obfuscate the common logic. There is much evidence that communities are ripe for action on such issues as tobacco and alcohol access among the young, and drunk driving at any age. Local regulations that effect such access through zoning and control of the numbers of retail outlets, billboard advertising restrictions, and so forth already exist. Beyond these issues there are policy options in many other areas of community health, such as in injury control (for sports and playground equipment), for institutional dining, and for public access to exercise facilities and smoke-free public areas. Community-based health promotion programmes could address all these options more effectively. Though community-based educational–motivational programmes that promote personal behaviour change should go on apace, they might now go on in parallel with these relatively neglected policy interventions at the community level. The whole concept of population risk versus individual risk must also be communicated more widely to help develop a broader constituency for public health (Rose 1985). Better methods are also needed to counter the tradition of 'rugged individualism' in health behaviour, returning rather to traditions that support the common good.

Research needed

Research in policy interventions is needed to define and evaluate links between policy, behaviour, and health outcomes in CVD-related issues and others, including drug use, injury, and cancer-related exposures. Research is needed to develop effective educational methods to reach the new 'target' populations for public policy, i.e. politicians, officials, merchants, and other 'gatekeepers', and to explore the complementary effects, at the community level, of both educational and policy approaches to behaviour change.

CONCLUSIONS

World-wide experience in community-based CVD prevention and health promotion programmes has much to offer future undertakings in public health. Little positive happens in communities, or nationally, in the absence of prevention policy and programmes, when, as affluence rises among previously deprived populations, disease rates also tend to rise. In industrial populations already at high risk, disease rates tend to remain high. But in many Western countries, the recent past has seen a rapid change of social norms and health practices as well as in disease rates. In the USA this is particularly evident in the decreased social acceptability of cigarette smoking. It is also seen in the remarkable advances made in hypertension control. New food products offered by industry and new government policies on production, labelling, and marketing have at long last built health concerns into American agri-economic policy. Moreover, public and private health agencies—local health departments, supported by the Centres for Disease Control, and voluntary associations such as the American Heart Association—are actively carrying out health promotion strategies. Industry is providing self-help programmes for its employees and modifying work environments, and grocery stores and restaurants are offering attractive choices.

In parallel, there is a broader base of informed citizens and more active involvement of health professions and government. A greater professional consensus on primary prevention, along with national and community-based promotional campaigns, are associated with important changes in community behaviour and risk levels, in preventive services, and in the marketing of good health. The process of community health promotion seems to leap ahead when the public begins to demand greater information, healthier products, and more preventive services, to which the medical system, industry, and government tend to respond quickly. This is particularly evident now in the medical care system in the USA, with greater demand for preventive services, with demands for environmental change at work sites, and in new commercial offerings in response to the market clamour for healthy products and information.

Central to future community health change, in the MHHP experience, is the formal organization of communities into health councils and task forces that provide local ownership of health programmes. Campaigns and environmental programmes in grocery stores, restaurants, schools, and work sites are recommended for the wide population exposure they provide. Risk factor screening and education, with systematic follow-up by the medical care system, remain an effective strategy for change where they can be afforded and conducted systematically. For the future, more cost-effective strategies for community interventions are needed, to include particularly needy audiences such as school children, senior citizens, and the culturally and economically disadvantaged. Finally, more cost-effective approaches are required for practical evaluations of community programme effects. These health innovations in communities will also create the need for more and accessible resources: health promotion resource centres, local expert consultation, materials, and training (Farquhar 1990).

Finally, let us consider some of the central lessons for epidemiologists from experience in community-based programmes. The difficulties and costs of risk factor and disease surveillance should be faced squarely, with concentration now on innovative designs to demonstrate links between intervention strategies and audience exposure and behaviour changes. We have demonstrated sufficiently that average population risk factor levels among community samples are less stable from year to year than imagined, and therefore are not the sensitive indicators of time trends or of comparative intervention effects that we anticipated. Greater epidemiological focus on the design of comparative intervention strategies that are free from requirements to demonstrate outcomes such as accelerated trends in risk factors or disease rates would allow greater power to make the more critically needed comparisons, i.e. of programme effectiveness. This focus would also facilitate more practical designs having relatively large numbers of randomized units and relatively small numbers in samples within them, thus enhancing power for detecting programme effect at a given cost. Innovative high and low intensity interventions might stimulate the public health scene to much needed progress in disease prevention and health promotion (Murray *et al.* 1990). Extending new methods to communities relatively untouched by intervention, and where risk is high, should prove particularly effective. Focus on proximal effects is promising because 'contamination' of control groups by social change over time is increasingly a major consideration. The recent experience in quasi-experimental design, using small numbers of non-randomized community units, should teach epidemiologists that we desert the time-tested mode of randomizing large numbers at considerable risk. We, and our expert colleagues in design and sampling, can no longer be confident that results in individual surveys or interventions can be transferred successfully to long-term community strategies, particularly in a rapidly changing society.

However, the complexity of interpreting the recent community study findings should not mitigate our attempts to achieve or detect community programme effects, nor should it reflect on the overall validity of public health strategies of health promotion. Rather, it dictates a return to original assumptions based on multiple 'natural experiments': the world *can* and *does* change; disease risk and disease rates *are* dynamic phenomena. It may be sufficient in future to demonstrate that health programmes achieve substantial new community exposure to positive health influences. But the link still required to be demonstrated is that between the educational programmes themselves, the exposure they achieve, and behavioural change in the population. The subsequent links to risk and disease may be safely assumed, based on well-established evidence. The recent community programme experience should therefore stimulate continued efforts towards a population strategy of prevention and public health promotion. The epidemiologist can contribute much to these efforts through improved designs for analysis of community health programmes. The public health should profit from intelligent commitment of epidemiologists to the task.

ACKNOWLEDGEMENTS

The Minnesota Heart Health Program (MHHP) Research Group has worked for more than a decade on the design, implementation, and evaluation of community-based programmes for the reduction of CVD risk. The conclusions herein are the author's alone, but the Research Group is responsible for the effort itself as well as for many advances in the population strategy of disease prevention and in health promotion for communities. The MHHP is fully supported by Grant R01-HL 25523 of the National Heart, Lung, and Blood Institute, US Public Health Service.

512   *Changing community behaviour*

REFERENCES

Bandura, A. (1977). *Social learning theory,* Prentice-Hall, Englewood Cliffs, NJ.
Blackburn, H. (1983). Research and demonstration projects in community cardiovascular disease prevention. *J. Public Health Policy,* **4,** 398–421.
Blackburn, H., Luepker, R. V., Kline, F. G., Bracht, N., Carlaw, R. W., Jacobs, D. R., *et al.* (1984). The Minnesota Heart Health Program: a research and demonstration project in cardiovascular disease prevention. In *Behavioural health: a handbook of health enhancement and disease prevention* (ed. J. D. Matarazzo), Wiley, New York, pp. 1171–8.
Bracht, N. (ed.) (1990). *Health promotion at the community level,* Sage, Newbury Park, CA.
Carleton, R. A., Lasater, T. M., Assaf, A. R., Lefebvre, R. C., and McKinlay, S. M. (1987). The Pawtucket Heart Health Program: I. An experiment in population-based disease prevention. *RI Med. J.,* **70,** 533–8.
Farquhar, J. (1978). The community-based model of lifestyle intervention trials. *Am. J. Epidemiol.,* **108,** 103–11.
Farquhar, J. W., Flora, J. A., Taylor, C. B., Haskell, W. L., Williams, P. T., Maccoby, N., and Wood, P. D. (1990). Effects of community-wide education on cardiovascular disease risk factors. The Stanford Five-City Project. *J. Am. Med. Assoc.,* **264**(3), 359–65.
Farquhar, J. W., Maccoby, N., and Wood, P. D. (1985). Education and communications studies. In *Oxford textbook of public health*, Vol. 3 (eds W. W. Holland, R. W. Detels, and G. Know), Oxford University Press, pp. 207–21.
Finnegan, J. R., Murray, D. M., Kurth, C., and McCarthy, P. (1989). Measuring and tracking education program implementation: the Minnesota Heart Health Program experience. *Health Educ. Q.,* **16,** 77–90.
Flora, J. A., Maccoby, N., and Farquhar, J. W. (1989). Communication campaigns to prevent cardiovascular disease: the Stanford Community Study. In *Public communication campaigns* (eds R. E. Rice and C. K. Atkin) (2nd edn), Sage, Newbury Park, CA.
Forster, J. L., Hourigan, M., and Weigum, J. (1990). The movement to resist children's access to tobacco in Minnesota. In *Proceedings of the Surgeon General's Inter-Agency Committee on Smoking and Health*, US Government Printing Office, Washington, DC.
Green, L. W. (1975). Diffusion and adoption of innovations related to cardiovascular risk behaviours in the public. In *Applying behavioural science to cardiovascular risk* (eds A. J. Enelaw and J. B. Henderson), American Heart Association, New York.
Hovland, C. I., Janis, I. L., and Kelley, N. H. (1953). *Communication and persuasion*, Yale University Press.
Jacobs, D. R., Luepker, R. V., Mittelmark, M. B., Folsom, A. R., Pirie, P. L., Mascioli, S. R., *et al.* (1986). Community-wide prevention strategies: evaluation design of the Minnesota Heart Health Program. *J. Chron. Dis.,* **39,** 775–88.
Jeffery, R. W., Forster, J. L., Schmidt, T. L., McBride, C. M., Rooney, B. L., and Pirie, P. L. (1990). Community attitudes towards public policies to control alcohol, tobacco and high fat food consumption. *Am. J. Prev. Med.,* **6,** 12–19.

Kottke, T. E., Blackburn, H., Brekke, M. L., and Solberg, L. I. (1987). The systematic practice of preventive cardiology. *Am. J. Cardiol.,* **59**(6), 690–4.

Luepker, R. V. and Rastam, L. (1990). Involving community health professionals and systems. In *Health promotion at the community level* (ed. N. Bracht), Sage, Newbury Park, CA.

Maccoby, N., Farquhar, J. W., Wood, P., and Alexander, J. (1977). Reducing the risk of cardiovascular disease effects of a community-based campaign on knowledge and behaviour. *J. Community Health,* **3**, 100–14.

McGuire, W. J. (1973). Persuasion, resistance and attitude change. In *Handbook of Communication* (eds I. DeSola and W. Schramm), Rand McNally, Chicago, IL.

Mittelmark, M. B., Luepker, R. V., Jacobs, D. R., Bracht, N. F., Carlaw, R. W., Crow, R. S., *et al.* (1986). Community-wide prevention of cardiovascular disease: education strategies of the Minnesota Heart Health Program. *Prev. Med.,* **15**, 1–17.

Mullis, R. M., Hunt, M. K., Foster, M., Hachfeld, L., Lansing, D., Snyder, P., *et al.* (1987). Environment support of healthful food behaviour: the Shop Smart For Your Heart grocery program. *J. Nutr. Educ.,* **19**, 225–8.

Murray, D. M., Luepker, R. V., Pirie, P. L., Grimm, R. H., Bloom, E., Davis, M., *et al.* (1986). Systematic risk factor screening and education: a community-wide approach to prevention of coronary heart disease. *Prev. Med.,* **15**, 661–72.

Murray, D. M., Kurth, C., Mullis, R. M., and Jeffery, R. W. (1990). Cholesterol reduction through low intensity interventions: results from the Minnesota Heart Health Program. *Prev. Med.,* **19**, 181–9.

NCEP (National Cholesterol Education Program) (1990). *Report of the Expert Panel on Population Strategies for Blood Cholesterol Reduction,* Publ. 90–3046, National Institutes of Health, Bethesda, MD.

Perry, C. L., Klepp, K. I., and Sillers, C. (1989*a*). Community-wide strategies for cardiovascular health: the Minnesota Heart Health Program youth program. *Health Educ. Res.,* **4**, 87–101.

Perry, C. L., Luepker, R. V., Murray, D. M., Hearn, M. D., Halper, A., Dudovitz, B., *et al.* (1989*b*). Parent involvement with children's health promotion: a one year follow-up of the Minnesota Home Team. *Health Educ. Q.,* **16**, 171–80.

Perry, C. L., Stone, E. J., Parcel, G. S., Ellison, R. C., Nader, P. R., Webber, L. S., *et al.* (1981). School-based cardiovascular health promotion: the child and adolescent trial for cardiovascular health (CATCH). *J. School Health,* **60**(8), 406–13.

Puska, P., Tuomilehto, J., Salonen, J., Nissinen, A., Virtamo, J., Björkqvist, S., *et al.* (1981). *Community control of cardiovascular diseases: the North Karelia Project,* WHO, Copenhagen.

Puska, P., Vartiainen, E., Pallonen, U., Salonen, J. T., Poyhia, P., Kosekela, K., *et al.* (1982). The North Karelia Youth Project: evaluation of two years of intervention on health behaviour and CVD risk factors among 13–15 year old children. *Prev. Med.,* **11**, 550–70.

Rose, G. (1981). Strategy of prevention. Lessons from cardiovascular disease. *Br. Med. J.,* **1**, 1847–51.

Rose, G. (1985). Sick individuals and sick populations. *Int. J. Epidemiol.,* **14**, 32–8.

Rothman, J. (1970). Three models of community organization practice. In *Strategies of community organization: a book of readings* (eds F. Cox, J. L. Erlich, J. Rothman, and J. E. Tropman), Peacock, Itasca, NJ.

Stone, E. J., Perry, C. L., and Luepker, R. V. (eds) (1989). Synthesis of cardiovascular behavioral research for youth health promotion. *Health Educ. Q.*, **16**(2), 155–68.

Viswanath, K. (1990). *Knowledge gap effects in a cardiovascular disease campaign: a longitudinal study of two community pairs,* Ph.D. Dissertation, University of Minnesota.

WHO (World Health Organization) Expert Committee (1982). *Primary prevention of coronary heart disease,* Tech. Rep. Ser. 678, WHO, Geneva.

WHO (World Health Organization) Expert Committee (1985). *Community prevention and control of cardiovascular diseases,* Tech. Rep. Ser. 732, WHO, Geneva.

35

Role of organized public health in cardiovascular disease prevention

R. D. Remington

Just what is public health? Surely that question is too basic, even trivial, to appear in a scholarly work devoted to improving the public health? Unfortunately, at least in the USA in the late twentieth century and probably in most of the world, the question is far from trivial. Moreover, the world finds itself urgently in need of an answer based on a working and workable consensus. In fact, the answer varies from discipline to discipline, from country to country, from time to time. To many respondents, public health consists of the assurance of a safe water supply accompanied by appropriate disposal of sewage and rubbish. To others, public health is best represented by the visiting nurse who attends a coronary heart disease (CHD) patient newly discharged from hospital. To still others, public health constitutes an enterprise charged with picking up the pieces left by the rest of the health care delivery system—pieces that represent those disenfranchised by the system, those for whom the system's rationing rules limit access, those in rural areas, or those unable to pay for services. To still others, public health constitutes an umbrella of concepts within which the health care system itself resides. In this latter view, public health includes medicine, dentistry, nursing, and the other health professions. It includes health aspects of the environment as well as the issues of cost, quality, and access to personal health services.

With this range of views, some commentators have suggested that public health is an inappropriate term. To date, however, no truly better alternative has caught hold, and we shall use the term here, while attempting to define it in a manner useful to the issues of cardiovascular disease epidemiology, prevention, and control under discussion in this volume.

The Institute of Medicine of the National Academy of Sciences of the USA recently released a report describing the findings and recommendations of a 2 year study of the future of public health (Remington *et al.* 1988). While the charge to the committee (chaired by the present author) was limited to the public health system of the USA, the findings and recommendations have substantially wider applicability. In the course of the investigation, committee members, who represented a range of professional backgrounds, solicited and received a great deal of information in written and oral form. Four public hearings were held—in Las Vegas, Boston, New Orleans, and Chicago. Intensive week-long site visits were made in the states of New Jersey, West Virginia, Mississippi, California, Washington, and South Dakota. Structured interviews were conducted with some 350 individuals.

As implied earlier, a wide variety of definitions of public health were provided by respondents. One of the committee's primary findings was that at present the public health system of the USA is in disarray, in part because of the lack of common understanding concerning the mission, functions, and definition of public health.

The committee proposed a new definition: 'Public health consists of all those things we as a society do collectively to assure the conditions in which people can be healthy'. This definition seems simple, but the simplicity is more apparent than real. In asserting that public health embraces 'all those things' we do collectively, the definition encompasses the health service delivery system, the environmental health system, sanitary and health regulations and statutes, the protection of food and water supplies, and by inference the systems of education and communication in so far as those systems relate to health. Considering the collective actions of society, we pass laws, we promulgate regulations, we develop standards, we systematically collect information on health status, we license practitioners, we control disease by the development of public programmes, and we evolve health-related policy. The notion that public health is involved in assuring 'the conditions in which people can be healthy' is similarly broad. Those conditions include access to personal health services at reasonable costs and of adequate quality, the ability to develop the skills needed to prevent disease and arrange life-styles consistent with such prevention, and the freedom from environmental hazards to health. The definition is much closer to the final broad alternative provided in the first paragraph of this chapter than to the other possible definitions. But the committee was convinced that no narrower definition is adequate to meet the challenges of a rapidly changing health environment—challenges including the re-establishment of control of infectious diseases such as measles formerly thought to be under adequate control at least in developed countries, provision of an adequately informed citizenry who can take advantage of continuously improving information concerning, for example, cardiovascular risk factors, and maintenance of a reasonable level of vigilance over environmental health risks.

The findings of cardiovascular epidemiology are, if they are to have wide community impact, susceptible to testing at the community level in a wide variety of situations. Such testing goes beyond the usual clinical trial with its narrow purpose and highly restrictive methodology. In an attempt to obtain a clear answer to a sharply defined question, that methodology often leads to the exclusion of many individuals (Remington 1989). Yet in the context of public health, none, or almost none, of these individuals can be excluded. All are part of their community, all contribute to the statistics on morbidity and mortality, and all will be used to provide a measure of the success of cardiovascular epidemiology as applied to the improvement of the health of the public. The realization of this fact probably accounts for the interest over the years in the first generation of observational and cohort studies such as those conducted in Framingham, Tecumseh, and other communities, and summarized by the Pooling Project Cooperative Group (1978). It probably accounts for the development of community-based trials like the Hypertension Detection and Follow-up Program (HDFP 1979*a*, *b*), and certainly accounts for the community-based intervention programmes like those in California (Farquhar *et al*. 1984, 1985), Minnesota (Blackburn *et al*. 1985; Jacobs *et al*. 1986), and Rhode Island (Elder *et al*. 1986; Lefebvre *et al*. 1987).

In summary, as epidemiology passes from aetiological investigations through longitudinal studies to community intervention programmes and evaluative trials of CHD control programmes, it recapitulates the several stages encompassed in this publication. The concern of this chapter is with the far end of that transition—the role of organized public health in applying the fruits of epidemiological investigation to cardiovascular disease prevention in the community. This transition from research to policy formation to application has received too little attention among epidemiologists and, for that matter, among professional public health workers. Yet the transition itself has much to do with the uses of epidemiology in improving community health. Put another way, in the language of the Institute of Medicine report, the substance of public health is considered to be 'organized community efforts aimed at the prevention of disease and promotion of health. (Public health) links many disciplines and rests upon the scientific core of epidemiology' (Remington *et al*. 1988, p. 41).

The Institute of Medicine Committee on the Future of Public Health defined three core functions for all public health agencies. These are assessment, policy development, and assurance. Epidemiology plays a key role in each of these core functions. Nowhere is that role more evident than in the first function, assessment.

Assessment was defined as follows:

Every public health agency (should) regularly and systematically collect, assemble, analyze, and make available information on the health of the community, including statistics on health status, community health needs, and epidemiologic and other studies of health problems. . . . This basic function of public health cannot be delegated. (Remington *et al*. 1988, p. 141)

The skills and experience of epidemiologists are fundamental to the assessment function, and in performing this function interdisciplinary relationships with biostatistics, data processing, and demography will often be necessary. In the case of cardiovascular disease prevention, the successful application of a public health programme will require knowledge of the incidence and prevalence of disease in the community, the variability of incidence rates among different sectors of the population, and time trends in those rates. Coverage by health services, for example the proportion of hypertensives in the community detected, treated, and controlled, will be important information which should be assessed in the population to which the public health control programme is to be applied.

The second core function of all public health agencies is policy development.

Every public health agency (should) exercise its responsibility to serve the public interest in the development of comprehensive public health policies by promoting use of the scientific knowledge base in decision-making about public health and by leading and developing public health policy. Agencies must take a strategic approach, developed on the basis of a positive appreciation for the democratic political process. (Remington *et al.* 1988, p. 141)

In a democratic society, policy development is a shared responsibility. Epidemiologists and other public health professionals want policy to be based to the maximum possible extent on current scientific information, and indeed that is often the case. In contrast, time and again the Institute of Medicine committee learned of instances in which public concerns and the specific interests of elected or appointed officials took precedence over such information. In fact, one of the most important barriers to forming and implementing effective public health policy in the USA today is the gulf that separates the scientific disciplines and professions related to public health from public policy specialists represented by elected and appointed officials. The committee frequently found that scientists were unwilling to accept the realities of community interests and needs in tempering their policy conclusions, while politicians and government officials were often ill equipped or unwilling to process scientific information and to act upon that information. In this case, the committee believed that there was a need for improved dialogue across the gulf separating these two areas and an increased level of appreciation of each side for the background, attitudes, and constraints of the other.

The third core function is assurance.

Public health agencies (should) assure their constituents that services necessary to achieve agreed upon goals are provided, either by encouraging actions by other entities (private or public sector), by requiring such action through regulation, or by providing services directly. (Remington *et al.* 1988, p. 142)

The assurance function is stated with substantial generality in order that it may apply to a variety of health service delivery systems. Whether a jurisdiction is part of a national or regional health insurance scheme, whether there is a national health service providing direct medical care services, or whether there is a patchwork system like that in the USA, Mexico, and many other countries, the assurance function must be provided by the public health apparatus. In the USA, for example, most medical care is delivered by the private sector, with a variety of special services such as those for the medically indigent, the elderly, mothers and children, veterans of military service, and other special groups. As is well known, this system leaves millions of Americans without even minimally adequate access to medical care.

Indeed, one of the largest challenges to organized public health in the USA today is the default position in which public health agencies are placed as providers of last resort. In fulfilling the assurance function, if no one else provides services, many public health agencies feel they must do so. This makes it difficult for those agencies to provide the appropriate oversight role that a more rational system entails. Further, the attention of these agencies is so directed towards the direct provision of one-to-one medical care that necessary community-level preventive and environmental health services are either de-emphasized or virtually ignored. This is sometimes exacerbated by the fact that the agency receives financial reimbursement for direct medical care but not for the latter services. However, even in jurisdictions with better access and coverage, the public health agency has often not attempted systematically to ensure the delivery of preventive and environmental health services. Ultimately, there can be no substitute for a public health agency that plays an important role in establishing health policy and then ensures that this policy is fulfilled. Provision of the assurance function then feeds back into the assessment function information concerning the delivery and receipt of specific services, preventive or therapeutic, for the population.

Another important recommendation by the Institute of Medicine committee was as follows:

The committee recommends that each public health agency involve key policy makers and the general public in determining a set of high-priority personal and communitywide health services that governments will guarantee to every member of the community. This guarantee should include subsidization or direct provision of high-priority personal health services for those unable to afford them. (Remington *et al.* 1988, p. 142)

At the time of writing (1991), out of the 50 states comprising the USA, exactly one (Michigan) is committed to providing exactly one high priority service (pre-natal care).

Although this recommendation is obviously cast in the American context, its message applies equally to other health service systems. Health policy must establish the necessary level, for example, of preventive services in the field of cardiovascular disease, and must then assess the coverage and ensure that those services are both delivered *and received*.

It has not been many years since the one-half of one-half of one-half rule characterized community high blood pressure control. This rule stated that half the hypertensives in a community were detected, of those detected half were treated, and of those treated half had their blood pressure controlled to within the normal range. This produced an overall level of high blood pressure control of approximately one in eight or 10–15 per cent of the population. These figures for hypertension control were apparently quite robust across different types of health service delivery systems. With, among other developments, the advent of the US National High Blood Pressure Education Program sponsored by the National Heart, Lung, and Blood Institute, this figure has been quadrupled, and now over half the hypertensives in the USA are detected, treated, and controlled.

If control of high blood pressure is one of the essential health services to be offered by organized public health, and most cardiovascular epidemiologists would probably believe it should be, then clearly we have much more to accomplish in virtually all nations and districts. Nothing short of a systematic approach involving assessment, policy development, and assurance seems likely to complete that task.

The public health agency of the future must accept an increased level of responsibility for the health of the population within its jurisdiction. Public health, as it meets the criteria of the Institute of Medicine report, guarantees that someone is 'watching the store', that someone is concerned for the health of all the people, that someone is working actively to improve the vital statistics that constitute the record of public health progress or lack thereof. Cardiovascular epidemiology has a major stake in this function. By providing the tools necessary for the assessment and assurance functions, and by constituting a source of unimpeachable data of high quality, epidemiology can, in its various applications and manifestations, assume a much more fundamental role in the future than it has been awarded in the past.

Taking another perspective on cardiovascular disease control in the community, there are three distinct intervention modalities that can be brought to bear. The first of these is the health services modality in which cases are diagnosed and treated. This is the classical medical care or health services approach, and in the USA approximately 97 per cent of all health expenditures are currently being allocated to this modality, with only 3 per cent remaining for public health and preventive measures. While other countries may have a more favourable balance of resource allocations to prevention, it seems doubtful that any nation can point with pride to its current posture. Medical care remains in the dominant position, and the health services modality will remain prominent relative to prevention for many more years.

Yet we know from the example of the US National High Blood Pressure Education Program that the availability of safe and effective pharmacological agents for the management of elevated blood pressure was insufficient to make a major impact on the one-half of one-half of one-half rule cited earlier. Something more was needed. In this case, the critically important component was improved communication and education. A four-fold increase in the percentage of hypertensives controlled resulted, in major part, from the development of improved education and communication. Thus health behaviour and health communication constitute the second important modality in controlling cardiovascular disease at the community level.

The third intervention modality is alteration of the environment to enhance health. The availability of low salt and low fat foods, the production and distribution of milk with a reduced butter fat content, the availability of improved occupational health services, the control and reduction of heavy metals in the atmosphere, water, and other sources of exposure, and the control of environmental tobacco smoke all play some role in reducing the burden of cardiovascular disease on the population.

Opinions may differ concerning the relative importance of these three intervention strategies, but one thing is clear. They involve entirely different skills and techniques, and unfortunately the last two areas, health behaviour and environmental health, are most often given short shrift in the preparation of physicians and other health professionals. In fact, too often they are given little recognition in the personnel rosters of public health agencies as well. Only in recent years has there been a rebirth of health education directed towards translating the findings of cardiovascular epidemiology into, for example, risk factor abatement in the general population. With the development of new tools, and here epidemiology's importance is well documented, a rebirth of educational, informational, and communications methodology has been seen in many countries and regions.

Other pieces of the heart disease control puzzle are falling into place. Important new and continuing investigations of the role of risk factors in early childhood, such as investigations in Muscatine (Schrott *et al.* 1979; Burns *et al.* 1989; Lauer and Clarke 1990) and Bogalusa (Srinivasan *et al.* 1986) have played a role in the American scene. Furthermore, investigations such as the Systolic Hypertension in the Elderly Program (SHEP 1988, 1991), now nearing conclusion, are providing insights at the other end of the life-cycle.

But many questions remain to be answered. For example, what is the role of blood pressure reduction in reducing the incidence of CHD? To what extent can the progress of evolution toward increased blood pressure be slowed by hygienic and preventive methods? What is the exact role of diet and its various constituents? How different in ultimate outcome are various antihypertensive agents affecting the blood pressure through vastly different modes of action?

Although hypertension has been selected as an example in this discussion, the situation concerning the interaction between epidemiology, disease control, and public health action for other cardiovascular conditions seems similar. Indeed, the roles of health services, health behaviour, and environmental health on the one hand and of assessment, policy development, and assurance on the other seem important in disease control across infectious and chronic diseases, across diseases of childhood and the elderly, and across racial, ethnic, cultural, and national groups.

In fact, public health, like medicine, may be the victim, to a degree, of its own intellectual success. That is, the accumulation of knowledge has inevitably and appropriately led to specialization. The problem is that medical specialization, public health specialization, and specialization of community programmes have taken very different directions, making communication leading to the development of effective policy more difficult. Even the separation of public health from other critical social programmes such as education and income maintenance has generated difficulties. Epidemiologists and community interventionists trying to assemble the risk factor pieces into a coherent picture of heart disease have too seldom taken literacy and poverty into account. Perhaps this is because these areas are too far removed from biology or medicine, or because public policy related to education and income maintenance was formed and implemented in areas of the bureaucracy distant from public health. Or perhaps, it was simply the working of an appropriate degree of modesty in delving into areas apparently far removed from one's own education or experience. Yet it has been shown repeatedly, for example, that literacy is one of the key determinants of health (Grosse and Auffrey 1989). The implication here seems clear. Public health, if it is to reach its full potential, cannot do so in isolation.

Surgeon General Koop was widely praised and heralded for distributing to every mail address in the USA an attractive and highly informative brochure describing the epidemiology, prevention, and control of human immunodeficiency virus (HIV) infection and AIDS. Yet, far too many Americans were unable to take advantage of this important information for a very simple reason—they could not read it. While percentage estimates of illiteracy in the adult population of the USA vary, commentators seem to agree that the number is shockingly high and has probably been increasing. If public health is to realize its full potential for maintaining the health of the community and for freeing people from the burdens of cardiovascular and other diseases, a new alliance between public health and education must be forged.

In many countries—Western, Eastern, First, Second, and Third World—health status relates closely to income and poverty. As was well known to public health pioneers, the conditions of life including income, housing, education and their concomitants, sanitation, nutrition, and access to health care are among the most important determinants of the health status of populations.

The message for policy-makers is clear. Not only must there be improved links between epidemiology and public health, but, even more difficult, there must be improved links between public health and education and income maintenance. This is not to imply a specific organizational structure combining health and welfare services in a single organizational unit. Attempts in that direction in the USA have seldom been successful. There seems to be no answer except for improved communication and a community health ethic that views populations from an epidemiological perspective, that notes the futility of basing all efforts on one-to-one medical care, that notes the absolute necessity of providing information and skills on a one-to-many basis (one information provider or educator providing information to many recipients), and that involves a respect for the impact of the environment (physical, biological, social, economic, and political).

The career of Geoffrey Rose has touched many of the issues outlined here. His important contribution to fundamental epidemiological measurement, to improved medical care, to education, to clinical and intervention trials, to the improvement of health and preventive services in industry, and to a better basis for the establishment of public health policy have been a positive example for this field. It is entirely fitting and proper that these contributions be honoured in the present volume.

REFERENCES

Blackburn, H., Grimm, R. H., Luepker, R. V., and Mittelmark, M. (1985). The primary prevention of high blood pressure: a population approach. *Prev. Med.,* **14**(4), 466–81.

Burns, T. L., Moll, P. P., and Lauer, R. M. (1989). The relation between ponderosity and coronary risk factors in children and their relatives: the Muscatine family study. *Am. J. Epidemiol.,* **129,** 973–87.

Elder, J. P., McGraw, S. A., Abrams, P. B., Ferreira, A., Lasater, T. M., Longpre, H., *et al.* (1986). Organizational and community approaches to community-wide prevention of heart disease: the first two years of the Pawtucket heart health program. *Prev. Med.,* **15**(2), 107–17.

Farquhar, J. W., Fortmann, S. P., Maccoby, N., Wood, P. D., Haskell, W. L., Taylor, C. B., *et al.* (1984). The Stanford Five-city Project: an overview. In *Behavioral health: a handbook of health enhancement and disease prevention* (ed. J. D. Matarazzo), Wiley, New York, pp. 1154–65.

Farquhar, J. W., Fortmann, S. P., Maccoby, N., Haskell, W. L., Williams, P. T.,

Flora, J. A., *et al.* (1985). The Stanford Five-city Project: design and methods. *Am. J. Epidemiol.*, **122**, 323–34.

Grosse, R. N. and Auffrey, C. (1989). Literacy and health status in developing countries. *Annu. Rev. Public Health*, **10**, 281–97.

HDFP (Hypertension Detection and Follow-up Program) Cooperative Group (1979*a*). Five-year findings of the hypertension detection and follow-up program. I. Reduction in mortality of persons with high blood pressure, including mild hypertension. *J. Am. Med. Assoc.*, **242**, 2562–70.

HDFP (Hypertension Detection and Follow-up Program) Cooperative Group (1979*b*). Five-year findings of the hypertension detection and follow-up program. II. Mortality by race, sex and age. *J. Am. Med. Assoc.*, **242**, 2572–7.

Jacobs, D. R., Luepker, R. V., Mittelmark, M. B., Folsom, A. R., Pirie, P. L., Mascioli, S. R., *et al.* (1986). Community-wide prevention strategies: evaluation design of the Minnesota heart health program. *J. Chron. Dis.*, **39**, 775–88.

Lauer, R. M. and Clarke, W. R. (1990). The use of cholesterol measurements in children for the prediction of adult hypercholesterolemia. The Muscatine study. *J. Am. Med. Assoc.*, **264**, 3034–8.

Lefebvre, R. C., Lasater, T. M., Carleton, R. A., *et al.* (1987). Theory and practice of health programming in the community: The Pawtucket heart health program. *Prev. Med.*, **16**, 80–95.

Pooling Project Cooperative Group (1978). Relationship of blood pressure, serum cholesterol, smoking habit, relative weight and ECG abnormalities to incidence of major coronary events: final report of the pooling project. *J. Chron. Dis.*, **31**, 201–306.

Remington, R. D. (1989). Potential impact of exclusion criteria on results of hypertension trials. *Hypertension*, **13** (Suppl.) I66–8.

Remington, R. D., Axelrod, D., Bingham, E., Boyle, J., Breslow, L., Citrin, J. A., *et al.* (1988). *The future of public health*, National Academy Press, Washington, DC.

Schrott, H. G., Clarke, W. R., Wiebe, D. A., Connor, W. E., and Lauer, R. M. (1979). Increased coronary mortality in relatives of hypercholesterolemic school children: the Muscatine family study. *Circulation*, **59**, 320–6.

SHEP (Systolic Hypertension in the Elderly Program) Cooperative Research Group (1988). Rationale and design of a randomized clinical trial on prevention of stroke in isolated systolic hypertension. *J. Clin. Epidemiol.*, **41**, 1197–208.

SHEP (Systolic Hypertension in the Elderly Program) (1991). Baseline characteristics of the randomized SHEP participants (eds H. Black, J. Curb, S. Pressel, J. Probstfield, and J. Stamler, for the National Cooperative SHEP Research Group). *Hypertension*, **17**(3).

Srinivasan, S. R., Freedman, D. S., Sharma, C., Webber, L. S., and Berenson, G. S. (1986). Serum apolipoproteins A-I and B in 2,854 children in a biracial community: Bogalusa heart study. *Pediatrics*, **78**, 189–200.

36

National strategies for dietary change

W. P. T. James and A. Ralph

Any discussion of national strategies for dietary change in the 1990s has to cope with philosophical and political perspectives on the prime role of government in encouraging changes in individual behaviour. In the UK and North America there is a substantial body of opinion which claims that behavioural patterns are a matter for individual choice and that the provision of information is the only role of government. During the 1980s the concept of a free market with dominant consumers making their own selection of commodities and life-styles became a major theme of the governing political parties in many countries and, in the UK, of such consumer organizations as the National Consumer Council and the Consumers' Association.

INDIVIDUAL FREEDOM VERSUS SOCIAL ENGINEERING

The desirability of informed choice alone dominating individual action cannot be sustained in any detailed discussion (James 1988). Even governments which aspire to minimum interference still impose limitations on behaviour to protect the rest of society. The drive for smoke-free public areas is justified on the grounds of the risk to passive smokers. The testing of hospital patients for human immunodeficiency virus (HIV) infections can be construed as a protective measure for hospital staff. Random breath-testing is further evidence of a societal demand to restrict individual liberties on the grounds of a recognized risk to others. Governments go further, however: for example, the wearing of seat-belts is becoming compulsory in the UK for rear-seated passengers, presumably because leaving the decision to the informed choice of passengers is insufficient to justify the cost to society of the injured. National policies are inevitably inconsistent as they evolve: the provision of alcohol in motorway restaurants and cafés is banned, but alcohol is acceptable in roadside public houses, presumably because patrons could walk there. Society imposes further restrictions to protect children or those unable to make informed choices and goes further with legislative restrictions reflecting societal concerns. Examples include limitations on the sale of tobacco and its heavy taxation, and new measures to promote higher environmental standards, for example in farm welfare and other aspects of agriculture. This then implies that society has a responsibility in a free-market consumer-dominated system for setting certain minimum standards which reflect the accepted cultural perceptions of the day.

The acquisition of behavioural habits in childhood depends on society's conditioning of the child. Yet children and young adults continue to be influenced by the promotional skills of numerous vested interests, for example in advertising where marketing agencies pay role models in public life to sell their wares. But some restrictions are imposed, for example on pornographic films, because the balance of influence on government favours those concerned with the public good. Most free-market thinkers come to consider the harsh taxation of cigarettes and perhaps alcohol as acceptable. Yet some individuals would baulk at the idea of selective food subsidies, classifying them as unacceptable social engineering. What is usually forgotten, however, by those who reject social engineering as a national strategy for inducing dietary change is that there are major structural, institutional, and financial pressures already in place which affect the nutritional quality and price of foods and people's perceptions of that food. The public is continually influenced by clear and covert pressures, few of which are recognized as operating against informed choice by the consumer. Those who advocate national strategies for inducing dietary change and improving public health must first set out for consumerists and free-marketeers the evidence of pressures which inhibit a truly 'informed' choice. National strategies are often required simply to modify the current national policies and subsidy systems which favour the consumption of inappropriate foods.

HOW DOES A NUTRITION POLICY DIFFER FROM A FOOD POLICY?

In 1976 the Pan American Health Organization (PAHO) noted that a nutrition policy is established for health reasons and involves many sectors of society (PAHO 1976). However, a food policy may be formulated on entirely different grounds, for example the current German and French desire to maintain small farmers in rural communities. Economic considerations are usually the priority. Thus cash-cropping has been encouraged, in the developing world not only to improve the food security of the rural poor, but also to generate foreign exchange so that governments can import commodities such as oil.

A recent analysis of food policies in the Third World (WHO 1990) shows that almost none incorporates a health priority. The unusual feature of UK and European food policies is that they include an implied health component based on the idea of food sufficiency. This implicit acceptance of a moral basis for current policies needs to be recognized if farmers, civil servants, and food manufacturers are to be understood when they react emotionally to criticism of their policies which they consider are not simply economic but incorporate a national priority to avoid starvation and maintain the health of the people.

PAHO's concern for a nutrition policy was probably based on a wish to combat infantile malnutrition in Central and South America. When nutritional problems in the Third World are being considered, it seems totally justifiable to control the allocation of resources to specific sectors and to integrate different ministry activities, for example in health, education, agriculture, and trade, to establish a coherent food policy which has a health component. The underlying health assumption is that the provision of enough food for everybody is fundamental. So important is this issue that historians have cited population pressures in relation to food supplies as one of the principal triggers to national expansion and major wars.

The present UK and European agricultural and food policies were originally based on similar concerns but now impose huge financial and organizational barriers to implementing a modern health-based nutrition and food policy. Some of these barriers reflect current financial obstacles; others reflect the consequences of previous financial manipulation of the food chain.

To understand why the UK and most other countries have this problem, we need to recognize the evolution of nutritional ideas during this century, and the resulting discordance between modern concepts of diet-related disease and current food policies. In effect there have been three revolutions since the turn of the century: the discovery of vitamins and the conquering of deficiency diseases, the development of new technologies in food production and food processing, and the recognition of the growing epidemic of chronic diet-related diseases. This evolutionary process has been described elsewhere (James and Ralph 1991). The World Health Organization (WHO) has recently produced an analysis of an integrated approach to all the major diet-related diseases of public health significance, relevant to both developing and developed countries (WHO 1990). These latest nutritional goals (Table 36.1) include an additional dietary goal relating to vegetable and fruit consumption to take account of new evidence on the potential protective value of these foods. This shift reflects recent research, some of which has been summarized elsewhere (US Surgeon General 1988; NRC 1989).

RESOLVING THE CONFLICT IN HEALTH AND AGRICULTURAL PRIORITIES

We are now in a position where the public health priorities are clear, but where the food policies of the government and of the farming and food

Table 36.1 Population nutrient goals

	Limits for population average intakes	
	Lower	Upper
Total energy[a]		
Total fat (% total energy)	15	30[b]
Saturated fatty acids (% total energy)	0	10
Polyunsaturated fatty acids (% total energy)	3	7
Dietary cholesterol (mg/day)	0	300
Total carbohydrate (% total energy)	55	75
Complex carbohydrate[c]	50	70
Dietary fibre[d]		
As NSP	16	24
As total dietary fibre	27	40
Free sugars[e]	0	10
Protein (% total energy)	10	15
Salt (g/day)	—[f]	6

[a] Energy intake needs to be sufficient to allow for normal childhood growth, for the needs of pregnancy and lactation, and for work and desirable physical activities, and to maintain appropriate body reserves of energy in children and adults. Adult populations on average should have a body mass index (BMI) of 20–22 (BMI = body mass in kg/(height in metres)^2).
[b] An interim goal for nations with high fat intakes; further benefits would be expected by reducing fat intake towards 15 per cent of total energy.
[c] A daily minimum intake of 400 g of vegetables and fruits, including at least 30 g of pulses, nuts, and seeds, should contribute to this component.
[d] Dietary fibre includes the non-starch polysaccharides (NSPs), the goals for which are based on NSPs obtained from mixed food sources. Since the definition and measurement of dietary fibre remain uncertain, the goals for total dietary fibre have been estimated for the NSP values.
[e] These sugars include monosaccharides, disaccharides, and other short-chain sugars produced by refining carbohydrates.
[f] Not defined.
Source: WHO 1990.

industries are geared to completely different goals. So entrenched is food production in the nutritional priorities of the 1950s that the farming community is now confronting the economic consequences of their 'success' in intensification. This success has led to agricultural surpluses, and the introduction of milk quotas and reduced production subsidies to try to cope with them. The growing demands on the farmer and the food producer for a healthier diet are only now being recognized as not simply a marketing opportunity for developing fat-reduced spreads.

However, no systematic analysis has yet been made of what would constitute a 'structural readjustment' for the Western World. In the Third World an analogous process of structural adjustment is underway with a reduction in food subsidies and the freeing of import–export markets. This is prejudicing the purchasing power and the availability of food to the poor in rapidly growing urban communities. Food riots and incipient revolution have followed, but the pressure persists to make food production and distribution more responsive to the market-place. The economic priorities established by the World Bank and the International Monetary Fund (IMF) in Asia, the Americas, and Africa are now being applied to Eastern Europe. Thus economic issues and the processes of structural adjustment dominate world agriculture.

A preliminary analysis of the potential conflict between health and economic priorities was included in the biennial Food and Agriculture (FAO) Regional Conference for European Ministers of Agriculture held in Venice in April 1990 (FAO 1990). This analysis was the first European FAO paper on nutritional issues in relation to agricultural policy for several decades and highlighted the need to reorganize production practices in the light of a deterioration in public health in Eastern Europe, the erosion of the health benefits of Mediterranean diets, and the modest improvements in cardiovascular morbidity and mortality in Northern Europe. All representatives (except the British) welcomed a re-examination of the priorities in agricultural policy to take account of the 'new' health needs of European populations. The UK delegation opposed this view on the grounds that the link between diet and conditions such as cardiovascular disease and cancers were too uncertain to warrant action. This isolated view is symptomatic of the way in which some government departments in practice ignore accepted official policy—in this case a ministerial acceptance by the Ministry of Agriculture, Fisheries, and Food (MAFF) of the report by the Committee on Medical Aspects of Food Policy (COMA) on preventing cardiovascular disease (COMA 1984). The view also reflects the perceptions of officials who have failed to recognize the new concepts of public health.

The financial burden of the current food policies became a matter of political concern in the early 1980s and can be illustrated by calculating the proportion of total production costs which are ascribable to central government or regional subsidies (Table 36.2). Producing food in the affluent world involves massive food subsidies. A report in *The Economist* (26 January 1991) assesses the European Community (EC) price of a tonne of butter as the equivalent of $4000, but the Russians are being asked to pay only $1000. Because of intensive competition in world trade, North America, the EC, and Australasia compete with each other in export subsidies, thereby depressing world food prices. Third World farmers then have little incentive to compete against these massively subsidized commodities, and so the developing countries fail to develop money-earning cash crops and thereby further reduce their income. Given their huge financial interests it is little wonder that the General Agreement on Tariffs and Trade (GATT) talks are stalled as European governments and the Japanese attempt to protect their own farming communities. Table 36.2 excludes the societal costs and financial burden of agriculture to the

Table 36.2 Producer subsidy equivalents (per cent) by commodity and country, average 1979–81

	USA	Canada	ECᵃ	Australia	Japan	New Zealand	Nordicᵇ	Mediter-ran*ᶜ	Austria	OECDᵈ
Dairy	48.2	66.5	68.8	20.8	83.3	18.0	70.8	68.4	77.9	63.5
Wheat	17.2	17.6	28.1ᵉ	3.4	95.8	-8.2	56.6	10.7	21.1ᶠ	21.5
Coarse grains	13.1	13.3	27.9	2.9	107.1	5.3	54.7	14.8	19.5	19.0
Beef & veal	9.5	13.1	52.7	4.0	54.9	12.5	61.6	17.6	42.9	30.0
Pig meat	6.2	14.5	21.7	2.7	14.0	7.4	23.5	16.7	32.2	16.5
Poultry meat	6.3	25.7	16.4	2.5	20.5	4.7	43.4	19.4	28.4	14.0
Sugar	17.1	12.5	25.0	-5.0	48.4	—	33.4	39.7	39.4	26.6
Rice	5.4	—	13.6	14.4	68.8	—	—	41.9	—	61.0
Sheepmeat	—	—	45.0	3.1	—	18.2	63.5	14.8	—	28.5
Wool	—	—	—	3.9	—	16.3	0.0	26.9	—	9.4
Soybeans	6.9	—	36.2	—	108.1	—	—	21.9	—	9.0
Average, all above commodities	16.0	23.9	42.8	4.7	59.4	15.5	56.1	26.1	42.8	32.1

— not calculated
Different combinations of commodities are included under the headings coarse grains and dairy for different countries.
ᵃ EC-10
ᵇ Finland, Iceland, Norway, Sweden, Switzerland.
ᶜ Portugal, Spain, Turkey.
ᵈ Based on national currencies converted to US dollars at prevailing exchange rates.
ᵉ Common and durum wheat.
ᶠ Wheat and rye.
Source: OECD 1987.

COMECON countries where the forced collectivization of farms has led to inflexible and inefficient farming and food distribution systems which are now being disrupted by the new drive to introduce market economies.

The latest estimate of the financial burden of farming in the EC amounts to approximately 32 billion ECU or, despite 10 years of political effort, nearly 60 per cent of the total EC budget! This EC spending on agriculture is not the total cost because consumers in Europe have to pay higher prices for non-EC foods as a special levy to discourage the entry and sale of imported foods and products. Thus the food production burden is intense, and we cannot object to a shift in price policies in favour of a more healthy diet on the basis of interference with a free market dominated by consumer choice because no such free market exists in the UK and European food chain.

PRACTICAL ASPECTS OF INAPPROPRIATE FOOD POLICIES IN THE UK

A comparison of WHO goals (Table 36.1) with the current UK diet shows that average food consumption in the UK is far from ideal. As Rose (1986) has emphasized, a preference for an intervention high risk strategy rather than a population approach ignores the recognition that the whole of the British population is at risk. Thus, even if we take the intermediate individual goals of 35 per cent fat and 15 per cent saturated fat, as enunciated by the 1984 COMA panel, then 70–80 per cent of all age groups can be shown to exceed this target. Individual small surveys are corroborated by governmental studies on the diets of school children and adults (Darke *et al.* 1980; Bingham *et al.* 1981; Thompson *et al.* 1982; Fehily *et al.* 1984; Nelson 1985; COMA 1989). Furthermore, studies by dietitians on how to persuade people to change their diet (Cole-Hamilton *et al.* 1986) show that reducing the fat intake seems to be the most difficult of all the nutritional manipulations (Black *et al.* 1984), a finding confirmed by the recent decline in saturated fatty acid intake but the unrelenting high total fat consumption by the British population (OPCS 1990). Of total fat intake, about 16 per cent comes from butter and margarines, 14 per cent from meat, 9 per cent from milk, 11 per cent from vegetables including chips and crisps, 12 per cent from other fats (e.g. confectionery and cooking oils), 10 per cent from meat products, 6 per cent from cheese, and a further 19 per cent from cakes, biscuits, and puddings (including ice-cream). Therefore the dairy, meat, and food manufacturing industries are key sources of inappropriate fat inputs into the food chain.

The UK dairy industry

The dairy industry is one of the success stories of the post-war years. Milk production rose rapidly in response to programmes designed to select animals for maximum productivity. The Milk Marketing Boards guaranteed to buy all milk at a fixed price, whatever the production level, and paid selectively high prices for high fat milk. There were penalties for low fat milk (<3.7 per cent fat) and national research strategies were designed to boost both total milk and milk fat output. Yields rose steadily, boosted by genetic selection programmes which identified bulls with high-milk-yielding progeny. The drive for increased efficiency led to a search for cheaper protein supplements and the introduction of recycled carcass waste and offals to enhance milk productivity. The disastrous consequences in terms of bovine spongiform encephalitis (BSE) are now well-recognized, and public anxiety has delayed the widespread introduction of bovine somatotrophin which is known to boost milk output by 20–30 per cent and therefore further cheapen milk production.

The guaranteed purchases of milk powder and butter by the EC ensured that prices for farmers remained artificially high so that they could be encouraged to produce more. This led to the milk powder and butter mountains of the early 1980s. Dairy surpluses in 1990 exceeded 0.5 million tonnes, despite the introduction of quotas. As Blaxter (1990) has pointed out, all this agricultural intensification is unsustainable because it is based on the misuse of cheap fossil fuel to produce cheap fertilizers and cheap spraying of growth promoters and pesticides at great cost in terms of soil degradation and other environmental damage.

The British have the highest milk consumption in Europe and a huge dairy industry which remains proud of its achievements and sensitive to any suggestion that milk or its products are hazardous. Those nutritional and scientific spokesmen who disbelieve the lipid hypothesis of heart disease are courted, and grants are given for research on areas such as calcium where human benefits of milk may emerge.

Advertising

Until recently, advertising has continued to promote full cream milk because the Milk Marketing Boards, who pay for the promotions, have mostly farmers on their management boards. The introduction of skimmed and semi-skimmed milk was resisted because it implied that full cream milk was a second-class product. Within 6 months of semi-skimmed milk's becoming available, retail sales of these lower-fat products had soared to 20 per cent of the market. The claims that the industry simply responds to consumer needs is therefore a selective view of what happens in practice. The Butter Information Council's first task is to promote butter sales, and the National Dairy Council has funds from both the Milk Marketing Board and the National Dairy Trade Federation to promote the consumption of milk and its products. Milk, butter, cheese, and cream continue to be advertised intensively in an attempt to maintain consumption, and farmers continue to depend on payment based on the fat content of their milk.

A new strategy?

Only in 1990 did research priorities change, with the Milk Marketing Boards in Scotland suggesting, but not implementing, a proposal that they should subsidise research on enhancing milk protein rather than fat production. Personal enquiry reveals little or no strategic analysis of what is required within the dairy industry or the Ministry of Agriculture if the public health goals, set out in the Canterbury Conference (1984) for example, are to be met. The Ministry's understandable concern is how to keep farming profitable in the face of a collapse in farm incomes, to which dairying makes a major contribution, and still limit food production by the imposition of new quotas and the setting aside of land. The progressive intensification of agriculture ensures that yields of both crops and animal-based commodities are likely to rise by at least 2 per cent per year for the foreseeable future. Therefore those with large vested interests hope that the total fat consumption in the UK will not decline too rapidly.

The meat trade

Beef, lamb, pork, and chicken were luxuries during the first half of this century, and continue to be in huge demand in Eastern Europe. The challenge for farmers world-wide has therefore been to produce more. Clearly, there are benefits in beef production in selecting for rapidly growing animals. New rearing practices for calves limited their growth retardation on weaning, and Preston's barley beef system at the Rowett allowed intakes to rise far above those achieved on high roughage diets. Fat marbling of the meat was perceived as a guarantee of tenderness, succulence, and taste, and so high fat steaks were the ultimate in luxury eating. Until the mid-1980s British butchers were selecting their carcasses for tenderness by buying animals with a fatty carcass, and the special marketing board, the Meat and Livestock Commission (MLC), helped to maintain a grading system which took account of the shape (or conformation) of the animal and its 'finish', which reflected fatness. Animals were bought and sold in livestock markets with premium prices set for those well-fattened animals chosen subjectively by MLC inspectors or by farmers themselves. Therefore the advantages of having a fat animal seemed immense, even though the actual feeding costs of putting on extra fat in a mature animal are substantial.

In the UK, with its huge dairy trade, almost 50 per cent of the carcasses used for beef were derived from the dairy herds and therefore had the extra fat characteristics of high-yielding dairy cows. If cows are to maintain not only beef cattle production, but also their own replacement, then male progeny will still be produced from artificial insemination derived from bulls with semen selected for its advantages in milk production systems. This explains why so much British beef is fatty and will continue to be so until the selection of the sex as well as the breed is guaranteed by semen separation or embryo selection techniques. This is an area of intense research competition with huge financial stakes. If male semen can be used selectively for lean continental breeds of beef animal, then the dairy cow is induced to lactate but her progeny is a bull calf of lean genetic type.

Bull beef production is hazardous in highly populated countries such as the UK if the bulls are not castrated, and so this has been routine practice despite the disadvantage of a more fatty animal. To counteract this, anabolic steroids were introduced to great effect and have become routine when rearing steers, i.e. castrates. Again, the beef industry was heavily sub-sidized directly and supported indirectly by a plethora of research, de-velopment, advisory services, and marketing surveys. When the UK joined the EC, guaranteed beef prices and the use of intervention stores ensured that farmers could invest in new beef-producing schemes with further govern-ment subsidies and a guaranteed market. Similar conditions applied to sheep production, so that huge quantities of sheep meat and fat became available.

It soon became apparent that the cost of pig-rearing was less than that for cattle and sheep production because the monogastric animal has a more efficient gastro-intestinal system. Pig production rose, costs plummeted, and pig meat sales soared. It then became apparent that intensive chicken production was even more efficient, so that cheaper chicken could be produced to compete with the other meats. Much of this greater efficiency depended on cheap cereal-feeding from new varieties and growing strategies with novel mechanization promoted by direct and indirect government subsidies. Indeed, the fat content of the intensively fed chicken has risen markedly, so that the whole bird is no longer the traditional low fat product provided by the free-range farm chicken.

Late in the 1970s consumers began to demand lean rather than fat meat, and so supermarkets responded by trimming the fat off the carcasses and demanding leaner bacon and pork. The enterprising Danish farmer re-sponded by new feeding and breeding strategies, thereby forcing the UK farmer to alter his pig husbandry. There has been a decline in pork fat production over the last 10 years, but little impact on the beef and sheep industries. This means that a huge amount of cattle and sheep fat cannot be sold directly to the consumer and therefore finds its way into the food chain in hidden form by being incorporated into meat products or other foods rich in fat. The consumer has responded to medical advice to reduce meat fat consumption only to find the fat reappearing in unrecognized form in other food products. Only if food labelling is understandable can this problem be overcome (see below).

Meat products, previously luxury items, are now the cheap food items favoured by the poorer sections of society. Sausages, meat pies, and salamis are all produced in huge volumes at prices which can now be lowered by using meat fragments recovered by special manufacturing techniques designed to produce colourful and organoleptically acceptable items in the daily diet.

Food processing

In many affluent societies the demand for convenience foods has led to a revolution in food processing, packaging, and marketing. In the UK about 70 per cent of products are now manufactured and/or packaged, and the principal sources of those nutrients of medical concern, i.e. fat, sugar, and salt, are to be found in poorly labelled packaged products set out in a myriad of varieties in huge supermarkets. Processing of simple foods, such as potatoes, has led to a huge increase in 'added value', i.e. profits from food processing. For example, crisps and chips with their extra fat content have increased their sales at the expense of potato sales. Thus, as consumers reduce their consumption of visible fat, they increase their intake of invisible fat. Similar trends have occurred in sugar intakes, with sales of table sugar falling as the sugar content of the diet, for example in soft drinks, rise. The hidden sugars now contribute the major source of refined sugars in the diet. Similarly, 85 per cent of salt intake is now derived from food products (James *et al.* 1987).

The dilemma of food labelling and consumer understanding

Although European consumers now demand more information on food labels, they do not understand current labelling. This is perhaps because until now there has been little effort made to present the nutritional content of foods in a coherent manner. Reliance on standardizing food ingredient composition has depended on the agreements of *Codex Alimentarius* which suggests that only the energy, protein, carbohydrate, and fat content of foods be specified. As is now apparent, this constitutes a very old-fashioned view of the nutritionally relevant components of the diet.

Extensive consumer surveys have shown that much better labelling is needed, but manufacturers, who currently make their profits on food products with a disproportionate amount of saturated fatty acids, sugar, and salt, are naturally reluctant to agree to any measure which might limit the sales of their product. Without compulsory standardized food labelling, however, the proposition that consumer choice currently operates in Europe can be considered not only fallacious but actually misleading.

Figure 36.1 shows the pressures to which the consumers are subject as

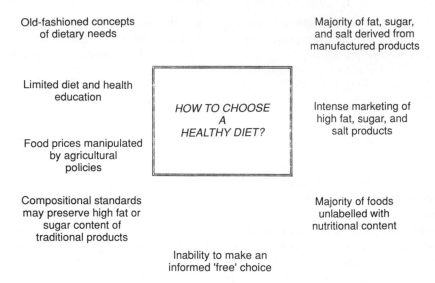

Old-fashioned concepts
of dietary needs

Majority of fat, sugar,
and salt derived from
manufactured products

Limited diet and health
education

*HOW TO CHOOSE
A
HEALTHY DIET?*

Intense marketing of
high fat, sugar, and
salt products

Food prices manipulated
by agricultural
policies

Compositional standards
may preserve high fat or
sugar content of
traditional products

Majority of foods
unlabelled with
nutritional content

Inability to make an
informed 'free' choice

Fig. 36.1 The consumer's dilemma.

they attempt to cope with the confusing pressures which determine their so-called 'free choice' of food products.

THE WAY FORWARD

This chapter concentrates on identifying the basis for our current problems because, without this understanding, policy-makers are likely to demand simplistic solutions on the assumption that the priority for dietary change to improve public health is self-evident, and the means to achieve it is straightforward. Only when the dimensions of the problem are recognized can a coherent strategy be developed.

A national or a European food protection agency?

It is little wonder, given all these issues, that there is such a widespread demand for some kind of independent food agency in the UK. This is now supported by the Consumer Association, the National Consumers' Council, the Retailers' Safety Advisory Bureau, and the Labour Party, and now by the National Farmers' Union as well.

The UK National Consumer Council has taken a lead and proposes that an agency might incorporate the following functions:

(1) formulation of a community food and nutrition policy;

(2) collection of food consumption and nutritional status data as a basis for policy-making;

(3) assessment and approval of food quality and conformity requirements;

(4) food safety monitoring;

(5) maintenance of a data-base on all legislation pertaining to food;

(6) review food regulations and advice to government on changes needed;

(7) involvement of consumers in community policy-making.

Agricultural strategies

The foregoing analysis highlights issues demanding changes in production policies, subsidy systems, priority setting for agricultural research, and new approaches to food manufacturing. All this needs to be integrated properly with up-to-date analyses involving producers, processors, and civil servants. Nothing will happen, however, until the health priorities are given proper consideration. Analyses of different policies suggest that health issues are readily squeezed out of discussion by economic and vested interests unless able promoters of the health issues are involved in the discussions. Whereas public health experts would consider themselves as suitable participants, at least as important are the consumer organizations and representatives of powerful interests in society, such as women's groups or trade union organizations. Their inclusion appears to be the *sine qua non* for action.

Practical agricultural strategies

The UK and European farmers can readily adapt to a new health-based agricultural strategy. Carcass fat can easily be reduced by new breeding techniques including embryo transfer, bull beef breeding with early slaughter could be more widespread, and immunocastration, which maintains a lower carcass fat than surgical castration, could be developed. Subsidy payments could be adjusted to give preference to lean animals, and feeding systems can help to reduce overfat sheep and cattle. These measures, and the use of carcass rather than live market grading, could all have a marked and rapid impact on the food chain.

Nutrition education

Modern concepts of healthy nutrition and methods of helping individuals to change their diets are not necessarily accepted or understood either by the public or the medical and educational professionals who seek to promote a better understanding and a preventive approach. A nutrition board could ensure that nutrition education is incorporated in the educational priorities of schools and in the professional training of teachers, doctors, nurses, and dietitians.

National surveys show that doctors are poorly taught in nutrition, and that dietitians themselves often had poor diets until recently and are trying to encompass new concepts to improve their care. The nursing profession also has almost no educational input on new approaches to healthy eating (Robertson and James 1991).

The medical professionals' own diet is beginning to improve, but few doctors know how to deal with dietary issues and have no practical understanding of what is involved. A recent proposal setting out novel approaches to coping with both healthy eating and the individual variation in energy requirements is presented elsewhere (James and Ralph 1990).

Food labelling

The British Coronary Prevention Group has recently produced a new system for food labelling which is based on a simple coding system for the key nutrients of current interest, i.e. fat, saturated fat, sugar, salt, and fibre, which are categorized as high, medium, or low by reference to WHO-defined nutrient goals expressed in terms of the energy content of the food (CPG 1990). This then allows both a small elderly woman and an active young sportsman with three times her energy requirement to identify suitable foods and balance their purchases to maintain an intake which complies with current recommendations. The only additionl requirement when balancing high, medium, and low items is that the individual has a very crude concept of the principal contributors to their dietary energy intake. This approach is in marked contrast to current systems which demand the impossible, i.e. a knowledge of one's own energy requirements and then a collation of all items purchased, having first calculated, for example, one's fat requirement in grams from the supposed figure for total energy needs. The new concept was incorporated in Appendix 6 of the global WHO report on diet and the prevention of chronic diseases (WHO 1990).

CONCLUSIONS

Dietary patterns are changing throughout Europe, but the whole of agricultural practice and food production is either promoted or constrained by government regulations or economic pricing systems which attempt to promote food production (in Eastern Europe) or limit specific commodity production (in Northern and Southern Europe). The problem of over-production of animal products and cereals for animal feeds is of major economic concern. Hitherto no health considerations to favour the development of a healthy diet have been included in agricultural policy. Medical understanding of the major public health problems in Europe now permits the development of appropriate agricultural practices. Agricultural research has developed new options in animal husbandry and crop production which favour a reduction in the total fat and saturated fatty acid production.

The present imbalance between consumer demand for low fat products and production policies leads to an excess of cheap products rich in fat which are selectively purchased by the poorer section of society to the disadvantage of their health.

The food industry has developed rapidly in most parts of Europe since the Second World War. These developments have proved to be both beneficial and detrimental. Unfortunately, food manufactured products are now major sources of fat, saturated fat, sugar, and salt intakes. The challenge is therefore to encourage the food industry to produce nutritionally more appropriate foods. This cannot be done in the free-market economy without a consumer-led demand for the healthier products.

Current labelling of food products is totally inadequate to allow people to choose a nutritionally appropriate diet. All evidence suggests that the educated consumer opts for a healthy diet. The lack of information and proper education of the consumer is a barrier to health in all parts of the European region. Compulsory nutritional labelling of all food products is needed if a coherent and effective food policy is to be developed.

REFERENCES

Bingham, S., McNeill, N. I., and Cummings, J. H. (1981). The diet of individuals: a study of a randomly chosen cross section of British adults in a Cambridgeshire village. *Br. J. Nutr.*, **45**, 23–35.

Black, A. E., Ravenscroft, C., and Sims, A. J. (1984). The NACNE report: are the dietary goals realistic? Comparisons with the dietary patterns of dietitians. *Hum. Nutr. Appl. Nutr.*, **38A**, 165–79.

Blaxter, Sir K. (1990). From hunting and gathering to agriculture. In *Planning for better nutrition in the 21st century*, Nestlé, Lausanne.

Canterbury Conference (1984). *Plans for action: Report of the Canterbury Conference*, London, Pitman.

Cole-Hamilton, I., Gunner, K., Leverkus, C., and Starr, J. (1986). A study among dietitians and adult members of their households of the practicalities and implications of following proposed dietary guidelines for the UK. *Hum. Nutr. Appl. Nutr.*, **40A**, 365–89.

COMA (Committee on Medical Aspects of Food Policy) (1984). *Dietary aspects of cardiovascular diseases. Report on health and social subjects* 28, HM Stationery Office, London.

COMA (Committee on Medical Aspects of Food Policy) (1989). *The diets of British school children. Report on health and social subjects* 36, Department of Health, London.

CPG (Coronary Prevention Group) (1990). *Nutrition banding. A scientific system for labelling the nutrition content of foods*, CPG, London.

Darke, S. J., Disselduff, M. M., and Try, G. P. (1980). Frequency distribution of mean daily intakes of food energy and selected nutrients obtained during nutrition surveys of different groups of people between 1968 and 1971 (Department of Health and Social Security). *Br. J. Nutr.*, **44**, 143–252.

FAO (Food and Agriculture Organization of the United Nations) (1990). *Policy changes affecting European agriculture. Proc. 17th Regional Conf. for Europe, Venice, April 1990*, Publ. ERC/90/INF/4, FAO, Rome.

Fehily, A. M., Phillips, K. M., and Sweetman, P. M. (1984). A weighed dietary survey of men in Caerphilly, South Wales. *Hum. Nutr., Appl. Nutr.*, **38A**, 270–6.

James, W. P. T. (1988). The implications of a change in diet. 1. Dietary reform: an individual or a national response? *R. Soc. Arts J.*, **136**, 373–87.

James, W. P. T. and Ralph, A. (1990). What is a healthy diet? *Med. Int.*, **82**, 3364–9.

James, W. P. T. and Ralph, A. (1991). National food policies. In *Human Nutrition. A continuing debate. An account of a Symposium Nutrition in the nineties*, (eds M. Eastwood, C. Edwards, D. Parry), 1–16. Chapman & Hall, London.

James, W. P. T., Ralph, A., and Sanchez-Castillo, C. P. (1987). The dominance of salt in manufactured food in the sodium intake of affluent societies. *Lancet*, **i**, 426–9.

Nelson, M. (1985). Nutritional goals from COMA and NACNE: how can they be achieved? *Hum. Nutr. Appl. Nutr.*, **36A**, 456–64.

NRC (National Research Council) (1989). *Diet and health: implications for reducing chronic risk*, National Academy Press, Washington, DC.

OECD (Organization of Economic Co-operation and Development) (1987). *National policies and agricultural trade*, OECD, Paris.

OPCS (Office of Population Censuses and Surveys) (1990). *The dietary and nutritional survey of British adults*, HM Stationery Office, London.

PAHO (Pan American Health Organization) (1976). Technical discussion on national food and nutrition policies. *PAHO Bull.*, **X.4**, 447–62.

Robertson, A. and James, W. P. T. (1991). Post-graduate education of dietitians and their potential role in medical education. *J. Hum. Nutr. Diet.*, **4**, 335–ff.

Rose, G. and Shipley, M. (1986). Plasma cholesterol concentration and death from coronary heart disease: 10 year results of the Whitehall study. *Br. Med. J.*, **293**, 306–7.

Thompson, M., Logan, R. C., and Sharman, M. (1982). Dietary survey in 40-year-old Edinburgh men. *Hum. Nutr. Appl. Nutr.*, **36A**, 272–80.

US Surgeon General (1988). *Report on nutrition and health*, US Government Printing Office, Washington, DC.

WHO (World Health Organization) (1990). *Diet, nutrition and the prevention of chronic diseases*, Tech. Rep. 797, WHO, Geneva.

Index